clinical
biomechanics
of the
lower extremities

clinical biomechanics of the lower extremities

Ronald L. Valmassy, DPM, MS

Professor and Past Chairman
Department of Podiatric Biomechanics
California College of Podiatric Medicine

Diplomate, American Board of Podiatric Orthopedics and
Primary Podiatric Medicine

Fellow and Former President
American College of Foot and Ankle Orthopedics and Medicine

Staff Podiatrist
Center for Sports Medicine
Saint Francis Memorial Hospital
San Francisco

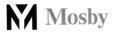 Mosby

An Affiliate of Elsevier

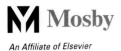

An Affiliate of Elsevier

Publisher: Don Ladig
Editor: James Shanahan
Developmental Editor: Susan Erikson
Project Manager: Linda Clarke
Senior Production Editor: Vicki Hoenigke
Designer: Ellen Dawson
Cover art: Christy Krames

Printed in the United States of America

Mosby, Inc.
11830 Westline Industrial Drive
St. Louis, Missouri 63146

Library of Congress Cataloging-in-Publication Data

Clinical biomechanics of the lower extremities / [edited by] Ronald L.
  Valmassy.
      p. cm.
    Includes bibliographical references and index.
    ISBN 0-8016-7986-9 (alk. paper)
    1. Leg—Mechanical properties. 2. Leg—Abnormalities—Patients—
Rehabilitation. 3. Gait disorders. I. Valmassy, Ronald L.
    [DNLM: 1. Biomechanics. 2. Leg—pathology. 3. Gait—pathology.
  4. Orthotic Devices.   WE 103 C64063 1996]
  RD779.C56 1996
  617.5'8—dc20
  DNLM/DLC
  for Library of Congress   95-35679
                                                                  CIP

ISBN 0-8016-7986-9

05 06 07 08 09 / 9

To my wife, Helen, and son, Paul,
who patiently tolerated the countless
weeknight and weekend hours which were
spent in the preparation of this work.

And to my parents, Gloria and Lou Valmassy,
for all the loving and caring support which
they have provided over the years.

foreword

Biomechanics is a necessary basic science for the field of Podiatry. No specialty in the field of medicine is more intimately involved, on an everyday basis, with the clinical application of biomechanics. The understanding of basic mechanics and biomechanics of the lower extremity can provide the Podiatrist with an invaluable diagnostic ability that cannot be otherwise matched. Many pathologic symptoms, particularly in the feet and legs, may be manifestations of either systemic disease or mechanical malfunction. The beauty of biomechanics is that there is such a logical and consistent correlation between various structural abnormalities and the symptoms they produce. A practitioner who is well trained in the field of lower extremity biomechanics can quickly determine whether there is a cause and effect relationship between a symptom and the mechanics of the extremity. If the symptom has an illogical relationship with the existing mechanics revealed during examination, the practitioner will immediately recognize that the symptom originates with a systemic condition that must be pursued medically rather than mechanically. The practitioner can then proceed with a medical workup sufficient to refer the patient to the proper specialist for further evaluation.

Biomechanics is also the most reliable basis for selecting the type of procedure when surgery is indicated. The understanding of biomechanics enables a surgeon to better recognize the cause and effect relationship between structural and functional abnormalities and the resulting symptoms. This in turn improves the results of the surgery.

An extensive basic training in biomechanics is likewise required for the orthopedic treatment of the abnormal foot and of some of the abnormal postural problems that result from the use of orthoses. Biomechanical knowledge enables the practitioner to ascertain just how much motion should be allowed by a functional orthosis to prevent postural problems. Examples of the importance of biomechanical training for the Podiatrist who prescribes orthoses are too numerous to mention in the space allotted here.

Biomechanics is first and foremost a necessary basic science for the field of Podiatry. As such, basic biomechanics should be taught by the science departments in our colleges. The application of biomechanics can be taught in the various clinical departments because that application also requires training in the arts of examination, casting, and surgery. Without sufficient basic scientific knowledge, however, the practitioner is unable to adequately apply all the arts required for differential diagnosis, surgery, and orthopedics.

A teacher can enjoy no greater pleasure than to be asked to write the foreword to a text compiled by a former student. Such was my pleasure when Dr. Valmassy requested that I write this foreword. Many of the subjects covered in this text have received little or no attention in prior podiatric literature. The subject of podiatric biomechanics should be considerably enhanced by this text.

Merton L. Root, BS, DPM, DSC
Professor Emeritus
California College of Podiatric Medicine

Former Chairman, Department of Podiatric Biomechanics,
California College of Podiatric Medicine

Fellow, American College of Foot and Ankle Orthopedics and Medicine

contributors

Richard Berenter, DPM
Associate Professor
Department of Podiatric Biomechanics, California
    College of Podiatric Medicine
San Francisco, California
Diplomate, American Board of Podiatric
    Orthopedics and Primary Podiatric Medicine

Richard L. Blake, DPM
Staff Podiatrist
Center for Sports Medicine, Saint Francis
    Memorial Hospital
San Francisco, California
Fellow and former President, American Academy
    of Podiatric Sports Medicine

Richard J. Bogdan, DPM
Past Chairman
Department of Podiatric Biomechanics, Ohio
    College of Podiatric Medicine
Cleveland, Ohio
Board certified by the American Board of Foot
    Surgery
Diplomate, American Board of Podiatric
    Orthopedics and Primary Podiatric Medicine

Notty Bumbo, PEDORTHIST
Co-Founder
Prescription Foot Orthotic Laboratory Association
Director of Quality Issues
KLM Laboratories
Valencia, California

Jane A. Denton, DPM
Staff Podiatrist
Center for Sports Medicine, Saint Francis
    Memorial Hospital
San Francisco, California
Fellow, American Academy of Podiatric Sports
    Medicine

Heather J. Ferguson, B. APP. SCI. (POD)
Podiatrist
The Alphington Sports Medicine Clinic
Northcote, Victoria, AUSTRALIA

Eric Arthur Fuller, DPM
Associate Professor
Department of Podiatric Biomechanics, California
    College of Podiatric Medicine
San Francisco, California
Diplomate, American Board of Podiatric
    Orthopedics and Primary Podiatric Medicine

Bart W. Gastwirth, DPM
Clinical Professor and Past Chairman
Department of Orthopedics, Scholl College
    of Podiatric Medicine
Chicago, Illinois
Diplomate, American Board of Podiatric
    Orthopedics and Primary Podiatric Medicine
Fellow, American College of Foot and Ankle
    Orthopedics and Medicine

Lester J. Jones, DPM, MS
Professor
Department of Podiatric Biomechanics, California
    College of Podiatric Medicine
San Francisco, California
Chief
Podiatric Section, VAMC
Long Beach, California
Former Dean
Clinical Education, Ohio College of Podiatric
    Medicine
Cleveland, Ohio
Diplomate, American Board of Podiatric
    Orthopedics and Primary Podiatric Medicine

Kevin A. Kirby, DPM
Assistant Clinical Professor
Department of Podiatric Biomechanics, California
    College of Podiatric Medicine
San Francisco, California
Diplomate, American Board of Podiatric
    Orthopedics and Primary Podiatric Medicine

Daniel K. Kosai, DPM
Assistant Professor
Department of Podiatric Biomechanics, California
    College of Podiatric Medicine
San Francisco, California
Diplomate, American Board of Podiatric
    Orthopedics and Primary Podiatric Medicine

James M. Losito, DPM
Professor
Department of Podiatric Biomechanics, Barry
   University School of Podiatric Medicine
Miami Shores, Florida
Diplomate, American Board of Podiatric
   Orthopedics and Primary Podiatric Medicine

Irene Minkowsky, MD
Director
Physicians' Back Institute
San Francisco, California
Attending Physician
Center for Sports Medicine, Saint Francis
   Memorial Hospital
San Francisco, California

Robert Minkowsky, MD
Assistant Clinical Professor of Medicine
University of California
San Francisco, California
Co-Director
Physicians' Back Institute
San Francisco, California

Jack L. Morris, DPM
Professor and Chairman
Department of Podiatric Biomechanics, California
   College of Podiatric Medicine
San Francisco, California
Diplomate, American Board of Podiatric
   Orthopedics and Primary Podiatric Medicine
Fellow, American College of Foot and Ankle
   Orthopedics and Medicine

William R. Olson, DPM
Assistant Clinical Professor
University of Osteopathic Medicine and Health
   Sciences
Des Moines, Iowa
Team Podiatric Physician
Department of Athletics, University of California
Berkeley, California
Staff Podiatrist
Center for Sports Medicine, Saint Francis
   Memorial Hospital
San Francisco, California
Diplomate, American Board of Podiatric
   Orthopedics and Primary Podiatric Medicine
Fellow, American Academy of Podiatric Sports
   Medicine

Paul R. Scherer, DPM
Professor
Department of Podiatric Biomechanics
Past Chairman
Department of Biomechanics
Past Vice President and Academic Dean
California College of Podiatric Medicine
San Francisco, California
Diplomate, American Board of Podiatric
   Orthopedics and Primary Podiatric Medicine
Board certified by the American Board of
   Podiatric Surgery

Michael O. Seibel, DO, DPM
Clinical Associate Professor
Stanford University
Stanford, California
Clinical Associate Professor
University of North Texas Health Science Center
Fort Worth, Texas
Director
Brain Injury Rehabilitation Program, Health South
   Rehabilitation Hospital
Forth Worth, Texas

Leon Paul Smith, MD
Clinical Professor of Pediatrics
University of California Medical Center
San Francisco, California
Marin General Hospital
Greenbrae, California
California College of Podiatric Medicine
San Francisco, California
Fellow, American Academy of Pediatrics

Charles C. Southerland, Jr., DPM
Associate Professor
Department of Podiatric Biomechanics
Barry University School of Medicine
Miami Shores, Florida
Diplomate, American Board of Orthopedics and
   Primary Podiatric Medicine
Board certified by the American Board of
   Podiatric Surgery
Fellow, American College of Foot and Ankle
   Orthopedics and Medicine
Fellow, American College of Foot and Ankle
   Surgeons

Russell G. Volpe, DPM
Associate Professor and Chairman
Division of Pediatrics
Associate Professor
Division of Orthopedic Sciences
New York College of Podiatric Medicine
New York, New York
East Coast Medical Director
The Langer Biomechanics Group
Deer Park, New York
Diplomate, American Board of Podiatric
  Orthopedics and Primary Podiatric Medicine
Fellow, American College of Foot and Ankle
  Orthopedics and Medicine

Justin Wernick, DPM
Professor
Division of Orthopedic Sciences
Clinical Instructor
Department of Pediatrics
New York College of Podiatric Medicine
New York, New York
Co-founder
The Langer Biomechanics Group, Inc.
Deer Park, New York
Diplomate, American Board of Podiatric
  Orthopedics and Primary Podiatric Medicine
Fellow, American College of Foot and Ankle
  Orthopedics and Medicine
Fellow, American Academy of Podiatric Sports
  Medicine

Stephen C. White, DPM
Assistant Professor
Department of Podiatric Medicine, California
  College of Podiatric Medicine
San Francisco, California
Private Practice
San Francisco, California

Ronald L. Valmassy, DPM, MS
Professor and Past Chairman
Department of Podiatric Biomechanics, California
  College of Podiatric Medicine
San Francisco, California
Staff Podiatrist
Center for Sports Medicine, Saint Francis
  Memorial Hospital
San Francisco, California
Diplomate, American Board of Podiatric
  Orthopedics and Primary Podiatric Medicine
Fellow and former President, American College
  of Foot and Ankle Orthopedics and Medicine

acknowledgments

A book of this scope and depth could not have been produced without the efforts of countless individuals. I would like to express my gratitude and appreciation to not only those individuals who contributed to the production of this work, but also to those who developed the basic foundation for the principles involved in the area of podiatric biomechanics.

Over the years, the Department of Podiatric Biomechanics at the California College of Podiatric Medicine has been fortunate to have had a number of instructors demonstrating a true dedication to the area of podiatric biomechanics. Not only have they educated countless numbers of today's practitioners, but they have also served to further the knowledge and understanding of lower extremity biomechanics for all those health care practitioners involved in assessing and improving human locomotion. The list of those individuals is headed by the names of Drs. Merton Root, John Weed, Tom Sgarlato, and Christopher Smith, all of whom spent long years of dedicated service in the area of podiatric biomechanics. The books produced by Drs. Root, Orien and Weed, namely, *Normal and Abnormal Function of the Foot,* along with a *Compendium of Podiatric Biomechanics* by Sgarlato, have served as classic texts on the subject for numerous years. As the years progressed, their ranks were joined by a number of other instructors, including Drs. Richard Bogdan, Joseph D'Amico, Harry Hlavac, Patrick Laird, John Marszalec, and Paul Scherer. On a national basis, countless others have dedicated their careers to this area. No list can be considered complete without mentioning the names of Drs. Larry Burns, Sheldon Langer, Richard Schuster, and Justin Wernick, and, in the area of podopediatrics and pediatric biomechanics, Drs. James Ganley and Herman Tax.

I am especially indebted to all those individuals who devoted countless hours of research and writing to produce this manuscript. Although it would have been easy to decline the invitation to participate in this work, the contributing authors all gave up a considerable amount of time from their professional and personal lives to bring this work to completion. For their dedication and willingness to participate in this work, I am most grateful.

The preparation of this work would not have been completed without the efforts of a number of other participants. They include those individuals who prepared the various chapters and diligently reworked each paragraph until the finished product was produced. They are Carole Glick, Margaret Raskowsky, and especially Betsy Cook, who has probably read more about the area of biomechanics than she ever thought she would. Special thanks are extended to Tricia Rubio and Chris Corpus, who graciously posed for a host of the clinical photographs used in this text. Because the production of this manuscript caused countless scheduling changes over the past three years, I must also acknowledge the patience of those individuals with whom I practice: Drs. Rodney Chan, Theresa Kailikole, Stephen White, Richard Blake, Jane Denton, and William Olson.

In the spring of 1992 I was contacted by James Shanahan of Mosby–Year Book to determine if a book could be produced dealing with the clinical practice of biomechanics. I am most grateful for that initial contact and the opportunity it brought with it to produce this text. The continued support and guidance of the editorial staff at Mosby–Year Book was provided by Mr. Shanahan, Ms. Anne Gleason, and Ms. Susan Eriksen. Their willing and professional assistance in proceeding through the various stages required for the production of such a book was a welcome resource. Finally, I must applaud the efforts and artistic skills provided by Jan Ruvido, the medical illustrator who prepared all of the wonderful line illustrations presented in this work. Her skills and attention to detail have added greatly to the overall presentation of this book.

preface

The study of lower extremity biomechanics allows today's practitioner to understand how and why the mechanical function of the lower extremity can lead to a wide variety of pathologic conditions. Once today's practitioners understand the normal and abnormal function of the lower extremities, they may then successfully implement a variety of treatment regimens specifically directed towards improving their patients' lower extremity mechanical function.

This book has been prepared to provide a sound combination of both didactic and clinical information pertaining to the treatment of lower extremity pathology. It is written for all health care practitioners and students interested in enhancing the function of patients suffering from gait-related problems. The book includes chapters dealing with the development of normal gait, as well as normal muscle and joint function. Additionally, a presentation on how deviation from this normal development will lead to the initiation of pathological conditions is covered. With this foundation in place, the subsequent chapters in this book then provide the necessary information required to clinically evaluate and treat the specific elements of lower extremity pathology.

Chapters range from the performance of straightforward clinical tests to determine muscle strength, joint range of motion, and evaluation of gait, to an explanation of how computer-assisted gathering of data may be effectively utilized in assessing the etiology of a patient's problem. The final chapters detail the use of various orthoses, shoes, braces, splints, and serial plaster immobilization techniques and provide the practitioner with an up-to-date resource on how to alter abnormal mechanical patterns. Specific considerations detailing appropriate evaluation and treatment techniques for the athlete and pediatric patient are discussed in their own chapters.

Although the area of lower extremity biomechanics has always played an integral part in improving the ambulatory status of our patients, its present-day role continues to expand. Accurately diagnosing and conservatively treating a multitude of lower extremity problems has never been more important, as an ever-increasing emphasis has been placed on the area of preventive and conservative management of medical problems.

Whether the study of lower extremity biomechanics is used to assess the effectiveness of a proposed surgical procedure, to alter the gait of a pediatric patient, or to maintain an improved level of comfort and health for the geriatric patient, the full appreciation and use of this particular discipline in one's practice cannot be overemphasized. My hope is that the information presented in this book will allow those individuals interested in this particular area of practice to treat their patients in an effective, efficient, and successful fashion.

Ronald L. Valmassy, DPM

contents

chapter 1 **Lower extremity function
and normal mechanics 1**
Justin Wernick and Russell G. Volpe

chapter 2 **Pathomechanics of lower extremity function 59**
Ronald L. Valmassy

chapter 3 **The classification of human foot types, abnormal foot function,
and pathology 85**
Paul R. Scherer and Jack L. Morris

chapter 4 **The spine, an integral part of the lower extremity 95**
Irene Minkowsky and Robert Minkowsky

chapter 5 **Biomechanical principles of running injuries 113**
Richard J. Bogdan

chapter 6 **Biomechanical examination of the foot and lower extremity 131**
Bart W. Gastwirth

chapter 7 **Gait evaluation in clinical biomechanics 149**
Charles C. Southerland, Jr.

chapter 8 **Computerized gait evaluation 179**
Eric Arthur Fuller

chapter 9 **Neuromuscular examination 207**
Michael O. Seibel

chapter 10 **Limp and the pediatric patient 223**
Leon Paul Smith

chapter 11 **Biomechanical evaluation of the child 243**
Ronald L. Valmassy

chapter 12 **Impression casting techniques 279**
James M. Losito

chapter 13 **Prescription writing for functional
and accommodative foot orthoses 295**
Lester J. Jones

chapter 14 **Orthotic materials 307**
William R. Olson

chapter 15 **Troubleshooting functional foot orthoses 327**
Kevin A. Kirby

chapter 16   **Utilizing footwear as a therapeutic modality**   349
Notty Bumbo

chapter 17   **Padding and taping techniques**   367
Stephen C. White

chapter 18   **Ankle-foot orthoses**   391
Notty Bumbo

chapter 19   **Serial plaster immobilization of congenital foot deformities**   405
Richard Berenter and Daniel K. Kosai

chapter 20   **Lower extremity treatment modalities for the pediatric patient**   425
Ronald L. Valmassy

chapter 21   **Athletic shoes**   453
Jane A. Denton

chapter 22   **The inverted orthotic technique:
Its role in clinical biomechanics**   465
Richard L. Blake and Heather Ferguson

lower extremity function and normal mechanics

Justin Wernick, DPM
Russell G. Volpe, DPM

General principles

Ankle joint
  Anatomy
  Ankle joint in function

The subtalar joint
  Anatomy
  The subtalar joint in function

The midtarsal joint
  Anatomy
  The midtarsal joint in function

The first ray
  Anatomy
  The first ray in function

The first metatarsophalangeal joint
  Anatomy
  First metatarsophalangeal joint in gait
  Axes of the first metatarsophalangeal joint
  First metatarsophalangeal kinetics in pathologic
    function
  Motion of the foot over the hallux in propulsion
  Range of motion
  Summary

Second, third, and fourth rays

The fifth ray
  Anatomy
  Axis of the fifth ray
  The fifth ray in function

Lesser metatarsophalangeal joints and digits

The gait cycle
  Three phases of walking
  Overview of the gait cycle
  The power of motion
  Phases of the gait cycle
    Contact phase
    Midstance phase
    Active propulsion
    Passive lift-off
    Swing

Introduction

The foot, at the interface between the body and the ground, is of great significance in human bipedal locomotion. It is a complex structure acted upon by hard, unyielding surfaces and by the rotations and translations of the trunk and leg necessary to advance the body forward. As the interface between the body and the ground, the foot is subject to tremendous stresses and loads during gait, making it a site of frequent pathologic disorders. The stresses and loads applied to the foot begin in a young child with earliest weightbearing and accumulate dramatically over a lifetime of walking. The ability of the foot to process these cumulative forces without developing pathologic changes and symptoms depends upon normal function.

Understanding the intricacies of the structure and function of the foot and leg under normal conditions is the necessary foundation for recognizing and treating pathomechanical function. This chapter covers normal function of the foot and leg in gait. We first introduce the principles of function at each of the key joints in the foot-ankle complex, and then integrate those principles into a discussion of the motions of the lower extremity throughout the phases of the gait cycle.

The role of the foot in gait as a passive organ acted on by the ground and the superstructure is emphasized. It is hoped that the normal function presented in this chapter enables the reader to appreciate the pivotal function of the foot in human locomotion.

General principles

The references for defining motion in the foot and leg are the cardinal body planes. These are known as the frontal, sagittal, and transverse planes. The sagittal plane divides the body into left and right halves. The transverse plane divides the body into top and bottom halves. The frontal plane divides the body into front and rear halves.

Motion at a joint is described as occurring about an axis. A joint axis is an imaginary line described as a point line about which motion occurs. It is the motion at the joint which defines the position or location of the joint axis. An axis is a point line which lies perpendicular to the direction of motion of a joint. The direction in which motion occurs at a given joint is called the plane of motion.

These axes in the body are not fixed in place as the motion at a given joint determines the axis position. It is only from understanding the type, direction, and amount of motion at a given joint that the position of a specific axis may be determined.

Certain axes change their location during func-

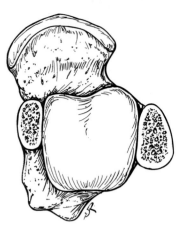

Fig. 1-1. Dorsal view of the talus. The lateral malleolus is larger than the medial malleolus and extends more distally.

tion, that is, axes are not stationary hinges. Axes in the lower extremity that shift position with motion include the knee joint and the first metatarsophalangeal joint.

Ankle joint

The ankle joint, or the tibiotalar joint, is the distal joint of the lower leg which serves as the connection between the leg and the foot. This is the major joint responsible for controlling sagittal plane movements of the leg relative to the foot. Sagittal plane motion at the junction of the leg and the foot is essential for bipedal ambulation over flat or uneven terrain.

Anatomy

The bones of the ankle joint include the distal articular surfaces of the tibia and the fibula and the trochlear surface of the talus. The trochlear surface of the talus is depressed centrally, is broader anteriorly than posteriorly, and corresponds to a reciprocally shaped surface on the inferior aspect of the tibia. The medial and lateral surfaces of the body of the talus are seated in the ankle mortise by the two malleoli. The lateral malleolus is larger than the medial malleolus and extends further distally than the medial malleolus. It also lies more posteriorly, which helps to determine the position on the ankle joint axis (Fig. 1-1). The lateral collateral ligaments and the medial collateral ligament, or deltoid ligament, establish the ligamentous integrity of the ankle joint. These ligaments serve to stabilize and limit the available range of sagittal plane motion at this joint. Plantarflexion at the ankle is limited by tension placed on the anterior talofibular ligament in this position, and by an osseous block produced when the posterior tubercle of the talus comes in

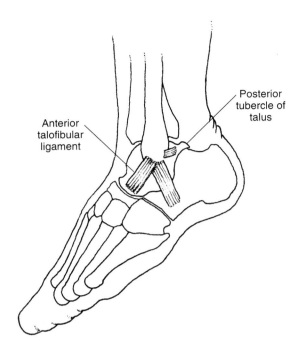

Fig. 1-2. Ankle plantarflexion (lateral view of the left ankle). The anterior talofibular ligament and the posterior tubercle of the talus limit range of motion. (From Michaud T: *Foot orthosis,* Baltimore, 1993, Williams & Wilkins.)

Anterior talofibular ligament

Posterior tubercle of talus

contact with the posterior margin of the tibia (Fig. 1-2). Dorsiflexion at the ankle is limited primarily by the limitations placed by stretch in the triceps surae muscle group, the posterior portion of the deltoid ligament, and the posterior talofibular ligament. Ankle joint dorsiflexion is also restricted by limitations placed on the range of motion, dictated by the point where the wider anterior portion of the trochlear surface of the talus comes in contact with the distal tibia and fibula (Fig. 1-3).

Ankle joint in function

Axis of the ankle joint

The axis of the ankle joint lies approximately 8 degrees from the transverse plane (or 82 degrees from the sagittal plane) and 20 to 30 degrees from the frontal plane.[31] The axis has been described as being directed laterally, posteriorly, and plantarly.[48] The plantar declination of the axis corresponds to the deviation of the axis from the midline of the tibia (or from the sagittal plane), while the posterior direction corresponds to the angulation of the malleoli (or deviation from the frontal plane). (Fig. 1-4) Inman described a hypothetical cone of which the trochlear surface of the talus forms a part (Fig. 1-5). The base of the cone is directed toward the fibula with a longer lateral than medial radius. The initial assumption, that the trochlear surface was cylindrical vs. the conical model, helps explain the minimal

deviation between the malleoli found during full excursion from plantarflexion to dorsiflexion.[31] As the longer radius is located laterally rather than medially there is a larger displacement of the fibula than of the tibial malleolus when the foot is in the closed kinetic chain and the leg moves over it.

Clinical approximation of the ankle joint axis has been described by Mann[42] as corresponding to an imaginary line running through the ankle, created by placing the ends of the examiner's index fingers at the distal bony tips of the malleoli (Fig. 1-6). Since the ankle joint axis lies close to the transverse and frontal planes, the principal motion available at this joint is in the sagittal plane (dorsiflexion-plantarflexion). The deviation from the transverse plane is responsible for the clinically significant motions of abduction coupled with dorsiflexion, and adduction coupled with plantarflexion, occurring at the ankle. This deviation from the transverse plane, which provides motion at the ankle capable of absorbing rotational motions from the leg, has had varying significance attributed to it. Inman[32] has stated that the deviation from the transverse plane may be as much as 23 degrees, and that the increase in abduction-adduction demonstrated with this deviation may be important in absorbing the rotational movements of the superstructure.[31] Root et al.[54] claim that increased deviation of the ankle joint axis from the transverse plane is relatively uncommon and is usually demonstrated as an adaptive change in the developing ankle joint of a person with limited subtalar joint motion present during skeletal growth.

Barnett and Napier[1] and Hicks published works in the 1950s suggesting that the ankle joint axis moves during plantarflexion and dorsiflexion. The axis of the ankle joint was said to deviate plantar and medially for plantarflexion, and to deviate plantar and laterally for dorsiflexion (Fig. 1-7).[1,27] Inman's work did not acknowledge significant deviations in the direction of the ankle joint axis from plantarflexion to dorsiflexion, describing the joint as a simple hinge.[31] A study by Lundberg et al.[40] in 1989 confirmed the earlier observations for varying angulations to the ankle joint axis in plantarflexion and dorsiflexion. The mean deviation in the position of the coronal plane axis was 37 degrees at a point between 10 and 30 degrees of dorsiflexion; the ankle joint axis was found to run parallel to a line drawn through the malleoli.

Motion at the ankle joint

The obliquely oriented ankle joint axis allows transverse plane motions to occur in the foot or leg with movements of the ankle. In open kinetic chain, with the leg fixed and the foot free, the obliquity of

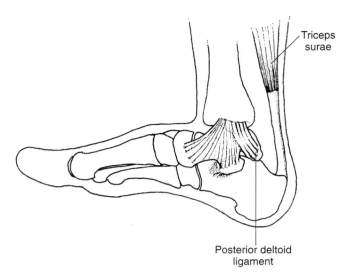

Fig. 1-3. Ankle dorsiflexion (medial view of right ankle). The triceps surae and posterior deltoid ligament limit range of motion. (From Michaud T: *Foot orthosis,* Baltimore, 1993, Williams & Wilkins.)

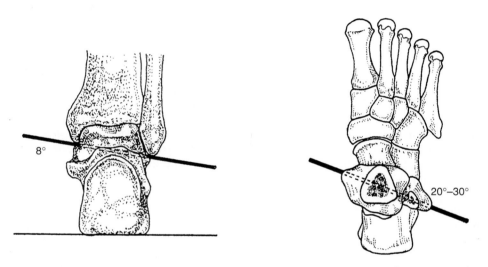

Fig. 1-4. Average axis of motion for the ankle joint. Note the direct relationship of the malleoli to the axis. (From Michaud T: *Foot orthosis,* Baltimore, 1993, Williams & Wilkins.)

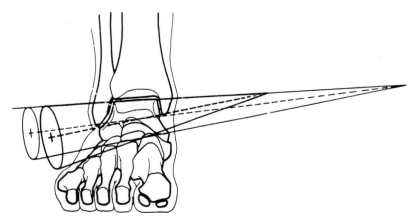

Fig. 1-5. Hypothetical cone of which the trochlea of the talus forms a part. Variation in the inclination of the ankle axis results from differences in the apical angle of the cone. (From Morris J: *Clin Orthop* 122:13, 1977.)

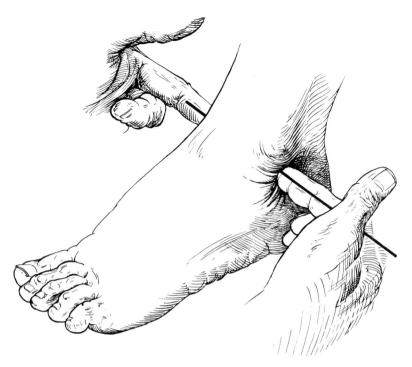

Fig. 1-6. Estimation of obliquity of the ankle axis by palpating the tips of the malleoli. (From Mann R: *Surgery of the foot,* ed 5. St Louis, 1986, Mosby–Year Book.)

the ankle joint axis causes the foot to abduct (deviate outward) on dorsiflexion and to adduct (deviate inward) on plantarflexion (Fig. 1-8). The amount of this transverse plane motion depends on the deviation of the axis from the transverse plane and the degree of sagittal plane motion.

Open kinetic chain

Movements at the ankle joint occur primarily in the sagittal plane and from a point of reference when the sole of the foot is perpendicular to the axis of the leg. Movement of the dorsal surface of the foot to approximate the anterior surface of the leg is known as flexion, referred to at this joint as dorsiflexion. Extension of the leg is movement of the dorsum of the foot away from the anterior surface of the leg. It is also known as plantarflexion at the ankle; however, technically, it cannot be considered a flexion motion, as flexion always requires approximation of segments of a limb to the trunk. Movements at the ankle joint are determined by the position of the axis of rotation for the joint. The shapes of the joint surfaces and their relationship to one another determine the movement at a given joint about the axis of rotation. Further, the motion at a joint is controlled by the integrity and stability of the joint surfaces. The collateral ligaments about a given joint such as the ankle stabilize and guide the movements about the axis of rotation by keeping the opposing joint surfaces in contact. When excessive laxity of

the collateral ligaments is present, the joint surfaces alter their relationship with one another, leading to shifts in the axis of rotation and variations in the types of motion available at that joint.

Closed kinetic chain

Motions occurring in the closed kinetic chain require that movements be described as occurring only in those structures whose motion is not restricted by the presence of the ground. A motion described in the open kinetic chain at a given joint produces an equal and opposite motion proximal to the joint in question in the closed kinetic chain. This concept is essential to describing and understanding normal function of the foot and leg in gait. As most motions of the foot in gait occur with the foot on the ground, we must rely on our ability to observe the classically described open chain motions of a given joint in the closed chain model with the distal segment bearing weight and the proximal segment moving relative to it.

In the case of the ankle joint, the greater amount of dorsiflexion required for normal function occurs during midstance, with the body passing over the foot. It is essential to visualize that the foot is not actually being brought toward the tibia as would be required for open kinetic chain dorsiflexion of the ankle, but is on the ground with the leg moving over it, thereby producing dorsiflexion of the foot relative to the leg (Fig. 1-9**A**, p.8). This means that the abduc-

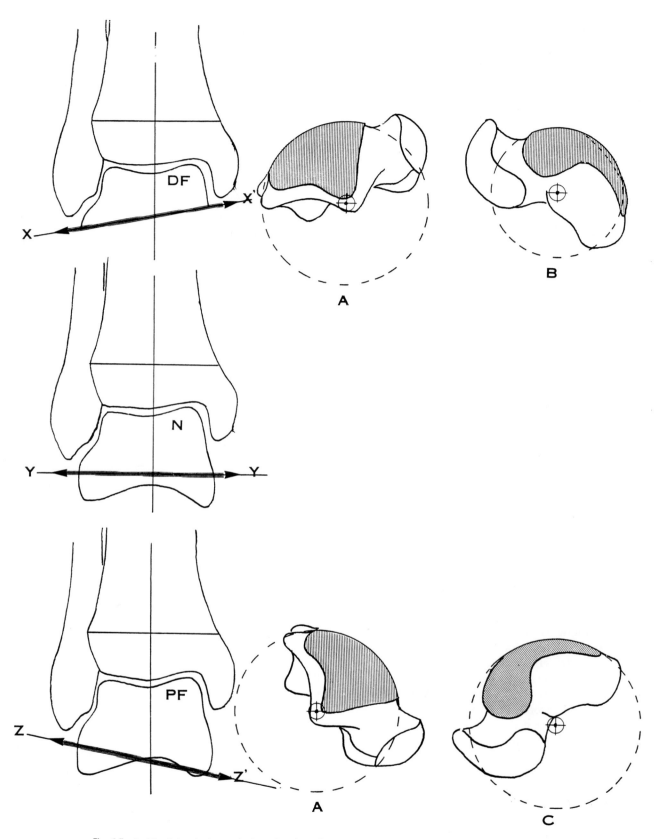

Fig. 1-7. Ankle joint axis variation. In dorsiflexion *(DF)*, the axis of motion *XX'* is inclined downward and laterally. In plantarflexion *(PF)*, the axis of motion *ZZ'* is inclined downward and medially. Near neutral *(N)*, the axis of motion *YY'* is almost horizontal. The lateral trochlear contour *(A)* is an arc of a true circle. The medial trochlear contour is more complex. Its anterior third of dorsiflexion arc *(B)* belongs to a smaller circle as compared with the posterior two thirds or plantarflexion arc *(C)*, which belongs to a large circle. (Adapted from Barnett CJ, Napier JR: *J Anat* 86:1, 1952.)

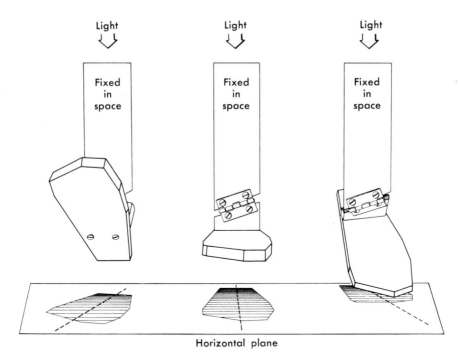

Fig. 1-8. Effect of obliquely placed ankle axis on rotation of the foot in the horizontal plane during plantarflexion and dorsiflexion, with the foot free. Displacement is reflected in the shadows of foot. (From Mann R: *Surgery of the foot*, ed 5. St Louis, 1986, Mosby–Year Book.)

tion (outward movement) of the foot that occurs with dorsiflexion in the open chain will manifest as inward movement or internal rotation of the leg on the foot.[31] As the heel lifts preparing for propulsion, the ankle joint plantarflexes with the forefoot stabilized against the ground.

This closed chain plantarflexion, occurring as the heel lifts and propulsion begins, actually represents an upward and backward motion of the tibia on the foot. The foot, which is already plantigrade throughout midstance, cannot plantarflex further without the tibia moving up and backward on the foot.

Thus, the adduction (inward movement) of the foot which occurs with plantarflexion in the open chain manifests as outward movement or external rotation of the leg on the foot.[1] (Fig. 1-9**B**). During the early portion of the stance phase, from heel contact until the foot is flat, open chain plantarflexion of the ankle occurs. This plantarflexion is accompanied by adduction, which can be seen as an in-toed or medial deviation of the foot on the leg during this portion of the stance phase (Fig. 1-10).

The degree of internal and external leg rotation occurring with sagittal plane ankle motions in the closed kinetic chain depends on the deviation of the ankle joint axis from the transverse plane, as well as the amount of concomitant sagittal plane motion. As more ankle dorsiflexion occurs, more

internal rotation of the leg proximal to the joint will occur.

Summary

1. The motion of the ankle joint occurs primarily in the sagittal plane, with slight transverse plane motion occurring as well. The average axis is 82 degrees from the sagittal plane and 8 degrees from the transverse plane, and corresponds closely to the angular deviation of the malleoli.

2. Sagittal plane plantarflexion is limited by the anterior talofibular ligament and the osseous block of the posterior talus against the tibia. Dorsiflexion is limited by the triceps surae muscle group, and the posterior deltoid and posterior talofibular ligaments.

3. The axis has been found to move with plantarflexion and dorsiflexion. It deviates plantarmedially with plantarflexion and plantarlaterally with dorsiflexion. It corresponds to a line through the malleoli at between 10 and 30 degrees of dorsiflexion.

4. Motion in the open chain is dorsiflexion with abduction and plantarflexion with adduction.

5. In closed kinetic chain motion, dorsiflexion with abduction appears as forward movement

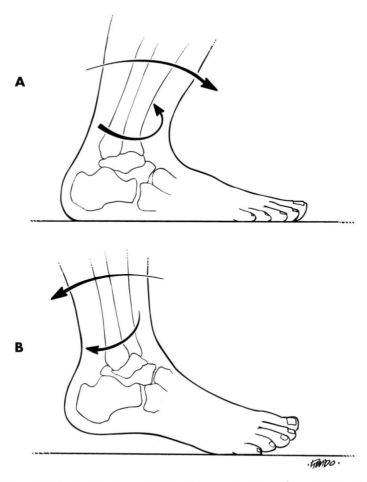

Fig. 1-9. A, Closed chain dorsiflexion with the tibia moving forward on the fixed foot. Internal rotation is associated with this movement. **B,** Closed chain plantarflexion. The tibia is moving backward along with external rotation.

of the leg on the foot, with internal rotation of the leg. Plantarflexion with adduction appears as backward movement of the leg on the foot with external rotation of the leg.

The subtalar joint

The ankle joint, while capable of some transverse plane motion, is not sufficient to translate the rotational relationships of the leg and foot to allow for smooth transmission of the body forward during ambulation. The subtalar joint, situated anatomically in close approximation to the ankle joint, is uniquely designed to allow the leg to undergo additional rotational movements in response to closed chain foot positions.

Anatomy

The subtalar, or talocalcaneal, joint is located between the talus and the calcaneus. It has been described as being composed of three facets on the

inferior surface of the talus articulating with three facets on the superior surface of the calcaneus. The posterior facet of the talus articulating with the broad, superior surface of the calcaneus is united by ligaments and a capsule so that the joint is anatomically distinct[4] (Fig. 1-11). The anterior and middle facets, while classically described as being separate, recently have been found to be a transitional two-facet configuration in which they appear to be merging or as a special two-facet configuration in which any distinction between the anterior and middle facets has been obliterated. Bruckner,[5] in his study of 32 cadaveric subtalar joints, noted that 20 specimens had two distinct articulations (either the transitional two-facet or the special two-facet configuration) and the remaining 12 had three separate articulations.

The ligaments of the subtalar joint are considered short and powerful structures well-adapted to the severe stresses applied to them during weightbearing activities. The main ligament is the interosseous

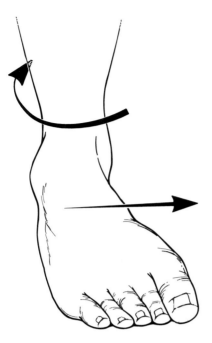

Fig. 1-10. Open chain plantarflexion of the ankle with associated adduction of the foot.

talocalcaneal ligament which consists of two bands occupying the sinus tarsi. The anterior band runs from the calcaneus superiorly, anteriorly, and laterally to insert on the inferior surface of the talar neck, just behind the edge of the articular facet of the head.[34] The posterior band originates just posterior to the anterior band and runs obliquely, superiorly, posteriorly, and laterally to insert just anterior to the posterior facet of the talus. The interosseous ligament has been described as limiting both inversion and eversion of the subtalar joint[7,29] as well as primarily limiting eversion.[63] The lateral talocalcaneal (or cervical) ligament runs from the lateral tubercle of the talus obliquely, inferiorly, posteriorly, and parallel to the intermediate band of the lateral collateral ligament of the ankle joint and inserts on the lateral surface of the calcaneus. This ligament, along with the inferior extensor retinaculum, limits inversion of the subtalar joint.[7] The last ligament is the posterior talocalcaneal ligament which courses from the posterolateral tubercle of the talus to the upper surface of the calcaneus and is of minor functional significance (Fig. 1-12).

The subtalar joint in function

Axis of the subtalar joint

The axis of the subtalar joint runs from posterior, plantar, and lateral, to anterior, dorsal, and medial. Manter[46] reported the angulation of the axis to have a 42-degree average inclination in a sagittal projection from the transverse plane (range, 29–47 de-

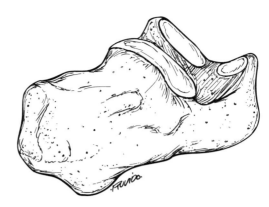

Fig. 1-11. Three facets on the calcaneus correspond with three facets on the talus. The posterior facet is broadest.

grees). Inman reported similar measurements: 42 degrees with an average deviation of ±9 degrees. Manter reported a 16-degree average medial deviation in a transverse projection from the sagittal plane (range, 8–24 degrees).[46] Inman reported an average 23-degree ±11 degrees medial deviation from the sagittal plane, or 23 degrees medially deviated from the axis of the foot, passing through the second interdigital space (Fig. 1-13).

Inman and Mann[43] have described the subtalar joint as a single-axis joint that acts like a mitered hinge, connecting the talus and the calcaneus. Figure 1-14A shows two boards joined by a hinge. If the axis of the hinge is at 45 degrees, a simple torque converter has been created and rotation of the vertical segment will result in equal rotation of the horizontal segment. Any alteration in the angulation of the hinge to bring it closer to one of the two planes alters this one-to-one relationship of upper segment motion to lower segment motion. A more horizontally placed hinge results in greater rotation of the horizontal segment for each degree of rotation of the vertical segment; the converse is true if the hinge is more vertically placed. In Figure 1-14B, the horizontal segment has been divided into a short proximal and a long distal segment with a pivot in between, which prevents the entire horizontal segment from displacing in response to rotation of the vertical segment. This allows the distal segment to remain stationary when vertical segment rotation produces corresponding rotation of the proximal horizontal segment. This pivot, which is located approximately one-third of the way distally on the horizontal segment, corresponds to the midtarsal joint of the foot, and enables rotations of the leg and hindfoot to occur without the forefoot leaving the ground.

Planal dominance

Just as Bruckner[5] described variations in the structure of the subtalar articulations, significant

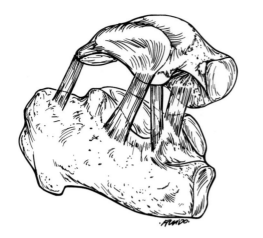

Fig. 1-12. Ligaments of the subtalar joint.

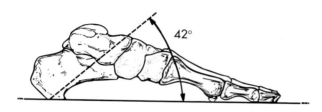

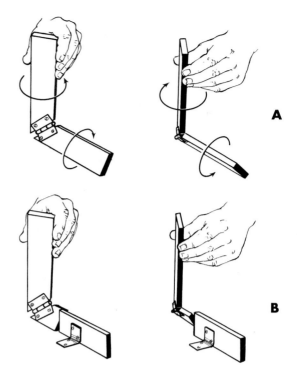

Fig. 1-14. Simple mechanism demonstrating functional relationships. **A,** Action of mitered hinge. **B,** Addition of a pivot between two segments of the mechanism. (From Mann R: *Surgery of the foot,* ed 5. St Louis, 1986, Mosby–Year Book.)

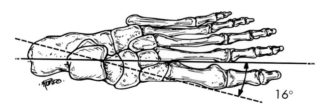

Fig. 1-13. Axis of the subtalar joint. The 16-degree deviation from the sagittal plane results in a smaller dorsiflexion-plantarflexion component of motion.

variations in the deviation of the axis also exist.[46] Manter and Inman both reported broad ranges for deviation of the axes, while several other investigators have noted both the frequency and the clinical significance of deviations of the subtalar axes from the stated averages.[16,21,22,54] Deviations from 20.5 to 68.5 degrees from the transverse plane and 4 to 47 degrees from the sagittal plane have been reported. The significance of these variations in the deviation of the axis can be appreciated by returning to the model of the mitered hinge. The mitered hinge model included a hinge deviated 45 degrees from the transverse plane. With the hinge at this angle, every 1 degree of rotation of the vertical segment produces 1 degree of rotation of the horizontal

segment. If the hinge is deviated approximately 70 degrees to the transverse plane, the amount of vertical segment rotation will greatly exceed horizontal segment rotation. If the hinge is deviated 20 degrees from the transverse plane, the amount of vertical segment rotation will be less than the amount of horizontal segment rotation. The deviations of the hinge in this model correspond to the effect of altered subtalar joint axes on the relationship of leg and foot displacement in function.

The person with a more vertical subtalar joint axis (further from the transverse plane) will have less corresponding subtalar joint inversion and eversion in response to rotation of the leg. Clinically, this may be the patient with more leg and postural complaints, as certain subtalar joint motions are decreased in response to vertical rotations. Conversely, the person with a more horizontal subtalar joint axis (closer to the horizontal plane) will have greater corresponding subtalar joint inversion and eversion in response to rotation of the leg. Clinically, this may be represented by the patient with severe foot abnormalities, as each degree of rotation of the leg is accompanied by greater amounts of subtalar joint inversion and eversion. Further, the deviation of the axis from the body planes also determines which components of pronation and supination will domi-

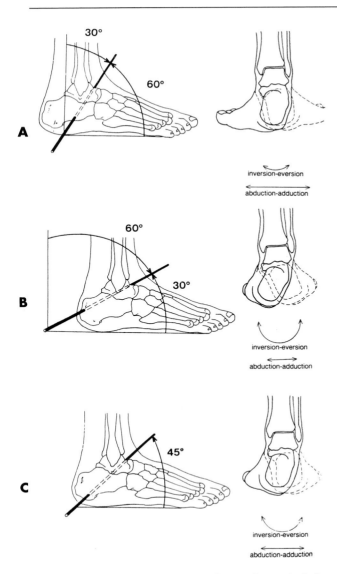

inversion-eversion

abduction-adduction

inversion-eversion

abduction-adduction

inversion-eversion

abduction-adduction

Fig. 1-15. A, When the axis is twice as close to the vertical plane as to the horizontal plane, twice as much motion occurs in the transverse plane as in the frontal plane. **B,** When the axis is twice as close to the horizontal plane as to the vertical plane, twice as much motion occurs in the frontal plane as in the transverse plane. **C,** When the axis is located halfway between the vertical and horizontal planes, equal amounts of transverse and frontal plane motion occur. (From Green D, Carol A: *J Am Podiatr Med Assoc* 74:98, 1984.)

nate in a given individual. In the foot in which the axes are deviated greatly from the transverse plane, horizontal or transverse plane motion of the subtalar joint will predominate. This may be seen as a foot with significant inversion or eversion displacements in function responding to deviation in axis orientation. This type of axis orientation and accompanying compensation profile is what occurs in the severe valgus flatfoot (Figs. 1-15**A, B,** and **C**).

The available motions in the average subtalar joint may be derived from the mean deviations for axis orientations at this joint. The average subtalar

joint axis deviates nearly equally from the transverse and frontal planes (42 degrees from the transverse plane, 48 degrees from the frontal plane). For all practical purposes, this axis deviation signifies that there are equal amounts of transverse and frontal plane motion at the subtalar joint. The average subtalar joint axis deviates only slightly from the sagittal plane (16 degrees from the sagittal plane), allowing only minimal motion in that plane. The 3:1 ratio of deviations of the axis on the frontal and transverse planes to deviation of the axis on the sagittal plane provides an easy formula for understanding the available motions in each body plane that may be expected in a normal subtalar joint. The deviation-of-axes ratio indicates that for every degree of sagittal plane motion there will be 3 degrees of transverse and frontal plane motion. The predominance of transverse and frontal plane motions at the subtalar joint, coupled with the sagittal plane motion available at the ankle joint, creates a rearfoot complex of two major joints in close proximity. Together, the joints have significant amounts of motion available in all three body planes to allow for smooth translation of the leg over the right-angled foot during gait.

Open kinetic chain

The motion available at the subtalar joint is triplanar, as the axis is deviated between all three body planes. The triplanar motions are known as pronation and supination. In open kinetic chain, with the foot free at the end of the leg, the components of supination are plantarflexion, adduction, and inversion. The resultant position of an open chain supinated subtalar joint is a foot pointing down, toward the midline, and facing inward (Fig. 1-16**A**). Open chain pronation consists of dorsiflexion, abduction, and eversion. The resultant position of an open chain pronated subtalar joint is a foot pointing up, away from the midline, and facing outward (Fig. 1-16**B**).[56]

Closed kinetic chain

Closed kinetic chain motion occurs at the subtalar joint throughout much of the stance phase of gait. Levens et al.[18] described the average rotation of the lower leg as 19 degrees, with a range of 13 to 26 degrees. In closed kinetic chain the foot is planted on the ground. Therefore, a mechanism must exist between the lower leg and the ground which allows these rotations to occur. While a severely oblique ankle joint would accommodate some of the leg rotation occurring over a planted foot, it is the subtalar joint which most accommodates this rotation. Using wooden models, Inman[31] described the capability of the subtalar joint to allow the leg above to rotate in the transverse plane while remaining

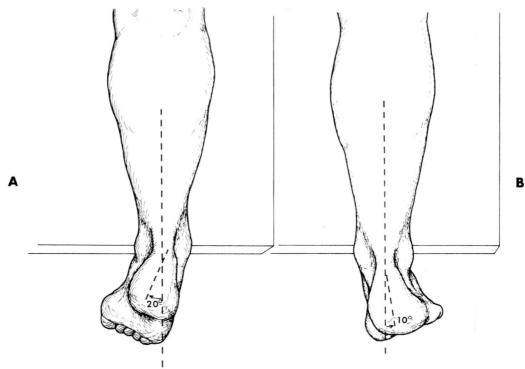

Fig. 1-16. A, Open chain supination of the subtalar joint. When the nonweightbearing foot is moved at the subtalar joint in the direction of supination, the talus is stable, and the calcaneus and foot move around the talus. The calcaneus and foot invert, plantarflex, and adduct. **B,** Open chain pronation of the subtalar joint. When the subtalar joint is moved into a pronated position in the nonweightbearing foot, the foot abducts, everts, and dorsiflexes around the stable talus. (From Root M, Weed J, Orien W: *Clinical Biomechanics Vol. II: Normal and abnormal function of the foot,* Los Angeles, 1977, Clinical Biomechanics Corp.)

vertical, and without adduction or abduction of the foot caused by slippage on the floor. Closed kinetic chain motion at the subtalar joint remains inversion with supination and eversion with pronation in the frontal plane. No limitations on frontal plane motion of the subtalar joint are placed on the foot with weightbearing; in other words, the subtalar joint and foot can easily invert and evert with the foot on the ground. Transverse and sagittal plane motions in closed kinetic chain are manifest with equal and opposite motions occurring proximal to the subtalar joint because of restrictions placed on these motions by the ground. The components of subtalar joint supination in the transverse and sagittal planes are plantarflexion and adduction. The friction from the ground in closed kinetic chain prevents the foot from plantarflexing and adducting, which are seen with dorsiflexion and abduction of the talus (which is just proximal to the subtalar joint) (Fig. 1-17**A**). The components of subtalar joint pronation in the transverse and sagittal planes are dorsiflexion and abduction. The friction from the ground as well as movement forward of the leg on the foot during stance prevents dorsiflexion and abduction of the foot on the leg. Therefore, in closed kinetic chain

pronation, equal and opposite plantarflexion and adduction of the talus just proximal to the subtalar joint is seen (Fig. 1-17**B**).

Closed kinetic chain supination consists of calcaneal inversion with talar abduction and dorsiflexion. This appears clinically as a foot facing inward, with a "stacking" of the talus over the calcaneus producing a "higher, thinner" appearance to the foot when viewed in the frontal plane. Conversely, closed kinetic chain pronation consists of calcaneal eversion along with talar adduction and plantarflexion (Fig. 1-18). This appears clinically as a foot facing outward, with a "lowering" of the talus from the calcaneus producing a "shorter, wider" appearance of the foot when viewed in the frontal plane.

Neutral position

Neutral position of a joint is a position from which a maximum excursion of the range of motion of the joint can occur in either direction. These neutral positions are purely reference points. Since the subtalar joint will affect the range and direction of motion of joints both proximal and distal to it, establishing the neutral position is functionally significant. Therefore, establishing neutral position

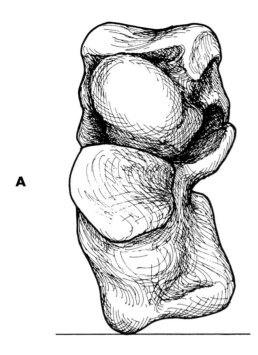

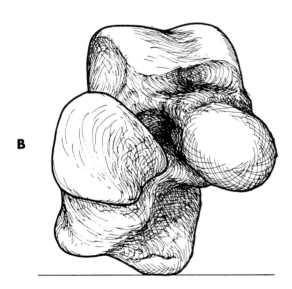

Fig. 1-17. A, Closed chain supination. Frontal plane view of the rearfoot showing calcaneal inversion with talar abduction and dorsiflexion. **B,** Closed chain pronation. Frontal plane view of the rearfoot showing calcaneal inversion with talar adduction and plantarflexion. (From Root M, Weed J, Orien W: *Clinical Biomechanics Vol. II Normal and abnormal biomechanics of the foot,* Los Angeles, 1977, Clinical Biomechanics Corp.)

prior to lower extremity assessment is required to obtain an accurate representation of the structures.

Root et al.[55] state that "the neutral position of the subtalar joint is that position of the joint in which the foot is neither pronated nor supinated." From this position, full supination of the normal subtalar joint inverts the calcaneus twice as many degrees as full pronation everts it. The average subtalar joint neutral position is a 0- to 3-degree inverted attitude of the calcaneus as measured relative to the lower one third of the leg.

Although it is common to find a 2:1 ratio of supination to pronation at the subtalar joint, it is not unusual for individuals to exhibit 3:1 or 4:1 ratios.

Range of motion of the subtalar joint

The reported normal range of motion of the subtalar joint is highly variable. Reported values of inversion and excursion range from 5 to 50 degrees. Reported values of eversion range from 5 to 26 degrees.[50] The average subtalar joint range of motion has been reported as 25 degrees (20 degrees inversion and 5 degrees eversion).[57] Root et al. report an average range of subtalar motion to be 30 degrees with two thirds (20 degrees) in the direction of inversion and one third (10 degrees) in the direction of eversion.[55]

Wright et al.[66] found that throughout the stance phase of gait, the average excursion of the subtalar joint was only 6 degrees and labeled this the "functional range" of motion. Root et al. state that normal locomotion requires an average minimum range of 4 to 6 degrees of inversion with supination and 4 to 6 degrees of eversion with pronation. Although there is some disagreement in regard to how much subtalar joint motion is required for normal locomotion, it appears that considerably less motion is actually required for normal function than is available in the average joint.

Summary

1. Articulation between the talus and the calcaneus involves three facets on the inferior surface of the talus articulating with three facets on the superior surface of the calcaneus. The anterior and middle facets form a transitional two-facet or special two-facet configuration.

2. Ligamentous attachments include the interosseous ligaments which primarily limit eversion, and the cervical ligament, which primarily limits inversion.

3. The average axis deviation is 42 degrees from the transverse plane and 16 degrees from the sagittal plane. There is three times as much

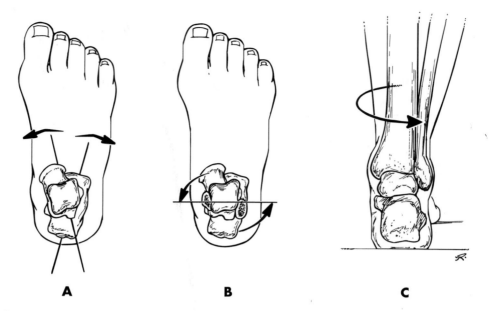

Fig. 1-18. Loading response of the subtalar joint. **A,** Adduction of the talus with foot pronation. **B,** The ankle axis *(solid line)* rotates medially *(arrows)* as the talus displaces with foot pronation. **C,** The tibia internally rotates with the talus.

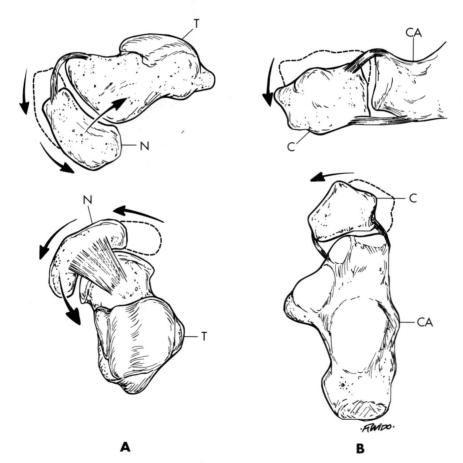

Fig. 1-19. Supination of the midtarsal joint. **A,** Plantar and medial movement of the navicular on the talus. **B,** Plantar and medial movement of the cuboid on the calcaneus. *N,* navicular; *T,* talus; *C,* cuboid; *CA,* calcaneus.

transverse and frontal plane motion as sagittal plane motion with average axis deviations.

4. Axes that deviate further from the transverse plane demonstrate less inversion or eversion and increased transverse plane motion. Axes that are closer to the transverse plane demonstrate more frontal plane motion and less transverse plane motion.

5. Open kinetic chain pronation of the subtalar joint consists of dorsiflexion, abduction, and eversion. Open kinetic chain supination consists of plantarflexion, adduction, and inversion.

6. Closed kinetic chain pronation consists of calcaneal eversion with equal and opposite motions in the proximal portion of the subtalar joint due to restrictions placed on open kinetic chain motions by the ground. This is manifested by talar adduction and plantarflexion. Closed kinetic chain supination consists of calcaneal inversion with equal and opposite motions in the proximal portion of the subtalar joint due to restrictions placed on open chain motions by the ground. This is manifested by talar abduction and dorsiflexion.

7. Average subtalar joint range of motion of 25 to 30 degrees has been reported. Approximately two thirds is inversion and one third, eversion.

8. Functional ranges of motion used in gait of 6 degrees total motion and 4 to 6 degrees of both inversion and eversion with supination and pronation, respectively, have been reported.

The midtarsal joint
Anatomy

The midtarsal joint (transverse tarsal joint, Chopart's joint) consists of the combined articulations of the talonavicular and calcaneocuboid joints. It represents the functional articulation between the hindfoot (talus and calcaneus) and midfoot (navicular and cuboid). These articulations have been described anatomically as "plane" or "gliding" joints.[22] The osseous movements of the midtarsal joint components when the subtalar joint is pronating and supinating have been described by Kapanji.[34] Medial and inferior movements of the navicular and cuboid, on the talus and the calcaneus, respectively, are described with supination. In pronation, lateral and superior movements of the navicular and cuboid, on the talus and calcaneus, respectively, may be expected (Fig. 1-19).

The ligamentous stability of the midtarsal joint is provided by the short and long plantar ligaments, the plantar calcaneonavicular ligament, and the bifurcate ligament.[58] The ligamentous structures contribute to limitations of pronation and supination at the midtarsal joint. Lewis[39] has stated that the plantar calcaneocuboid (short plantar) ligament and the calcaneocuboid component of the bifurcate ligament are tightened with pronation of the rearfoot and supination of the midtarsal joint. It has also been noted that the principal resistance to supination at this joint is provided by tension from the ligamentous structures.

The midtarsal joint in function
Axis of the midtarsal joint

Although the midtarsal joint is actually composed of two separate anatomic articulations, the transverse tarsal region is described as a single functional unit. Manter[46] has described its movement as a segment rotating about two distinct axes of the midtarsal joint: the longitudinal and the oblique (Fig. 1-20). Unlike the axes of the ankle and subtalar joints, these axes bear little relationship to anatomic landmarks. Rather, these axes are posited to understand the functional behavior of the joint.[50] The longitudinal axis is directed from proximal, plantar, and lateral to distal, dorsal, and medial. It deviates an average of 15 degrees from the transverse plane and 9 degrees from the sagittal plane.[46] The longitudinal axis, because of its close proximity to the transverse and sagittal planes, primarily allows the frontal plane motions of inversion and eversion. The presence of frontal plane motion on the longitudinal axis of the midtarsal joint enables the midfoot to respond well to significant frontal plane variations in rearfoot position caused by subtalar joint motions. This plays an important role in maintaining the forefoot on the ground during closed kinetic chain function. The ability of the axis to allow frontal plane motion to function separately from the other axis of the midtarsal joint is crucial in allowing opposing positions of the forefoot and rearfoot when walking on uneven terrain.

The oblique axis of the midtarsal joint also runs from proximal, plantar, and lateral to distal, dorsal, and medial. It is oriented more steeply and obliquely from the foot as it deviates an average of 52 degrees from the transverse plane and 57 degrees from the sagittal plane.[46] This significant average deviation from the transverse and sagittal planes provides the oblique axis with increased amounts of motion in these planes. The principal motions demonstrated at the oblique axis are dorsiflexion coupled with abduction, and plantarflexion coupled with adduction. The significant amounts of sagittal plane motion in addition to transverse plane motion available at this axis have earned it the name of "secondary ankle joint," as limitations of motion at

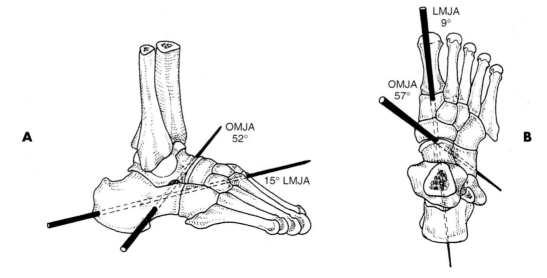

Fig. 1-20. The midtarsal joint axes of motion. **A,** The oblique midtarsal joint axis *(OMJA)*. **B,** The longitudinal midtarsal joint axis *(LMJA)*. (From Michaud T: *Foot orthosis,* Baltimore, 1993, Williams & Wilkins.)

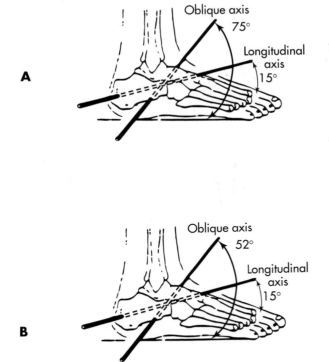

Fig. 1-21. Effects of axis deviation on midtarsal joint motion. **A,** Increased deviation of the oblique axis from the transverse plane results in a greater abduction and adduction component of the motion. **B,** Increased deviation of the oblique axis from the sagittal plane results in a greater dorsiflexion-plantarflexion component of the motion. (From Green D, Carol A: *J Am Podiatr Med Assoc* 74:98, 1984.)

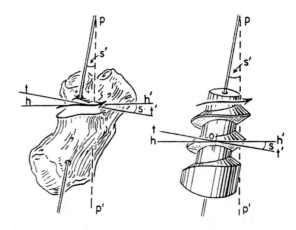

Fig. 1-22. Comparison of the posterior calcaneal facet of the right subtalar joint with a right-handed screw. The *arrow* represents the path of a body following the screw; *hh′* is the horizontal plane in which motion is occurring; *tt″* is a plane perpendicular to the axis of the screw; *n* is the helix angle of the screw, equal to the angle *s′* which is obtained by dropping a perpendicular *(pp′)* from the axis. (From Manter JT: *Anat Rec* 80:402, 1941.)

the ankle joint are often compensated at the oblique axis of the midtarsal joint.

Planal dominance

Planal dominance, or alteration in the motions found in individual joints due to axis deviations, plays a significant role in midtarsal joint function. Root et al. reported that in some persons the oblique axis deviates more than 52 degrees from the transverse plane (Fig. 1-21). This allows dominance of abduction and adduction movements over dorsiflexion and plantarflexion movements. If an altered axis is present, normal midtarsal joint oblique axis pronation, which occurs as the forefoot begins to bear weight, results in excessive abduction of the forefoot with relative rearfoot adduction. This midfoot and talar adduction causes the leg to be medially displaced above the calcaneus. The forces of body weight in these persons fall medial to the sagittal plane of the calcaneus, thereby creating a large lever arm which everts the calcaneus and pronates the subtalar joint. This foot type may manifest itself clinically by an increased cuboid abduction on the calcaneus, or rearfoot adduction on loading of the forefoot during stance. This may be seen when observing the foot from above in weightbearing, as well as posterior to the calcaneus during static stance. This foot type, with body weight producing a large lever arm to pronate the subtalar joint, may be very difficult to control with a functional foot orthosis, which must oppose these forces.

Interdependence of the subtalar and midtarsal joints

Manter,[46] in his pioneering work on the subtalar and midtarsal joints, described the interdependence of these two joints in function. He described a helical screwlike motion to the subtalar joint which produces forward displacement of the talus with pronation (Fig. 1-22). He also attributed screwlike motion to the longitudinal axis of the midtarsal joint. He described the screw effect of the longitudinal axis as opposite to that found in the subtalar joint. His model for the subtalar joint was for a right-handed screw in the right subtalar joint and the reverse on the left side. The longitudinal axis screw is said to be opposite to the subtalar screw motion. That is, the talonavicular screw is left-handed in the right foot with a right-handed subtalar joint screw. In the left foot, the talonavicular screw is right-handed. In this model, the subtalar and midtarsal joints have been described as dual screws connected to the talonavicular joint in opposite directions. This model introduced the concept that the midtarsal joint range of motion was under the control of the position of the subtalar joint. Manter described an oblique axis without a screwlike mechanism with motion limited by the action of ligaments and muscles.[46]

Hicks[27] expanded the concept initially proposed by Manter. He described the interrelationship of the subtalar and midtarsal joints providing full pronation and supination motions through the foot. The axes are interrelated in their function due in part to their all passing through the center of the head of the talus. Hicks based most of his concepts on talona-vicular joint function, which he believed to be a ball-and-socket type of joint that demonstrated hinge joint function with 3 degrees of freedom.

Role of axis orientation in determining flexibility and stability

Elftman[15] contributed important work on the role of axis orientation in determining flexibility or stability of the midtarsal joint. He described the calcaneocuboid joint as the key to the midtarsal joint. He noted that although they are not fully attached, the cuboid and navicular function as a unit. He described two axes for the calcaneocuboid joint. The first lies within the calcaneus, is projected upward, and passes through the head of the talus. The second lies in the cuboid at a right angle to the first axis. The resultant axis of the two axes intersects the perpendicular line uniting both axes and runs just below the sustentaculum tali and through the talus. The resultant axis of the calcaneocuboid joint as described by Elftman closely approximates the oblique axis described by Manter and Hicks. This model also describes two axes for the talonavicular joint with a resultant axis approximating the longitudinal axis.

Elftman's greatest contribution to understanding midtarsal joint function was his description of the relationship of the major axis of the calcaneocuboid joint to the major axis of the talonavicular joint in response to subtalar joint position. In a significantly pronated subtalar joint, these axes of the midtarsal joint take a more parallel orientation to each other, facilitating increased range of motion of the forefoot on the rearfoot. In a supinated subtalar joint, this parallel relationship is lost, and movements of the midtarsal joint about both axes are decreased. In 1964, Mann and Inman[43] also wrote of the orientation of the two midtarsal joint axes in response to the position of the subtalar joint. The two axes, when seen in a frontal plane view of the midfoot with the forefoot missing, pass obliquely through the calcaneus and talus respectively. In a foot with a pronated subtalar joint, with the talus plantarflexing and adducting on an everted calcaneus, the orientation of the two midtarsal axes becomes more parallel. This facilitates "unlocking" or easy movement of the midfoot on the hindfoot under these conditions. These axes diverge in a foot with a supinated subtalar joint, with the talus dorsiflexing and abducting on an inverted calcaneus (Fig. 1-23). This significantly restricts movement of the midfoot on the hindfoot and produces a decrease in available midtarsal joint range of motion.

Locking mechanism of the midtarsal joint

The midtarsal joint has been described as similar to the subtalar joint in that it also possesses an

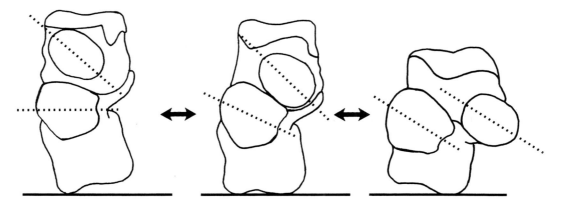

Fig. 1-23. When the subtalar joint (STJ) is in its maximally pronated position *(far right)*, the longitudinal axes of the articular facets are lined up approximately parallel with one another. In the STJ neutral position, the angulation between the longitudinal axes has increased. Further divergence of the axes is noted on the *far left* with the STJ in its maximally supinated position. (From Seibel M: *Foot function, a programmed text*, Baltimore, 1988, Williams & Wilkins.)

osseous locking mechanism to prevent excessive motion.[2] In this theory, the calcaneocuboid joint is described as a concave-convex joint, not shaped as a saddle, as previously described, but as half of an hourglass. This structure facilitates rotation of the cuboid on the calcaneus with the calcaneal process serving as a pivot. Bojsen-Møller[2] described pronation of the calcaneocuboid joint as dorsal movement of the tonguelike inferior lateral extension of the cuboid joint surface until the joint reached a closely packed position, resulting in maximum joint surface congruence and stability. The overhanging dorsolateral calcaneus prevents overpronation at this joint when the superoproximal border of the rotating cuboid comes into contact with it (Fig. 1-24). The ligaments of the midtarsal joint, which tighten in this pronated position, prevent further pronation beyond the osseous locking point. Subluxation of the calcaneocuboid joint with overstretching of the restraining ligaments would result, with midtarsal joint pronation beyond this point.[39]

On the other hand, supination of the calcaneocuboid joint is limited only by the tightening of ligaments. In this position the joint is not closely packed, with the articular surfaces only partially contacting one another, so osseous locking is not present. Bojsen-Møller's description of the osseous locking mechanism of the midtarsal joint helps explain the pronated position of this joint as the position of stability in gait. Both the subtalar and midtarsal joint locking mechanisms have been described by Manter[46] as uniquely human traits allowing for improved bipedal ambulation. The midtarsal joint's locking mechanism is assisted in late midstance and propulsion as the lesser tarsal bones are stabilized by the synergistic action of the posterior tibial and peroneus longus and peroneus

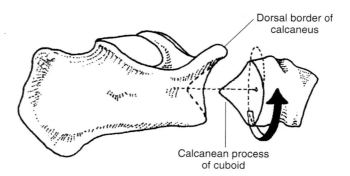

Dorsal border of calcaneus

Calcanean process of cuboid

Fig. 1-24. The pronating cuboid pivots about the calcaneal process until its dorsal border contacts the overhanging calcaneus. (Adapted from Bojsen-Møller F: *J Anat* 129:165–176, 1979.)

brevis muscles.[12] Plantar insertions of the posterior tibial into the navicular, the three cuneiforms, the three central metatarsal bases, and the cuboid provide it with a posterior and medial stabilizing effect on the lesser tarsus. The peroneus longus, with its oblique insertion into the lateral aspect of the base of the first metatarsal, exerts a posterior and lateral stabilizing effect on the lesser tarsus. These tendons cross under the lesser tarsus and create broad stability when contracting with their posterior and cruciform action. The peroneus brevis, with its insertion into the fifth metatarsal base, assists the peroneus longus in providing lateral stabilization of the lesser tarsus[56] (Fig. 1-25).

Clinically, the locking position of the midtarsal joint may be approximated by placing the subtalar joint in its neutral position and applying a dorsiflexion force on the fourth and fifth metatarsal heads to resistance. This dorsiflexion force approximates the effect of the ground reaction force on the lateral

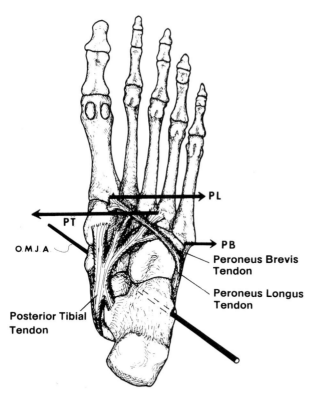

Fig. 1-25. The peroneus longus muscle courses around the stable cuboid to insert into the plantar-medial aspect of the base of the first ray. Contraction of the peroneus longus muscle exerts an abduction force *(arrow PL)*, which stabilizes the first ray against the lesser tarsus. Contraction of the posterior tibial muscle exerts an adduction force on the lesser tarsus *(arrow PT)*. The simultaneous contraction of these two muscles stabilizes the lesser tarsus transversely by compressing the lesser tarsal bones against one another. (From Root M, Weed J, Orien W: *Clinical Biomechanics Vol. II Normal and abnormal function of the foot,* Los Angeles, 1977, Clinical Biomechanics Corp.)

forefoot during terminal midstance. This position enables the examiner to determine the forefoot-to-rearfoot relationships when the osseous locking mechanism is engaged. This is the position recommended for off-weightbearing impression casting for foot orthoses (Fig. 1-26).

Open kinetic chain

Throughout the contact period of gait, the oblique axis of the midtarsal joint is pronated and the longitudinal axis is supinated. This represents an open kinetic chain position created by the pull of the muscles of the anterior compartment, which are eccentrically contacting to decelerate plantarflexion of the ankle after heel-strike. Contraction of the anterior tibial, which inserts medial to the long axis of the foot, will invert or supinate the midtarsal joint about the longitudinal axis. Contraction of the extensor digitorum longus and peroneus tertius, which insert lateral to the long axis of the foot,

abduct and dorsiflex, or pronate, the midtarsal joint about the oblique axis. Throughout the contact period, with the subtalar joint pronating to absorb shock, the longitudinal axis remains inverted to maintain the foot in a plantigrade position. Forefoot loading through contact, beginning on the lateral side of the foot, enables ground reaction forces to maintain the midtarsal joint's oblique axis in its maximally pronated position.

Closed kinetic chain

Continued loading of the forefoot throughout midstance maintains the oblique axis in a pronated position as ground reaction forces apply a dorsiflexion and abduction force about this axis. Recall the effect of a more obliquely oriented axis of this joint described earlier. Here, with the axis angle farther from the transverse plane, motion is increased in that plane, and the effect of ground reaction forces during midstance is primarily to adduct the rearfoot with a resultant abduction of the forefoot. This leads to medial displacement of the leg over the rearfoot and a resulting greater lever arm for pronation at the subtalar joint[56] (Fig. 1-27).

In midstance, the longitudinal axis begins to evert or pronate in response to subtalar joint supination which occurs throughout midstance. Therefore, by the end of midstance, closed kinetic chain pronation occurs about both axes of the midtarsal joint. Ideally, pronation about the longitudinal axis locks the joint as the cuboid comes in contact with the dorsal border of the overhanging calcaneus creating a position of stability for propulsion.[2] In closed kinetic chain function, the distal segment is on the ground. Motions in the "grounded" distal segments are seen as equal and opposite motions of the proximal joint. In the case of midtarsal joint pronation about both axes during midstance, the rearfoot (subtalar joint) supinates with a stable forefoot. Therefore, pronation of the midtarsal joint axes, under the closed chain circumstances of midstance, is demonstrated as supination of the rearfoot, since the distal segment is fixed on the ground (Fig. 1-28**A,** p. 21). This explains why, in the locked position, the midtarsal joint is pronated about both its axes. Under the closed kinetic chain circumstances of gait, the midtarsal joint is pronated and in a stable position, while the subtalar joint is supinated. Although the oblique axis is pronated throughout midstance, it becomes relatively less pronated as the midstance period ends. Conversely, a supinated position of the midtarsal joint, present with a pronated rearfoot in the closed kinetic chain, represents an unlocked or unstable position in function (Fig. 1-28**B,** p. 21).

This connection between a supinated position of the midtarsal joint's longitudinal axis and a pro-

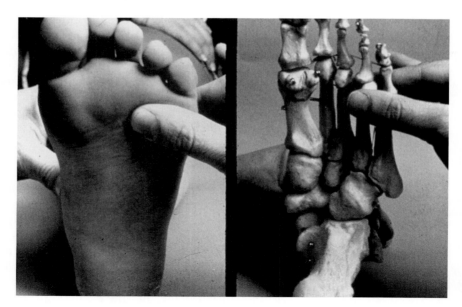

Fig. 1-26. Position for locking the midtarsal joint. The subtalar joint is maintained in the neutral position, and a dorsiflexion force is applied to the fourth and fifth metatarsal heads.

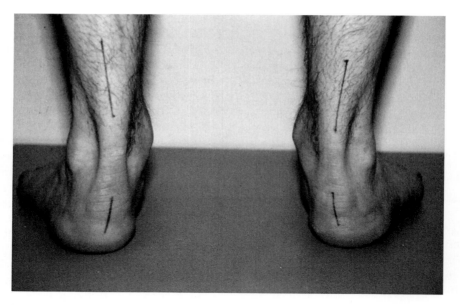

Fig. 1-27. Closed chain, midtarsal joint, oblique axis pronation. The leg is medially displaced as the foot slips from under the tibia. Adduction of the rearfoot provides "apparent abduction of the forefoot."

nated subtalar joint helps explain the "supinatus-"deformity of the forefoot. Classically, a supinatus deformity occurs when the heel everts beyond the perpendicular. More commonly, however, a supinatus, or acquired, inverted position of the forefoot on the rearfoot, results when the subtalar joint has not adequately resupinated after heel-lift. This relatively pronated rearfoot will have an unlocked supinated midtarsal joint longitudinal axis accompanying it during this most destructive period of the

gait cycle, that is, immediately after the heel has lifted off the ground. Repeated functioning in this position causes the midtarsal joint to "acquire" this inverted position over time, thereby leading to a supinatus deformity. This helps explain the frequency with which this deformity is demonstrated in feet whose heels do not pronate beyond the perpendicular, once thought to be the mechanism of action for the creation of a supinatus deformity (Fig. 1-29, p. 22). The longitudinal axis of the midtarsal

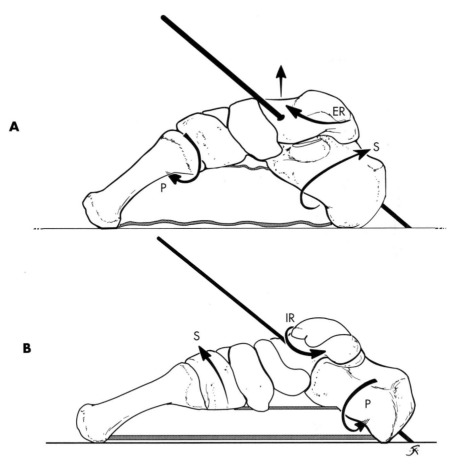

Fig. 1-28. A, External rotation and vertical loading of the foot by the tibiotalar column. The arch is higher and shorter. The plantar aponeurosis and plantar ligaments are relaxed. The rearfoot is supinated (varus) and the forefoot is pronated. Without pronation the forefoot will be off the ground on the medial side. *ER,* external rotation; *P,* pronation; *S,* supination. **B,** Internal rotation and vertical loading of the foot by the tibiotalar column. The arch is lower and longer. The plantar aponeurosis and the plantar ligaments are under tension. The rearfoot is pronated (valgus) and the forefoot is supinated. Without supination the forefoot will be off the ground on the lateral side. *IR,* internal rotation; *P,* pronation; *S,* supination. (Adapted from Serrafian SK: Functional characteristic of the foot and plantar aponeurosis under tibiotalar loading, *Foot & Ankle* 8:14-16, 1987.)

joint remains pronated during propulsion. This everted position enables the efficient pull of the peroneal muscle group which is helping to shift weight medially across the foot and, eventually, to lift the lateral side of the foot off the ground. A midtarsal joint that is not pronated about the longitudinal axis prior to propulsion will contribute to an inefficient pull of the lateral muscles of the leg, as the joint axis must first be everted before the muscles can begin to lift the lateral side of the foot off the ground. Over time, these circumstances will produce fatigue and overuse of the peroneal muscle group. Propulsion is accompanied by marked external leg rotation, supination of the rearfoot, and lifting of the heel off the ground. This raises and abducts the rearfoot away from the planted forefoot during this phase. The

oblique axis of the midtarsal joint supinates during propulsion. This relative adduction and plantarflexion of the forefoot in the closed kinetic chain is actually abduction and dorsiflexion of the rearfoot facilitated by external leg rotation, subtalar joint supination, and heel lift[56] (Table 1-1).

Windlass effect

Supination of the oblique axis of the midtarsal joint during propulsion is aided by the contraction of the intrinsic muscles of the foot originating on the medial calcaneus[47] and by the windlass effect of the plantar aponeurosis.[28] Hicks[28] described a strong distal attachment for the plantar aponeurosis through the plantar pads of the metatarsophalangeal joints. During dorsiflexion or extension of

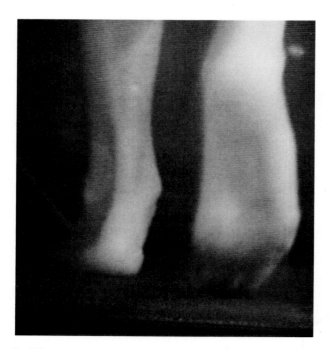

Fig. 1-29. Development of forefoot supinatus at heel-lift. The calcaneus is everted (subtalar joint pronation) to the plane of the forefoot. The floor maintains the horizontal position of the forefoot, resulting in an inverted position of the forefoot relative to the rearfoot about the longitudinal metatarsophalangeal joint.

the toes, the plantar pads and, hence, the aponeurosis are pulled forward around the heads of the metatarsals "like a cable being wound onto a windlass." This causes the rearfoot to supinate as the pull of the aponeurosis causes the distance between the metatarsal heads and the calcaneus to shorten. Hicks further described that as dorsiflexion of the toes is forced by the forward momentum of the body, and as the arch height is increased by the ligamentous mechanism of the windlass, these activities are accomplished without the direct action of any muscle[28] (Fig. 1-30). Sarrafian[59] described the foot as having the structural and functional characteristics of a beam and a truss. The truss is made possible by the plantar aponeurosis which, when placed under tension, relieves the tensile forces from the plantar surfaces of the skeleton, which is then subjected only to compressive forces. Vertical loading and forward movement of the leg increase the tension on the aponeurosis and initiate the truss phenomenon. Serrafian describes the effect of an externally rotated leg, with a supinated rearfoot and pronated forefoot, as producing relaxation of the plantar aponeurosis about which extension of the toes can occur. Conversely, an internally rotated leg, with a pronated rearfoot and supinated forefoot, places the aponeurosis under increased tension and mark-

edly limits extension of the metatarsophalangeal joints.

Range of motion of the midtarsal joint

Hicks[27] described the average range of motion of the two midtarsal joint axes. The oblique axis has an average range of motion of 22 degrees; the longitudinal axis has an average range of motion of 8 degrees. Root et al.[55] stated that the minimum amount of oblique axis motion needed for normal ambulation is unknown. The authors concluded, however, that the minimum amount of longitudinal axis motion required for normal gait is 4 to 6 degrees. This longitudinal axis motion is required to keep the foot plantigrade when the subtalar joint is pronating to an equal extent during the contact phase of gait.

In 1983, Phillips and Phillips[53] verified and quantified the relationship between midtarsal joint range of motion and subtalar joint position. They studied the effect of a supinated, neutral, and pronated subtalar joint on midtarsal joint range of motion and the maximum locked position of the joint. When the subtalar joint moved from a supinated to a neutral position, the locked position of the midtarsal joint gained an average of 11.6 degrees of pronation. As the subtalar joint moved from a supinated to a pronated position, the locked position became progressively more pronated. The increase in midtarsal joint pronation for each degree of subtalar pronation was found to be exponential, not linear. Understanding the midtarsal joint's locking mechanism, and control of range of motion, confirms that as the subtalar joint becomes progressively more supinated, the maximally pronated position of the midtarsal joint moves in the direction of supination. As this more supinated position for end range of pronation is achieved, the midtarsal joint progressively locks, becoming more stable. Therefore, the more supinated the midtarsal joint is at the end range of pronation motion, the more stable the joint will be when locked.

Summary

1. The midtarsal joint consists of two separate anatomical articulations, the talonavicular and calcaneocuboid joints, which together make up the transverse tarsal region and function as a single unit.

2. Restrictions of joint motions are provided by an osseous locking mechanism aided by ligamentous attachments with pronation and with supination.

3. The average longitudinal axis deviates 15 degrees from the transverse plane and 9 degrees from the sagittal plane. Motion about this axis

Table 1-1
Normal motions during gait

	Subtalar joint	Midtarsal longitudinal axis	Midtarsal obl. axis
Contact	Pronation	Supination	Pronation
Midstance	Supination	Pronation	Pronation
Propulsion	Supination	Pronation	Supination
Swing	Pronation/supination	Pronation/supination	Supination/pronation

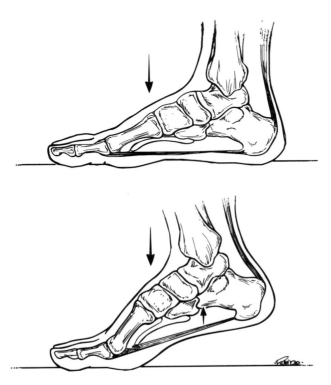

Fig. 1-30. The plantar aponeurosis reaches from the calcaneus to the proximal phalanges of the toes. It acts as a tie for the longitudinal arch held in reserve while standing, but becomes tensed when the heel is lifted, and the toes wind its distal part around the metatarsal heads. As the heel lifts, the calcaneus is brought closer to the forefoot, raising the arch. (Modified from Bojsen-Møller F, Lamoreux L: *Acta Orthop Scand* 50-411– 479, 1979.)

is primarily in the frontal plane, enabling the forefoot to remain plantigrade while accommodating the positions of the rearfoot during gait.

4. The average oblique axis deviates 52 degrees from the transverse plane and 57 degrees from the sagittal plane. Motions about this axis occur primarily in the transverse and sagittal planes. It is functionally significant in persons lacking sufficient sagittal plane motion of the ankle to help move the leg over the planted foot in gait. These persons may compensate for this deficiency at this "secondary ankle joint."

5. The range of motion of the midtarsal joint is controlled by subtalar joint position. In a pronated subtalar joint, the two axes of the midtarsal joint are in a more parallel orientation increasing the range of motion. In a supinated subtalar joint, the two axes of the midtarsal joint are in a more oblique orientation, decreasing the range of motion.

6. The calcaneocuboid joint provides the midtarsal joint with an osseus locking mechanism in gait. Excessive pronation is blocked when the rotating cuboid abuts the dorsolateral calcaneus. This locking mechanism is assisted by compression of the lesser tarsus by the synergistic action of the posterior tibial, peroneus brevis, and peroneus longus muscles during the late midstance and propulsive phases of gait.

7. The normal positions of the midtarsal joint in stance are as follows: The longitudinal axis is supinated in the contact phase of gait and pronated in both the midstance and propulsive phases of gait. The oblique axis is pronated in the contact and midstance phases of gait and supinated in the propulsive phase of gait.

8. The windlass effect of the plantar aponeurosis, activated with heel-lift, aids with supination of the oblique axis during propulsion. With dorsiflexion at the metatarsophalangeal joints, the plantar aponeurosis is pulled around the heads of the metatarsals, shortening the distance between the metatarsal heads and calcaneus. This aids subtalar and oblique midtarsal joint supination during propulsion.

9. A minimum of 4 to 6 degrees of longitudinal axis motion in gait is needed to maintain the foot plantigrade when the subtalar joint pronates to that degree during the contact phase of gait.

The first ray

Under normal conditions, the movements of the first ray in midstance and propulsion flow smoothly into continued forward movement of the foot over the planted hallux during first metatarsophalangeal joint function. Creating stabilization of the first ray for propulsion enables forward movement of the body to occur at the first metatarsophalangeal joint leading to toe-off. Viewing these two joints as a functional unit is essential to understanding movement of the body over the foot in gait.

Anatomy

The first ray is a functional unit consisting of the first metatarsal and the medial (first) cuneiform. The first metatarsal base and medial cuneiform are tightly bound together by ligaments. A large, thick dorsal ligament attaches the base of the first metatarsal to the medial cuneiform. At the plantar aspect a broad, rectangular ligament links the two bones. There are also attachments between the lateral side of the first cuneiform and the base of the second metatarsal. These include the plantar and dorsal ligaments, as well as the interosseous ligaments. The first ray is united to the navicular by a dorsal and plantar ligament. In addition, the medial cuneonavicular ligament unites the base of the cuneiform medially to the navicular.[58]

The first ray in function

Axis of the first ray

In 1954, Hicks[27] published the first scientific examination of motion at the first ray in his investigation of the axes of motion for many of the pedal articulations. His experiments were performed on five anatomic specimens under laboratory conditions. These circumstances may suggest that his findings do not correspond to certain joint motions in actual, closed kinetic chain function. Hicks described an axis for the first ray that runs from posterior, medial, and dorsal to anterior, lateral, and plantar (Fig. 1-31). The axis deviates approximately 45 degrees from the frontal and sagittal planes with very slight deviation from the transverse plane. Because this axis runs in the opposite direction to the subtalar and midtarsal axes, their motions are different from those at the latter joints. The motion is uniaxial and triplanar without pronation and supination.[50] At this axis, dorsiflexion is coupled with inversion and adduction in pronation, and plantarflexion is coupled with eversion and abduction in supination.

Closed kinetic chain

There have been conflicting reports in the literature regarding the function of the first ray. The importance of the first ray as a functional unit has long been recognized. It plays an important role in responding to varying positions of the rearfoot

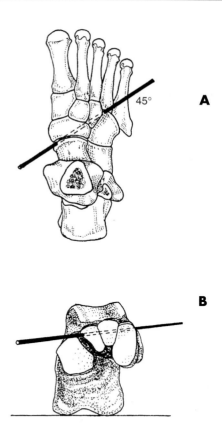

Fig. 1-31. Axis of motion for the first ray. **A,** Anterior view (sectioned at the cuneiforms). **B,** Dorsal view. (From Michaud T: *Foot orthosis,* Baltimore, 1993, Williams & Wilkins.)

throughout gait so that the forefoot remains plantigrade. It also plays a major role in allowing the hallux to dorsiflex adequately during gait to enable effective propulsion.

Broca,[4] writing in 1852 about the development of hallux valgus, referred to changes in the first ray "in the direction of the longitudinal axis and around it." The rotational component he referred to seemed to indicate an eversion of the metatarsal with dorsiflexion. Kelikian,[35] in his review of the development of hallux valgus, stated that the first metatarsal head inverts with pronation. He quoted Stein and Hauser as stating that the first metatarsal inverts in relation to both the hallux and the ground during pronation.

In 1968 Ebisiu[14] confirmed the conclusions of Hicks, that "the overall effect of a severe pronatory force is the extension (dorsiflexion) and inversion of the first ray." Sgarlato,[62] as well as Root et al.,[56] described dorsiflexion with inversion of the first ray. D'Amico and Schuster,[8] in 1979, suggested that the conclusions of Hicks did not seem to apply to a loaded foot in function. Their study began to focus interest on the differences between describing isolated positions of the ray under experimental conditions and the net effect on the first ray on overall forefoot positions. The authors illustrated this point by concluding that "we were unable to demonstrate the accepted understanding of inversion of the first ray with dorsiflexion accompanying pronation with closed-kinetic chain pronation." They concluded that "there is a noted dorsiflexion and eversion of the first ray accompanying pronation." D'Amico and Schuster suggested that after heel-off, with ground reaction force loading the forefoot, some relative inversion of the first ray may occur from a markedly everted position.[8] It is this notion that may help to clarify the apparent discrepancies throughout the literature regarding the frontal plane motions of the first ray. Descriptions of isolated rays inverting with dorsiflexion and the first ray everting with the rest of the forefoot with pronation may actually be consistent and explainable when examined closely.

Oldenbrook and Smith,[51] studying metatarsal head motion secondary to rearfoot position, concluded that with subtalar joint pronation, the first metatarsal everts relative to the ground, but that it everts less than the lesser metatarsal heads. They studied motions of the individual metatarsals with the subtalar joint pronated and found less frontal plane motion of the first metatarsal compared to the second, but more sagittal plane motion of the first metatarsal compared to the second. As the first ray axes pass opposite to the pronation-supination axis, motion is dorsiflexion with inversion and plantarflexion with eversion. The inversion of the first ray, while relatively small, is subtracted from the larger amount of eversion of the forefoot occurring with rearfoot pronation, leaving a net eversion of the first ray relative to the ground. The authors' study further clarifies that, while the first ray dorsiflexes with inversion, the forefoot everts substantially with pronation, leaving a net dorsiflexed and everted first ray relative to the ground (Fig. 1-32). This concept is also illustrated by pathologic function. Excessive pronation of the rearfoot is accompanied by inversion of the longitudinal axis of the midtarsal joint. This axis has a relatively small range of motion and is unable to compensate for significant eversion of the forefoot. Further inversion of the medial column occurs with dorsiflexion of the first ray to accommodate this severe pronation deformity. Although first-ray dorsiflexion and inversion occur in the valgus foot type, a net everted first ray and forefoot, relative to the ground, still occurs.

On examination of cadaveric specimens with hallux abducto valgus, Grodel and McCarthy[23] found anatomical changes consistent with first-ray dorsiflexion and eversion with pronation in function. Root et al.[56] studied the range and direction of first-ray motion in cadaveric specimens. Their data

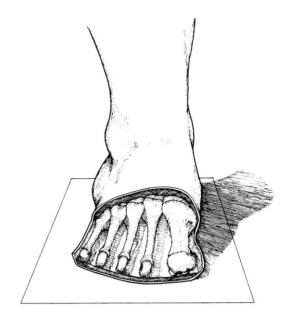

Fig. 1-32. Eversion of the foot that occurs with subtalar joint pronation will also evert the forefoot. When the forefoot everts in relation to the ground, vertical ground reaction forces against the first metatarsal cause the first ray to evert less than the lesser metatarsals. Dorsiflexion with inversion of the first ray results in a less everted position of the ray. (From Root M, Weed J, Orien W: *Clinical Biomechanics Vol. II Normal and abnormal function of the foot*, Los Angeles, 1977, Clinical Biomechanics Corp.)

revealed that the first-ray axis caused inversion with dorsiflexion locally, as long as the rearfoot was immobilized.

Mason (unpublished) utilized a mechanical model of the foot to confirm the effects of rearfoot position on the first-ray motion previously reported. With rearfoot eversion, the first ray was found to be everted relative to the ground, but less everted than the other metatarsals. When the subtalar joint was set in supination, the first ray was inverted relative to the ground, but less inverted than the other metatarsals. Mason also discussed shifting of the first-ray axis with motions of the rearfoot. In a pronated rearfoot, the first-ray axis angulates more with the transverse plane, increasing adduction of the first metatarsal. He hypothesized that the increased obliquity of the first-ray axis in pronated feet may play a role in the development of metatarsus primus adductus as a component of hallux abducto valgus. The axis shift with pronation places the first-ray axis closer to the frontal plane. The overall eversion of the first metatarsal to the ground with pronation is greater, as change in the first ray axis decreases available frontal plane inversion with dorsiflexion.

First ray in gait

The first ray begins the stance phase in a maximally dorsiflexed position due to the pull of the anterior tibial muscle which acts after heel-strike to decelerate plantarflexion of the ankle. After the anterior tibial relaxes throughout contact, the first ray plantarflexes toward the supporting surface. Later in stance, as the subtalar joint supinates, the longitudinal axis of the midtarsal joint pronates in response. Concurrently, passive plantarflexion of the first ray occurs to maintain the metatarsal head on the ground. Once heel-lift has occurred, the first ray continues to plantarflex until the end of its range of motion is reached. This plantarflexion of the first ray after heel-lift is essential for normal first metatarsophalangeal joint function during propulsion. The literature states that the first ray is required to plantarflex 10 degrees to facilitate first metatarsophalangeal joint dorsiflexion in gait. First-ray plantarflexion limits the amount of compression at the first metatarsophalangeal joint during propulsion.[36]

The ability of the first ray to plantarflex during propulsion is established by the supinated positions of the subtalar joint and midtarsal joint oblique axis, which stabilize the lateral column of the foot. This position increases the transverse arching of the lesser tarsus and the effective fulcrum of pull of the peroneus longus after it enters the plantar surface of the foot through the cuboid notch. The peroneus longus stabilizes the first ray posteriorly against the lesser tarsus and the first metatarsal head against the ground in midstance.[36] The peroneus longus also contributes to the transfer of body weight medially across the forefoot after heel-lift when it is exerting its lateral pull against a firmly planted first metatarsal head. While it is clear that the peroneus longus is a major stabilizer of the lesser tarsus and contributes to the medial shift of body weight, its role as a plantarflexor of the first ray has been questioned. Kravitz et al.[36] noted that the lever arm of the peroneus longus to plantarflex the first ray is relatively poor. Root et al.,[55] however, citing Hicks, attributed to the peroneus longus a "strong plantarflexion force to the base of the first metatarsal" in midstance and propulsion. In describing the lever arm of this muscle as relatively poor for plantarflexion, Kravitz et al.[36] attributed "stabilization of the medial column in a plantarflexory direction" as the primary function of the peroneus longus. The effect of the intrinsic musculature of the medial side of the foot, most notably the abductor hallucis brevis, to plantarflex the first ray in gait has been described.[27,36] With the tibial sesamoid planted on the ground during propulsion, the abductor hallucis is in a good position to develop an effective lever arm to plantarflex the first ray. Contraction between its attachment into the fixed tibial sesamoid and its origin from the calcaneus initiates a nutcracker

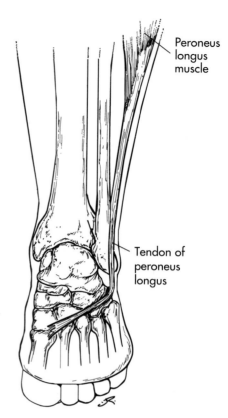

Fig. 1-33. The tendon of the peroneus longus passes obliquely across the sole of the foot, stabilizing the first ray in a lateral and posterior direction.

effect of the lesser tarsus with a resultant plantarflexion force to the first ray[36] (Fig. 1-33).

The abductor hallucis brevis passes under and nearly 45 degrees to the first-ray axis, providing it with an effective lever arm for plantarflexion of the first ray. The flexor hallucis brevis, with its origin on the plantar-medial cuboid and the lateral cuneiform, may also exert a plantarflexion effect on the ray.

Kravitz et al.,[36] citing a communication with G. Hice, D.P.M., attributed a retrograde force from the hallux on the ray to plantarflex it during first metatarsophalangeal joint dorsiflexion. This effect is greatest at end-stage propulsion, when the base of the proximal phalanx of the hallux is articulating with the head of the metatarsal, thereby increasing its retrograde force.

Summary
The first ray consists of the first metatarsal and medial cuneiform, tightly bound by ligamentous attachments. The axis of the first ray is deviated 45 degrees from the frontal and sagittal planes, with principal motions in those planes. Plantarflexion of the first ray during midstance and propulsion is necessary for sufficient first metatarsophalangeal joint dorsiflexion to occur in toe-off. The supinated

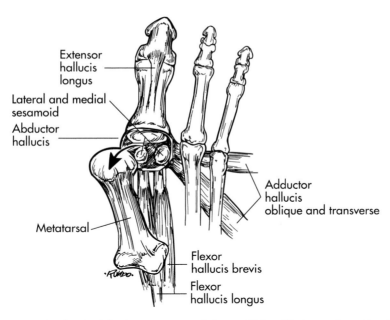

Extensor
hallucis
longus

Lateral and medial
sesamoid

Abductor
hallucis

Adductor
hallucis
oblique and transverse

Metatarsal

Flexor
hallucis brevis

Flexor
hallucis longus

Fig. 1-34. "Hammock effect" of the first metatarsophalangeal joint. (Redrawn from *Grant's Atlas of Anatomy*, ed 7, Baltimore, 1978, Williams & Wilkins.)

subtalar joint, along with a stable midtarsal joint, enables plantarflexion of the first ray. The peroneus longus contributes to this plantarflexion by stabilizing the lesser tarsus and the first metatarsal against the ground. The active muscular plantarflexion of the metatarsal appears to come from the intrinsics, most notably the abductor hallucis brevis muscle.

When the first ray is considered as an isolated unit, the frontal plane motions are dorsiflexion coupled with inversion, and plantarflexion coupled with eversion. In function, when the entire forefoot is everted with pronation and dorsiflexion of the ray has occurred, the isolated inversion of the first ray is hidden within the global eversion. When the foot is considered as a unit in function, pronation of the rearfoot leads to a net everted position of the first ray. The degree of eversion of the first ray, when compared with that of the lesser metatarsals, is less, owing to the local inversion of the ray, which has been described.

The first metatarsophalangeal joint
Anatomy

The first metatarsophalangeal joint incorporates the articular facets of four bones within a single synovial joint capsule[13]: the first metatarsal head, the base of the proximal phalanx, and the superior surfaces of the medial and lateral sesamoid bones. Since the metatarsophalangeal joints are condylar, both sagittal and transverse plane motions are mechanically possible. Although the main motion of

this joint is in the sagittal plane (dorsiflexion and plantarflexion), the proximal phalanx also has some passive transverse plane mobility on the metatarsal head.[13]

Function of the first metatarsophalangeal joint is best understood by considering the soft tissue structures surrounding this joint as constituting a "hammock."[35] The hammock is composed of the concavity of the proximal phalanx base with its multiple soft tissue insertions. The sesamoids, with soft tissue and muscle tendons, form the plantar pad of the joint.[24] The anatomy of this joint is a concentration of soft tissue attachments to the proximal phalanx, with a ball-and-socket type of motion of the first metatarsal head within it. This hammock, with rolling of the metatarsal head within it, has been aptly described by Heatherington et al.[24] as a "dynamic acetabulum" (Fig. 1-34).

The medial and lateral stability of the first metatarsophalangeal joint is provided by a triangular arrangement of ligaments reinforcing the capsule.[13] The collateral ligaments, the suspensory sesamoid, and the plantar sesamoid ligaments make up the three arms of the triangle on either side of the joint. In addition, a ligament is transversely attached between the two sesamoids and the deep transverse metatarsal ligament (medial segment), which, with the other intermetatarsal segments, forms a "strap"[35] that resists separation of the joints under loading stress.

It is important to note that this complex support structure, or hammock, which allows the metatarsal head to move within it, contributes as well to medial and lateral stability of the joint. Under pathologic conditions, such as those seen in hallux abducto valgus, frontal plane motion of the hammock occurs as the proximal phalanx of the hallux rotates into valgus angulation. Consequently, the medial arm of the hammock, which provided medial stability against the metatarsal head, has shifted plantar, enabling the medial deviation (escape) of the first metatarsal that is associated with this deformity.

First metatarsophalangeal joint in gait

The first metatarsophalangeal joint, along with the lesser metatarsophalangeal joints, undergoes active dorsiflexion in the late swing phase just before heel contact, continuing until after the ball of the foot contacts the ground. The action of the extensor hallucis longus, a secondary ankle dorsiflexor, is primarily responsible for this effect. The lesser metatarsophalangeal joints plantarflex to the ground prior to the first in late contact phase. During forefoot contact, loading of the forefoot from lateral to medial maintains the hallux in a dorsiflexed position for the longest period of time. The first metatarsophalangeal joint undergoes dorsiflexion again after heel-lift. This is a passive dorsiflexion as the toes are forced dorsally by the weight of the body with forward movement.[3] After toe-off, the digits plantarflex, so they are slightly dorsiflexed during swing phase before beginning active contraction again with the next gait cycle.

The first metatarsophalangeal joint is a ginglymoarthrodial joint. Its motion is determined by the degree of hallux dorsiflexion. It is a ginglymus, or hinge joint, for the first 20 to 30 degrees of hallux dorsiflexion. At this point, the first ray begins to plantarflex, resulting in a shift in the transverse axis dorsally and proximally, resulting in arthrodial motion for the remainder of propulsion. Heatherington et al.[24] reported that an average of approximately 34 degrees of dorsiflexion of the hallux was obtained before plantarflexion of the first metatarsal could be observed or palpated. Plantarflexion of the first ray requires heel-lift, subtalar joint supination, normal sesamoid function, and a second metatarsal longer than the first.[56] As more plantarflexion of the first metatarsal occurs, the metatarsal head moves in a posterior direction on the sesamoids, and the sesamoids are positioned under the distal articular surface of the first metatarsal head during final propulsion. Shereff et al.[61] described approximately 50 degrees of motion of the medial sesamoid in the sagittal plane in open chain kinetics.

During propulsion, the body weight is moving forward over the planted hallux, creating relative dorsiflexion of the first metatarsophalangeal joint. This occurs with the hallux planted firmly on the ground and with the heel lifting for propulsion. This is a closed kinetic chain phenomenon created by the 35 degrees of flexion which occurs at the knee and the 20 degrees of plantarflexion which occurs at the ankle at this point in the gait cycle.[52] Therefore, during terminal propulsion the hallux is dorsiflexed 50 to 60 degrees relative to the longitudinal axis of the first metatarsal.

Axes of the first metatarsophalangeal joint

The first metatarsophalangeal joint has two distinct axes of motion or degrees of freedom.[56] The transverse or horizontal axis provides pure sagittal plane motion, and the vertical axis provides pure transverse plane motion. The transverse axis of the first metatarsophalangeal joint is an axis whose position moves with sagittal plane motion of the joint. As arthrodial motion of the joint begins at 20 degrees of dorsiflexion, the transverse axis shifts dorsally and proximally within the metatarsal head. The vertical axis lies in the sagittal and frontal planes; hence, only transverse plane motion will occur about it. No normal frontal plane motion of the first metatarsophalangeal joint is said to exist.

Heatherington et al.,[24] in a study of first metatarsophalangeal joint motion, examined in conditions of simulated closed chain kinetics, found four centers of motion (Fig. 1-35). These four points fall within the metatarsal head, forming somewhat of an arc. The first center is located near the joint surface, suggesting a rolling motion initially. The next two centers are situated more in the center of the metatarsal head and produce velocity tangential to the joint surface. This is characteristic of a sliding motion. The authors postulated that the sliding motion occurs simultaneously with plantarflexion of the first ray. The final center is situated more dorsally in the metatarsal head with a vector entering the proximal phalanx of the hallux. This is characteristic of a compressive force at the end of the range of motion (Fig. 1-36). Shereff et al.[61] studied first metatarsophalangeal joint kinematics in the open kinetic chain. The authors found no rolling motion, but they did note a sliding motion with compression at the end of the range of motion. The centers of rotation were also all within the metatarsal head in this study, but they were in a quite different arrangement and were more suggestive of a ring than the arc described by Heatherington et al. Heatherington et al. also noted that the centers of rotation appeared to fall behind the area of the densest trabecular bone within the metatarsal head. This area corresponded to the area of greatest compressive forces when motion of the first metatarsal occurred in normal function. Shereff et al. emphasized the displacement of the sesamoid bones with joint motion. They reported 10 to 12 mm of

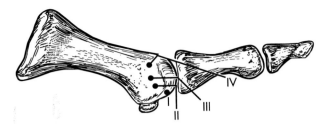

Fig. 1-35. Constructed from the vectors of the instant centers of velocity, this drawing demonstrates the character of motion occuring at the first metatarsophalangeal joint for each center. Center *I* falls on the joint surface and indicates rolling motion. Centers *II* and *III* are velocity vectors that are tangential to the joint surface, indicating that sliding is occurring. Center *IV* demonstrates that compression from the velocity vector is directed into the base of the proximal phalanx.

motion.[61] The closed chain study of Heatherington et al. found no significant motion of the sesamoids, but rather motion of the first metatarsal head on the stationary sesamoids.[24]

First metatarsophalangeal kinetics in pathologic function

Shereff et al.[61] studied centers of rotation of the first metatarsophalangeal joint in patients with hallux abducto valgus and hallux rigidus as well as in normal patients. With dorsiflexion of the hallux in a stable metatarsal, occurring in open kinetic chain models, the authors noted widely dispersed centers of rotation throughout the metatarsal head with hallux valgus. Additionally, moderate distraction during early motion, followed by a short interval of sliding, and finally jamming during maximum dorsiflexion, was also noted. A decrease in the sliding component of first metatarsophalangeal joint motion corresponds to the first-ray dorsiflexion associated with the development of this deformity. Under normal conditions, the sliding motion during the greater part of the dorsiflexion arc at this joint is facilitated by first-ray plantarflexion, thereby reducing compressive forces during the jamming phase of motion. The hallux valgus foot, with increased jamming associated with loss of sliding from first-ray dorsiflexion, will experience significant compressive forces at the first metatarsophalangeal joint at the end of its range of motion. The hallux rigidus foot displayed centers of rotation outside the metatarsal head and jamming motion throughout the arc of motion.

Motion of the foot over the hallux in propulsion

Dorsiflexion of the toes has an effect on the soft tissues of the ball of the foot. This dorsiflexion causes the ball of the foot to become *"tense, firm and pale,"* according to Bojsen-Møller,[3] with reduction in the mobility of the skin. This stiffening ensures that shear forces are not carried by the skin alone,

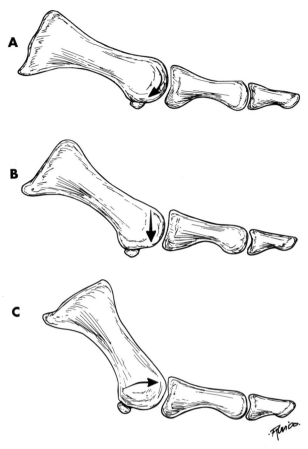

Fig. 1-36. Motion of the first metatarsophalangeal joint. **A,** Rolling motion. **B,** Sliding associated with first-ray plantarflexion. **C,** Compression at the end of the range of motion.

but are taken up by the "underlying connective tissue frame and transferred to the *skeleton.*"

According to Root et al. the propulsive function of the hallux requires three conditions: (1) stability and plantarflexion of the first ray, (2) normal sesamoid function, and (3) normal function of the muscles responsible for hallux and first metatarsophalangeal joint stability. The role of stability and plantarflexion of the first ray has been discussed. Normal sesamoid function is necessary for stabilization of the first metatarsophalangeal joint during propulsion. The sesamoids, placed directly under the metatarsal, serve as pulleys for the muscles, which stabilize the hallux against the ground during propulsion.[47] As the heel lifts and the limb moves forward, the first metatarsal moves posteriorly with plantarflexion, while the sesamoids reach a position underneath the anterior articular surface of the metatarsal head. The sesamoids determine the angle of insertion of the tendons, investing the first metatarsal in the course of the insertion of the tendons on the hallux. With the heel lifted and the hallux dorsiflexed, the flexor hallucis brevis utilizes

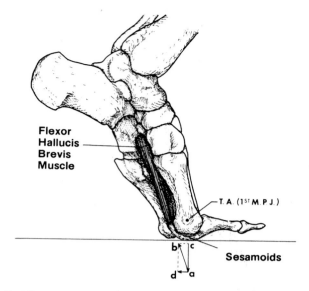

Fig. 1-37. During propulsion, as the heel becomes elevated, the sesamoids and first metatarsal head combine to form a pulley for function of the long and short hallux flexors. The first metatarsal head moves posteriorly on the sesamoids, and they become positioned over the anterior aspect of the first metatarsal head. The flexor muscles exert a plantarflexion force on the hallux (*arrow c–a*). They provide a weak posterior force to stabilize the hallux against the first metatarsal head (*arrow a–d*). (From Root M, Weed J, Orien W: *Clinical Biomechanics Vol. II Normal and abnormal function of the foot,* Los Angeles, 1977, Clinical Biomechanics Corp.)

the sesamoids as a pulley placed below the anterior articular surface of the metatarsal head to angle more obliquely up to its insertion on the base of the proximal phalanx (Fig. 1-37). This provides a lever arm for a plantarflexion force of the hallux against the ground. With the heel on the ground, the pull of the flexors will not "wind around the pulley" to increase their obliquity up to the insertion. Flexors pulling without the pulley effect of the sesamoids under the plantarflexed metatarsal head will primarily stabilize the hallux against the metatarsal head, not the ground.

The muscular effect on the hallux includes the effect of the extensor hallucis brevis to stabilize the lesser tarsus and the metatarsal bases in a posterior and dorsiflexory direction in midstance and propulsion. The extensor hallucis longus does not contract until late in propulsion and appears to function primarily in preparation for swing phase. It appears to provide only a minor role in stabilizing the hallux during propulsion. Plantar stability of the hallux against the ground during propulsion is provided by the flexor hallucis longus and flexor hallucis brevis muscles.[55] The flexor hallucis longus is active from the end of the contact phase through most of the propulsive phase. It provides a strong plantar force to the hallux as it passes around the sesamoid apparatus and firmly stabilizes the hallux on the

ground. The transverse stability of the joint is provided by the adductor and abductor hallucis muscles. As Kelikian described it earlier, the balanced position of these muscles around the hallux make up the "fibers" of the hammock.[35] Even the pull of the dorsal-plantar and medial-lateral "fibers" of the hammock maintains stability for rolling of the metatarsal head to occur during propulsion. Valgus rotation of the hallux associated with pathologic function of this joint leads to uneven pull of the medial and lateral fibers of the hammock leading to a mechanical advantage for the laterally placed adductor, hallux and a progressive transverse plane deformity of the hallux.[41]

Stokes et al.[64] estimated that 40% of body weight is imposed on the great toe in "the final stages of forefoot contact." This load is dissipated by tension in the flexor tendons. The resultant force produced is about 600 Newtons for the hallux. It is initially a ground reaction force followed by a compressive metatarsophalangeal joint force. Hutton and Dhanendran[30] found the force acting across the first metatarsophalangeal joint to approximate body weight. Hallux and first metatarsal loads peak at the same time, highlighting the importance of the hallux in complementing the load-bearing function of the first metatarsal.

Range of motion

Much variation has been reported in the literature on the available range of motion of the first metatarsophalangeal joint in the sagittal plane. The transverse plane motion is very slight, and it is passive motion that is rarely subject to voluntary control. Transverse plane motion, after evolutionary changes from our arboreal ancestors, no longer appears functionally significant for human locomotion.

Joseph et al.[33] reported a mean average for total range of motion of active dorsiflexion plus passive additional dorsiflexion as 75 degrees from the relaxed stance position. Kelikian[35] stated that the average range of motion of the first metatarsophalangeal joint is 70 degrees of dorsiflexion and 5 degrees of plantarflexion. He did not describe a neutral position. Mann[45] stated that 70 to 90 degrees of passive dorsiflexion is available at this joint, depending on individual flexibility. Giannestras[18] reported average values of 70 degrees of dorsiflexion from a neutral position and 45 degrees of plantarflexion from a neutral position. Sgarlato,[62] in a study in which the first metatarsal was stabilized, found 50 to 80 degrees of dorsiflexion from the straight-line position. Root et al.[55] referred to 65 to 75 degrees of dorsiflexion as the minimum necessary for proper functioning of this joint. Gerbert,[17] using anatomical landmarks, stated that if the hallux is not allowed to dorsiflex 60 to 65 degrees at toe-off, jamming, with resultant articular damage, will occur. With precise identification of surface landmarks, Buell et al.[6] clinically identified an average unassisted dorsiflexion of 77 degrees and an average assisted dorsiflexion of 82 degrees from the straight-line position. The average assisted plantarflexion was 17 degrees from the straight-line position. The authors reported that their findings for first metatarsophalangeal joint range of motion are close to those reported earlier by Joseph.

Necessary dorsiflexion of the first metatarsophalangeal joint during gait has been studied as well. Heatherington et al.[25] reported that values of "functional dorsiflexion" appear lower than those obtained by measuring assisted dorsiflexion off weightbearing. This study, of functional dorsiflexion required in gait, revealed a mean of 50.56 degrees. Bojsen-Moller and Lamoreux,[3] in a similar study of dorsiflexion of the first metatarsophalangeal joint in gait, reported a mean of 58 degrees.

Summary

The first metatarsophalangeal joint is composed of the first metatarsal head, the base of the proximal phalanx, and the superior surfaces of the medial and lateral sesamoids within a single synovial joint capsule. The soft tissue attachments insert medially and laterally into the proximal phalanx, with the plantar plate containing the sesamoids. They constitute a hammock in which rolling of the metatarsal head can occur. This creates a "dynamic acetabulum."

The first metatarsophalangeal joint has two distinct axes of motion. The vertical axis allows passive transverse plane mobility of the proximal phalanx. A ginglymoid or hinge motion occurs for the first 20 degrees of dorsiflexion. Arthrodial motion begins at 20 degrees, with the transverse axis shifting dorsally and proximally within the metatarsal head. Plantarflexion of the first ray with heel-lift, subtalar joint supination, normal sesamoid function, and a second metatarsal longer than the first is necessary for normal function of the arthrodial portion of the dorsiflexion at the first metatarsophalangeal joint. During propulsion, first metatarsophalangeal joint dorsiflexion occurs with the hallux planted on the ground, the knee flexed 35 degrees, and the ankle plantarflexed 20 degrees.

First metatarsophalangeal joint kinetics include four centers of motion forming an arc. Rolling motion occurs around the first center corresponding to the hinge motion of the joint. Sliding motion occurs around the second and third centers, facilitated by first-ray plantarflexion, corresponding to the arthrodial motion of the joint. The fourth center lies more dorsally and produces a compressive force at the end of the range of motion. Plantar soft tissue stiffening with dorsiflexion causes the dampening of shear forces in propulsion.

The propulsive function of the hallux requires stability of the first ray, normal sesamoid function, and normal function of the muscles, providing first metatarsophalangeal joint stability. The sesamoids serve as a pulley to increase the lever arm of the flexor hallucis brevis in stabilizing the hallux against the ground. Plantar stability of the hallux against the ground in propulsion is provided by the flexor hallucis longus and brevis. Unassisted dorsiflexion of the first metatarsophalangeal joint has been found to be on average, 77 degrees with precisely identified surface landmarks. Average assisted dorsiflexion is 82 degrees. In dynamic studies, necessary dorsiflexion of the first metatarsophalangeal joint during gait has been found to be 50 to 60 degrees.

Second, third, and fourth rays

The second and third rays consist of the second metatarsal with the intermediate cuneiform and the third metatarsal with the lateral cuneiform. These articulations have dense ligaments between them uniting them as a functional unit. The fourth ray is the fourth metatarsal alone. Root et al.[55] described the axes of these rays as most likely to be present in the transverse and frontal planes, just proximal to the tarsometatarsal articulations. Motion about this axis would be pure sagittal plane dorsiflexion-plantarflexion. Some plantarflexion movement of the rays is required for lesser metatarsophalangeal joint dorsiflexion to occur. However, the exact nature of this motion has not been reported.

The fifth ray

Anatomy

The fifth ray consists of the fifth metatarsal only.[27] Its motions occur at the articulation of the base of the fifth metatarsal and the cuboid. The fifth metatarsal base is connected to the cuboid by a ligament that lies dorsolateral to the base. In some individuals, a transverse band extends from this ligament to the dorsum of the third cuneiform.[58]

Axis of the fifth ray

The axis of the fifth ray lies at an angle of approximately 20 degrees from the transverse plane and 35 degrees from the sagittal plane. It is a triplanar axis that runs in a similar direction to the axis of the subtalar joint, that is, from proximal, plantar, and lateral, to distal, dorsal, and medial. This orientation allows for pronation and supination. Specifically, dorsiflexion is coupled with abduction and eversion with pronation, while plantarflexion is coupled with adduction and inversion

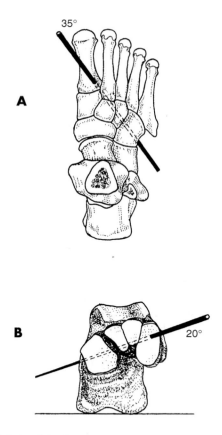

Fig. 1-38. Axis of the fifth ray. **A,** Anterior view. **B,** Dorsal view. (From Michaud T: *Foot orthosis*, Baltimore, 1993, Williams & Wilkins.)

with supination. The fifth-ray axis deviates principally from the frontal and sagittal planes, with only slight deviation from the transverse plane (Fig. 1-38). Consequently, triplanar motion of the fifth ray is mostly dorsiflexion and eversion with pronation, and plantarflexion and inversion with supination. Abduction and adduction of this ray are considered clinically negligible.

The fifth ray in function

Root et al. described equal ranges of plantarflexion and dorsiflexion at the fifth-ray axis as it is pronated and supinated. He stated that the minimum range of fifth-ray motion necessary for locomotion is unknown. However, as was the case for the first ray, it seems likely that plantarflexion of the fifth ray is necessary to facilitate dorsiflexion of the fifth metatarsophalangeal joint. Less fifth metatarsophalangeal joint dorsiflexion is needed in gait since the fifth metatarsal leaves the ground first. Therefore, less than the 10 degrees of plantarflexion required for the first ray may be needed by this most lateral metatarsal.

Lesser metatarsophalangeal joints and digits

The second, third, fourth, and fifth metatarsophalangeal joints have transverse and vertical axes similar to those of the first metatarsophalangeal joint. Motion at these joints includes active sagittal plane motion about the transverse axis, and passive transverse plane motion about the vertical axis.[56] While significant dorsiflexion is needed at these joints to complete propulsion, less dorsiflexion is needed than at the first metatarsophalangeal joint, with the least amount required by the fifth metatarsophalangeal joint, which leaves the ground first as body weight is transferred medially.

Stabilization of the lesser digits against the ground for propulsion at the metatarsophalangeal joints is provided mainly by the flexor digitorum longus and flexor digitorum brevis tendons, which insert into the distal and middle phalanges, respectively. It is assisted in this function by the much weaker lumbricales and interossei.[60] Dorsiflexion of the lesser metatarsophalangeal joints is accomplished by the action of the extensor digitorum longus through the extensor sling which supports the proximal portion of the proximal phalanx. Extension (dorsiflexion) of the middle and distal phalanges of the lesser digits is mediated through an extensor hood, and is controlled by the lumbricales and interossei.

THE GAIT CYCLE

Human gait is a very complicated, coordinated series of movements that involve both the upper and lower extremities. Winter states: "The sole purpose of walking or running is to transport the body safely and efficiently across the ground, on the level, uphill and downhill with a minimal expenditure of energy. The neuromuscular control system must also provide appropriate shock absorption, prevent collapse, and maintain balance of the upper

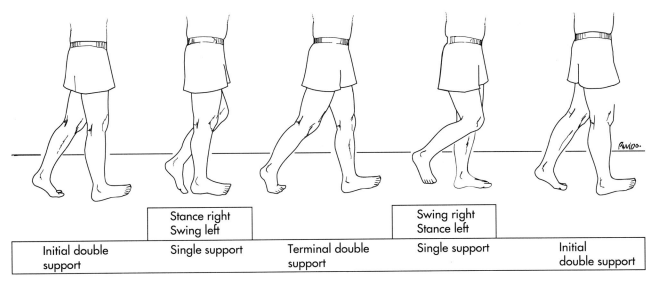

Fig. 1-39. Subdivisions of stance, swing, and single and double support. (*Note:* The swing phase of one limb comprises the entire single support period of the opposite limb.)

extremity."[65] Human gait in adults is the erect bipedal gait. It is a learned process, not the result of inborn reflexes. It takes time and proper conditions to develop and mature propulsive gait is not attained until approximately 4 years of age.

Three phases of walking

Walking is divided into three phases. The *development phase* is that time when we initiate movement from a resting state and accelerate up to a walking speed. Once the acceleration has stopped, and we have attained a steady speed, we enter into the rhythmic phase. The *rhythmic phase* is a series of cyclic, repetitive motions that dominate the greatest part of our walking. The *decay phase* is that phase of walking at which we decelerate as we prepare to stop. The rhythmic phase is the phase during which almost all gait-related complaints are derived. It is for this reason that most of this discussion of gait is concentrated on the rhythmic phase.

Overview of the gait cycle

When we walk, we progress through a series of repetitive events. Our feet are picked up and swung forward, placed on the ground, walked over, and picked up and swung forward again. The rhythmic phase of walking is merely a series of these repetitive motions strung together. Each of these repetitive motions is termed a *gait cycle*. One gait cycle is measured from floor contact of the heel to the following heel contact of the same limb. Each gait cycle is divided into two parts. The *swing* phase is that pe-

riod of time in which the foot does not touch the ground and is swung forward. The swing phase occupies approximately one third of a total gait cycle (38%–42%). The stance phase of the gait cycle is that period of time when the foot makes contact with the ground. The stance phase is approximately two thirds of the gait cycle (51%–62%). Both the start and end of stance phase involve a period of bilateral foot contact with the floor. This is called double support, or double stance, and each period occupies 8% to 12% the cycle. One gait cycle will last approximately 1 second, with 0.6 second occurring in stance (Fig. 1-39).

Stance phase

The *stance phase* is the weightbearing portion of each gait cycle. It is initiated with heel contact and ends with toe-off of the same foot. This period of time when the foot is in contact with the ground is divided into four functional phases, further subdividing the traditional three subphases of stance. This is due to the fact that there are two distinct periods during the heel-lift stage: heel-lift without and with the opposite limb on the ground. The function of the foot in these two distinct periods after heel-lift is profoundly different and requires that they be identified individually for clarity.

1. The *contact phase* is the period initiated by initial floor contact of the heel to toe-off of the opposite limb. It occupies 10% of the gait cycle and 18% of the stance phase.

2. *Midstance phase* is that period from opposite side toe-off to heel-lift of the support foot.

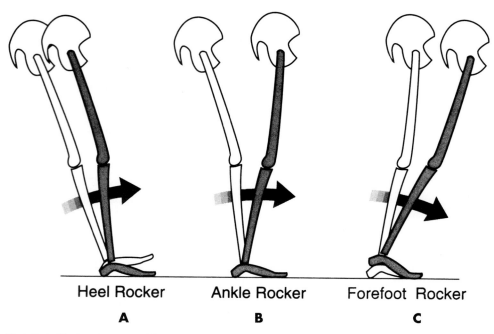

Heel Rocker   Ankle Rocker   Forefoot Rocker

A   B   C

Fig. 1-40. **A,** Heel rocker. **B,** Ankle rocker. **C,** Forefoot rocker. (From Perry J: *Gait analysis,* 1992, Slack, Inc., Thorofare, NJ.)

It occupies 20% of the gait cycle and 30% of the stance phase.

3. *Active propulsion* is that period from heel-off of the support limb to full strike of the opposite limb. It occupies 20% of the gait cycle and 30% of the stance phase.

4. *Passive lift-off* is that period from opposite-side heel contact to toe-off of the support side. It occupies 10% of the gait cycle and 20% of the stance phase.

These subphases help advance the body in a smooth progression while providing stability to the trunk. Perry states, "The essential element for progression over the stance limb is rocker action by the foot and ankle."[52] Each provides a specific function during each stance phase.

With contact phase, the *heel rocker* serves as a fulcrum to roll the foot into plantarflexion so that it is in full contact with the ground. This facilitates progression of the limb and redirects force from a vertical direction toward forward momentum (Fig. 1-40**A**). During midstance, the *ankle rocker,* with the ankle joint acting as the fulcrum, allows the tibia to roll forward. This advances the body weight from behind the ankle to the forefoot (Fig. 1-40**B**). During active propulsion and passive lift-off, the *forefoot rocker,* with the metatarsophalangeal articulation acting as a fulcrum, accelerates progression of the limb over the forefoot and expedites heel-lift (Fig. 1-40**C**).

Swing phase

Swing phase is initiated with toe-off of the support limb and ends with heel contact of the same limb. It is the nonweightbearing portion of the gait cycle. Swing phase provides the actual step which moves us from one location to another, and the power necessary to pull the body forward.[9,52]

Double limb support

During the gait cycle there are two periods when both feet are on the floor at the same time.

Initial double support, or double stance, occurs from heel contact of one limb to toe-off of the opposite limb. This period has often been referred to as the *period of reception, weight acceptance,* or the *braking period.* During this phase, the body decelerates in preparation for stability and support by the limb that has just completed swing. Once this is accomplished, the opposite limb leaves the floor.

Terminal double support, or double stance, occurs from opposite-limb heel-strike to support-limb toe-off. This period has often been referred to as *thrusting double support, preswing,* or *weight release.* Once again, there is a deceleration of the body as weight is transferred to the opposite limb. Once unloaded, it prepares for toe-off and the swing phase.

Single limb support

Single limb support, or single stance, is initiated by opposite-foot toe-off and terminates with opposite-

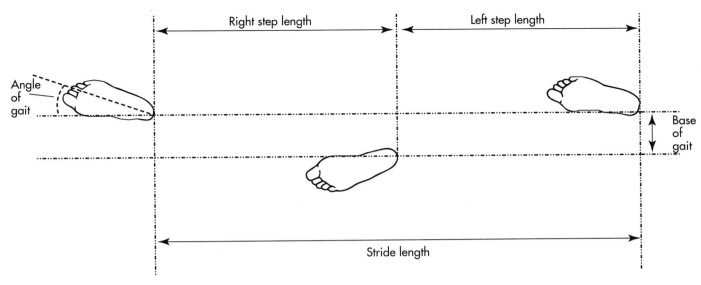

Fig. 1-41. Subdivision of stride length, step length, angle, and base of gait.

side heel-strike. Therefore, single limb support is identical to the period of swing of the opposite limb and so is responsible for support of the entire body. The duration of single limb stance is often a measure of an individual's capability to stabilize and support the body.

Cadence

Cadence, or step rate, is defined as the number of steps per minute when a person walks. Most people will select a natural or free cadence. The average cadence ranges from 101 to 122 steps per minute.[11,65] Women have a faster cadence than men (117 vs. 111 steps per minute). Cadence generally slows down with age. It should be noted that as cadence increases, both stance and swing time decrease, but stance phase decreases 3.5 times as rapidly as swing phase.[49] In addition, an increase in cadence shortens both double support periods.

Murray et al.,[49] in a study of older men, included subjects up to 87 years old and noted that for those older than 65, both cadence and stride length decreased.

Stride

Stride length is defined as the distance between two consecutive contacts of the same foot. Therefore, it is measured from heel contact of one limb to heel contact of the same limb. The average stride length for normal persons is 1.41 m (4.5 ft). Men have a 14% longer stride length than women.[52]

Step

Step is defined as the period from heel contact of one limb to heel contact of the opposite limb. Each stride consists of two steps, usually of equal length (Fig. 1-41).

In pathologic gait, it is possible for the step lengths to be unequal. That is, if one foot is moved forward and the other is brought up to it but does not advance in front of it, it is considered a 0 step length.

Lamoreux[37] noted that between a cadence of 80 and 120 steps per minute, stride length and cadence have a linear relationship. Thus, up to 120 steps per minute, speed increases are achieved both by increasing the stride length and the cadence. Individuals generally have a maximum stride length. After this is achieved, velocity can only occur by increasing cadence. Therefore, above 120 steps per minute, the stride length levels off and only cadence increases.[37]

Base of gait

Base of gait is defined as the horizontal distance from one heel-strike to the next heel-strike. The average base of gait is 3.5 in. in order for the lateral shift of the body to be properly accepted by the limb.

Angle of gait

Angle of gait is defined as the angle formed by the longitudinal axis of the foot and the line of progression (sagittal plane). It is measured by a line bisecting the center of the heel and the first interspace with the sagittal plane. The average gait angle is 7 degrees toe-out per side, or an average of 12 to 15 degrees total. Torsional or positional changes in the hip, femur, and tibia have a major influence on this position (see Chapter 11).

The power of motion

In order to understand the gait cycle in its totality, the way the body develops the power necessary for walking must be described. Inman[31] initially described this power generation as concentric muscular contraction, which created force moments across joints, which in turn created motion. Unfortunately, this particular model for power generation found a 6% discrepancy between peak power and peak demand. Mann et al.,[44] in a study of muscle function during more forceful activity, such as running and jogging, described a different role for muscle function. The authors stated that muscle power appeared to be directed at the swinging, rather than the weightbearing limb. They demonstrated that muscle action of the weightbearing leg was actually "turned off" during the push-off phase.[44]

Dananberg, in 1986 and 1993, described a different mechanism for creating the power of motion.[9,10] He discussed how the body appeared to pull itself through swing, rather than directly push (Fig. 1-42). This creates a more efficient method that is capable of permitting motion on a near-perpetual basis. He listed four specific actions which collectively created the power of motion. These included (1) the pull created by the swing limb, (2) momentum of the center of mass, (3) gravity's action on the center of mass, and (4) elastic tissue response. When combined, these actions create the sufficient aggregate force necessary for walking.

Herman et al.,[26] evaluating neurologically normal subjects, showed that swing phase action appeared as a constant motion. The angular displacements of the hip, knee, and ankle appear remarkably similar across subjects regardless of age, body morphology, or sex. The motion of swing phase also appears as an instinctive reflex, which newborns demonstrate when held erect with the stepping reflex.[26] During gait, the motion of the swing limb appears to be related to the interrelationship between the muscular action of the iliopsoas and an energy storage and return phenomenon in the spine. As the arms and legs swing in reciprocal motions, energy is stored within the fascia, muscles, and ligaments in the back. This is visible as reverse rotations between the shoulder and pelvic girdles (Fig. 1-43). Once sufficient tension is applied, the shoulders and pelvis reverse rotations as this stored energy is returned. This motion creates the necessary pelvic motion to initiate the swing phase action. Since the trailing limb has just assumed a point that is extended from under the hip joint, it is like a cocked trigger waiting to be released. As the energy is returned from the spine, the femur accelerates (as the hip flexes) to a point under the torso. The iliopsoas then fires to continue this motion, and the now swinging limb advances forward.[20]

When this swing phase motion occurs, it establishes a pulling moment on the center of mass of the

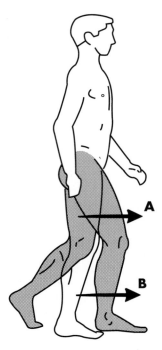

Fig. 1-42. A progressional force (arrow) is provided by the swing limb.

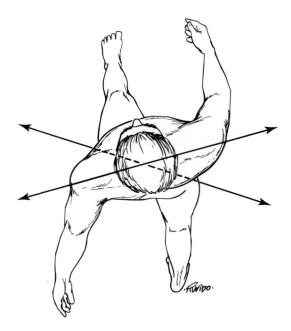

Fig. 1-43. As the shoulder girdle advances, the pelvis and limb trail behind. With each step this is reversed.

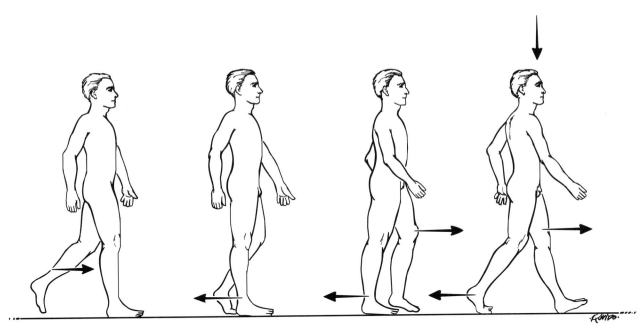

Fig. 1-44. With the center of gravity forward of the hind limb, a reverse thrust is created. This assists in forward movement.

body. As the center of the body is pulled forward, the weightbearing limb serves as a lever. As the body is pulled forward, this lever effect thrusts the ground backward. Forward motion must therefore take place (Fig. 1-44). The muscles of the weight-bearing limb act to stabilize it under the single support load of the body. They can then function in the eccentric mode of contraction. This eccentric contraction permits an efficient utilization of muscle function while simultaneously taking advantage of the pull action of the swing limb. Once the center of mass is pulled beyond the weightbearing foot, gravity continues to act to pull it toward the ground. In effect, this creates the final thrust against the ground. This action takes advantage of one's own body mass as a prime mover. When combined, these actions create efficient forward motion.[9]

Perry[52] states:

Forward swing of the contralateral limb provides a second pulling force. This force is generated by accelerated advancement of the limb and its anterior alignment. The sum of these actions provides a propelling force at the time residual momentum in the stance limb is decreasing. It is particularly critical in mid stance to advance the body vector past the vertical and again create a forward fall position. At the end of the step, the falling body weight is caught by the contralateral swing limb, which by now has moved forward to assume a stance role. In this manner a cycle of progression is initiated that is serially perpetuated by reciprocal action of the two limbs.

Phases of the gait cycle (Table 1-2)
Contact phase (Fig. 1-45, p. 39)
This is represented by a double support period which begins with heel contact and terminates with forefoot loading and opposite-side toe-off. This initial phase of floor contact requires the foot to aid in shock absorption, adapt to the surface terrain, assist the hip to undergo its normal transverse plane rotation, and continue the progression.

Ground reaction forces

Vertical load. (Fig. 1-46, p. 39) Just prior to heel contact, the body weight is forward of the opposite forefoot while the advancing leg (contact leg) is falling toward the floor. This results in an abrupt initial loading of the heel with an acceleration of the body weight. Ground reaction forces are approximately 110% to 125% of body weight during this period. Speed of walking has an effect on vertical loads, that is, faster cadence results in higher peaks and lower valleys.

Anteroposterior shear. (Fig. 1-47, p. 39) In addition to the vertical load, there is also a deceleration of the horizontal movement of the limb, which will result in a posterior shear force. This is the result of the anterior movement of the foot being interrupted by friction from the ground at contact.

Horizontal plane (Table 1-3, p. 39)
The pelvis, femur, and tibia have advanced forward of the support limb, which is undergoing

Table 1-2
Gait cycle

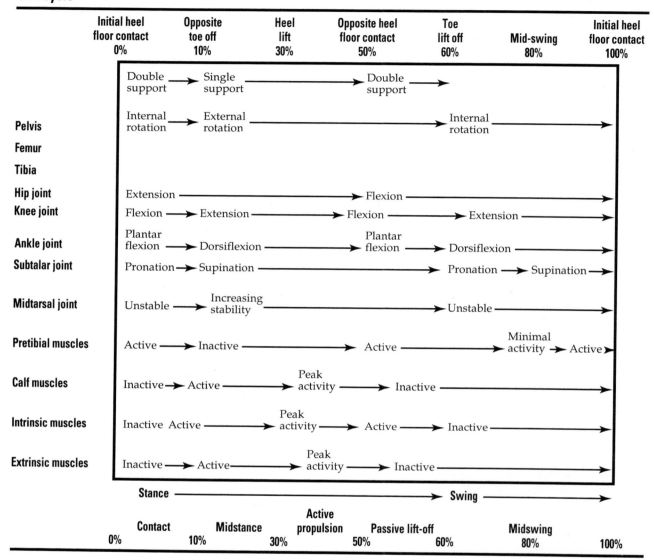

	Initial heel floor contact 0%	Opposite toe off 10%	Heel lift 30%	Opposite heel floor contact 50%	Toe lift off 60%	Mid-swing 80%	Initial heel floor contact 100%
	Double support → Single support ─────────── → Double support →						
Pelvis	Internal rotation → External rotation ───────── → Internal rotation ─────						
Femur							
Tibia							
Hip joint	Extension ──────────── → Flexion ─────						
Knee joint	Flexion → Extension ───── → Flexion ── → Extension ─────						
Ankle joint	Plantar flexion → Dorsiflexion ────			Plantar flexion → Dorsiflexion ────			
Subtalar joint	Pronation → Supination ───────── → Pronation → Supination →						
Midtarsal joint	Unstable → Increasing stability ──── → Unstable ────						
Pretibial muscles	Active → Inactive ───── → Active ──── → Minimal activity → Active ▸						
Calf muscles	Inactive → Active ──── → Peak activity → Inactive ────						
Intrinsic muscles	Inactive Active ──── → Peak activity ── → Active ── → Inactive ────						
Extrinsic muscles	Inactive → Active ── → Peak activity ── → Inactive ────						
	Stance ────────────────── → Swing ─────						
	Contact 0%	Midstance 10%	Active propulsion 30%	Passive lift-off 50% 60%		Midswing 80%	100%

external rotation. Rotation about this limb results in internal rotation, which continues after heel contact until the opposite limb leaves the floor. Internal rotation has an adduction effect on the foot, which occurs briefly until the forefoot contacts, with friction then preventing any further movement. The continuation of internal rotation of the limb is manifested as pronation (talar adduction) of the subtalar joint.

Hip joint (Table 1-4)

The hip is flexed about 30 degrees and experiences a flexor torque at contact, which is resisted by the gluteus maximus and adductor magnus. Extension is produced as the knee and ankle plantarflex, which advances the femur forward faster than the pelvis, resulting in a relative extension. Motion at the pelvis is minimal so as to stabilize the trunk over the limb.

Knee joint (Table 1-5)

Knee flexion is the main shock-absorbing mechanism during this phase. As the heel strikes, plantarflexion at the ankle rapidly moves the tibia forward while the femur lags behind, resulting in flexion of the knee. The quadriceps restrains rapid flexion as the hamstrings resist hyperextension. Together they dampen impact load while maintaining stability of the joint. In addition, pronation at the subtalar joint permits faster internal rotation of the tibia to continue, resulting in medial rotation of the femur and further unlocking of the knee.

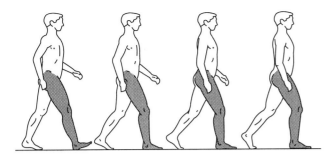

Fig. 1-45. Contact phase.

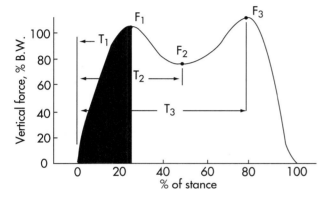

Fig. 1-46. Vertical load.

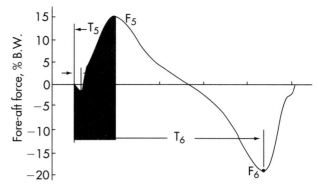

Fig. 1-47. Anteroposterior shear.

Ankle joint (Table 1-6)

At heel contact, the ground reaction force (vector) is directed behind the ankle joint, which applies a vertical force on the heel, resulting in rapid plantarflexion of the forefoot. The heel serving as a rocker expedites this action. This rapid plantarflexion occurs until the pretibial muscles (eccentrically contracting) gain sufficient strength to effectively resist this movement. The slow deceleration action of the muscles serves to absorb some of the ground reaction force. Once this occurs, the movement is slowed, and even weight distribution takes place. This early "free fall" of the ankle, associated with rapid ankle plantarflexion, serves to absorb impact from the ground as the center of the ankle joint drops.[52] Plantarflexion ends with full loading of the forefoot, which applies a dorsiflexion force to the rearfoot as well as the forefoot.

Subtalar joint (Table 1-7)

Pronation at the subtalar joint during this period is a passive event. Plantarflexion of the ankle is resisted by contraction of the pretibial muscle group. This supinates the longitudinal axis of the midtarsal joint, which in open chain (swing) supinates the subtalar joint. This results in an inverted attitude of the calcaneus relative to the floor. On

Table 1-3
Horizontal plane

	Position	Motion
Pelvis	0-2 degrees internal	4-5 degrees internal rotation
Femur	0 degrees neutral	6 degrees internal rotation
Tibia	2 degrees internal	9 degrees internal

Table 1-4
Hip joint

	Position	Motion
Hip joint	Flexed 30-40 degrees	Flexion 20 degrees

Table 1-5
Knee joint

	Position	Motion
Knee joint	Flexed 0-5 degrees	Flexion 15-18 degrees

Table 1-6
Ankle joint

	Position	Motion
Ankle joint	Neutral 0 degrees	Plantarflexion 8 degrees

Table 1-7
Subtalar joint

	Position	Motion
Subtalar joint	Supinated 2-4 degrees	Pronation 4-6 degrees

Table 1-8
Midtarsal joint

	Position	Motion
Longitudinal midtarsal joint	Supinated	Supination
Oblique midtarsal joint	Pronated	Pronation

Table 1-9
Pretibial muscles

	Ankle joint	Subtalar joint	Midtarsal joint Longitudinal axis	Midtarsal joint oblique axis
Anterior tibal	Dorsiflex	Supination	Pronation	Supination
Extensor digitorum longus	Dorsiflex	Pronation	Pronation	Pronation
Extensor hallucis longus	Dorsiflex	Supination	Pronation	Supination

Table 1-10
Calf muscles

	Femur	Tibia	Ankle joint	Subtalar joint
Gastrocnemius	Flexion external rotation	—	Plantflexion	Supination
Soleus	—	Extension external rotation	Plantflexion	Supination

contact, the ground reaction force attempts to reverse this by applying an everting force to the lateral condyle of the calcaneus, resulting in pronation.

Pronation assists internal rotation of the limb, which results in an adduction force on the foot. Friction stops the foot from adducting, which occurs at forefoot contact and manifests as talar adduction (subtalar joint pronation). The ability to convert horizontal plane influences from the pelvis and limb is an essential function of the subtalar joint.

In addition, body weight has not yet fully moved over the new weightbearing limb so that the center of gravity falls medial to the subtalar joint axis. This places a pronation effect on the joint.

Pronation is normally limited by the congenital placement of the subtalar and midtarsal joint axes, the anatomy of their articulating surfaces, and their ligamentous attachments. Muscle activity primarily allows for deceleration of this movement to allow an orderly distribution of weight to the medial aspect of the foot.

Midtarsal joint (Table 1-8)

As the subtalar joint pronates, the range of motion of the midtarsal joint increases.

Longitudinal axis

The longitudinal axis of the midtarsal joint supinates owing to contraction of the anterior tibial and extensor digitorum longus, which insert medial to the axis. Since supination of the longitudinal axis of the midtarsal joint is accompanied by subtalar pronation, joint instability occurs, and adaptation to the floor surface is expedited. An inverted attitude about this axis permits normal excursion of subtalar joint pronation.

Oblique axis

Oblique axis midtarsal joint pronation occurs as a result of contraction of the pretibial muscles, which insert lateral to the axis. In addition, the dorsiflexory force of the ground against the metatarsal heads pronates the joint to the end of its range. As this increases, a mild degree of arch collapse occurs. This action assists in absorbing impact load from the floor.

Pretibial muscles (Table 1-9)

Anterior tibial—active
Extensor digitorum longus—active
Extensor hallucis longus—active

Table 1-11
Extrinsic muscles

	Tibia	Ankle joint	Subtalar joint	Midtarsal joint long. axis	Midtarsal joint obliq. axis
Posterior tibial	Extension ext. rotation	Plantarflexion	Supination	—	—

Function

1. Decelerate plantarflexion of the ankle
2. Decelerate pronation and provide even weightbearing from the lateral to the medial side of the foot
3. Provide an unstable midtarsal joint for shock absorption and adaptation
4. Absorb impact loads from the floor

At contact, all the muscles are active and reach their peak activity prior to foot flat. Perry[52] states that the anterior tibial generates the largest torque around the ankle joint, followed by the extensor digitorum longus and the extensor hallucis longus. At heel contact, the subtalar joint is supinated. The anterior tibial assists in the deceleration of subtalar joint pronation.

Calf muscles (Table 1-10)

Soleus—active
Gastrocnemius—active

Function

1. The soleus decelerates internal rotation of the tibia.
2. The soleus provides mild deceleration of calcaneal eversion.
3. The soleus decelerates forward movement of the tibia.
4. The gastrocnemius provides mild flexion of the knee to prevent hyperextension.

Both muscles initiate activity midway through this phase and therefore do not develop sufficient torque to control subtalar joint function. With the foot on the floor, the soleus exerts a force from the heel to its tibial insertion, resisting forward movement of the tibia due to momentum. The gastrocnemius insertion on the femur creates flexion tension on the knee to resist hyperextension.

In addition, the tendon of the gastrocnemius and soleus inserts medial to the subtalar joint axis, thereby introducing a supination effect on the subtalar joint which assists in decelerating its pronation movement.

Intrinsic muscles and extrinsic muscles (Table 1-11)

The intrinsic muscles are inactive. The extrinsic muscles include the following:

Posterior tibial—active
Peroneus longus—inactive
Peroneus brevis—inactive
Flexor digitorum longus—inactive
Flexor hallucis longus—inactive

Function of the posterior tibial muscle

1. Decelerates pronation at the subtalar joint
2. Decelerates anterior movement of the tibia
3. Decelerates internal rotation of the tibia

The posterior tibial has a prime effect on decelerating subtalar joint pronation owing to its perpendicular angle relative to the subtalar joint axis combined with its long lever arm. The posterior tibial has approximately twice the muscle leverage to supinate the subtalar joint as does the soleus.[52] Electromyographic studies show that this muscle exhibits two peaks, one during the contact phase of gait and the other during active propulsion. Since the muscle inserts proximally on the leg, it has a substantial effect on decelerating internal rotation and forward movement of the tibia.

Summary

This phase concludes with full forefoot loading and toe-off of the opposite limb (see Table 1-2).

1. The limb is internally rotating with associated subtalar joint pronation.
2. Sagittal plane motion at the knee and ankle is in flexion and available for prime shock absorption.
3. The rearfoot and midfoot are unstable and available for adaption to the terrain.
4. The pretibial muscles are primarily active to decelerate plantarflexion and pronation of the foot.
5. Ground reaction force exceeds body weight due to dropping of the center of gravity.
6. The limb and foot decelerate at this time.

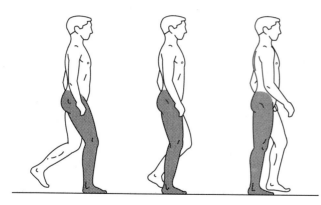

Fig. 1-48. Midstance phase.

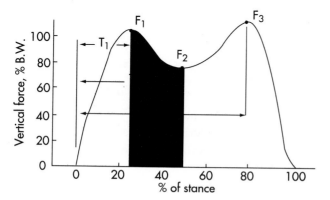

Fig. 1-49. Vertical load.

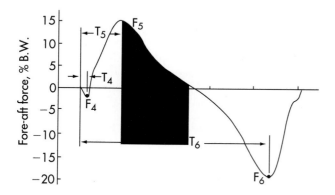

Fig. 1-50. Anteroposterior shear.

7. A period of initial double support occurs until opposite-side toe-off.

Midstance phase (Fig. 1-48)

This is the initial single support period which begins with opposite-side toe-off and full forefoot loading, and terminates with heel-lift. This phase occurs

Table 1-12
Horizontal plane

	Position	Motion
Pelvis	4-5 degrees internal	4-5 degrees ext. rotation
Femur	6 degrees internal	6 degrees external rotation
Tibia	9 degrees internal	6 degrees external rotation

when one limb is responsible for supporting body weight. Stability of the limb and trunk is required as the swing leg passes from a posterior position to an anterior position relative to the single support limb. The foot is now required to become more stable in anticipation of heel-lift and increased ground reaction force. Progression of the body needs to be preserved.

Ground reaction forces

Vertical load. (Fig. 1-49) At this point, the knee is extending, causing a rise in the center of gravity. The trunk climbs to its highest point, approximately 25 mm above its mean level. This rise is accentuated by the body passing over the stationary foot, which effectively decelerates body weight. The ground reaction forces can fall to approximately 75% of body weight during this period.

Anteroposterior shear. (Fig. 1-50) At this time the deceleration has stopped. As the swing limb now advances, acceleration against the floor increases.

Horizontal plane (Table 1-12)

At this point, the opposite limb has lifted from the floor, initiated swing, and is advancing forward. This motion, along with momentum, creates an external rotary force on the support limb, a reversal of the previous internal rotation influence. This external rotary effect is initiated at the pelvic level and continues down the limb. Rotation of the swing limb is countered by the arm swing on the support side. With the foot fixed on the ground, external rotation of the limb has a supination effect on the subtalar joint.

Hip joint (Table 1-13)

During this period, the abductor muscle stabilizes the pelvis in a level posture. The hip continues to extend as momentum carries the pelvis forward over the thigh. As this occurs, the body vector moves from anterior through the center of the joint. At the end of midstance it will be slightly posterior, resulting in minimal extensor muscle control.

Knee joint (Table 1-14)

At the end of contact, the knee reaches its maximum flexion and now begins to extend. At this

Table 1-13
Hip joint

	Position	Motion
Hip joint	Flexed 20 degrees	Flexion 20 degrees

Table 1-14
Knee joint

	Position	Motion
Knee joint	Flexed 15-18 degrees	Extension 12 degrees

Table 1-15
Ankle joint

	Position	Motion
Ankle joint	Plantarflexed 7 degrees	Dorsiflexion 7-10 degrees

Table 1-16
Subtalar joint

	Position	Motion
Subtalar joint	Pronated 4-6 degrees	Supination 4 degrees

Table 1-17
Midtarsal joint

	Position	Motion
Longitudinal midtarsal joint	Supinated	Pronation
Oblique midtarsal joint	Pronated	Pronation

time the quadriceps are active, assisting in knee extension while also resisting excessive knee flexion. In addition, the soleus is decelerating forward advancement of the tibia, and allowing the femur to advance more rapidly, thereby creating extension at the knee.

Ankle joint (Table 1-15)

With the foot flat on the ground, the knee extending, and the opposite limb in swing, the fulcrum for forward progression of the trunk and limb is now located at the ankle joint. As the knee extends along with forefoot loading, the tibia advances over the fixed foot, causing ankle joint dorsiflexion. Excessive dorsiflexion is resisted by the action of the soleus on the tibia.

Subtalar joint (Table 1-16)

With external rotation of the limb, the talus abducts in the ankle mortise, resulting in supination of the subtalar joint. The ability of the subtalar joint to supinate depends on how well pronation was controlled during contact phase. With supination of the subtalar joint, the external rotary torque at the ankle is reduced, preventing impingement.

Midtarsal joint (Table 1-17)

With supination of the subtalar joint a decrease in range of motion occurs in the midtarsal joint. In addition, the parallelism of the axes changes, moving toward a more oblique relationship and an increasingly stable joint.

Longitudinal axis

Supination of the subtalar joint has an inverting effect on the forefoot. Since the ground loading the lateral forefoot prevents the forefoot from inverting along with the rearfoot, pronation (eversion) of the forefoot results. This occurs about the longitudinal axis of the midtarsal joint and is a passive motion facilitated by subtalar joint motion.

In addition, this pronation motion assists the dorsal surface of the cuboid to rotate under the dorsal calcaneal ledge and "lock up" the midtarsal joint, thereby creating stability.[2] This occurs at the end of midstance.

Oblique axis

With supination of the subtalar joint, the ground reaction force acting on the forefoot continues to provide a pronatary force to the joint. This continues until the heel lifts from the ground, and so maintains a locked position of the joint.

Pretibial muscles

Anterior tibial—inactive

Extensor digitorum longus—inactive

Extensor hallucis longus—inactive

Recent studies have shown that persons who pronate into midstance phase have continued anterior tibial participation.

Calf muscles (Table 1-18)

Soleus—active

Gastrocnemius—active

Function

1. The soleus resists excessive dorsiflexion provided by the tibia as it advances over the ankle and assists in heel-lift.

Table 1-18
Calf muscles

	Femur	Tibia	Ankle joint	Subtalar joint
Gastrocnemius	Flexion external rotation	—	Plantarflexion	Supination
Soleus	—	Extension external rotation	Plantarflexion	Supination

Table 1-19
Intrinsic muscles

	Midtarsal oblique axis	1st MP joint	Lessor MP joints
Extensor digitorum brevis	Pronation	—	Extension
Interossei	—	—	Extension
lumbricales	—	—	Plantflexion abduction-adduction

2. The gastrocnemius assists in supination of the subtalar joint along with external rotation of the femur.
3. The gastrocnemius exerts a flexion force on the femur to allow for smooth extension of the knee. This is assisted by the action of the soleus, which extends the leg.
4. The soleus stabilizes the lateral aspect of the forefoot against the ground.
5. The soleus assists the other muscles in accelerating external tibial rotation.
6. As the gastrocnemius arises from the femur, its effect will be to flex the knee.
7. The soleus affects the tibia by slowing forward momentum, thereby extending the tibia. Together they assist in extension of the knee.
8. The soleus has a long lever arm with the subtalar joint axis, thereby placing a supination effect on the joint. This results in stabilizing the lateral column of the foot, which provides a stable segment for normal peroneus longus function around the cuboid.

Intrinsic muscles (Table 1-19)

Extensor hallucis brevis—inactive
Abductor hallucis—inactive
Adductor hallucis—inactive
Flexor hallucis brevis—inactive
Flexor digitorum brevis—inactive
Interossei and lumbricales—active
Extensor digitorum brevis—active

Function

1. The extensor digitorum brevis primarily stabilizes the three central metatarsals against the tarsal region.
2. The lumbricales primarily stabilize the proximal and middle phalanges in anticipation of propulsion.

Extrinsic muscles (Table 1-20)

Posterior tibial—active
Peroneus longus—active
Peroneus brevis—active
Flexor digitorum longus—active
Flexor hallucis longus—active

Function

1. Because of its long lever arm relative to the subtalar joint axis, the posterior tibial muscle strongly assists in subtalar joint supination along with external rotation of the leg. It also weakly assists with deceleration of the forward momentum of the leg.
2. The posterior tibial tendon is a strong supinator of the oblique axis of the midtarsal joint and acts in concert with the peroneus longus to compress the tarsus and stabilize the midfoot.
3. The peroneus longus is a prime antagonist of the posterior tibial in the direction of pronation.
4. The peroneus longus initiates its contraction during the middle of midstance phase. It

Table 1-20
Extrinsic muscles

	Ankle joint	Subtalar joint	Midtarsal joint longitudinal axis	Midtarsal joint oblique axis
Posterior tibial	Plantarflexion	Supination	—	Supination
Peroneus longus	Plantarflexion	Pronation	Pronation	—
Peroneus brevis	Plantarflexion	Pronation	Pronation	Pronation
Flexor digitorum longus	Plantarflexion	Supination	—	Supination
Flexor hallucis longus	Plantarflexion	Supination	—	Supination

has a significant lever arm for pronating the midtarsal joint and therefore stabilizes the entire medial forefoot against the ground.

5. The peroneus longus is a primary stabilizer of the first ray in the posterior, lateral, and plantar direction. In addition, it maintains the stability of the midfoot along with the posterior tibial by compressing the tarsus.

6. The peroneus brevis exerts an effective pronatory lever arm on the subtalar joint, which assists in a smooth gradual supinatory motion. It also exerts an abduction influence on the forefoot, and assists in stabilizing the lateral column of the foot. This enhances peroneus longus function.

7. The flexor digitorum longus assists with supination of the subtalar joint, along with deceleration of forward momentum and external rotation of the tibia. It also stabilizes the digits against their respective metatarsal heads in preparation for heel-lift.

8. The flexor hallucis longus assists the posterior tibial, soleus, and flexor digitorum longus with acceleration of supination of the subtalar joint and external rotation of the leg.

9. The flexor hallucis longus also acts to stabilize the hallux against the first metatarsal head in a posterior direction in anticipation of heel-lift.

Summary
This phase ends with heel-lift of the support limb (see Table 1-2).

1. Toe-off and advancement of the swing leg initiate external rotation of the support limb along with supination of the subtalar joint.

2. Deceleration of forward momentum of the tibia by the extrinsic muscles contributes to extension at the knee.

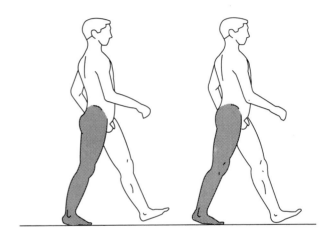

Fig. 1-51. Active propulsion.

3. Contraction of the peroneus longus, flexor digitorum longus, flexor hallucis longus, soleus, and gastrocnemius assists in supination of the subtalar joint.

4. Supination of the subtalar joint, compression of the calcaneal cuboid articulation, and talonavicular congruence all contribute to stabilizing the midfoot. Additionally, eccentric contraction of the posterior tibial and the peroneus longus assists in compressing the tarsus.

5. Ground reaction forces drop below body weight as the center of gravity is raised with knee extension.

6. Acceleration of the leg and trunk over the foot occurs as the swing limb passes from a posterior position to an anterior position relative to the single support limb.

7. Ankle joint dorsiflexion occurs with forward movement of the tibia and eventually initiates heel-lift.

8. A period of single support continues after heel-lift.

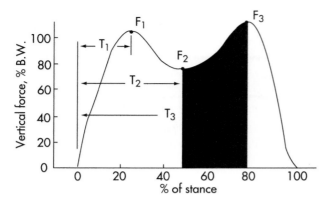

Fig. 1-52. Vertical load.

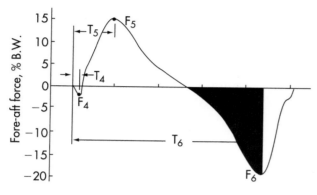

Fig. 1-53. Anteroposterior shear.

Table 1-21
Horizontal plane

	Position	Motion
Pelvis	Neutral	2-4 degrees external rotation
Femur	Neutral	4 degrees external rotation
Tibia	0-3 degrees internal	3-4 degrees external rotation

Active propulsion (Fig. 1-51)

This is a continuation of the single support period which begins with support-side heel-lift and ends with opposite-side heel-strike. This is the period when the greatest vertical and horizontal forces are directed against the foot. This phase allows smooth progression of the body beyond the supporting foot. In addition, the metatarsophalangeal joint becomes the active center of rotation for the foot.

Ground reaction forces (Fig. 1-52)

Vertical load. As the heel lifts, the body weight is now forward of the support limb and the center of

Table 1-22
Hip Joint

	Position	Motion
Hip joint	Neutral	Extension 20 degrees

Table 1-23
Knee joint

	Position	Motion
Knee joint	Flexed 3-5 degrees	Extension 5-7 degrees

gravity is falling. As the body weight drops over the forefoot rocker, there is a downward acceleration which results in the highest vertical force received by the body.

Anteroposterior shear. (Fig. 1-53) The acceleration of the leg forward of the ankle, associated with lifting of the heel, results in a posterior shear against the ground. This reaches its highest amplitude at heel-strike of the opposite limb. The combination of high vertical load and high and posterior shear provides an environment which may cause the greatest damage during the gait cycle.

Horizontal plane (Table 1-21)

The pelvis, femur, and tibia rapidly externally rotate with further advancement of the swing limb. The tibia rotates farther and faster than the thigh, with resultant external knee rotation. The thigh rotates further and faster than the pelvis, producing external rotation at the hip.[56]

Hip joint (Table 1-22)

With further advancement of the swing limb, the body weight moves forward over the forefoot, which increases the posterior position of the support limb. This results in a hyperextension at the hip in relation to the erect trunk and pelvis.[52]

Knee joint (Table 1-23)

Knee extension continues from midstance and extends to a position of 3 degrees of flexion (the knee never fully extends). Knee extension prevents excessive lowering of the center of mass associated with the anterior movement of the body weight. It is important that the knee function in extension during this phase, as the limb experiences high vertical loads. Extension of the knee also contributes to increasing stride length. At the end of this phase, the posterior muscle group releases the tibia so that knee flexion can be initiated.

Table 1-24
Ankle joint

	Position	Motion
Ankle joint	Dorsiflexed 5-7 degrees	Dorsiflexion 5 degrees

Ankle joint (Table 1-24)

This phase is initiated by heel-lift. With the active contraction of the soleus and gastrocnemius resisting dorsiflexion, the tibia moving forward in the ankle mortise, and the pelvis advancing forward over the forefoot, the heel is pulled off the ground. Perry states[52]

> ... the combination of ankle dorsiflexion and heel rise in terminal stance places the body centre of gravity anterior to the source of foot support. As the center of pressure moves more anterior to the metatarsal head axis, the foot rolls with the body, leading to greater heel rise. The effect is an ever-increasing dorsiflexion torque. This creates a full forward fall situation that possibly generates the major progression force used in walking. The signs of effective ankle function during active propulsion are heel lift, minimal joint motion and a nearly neutral ankle position.

It is important to note that a stable midfoot is essential for normal sequencing of heel-lift. The primary force on the ankle is dorsiflexion. During the early part of this phase, the tibia advances with heel-lift, causing the foot to plantarflex. Once the heel has lifted sufficiently off the ground, knee flexion can occur, which subsequently releases the foot to plantarflex.

Subtalar joint (Table 1-25)

With the heel off the ground, the external rotating influence from the limb is now free to rapidly supinate the subtalar joint. The entire rearfoot abducts as it pivots over the metatarsophalangeal joint articulation. Dynamic locking of the midtarsal joint mechanisms increases as the subtalar joint continues to supinate.

Midtarsal joint (Table 1-26)

Maximum control of the midtarsal joint is required as body weight has now reached its highest level and is advancing over the metatarsal heads. This is accomplished by several mechanisms.

The windlass effect is incorporated as the heel lifts and the plantar fascia winds itself around the drum of the metatarsal heads. Since the diameter of the first metatarsal head is larger than those of the lesser metatarsals, the medial band of the fascia demonstrates a greater effect in pulling the calcaneus toward the forefoot. This results in a higher

Table 1-25
Subtalar joint

	Position	Motion
Subtalar joint	Pronated-neutral	Supination 4 degrees

Table 1-26
Midtarsal joint

	Position	Motion
Longitudinal axis midtarsal joint	Pronated	Pronation
Oblique axis midtarsal joint	Pronated	Supination

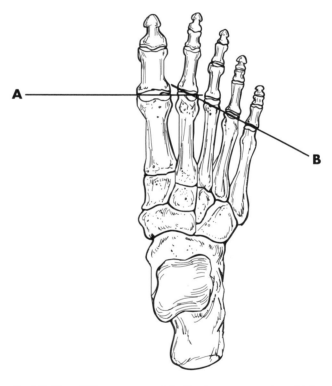

Fig. 1-54. Two different axes exist—the transverse axis, which corresponds to the high-gear axis (A), and the oblique axis, which corresponds to the low-gear (B). (*Redrawn from Bojsen-Møller, Clin Orthop 14:11, 1978.*)

arch along with supination of the subtalar joint.[28]

Bojsen-Møller[2] described a high-gear and low-gear mechanism by which the heel-lift period creates efficient propulsion for the foot. He described two axes, the transverse axis composed of the first and second metatarsals, and the oblique axis composed of the second to fifth metatarsals (Fig. 1-54). The high gear is consistent with the transverse axis

Table 1-27
Calf muscles

	Knee	Femur	Tibia	Ankle joint	Subtalar joint
Gastrocnemius	Flexion	Flexion external rotation	—	Plantarflexion	Supination
Soleus	—	—	Extension external rotation	Plantarflexion	Supination

and the low gear is consistent with the oblique axis. Since the distance from the ankle joint axis to the oblique axis is shorter, this axis is used first on heel-lift before the shift to the high-gear position. Function across the high-gear push-off results in a pronated forefoot-to-rearfoot position, a tight plantar aponeurosis, and increased weightbearing under the medial forefoot. The peroneus longus assists in further elevating the lateral aspect of the foot, thereby expediting the high-gear mechanism.

Longitudinal axis

Pronation of the longitudinal axis of the midtarsal joint continues with the aid of subtalar joint supination and body weight. Body weight holds the metatarsal heads firmly against the ground, while the subtalar joint supinates. This results in pronation of the longitudinal axis. In addition, the lateral column of the foot, which has been held firmly against the ground by the soleus, can now elevate with the aid of the peroneus longus, thereby shifting body weight medially.

Oblique axis

As the heel lifts, the leg continues to rotate externally, abducting and dorsiflexing the talus. This motion, occurring proximal to the fixed forefoot, results in supination of the oblique axis of the midtarsal joint. Since the main components of oblique axis midtarsal joint supination are adduction and plantarflexion, the arch height of the foot is increased, thereby compressing the tarsus and creating further stability.[56]

Pretibial muscles

Anterior tibial—inactive
Extensor digitorum longus—inactive
Extensor hallucis longus—inactive

Calf muscles (Table 1-27)

Soleus—active
Gastrocnemius—active

Function

1. Strong gastrocnemius-soleus action is required to stabilize the tibia at the ankle as ground reaction forces increase.

2. The gastrocnemius is free to assist with flexion of the knee as the heel is released from the ground and the tibia advances.

3. The gastrocnemius assists with active plantarflexion of the ankle, which occurs with flexion of the knee.

4. The soleus diminishes its activity, reducing its ability to stabilize the lateral side of the foot. Peroneal muscle action is now free to direct body weight medially as it lifts the lateral side of the foot.

5. As the gastrocnemius assists in ankle plantarflexion and knee flexion, it applies an upward and forward momentum on the knee that assists in hip flexion.

Intrinsic muscles (Table 1-28)

Function

1. The abductor and adductor hallucis brevis stabilize the proximal phalanx of the hallux against the ground.

2. The abductor hallucis brevis assists in plantarflexing the first ray and supinating the oblique axis of the midtarsal joint.

3. The adductor hallucis brevis resists splay of the metatarsal heads through its origin from the proximal phalanx of the hallux and insertion into the lesser metatarsals.

4. The flexor hallucis brevis is a major stabilizer of the proximal phalanx of the hallux and assists in compressing the first metatarsophalangeal joint at the end of its range of motion.

5. The flexor digitorum brevis assists in compressing the lesser metatarsophalangeal joints, so they act to supply effective ground contact of the forefoot as the heel lifts.

6. The interossei maintain transverse stability of the lesser metatarsophalangeal joints and assist in compressing the proximal phalanx against the metatarsal heads.

7. The lumbricales apply an adduction force to the lesser digits and assist in compressing the middle and distal phalanges to resist vertical ground reaction force.

8. The lumbricales and interossei together func-

Table 1-28
Intrinsic muscles

	Midtarsal oblique axis	1st MP joint	Lessor MP joints
Extensor digitorum brevis	—	—	—
Abductor hallucis	Supination	Adduction	—
Adductor hallucis	—	Abduction	Adduction
Flexor hallucis brevis	—	Flexion	—
Flexor digitorum brevis	Supination	—	Flexion
Interossei	—	—	Extension
Lumbricales	—	—	Plantarflexion abduction-adduction

Table 1-29
Extrinsic muscles

	Tibia	Ankle joint	Subtalar joint	Midtarsal joint longitudinal axis	Midtarsal joint oblique axis
Posterior tibial	Extension/external rotation	Plantarflexion	Supination	—	Supination
Peroneus longus	Extension/internal rotation	Plantarflexion	Pronation	Pronation	—
Peroneus brevis	Extension/internal rotation	Plantarflexion	Pronation	Pronation	Pronation
Flexor digitorum longus	Extension/external rotation	Plantarflexion	Supination	—	Supination
Flexor hallucis longus	Extension/external rotation	Plantarflexion	Supination	—	Supination

tion to maintain extensor rigidity of the digits during propulsion.

In general, the intrinsic muscles of the foot during this stage assist in compressing not only the digits but the tarsal joints as body weight shifts forward with heel lift.

Extrinsic muscles (Table 1-29)

Posterior tibial—active
Peroneus longus—active
Peroneus brevis—active
Flexor digitorum longus—active
Flexor hallucis longus—active

Function

1. The function of the posterior tibial diminishes as the heel lifts, and only marginally participates in ankle plantarflexion.
2. The peroneus longus provides a transverse and compressive force to the tarsal joints as it functions in unison with the posterior tibial muscle.
3. The peroneus longus primarily stabilizes the first ray posteriorly and laterally against the tarsus. It also plantarflexes the first ray and exerts a major force in resisting dorsiflexion of the first ray by ground reaction force.
4. The peroneus longus, along with the peroneus brevis, elevates and everts the lateral column of the foot, and assists in directing body weight medially.
5. The peroneus brevis continues to compress the cuboid into the calcaneus, contributing to lateral column stability.
6. The flexor digitorum longus assists in plantarflexion of the ankle and primarily stabilizes the digits against the ground. It helps compress the lesser metatarsophalangeal joints and provides a stable rocker for forward progression of the trunk.
7. The flexor digitorum longus also is a supinator of the oblique axis of the midtarsal joint.
8. The flexor hallucis longus develops a strong plantarflexion force on the hallux, which assists in resisting ground reaction force.
9. The flexor hallucis longus also assists in supination of the oblique axis of the midtarsal joint and is a strong plantarflexor of the ankle.

The extrinsic muscles of the foot and leg play a significant role in creating stability of the midfoot and forefoot during this phase of gait.

Summary

This phase ends with heel contact of the opposite limb (see Table 1-2).

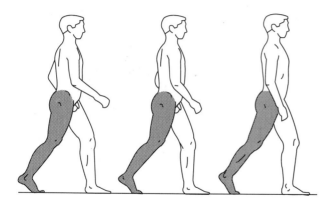

Fig. 1-55. Passive lift-off.

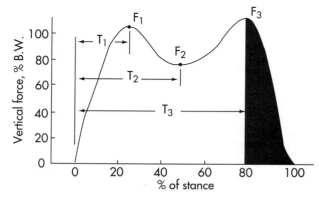

Fig. 1-56. Vertical load.

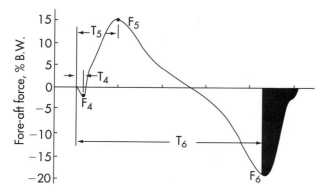

Fig. 1-57. Anteroposterior shear.

1. The rocker action of the foot has moved from the ankle joint to the metatarsophalangeal joints.
2. Momentum, the pull of the swing leg, and dropping of the center of gravity make the largest contribution to the amplitude of vertical load and anteroposterior shear.
3. Maximum range of hyperextension is reached at the hip and pelvis.

4. Knee extension resists excessive lowering of the center of body mass.
5. Ankle joint dorsiflexion continues to stabilize the foot during heel-lift. Once this occurs, rapid plantarflexion may take place.
6. Continued supination of the subtalar joint contributes to increased midtarsal joint stability.
7. The concentration of vertical load has shifted to the midfoot and forefoot. Longitudinal midtarsal joint pronation, oblique axis midtarsal supination, the windlass effect, and the low- and high-gear push all contribute to maximum midfoot and forefoot stability.
8. Shift of body weight medially prepares for heel contact of the opposite limb and acceptance of body weight.
9. This period of single support ends with opposite heel-strike.

Passive lift-off (Fig. 1-55)

This is a second period of double support which begins with opposite-side heel contact and terminates with support-side toe-off. The foot and limb prepare for the swing phase and advancement of the limb. This is a passive event as momentum carries the limb forward.

Ground reaction forces

Vertical load. (Fig. 1-56) There is a rapid drop-off in body weight as it is transferred to the opposite, contacting limb. By the end of this phase the vertical load has completely diminished.

Anteroposterior shear. (Fig. 1-57) As heel-lift increases and the opposite limb contacts, there is a deceleration of forward movement or a posterior shear. This slows the limb down momentarily until it lifts for swing phase.

Horizontal plane (Table 1-30)

The pelvis, femur, and tibia continue to externally rotate as the opposite-side pelvis advances. Maximum external rotation occurs during this phase. This external influence from the limb places an abduction effect on the foot and is manifested as subtalar and oblique midtarsal joint supination.

Hip joint (Table 1-31)

Extension of the hip is reversed and rapid flexion is initiated reaching a neutral position by toe-off. This action is the result of an increase in knee flexion due to ankle joint plantarflexion. This combined action provides an upward movement to the trunk, assisting in hip flexion. In addition, rectus femoris restraint of knee flexion provides direct hip flexion. This is the beginning of leg acceleration.[52]

Table 1-30
Horizontal plane

	Position	Motion
Pelvis	2-4 degrees external	2 degrees external rotation
Femur	4 degrees external	4 degrees external rotation
Tibia	3-4 degrees external	3-4 degrees external rotation

Table 1-31
Hip joint

	Position	Motion
Hip joint	20 degrees extended	10-20 degrees flexion

Table 1-32
Knee joint

	Position	Motion
Knee joint	Flexed 3-5 degrees	Flexion 35-40 degrees

Table 1-33
Ankle joint

	Position	Motion
Ankle joint	Dorsiflexed 5-7 degrees	Plantarflexion 20 degrees

Table 1-34
Subtalar joint

	Position	Motion
Subtalar joint	Supinated 4 degrees	Supination 2-4 degrees

Table 1-35
Midtarsal joint

	Position	Motion
Longitudinal axis midtarsal joint	Pronated	Pronation
Oblique axis midtarsal joint	Supinated	Supination

Table 1-36
Pretibial muscles

	Hallux	Lesser digits
Extensor digitorum longus	Extension	—
Extensor hallicus longus	—	Extension

Knee joint (Table 1-32)

The knee continues to rapidly undergo flexion, reaching 40 degrees at toe-off. This is a passive event which occurs as a result of ankle plantarflexion and movement of the tibia forward. This, in conjunction with gastrocnemius action, flexes the knee and provides adequate toe clearance.

Ankle joint (Table 1-33)

The ankle continues to rapidly plantarflex, reaching 20 degrees at toe-off. The residual action of the gastrocnemius and the soleus propel the tibia forward while the foot rolls over the forefoot rocker at the metatarsophalangeal joint. This places the ground reaction force behind the knee creating knee flexion and continued ankle plantarflexion.

Subtalar joint (Table 1-34)

Supination of the subtalar joint continues, but not as rapidly as during active propulsion. As heel-lift increases, external rotation of the tibia is partially absorbed by ankle plantarflexion and abduction of the entire rearfoot. Since the heel is off the ground the rearfoot is free to do this. Supination continues until swing phase, when the long digital extensors initiate pronation.[56]

Midtarsal joint (Table 1-35)

External rotation of the limb and muscle action are the primary factors in controlling midtarsal joint function.

Longitudinal axis

Since body weight has transferred medially, and the lateral side of the foot has lifted from the ground, the longitudinal axis of the midtarsal joint continues to pronate. This continues to provide a stable midfoot and maintains osseous stability for intrinsic muscle action.

Oblique axis

External rotation of the leg is the major factor in maintaining supination of the oblique axis of the midtarsal joint. Since the forefoot is fully weight-bearing, rotation of the limb is manifested as dorsiflexion and abduction of the talus, resulting in a plantarflexed and adducted forefoot. This represents supination of the oblique axis of the midtarsal joint. This position of the joint, along with intrinsic

Table 1-37
Calf muscles

	Knee	Femur	Tibia	Ankle joint	Subtalar joint
Gastrocnemius	Flexion	—	—	Plantarflexion	—
Soleus	—	—	—	Plantarflexion	—

Table 1-38
Intrinsic muscles

	Midtarsal oblique axis	Hallux	Lesser digit
Extensor digitorum brevis	—	—	Dorsiflexion
Abductor hallucis	Supination	Plantarflexion/adduction	—
Adductor hallucis	—	Plantarflexion/abduction	Adduction
Hallucis flexor brevis	—	Plantarflexion	—
Digitorum flexor brevis	Supination	—	Plantarflexion
Interossei	—	—	Extension
Lumbricales	—	—	Plantarflexion abduction/adduction

and extrinsic muscle contraction, maintains stability of the forefoot until toe-off.[56]

Pretibial muscles (Table 1-36)

Anterior tibial—inactive-active
Extensor digitorum longus—active
Extensor hallucis longus—active

Function

1. The extensor hallucis longus acts on the hallux to extend the interphalangeal joint, stabilize the joint, and assist the plantarflexors in maintaining ground contact.
2. The extensor digitorum longus stabilizes the lesser toes so that ground contact can be maintained by the long and short flexors.

The primary purpose of the anterior group during this phase is to maintain the digits in extension so that the plantarflexors may maintain the toes against the ground reaction force.

Calf muscles (Table 1-37)

Soleus—active-inactive
Gastrocnemius—active-inactive

Function

1. The soleus has a mild plantarflexory effect on the ankle.

2. The gastrocnemius has a mild effect on knee flexion.

Both muscles rapidly diminish their activity during this phase. Their main contribution is releasing the tibia to advance forward to provide ankle plantarflexion and knee flexion.

Intrinsic muscles (Table 1-38)

Extensor digitorum brevis—active
Abductor hallucis brevis—active
Adductor hallucis brevis—active
Flexor hallucis brevis—active
Flexor digitorum brevis—active
Interossei—active
Lumbricales—active

Function

1. The extensor digitorum brevis continues to reinforce the stability of the digits by assisting in extending the toes.
2. The abductor hallucis functions to plantarflex the first ray and stabilizes it against the ground. It also assists in supinating the oblique axis of the midtarsal joint.
3. The adductor hallucis functions to stabilize the proximal phalanx of the hallux in the direction of adduction and plantarflexion.
4. The combined action of the abductor and

Table 1-39
Extrinsic muscles

	Ankle joint	Midtarsal joint oblique axis	Hallux	Lesser digit
Flexor digitorum longus	Plantarflexion	Supination	—	Flexion
Flexor hallucis longus	Plantarflexion	Supination	Flexion	—

adductor hallucis brevis stabilizes the proximal phalanx in a posterior direction against the first metatarsal head.

5. The flexor hallucis brevis primarily stabilizes the proximal phalanx of the hallux against vertical ground reaction forces.

6. The flexor digitorum brevis primarily stabilizes the phalanges of the digits against vertical ground reaction forces. It also assists in supination of the oblique axis of the midtarsal joint axis.

7. The flexor digitorum brevis plantarflexes the lesser metatarsal heads.

8. The interossei continue to maintain transverse stability of the lesser metatarsophalangeal joints and help compress the proximal phalanx against the metatarsal heads.

9. The lumbricales continue to help compress the middle and distal phalanges to resist vertical ground reaction forces.

The intrinsic muscles continue to provide stability for the digits so that vertical ground reaction forces will not sublux them. In addition, the digits provide a stable buttress which facilitates rotation of the metatarsal head around them.

Extrinsic muscles (Table 1-39)

Posterior tibial—inactive
Peroneus longus—inactive
Peroneus brevis—inactive
Flexor digitorum longus—active
Flexor hallucis longus—active

1. The flexor hallucis longus maintains stability of the hallux to resist vertical ground reaction forces.

2. The flexor hallucis longus assists in supination of the oblique axis of the midtarsal joint.

3. The flexor digitorum longus maintains stability of the phalanges relative to one another and resists vertical ground reaction forces.

4. The flexor digitorum longus assists in supination of the oblique axis of the midtarsal joint.

5. The flexor digitorum longus and flexor hallucis longus both assist in ankle plantarflexion. The primary action of both muscles is to provide a stable digital platform which elongates the forefoot support area without negatively influencing the rocker action.

Summary
This phase concludes with final toe-off (see Table 1-2).

1. There is a rapid drop-off of the vertical load and a reverse of the anteroposterior shear to decelerate motion.

2. The limb continues to externally rotate until toe-off.

3. The hip rapidly changes from extension to flexion.

4. There is rapid knee flexion and ankle plantarflexion.

5. Subtalar joint supination, along with midtarsal joint stability, maintains the integrity of the foot.

6. Primary muscle function is represented mainly by the intrinsic muscle group, which along with the long flexors and extensors, maintains digital stability.

7. A period of double support ends with toe-off.

Swing (Fig. 1-58)
This is a period of nonsupport which begins with toe-off and terminates with heel-strike of the same limb. This is a period when the limb advances from a trailing position to a position anterior to the trunk. Foot clearance off the floor is facilitated by hip and knee flexion.

Ground reaction forces
There are no ground reaction forces acting on the limb during this phase.

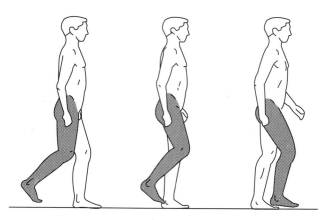

Fig. 1-58. Swing.

Horizontal plane (Table 1-40)

Reversal of external rotation begins as the foot leaves the ground and the swing limb now rotates around the opposite support limb. This begins as external rotation but the foot will internally rotate by the time of heel contact.

Hip joint (Table 1-41)

Flexion continues with the aid of momentum generated from the passive lift-off phase and the assistance of the hip flexor muscles. Mild activity of the gracilis and sartorius help with flexion. As the leg nears the end of swing, the hamstrings control the limb and reduce flexion at the hip in preparation for heel-strike.

Knee joint (Table 1-42)

Knee flexion increases, as this is the primary motion for lifting the foot, allowing toe clearance, and advancing the limb. A minimum of 60 degrees of knee flexion is required, since the ankle is in plantarflexion and so positions the digits to strike the ground. This is accomplished by flexion initiated during passive lift-off, momentum from hip flexion, and the action of the biceps femoris. By midswing, the foot is forward of the hip and extension is initiated. Further knee extension is assisted by momentum, but hyperextension is controlled by the action of the hamstrings. The limb is now prepared for heel contact.[52]

Ankle joint (Table 1-43)

At toe-off, the ankle is in 20 degrees of plantarflexion. With the foot trailing behind the leg, dorsiflexion of the digits and the ankle is initiated by contraction of the anterior muscle group. This continues until midswing when the ankle is slightly plantarflexed. By this time, adequate ground clearance has occurred and the anterior muscle group briefly becomes inactive. Just prior to heel contact,

Table 1-40
Horizontal plane

	Position	Motion
Pelvis	2 degrees external	2 degrees internal rotation
Femur	4 degrees external	4 degrees internal rotation
Tibia	3-4 degrees external	6 degrees internal rotation

Table 1-41
Hip joint

	Position	Motion
Hip joint	Neutral	30-40 degrees flexion

Table 1-42
Knee joint

	Position	Motion
Knee joint	Flexed 35-40 degrees	Extension 35-40 degrees

Table 1-43
Ankle joint

	Position	Motion
Ankle joint	Plantarflexed 20 degrees	Dorsiflexion 20 degrees

the anterior muscle group fires and further dorsiflexes the ankle in preparation for the contact phase.

Subtalar joint (Table 1-44)

As the foot leaves the ground, the subtalar joint now functions as an open chain unit. Only muscular action will affect the joint. Because of extensor digitorum longus activity, the subtalar joint pronates initially after toe-off. Pronation of the subtalar joint brings the plantar surface of the foot closer to the horizontal plane and so ensures greater foot clearance to the ground. Then, as the anterior tibial and extensor digitorum longus are recruited, the joint resupinates in preparation for heel contact.[47,56]

Midtarsal joint (Table 1-45)

Like the subtalar joint, the midtarsal joint also functions as an open chain unit.

Longitudinal axis

At toe-off, the joint is maximally pronated. After midswing, the action of the anterior tibial resupi-

Table 1-44
Subtalar joint

	Position	Motion
Subtalar joint	Supinated 4-6 degrees	Pronation-supination

Table 1-45
Midtarsal joint

	Position	Motion
Longitudinal midtarsal joint	Pronated	Supination
Oblique midtarsal joint	Supinated	Pronation

Table 1-46
Pretibial muscles

	Ankle joint	Subtalar joint	Midtarsal longitudinal axis	Midtarsal oblique axis
Anterior tibial	Dorsiflex	Supination	Supination	—
Extensor digitorum longus	Dorsiflex	Pronation	Pronation	Pronation
Extensor hallucis longus	Dorsiflex	—	—	—

nates the longitudinal axis of the midtarsal joint, and subsequently the subtalar joint.

Oblique axis

At toe-off, the oblique axis of the midtarsal joint is supinated. With activity of the extensor digitorum longus, the joint then pronates and remains pronated during the entire swing phase.

Pretibial muscles (Table 1-46)

Anterior tibial—active-inactive-active

Extensor digitorum longus—active-inactive-active

Extensor hallucis longus—active-inactive-active

Function

1. The anterior tibial assists with dorsiflexion of the foot at toe-off and toe clearance at midswing.
2. The anterior tibial assists in supinating the subtalar joint in anticipation of heel-strike.
3. The anterior tibial acts to resist excessive pronation of the foot initiated by extensor digitorum longus function.
4. The extensor digitorum longus assists in dorsiflexion of the foot for toe clearance and prevents excessive supination.
5. The extensor hallucis longus is a strong dorsiflexor of the foot, flexing the ankle immediately after toe-off.
6. The extensor hallucis longus assists in toe clearance by dorsiflexing the hallux and maintaining this position during the early swing period.

With the foot in a plantarflexed position at toe-off, active pretibial muscle action must take place to rapidly dorsiflex both the toes and the foot. The extensor hallucis longus is mostly responsible for this rapid dorsiflexion. The mechanism for this is expedited by the anterior tibial muscle contracting and dorsiflexing the first ray. This reduces the dorsiflexion range of the first metatarsophalangeal joint, so that the extensor hallucis longus now has a longer lever arm to act on the foot. Dorsiflexion momentum carries the foot into midswing at which the pretibial muscles become inactive. After a brief period, they again become active to maintain the foot in dorsiflexion in preparation for heel-strike.

Calf muscles—inactive

Intrinsic muscles—inactive

Extrinsic muscles—inactive

Summary

This phase concludes with heel-strike (see Table 1-2).

1. The limb briefly continues external rotation and then internally rotates for the balance of the phase.
2. The hip, knee, and ankle all dorsiflex to shorten the limb. This allows it to pass smoothly from posterior to anterior relative to the support limb.
3. Only muscle action acts on the foot, which results first in pronation and then supination of the subtalar joint.
4. Step length is determined by the excursion of the swing limb.

References

1. Barnett CH, Napier JH: The axis of rotation of the ankle joint in man. Its influence upon the form of the talus and the mobility of the fibula, *Anatomy* 86:1–8, 1952.

2. Bojsen-Møller F: Calcaneocuboid joint and stability of the longitudinal arch of the foot at high and low gear push off, *J Anat* 129:165–176, 1979.

3. Bojsen-Møller F, Lamoreux L: Significance of free dorsiflexion of the toes in walking, *Acta Orthop Scand,* 50:411–479, 1979.

4. Broca P: Des difformités de la partie antérieure des pied produite per l'action de la chaussure, *Bull Soc Anat,* 27:60, 1852.

5. Bruckner J: Variations in the human subtalar joint, *J Orthop Sports Phys Ther* 8:489–494, 1987.

6. Buell T, Green D, Risser J: Measurement of the first metatarsophalangeal joint range of motion, *J Am Podiatr Med Assoc* 78:439–448, 1988.

7. Cahill DR: The anatomy and function of the contents of the human tarsal sinus and canal, *Anat Rec* 153:1, 1965.

8. D'Amico JC, Schuster RO: Motion of the first ray, *J Am Podiatr Med Assoc* 69:17–23, 1979.

9. Dananberg HC: Functional hallux limitus and its relationship to gait efficiency, *J Am Podiatr Med Assoc* 76:6–18, 1986.

10. Dananberg HC: Gait styles as an etiology to chronic postural pain, Part II, *J Am Podiatr Med Assoc* 83:615–624, 1993.

11. DuChatinier K, Molen NH, Rozendale RH: Step length, step frequency and temporal factors of the stride in normal human walking, *Proc Kon Ned Akad Wat C* 73:214–226, 1970.

12. Dykyj D: Anatomy of motion, *Clin Podiatr Med Surg* 5:447–490, 1988.

13. Dykyj D: Pathologic anatomy of hallux abducto valgus, *Clin Podiatr Med Surg* 6:1-14, 1989.

14. Ebisui JM: The first ray axis and the first metatarsophalangeal joint: an anatomical and pathomechanical study, *J Am Podiatr Med Assoc,* 58:160–168, 1968.

15. Elftman H: The transverse tarsal joint and its control, *Clin Orthop* 16:41, 1960.

16. Englesberg JR, Andrews JG: Kinematic analysis of the talocalcaneal/talocrural joint during running support, *Med Sci Sports Exerc* 3:275–284, 1987.

17. Gerbert J editor: *Textbook of bunion surgery,* Mt. Kisco, NY, 1981, Futura.

18. Giannestras N: *Foot disorders, medical and surgical management,* Philadelphia, 1973, Lea & Febiger.

19. Goss CM, editor: *Anatomy of the human body by Henry Gray, FRS,* Philadelphia, 1973, Lea & Febiger, pp 356–367.

20. Gracovetsky S: *The spinal engine,* Vienna, 1988, Springer-Verlag.

21. Green D, Carol A: Planal dominance *J Am Podiatr Med Assoc* 74:98, 1984.

22. Green DR, Whitney AK, Walter P: Subtalar joint motions, *J Am Podiatr Med Assoc* 61:83, 1979.

23. Grodel SE, McCarthy DJ: The anatomical implications of hallux abducto valgus, *J Am Podiatr Med Assoc* 70:11, 1980.

24. Heatherington VJ, Carnelt J, Patterson B: Motion of the first metatarsophalangeal, *J Foot Surg* 28:13–19, 1989.

25. Heatherington VJ, Johnson R, Arbritton J: Necessary dorsiflexion of the first metatarsophalangeal joint during gait, *J Foot Surg* 29:218–222, 1990.

26. Herman R, Wirta R, Perry: *Human solutions for locomotion.* New York, 1976, Plenum Press, pp 13–76.

27. Hicks JH: The mechanics of the foot I. The joints, *J Anat* 88:345–357, 1954.

28. Hicks JH: The mechanics of the foot II. The plantar aponeurosis and the arch, *J Anat* 88:25–30, 1954.

29. Huson A: *Ein ontleed kundig-functional onderzoek van de voetwortel [An anatomical and functional study of the tarsal joints],* Leiden, Netherlands, 1961, Luctor et Emergo.

30. Hutton WC, Dhanendran M: The mechanics of normal and hallux valgus feet of a quantitative study, *Clin Orthop* 157:7–13, 1981.

31. Inman V: *Human walking,* Baltimore, 1981, Williams & Wilkins.

32. Inman VT: *The joints of the ankle,* Baltimore, 1976, Williams & Wilkins.

33. Joseph J: Range of movement of the great toe in men, *J Bone Joint Surg [Br],* 36:450, 1954.

34. Kapanji IA: *The physiology of joints: lower limb,* vol 2: Edinburgh, Scotland, 1970, Churchill Livingston.

35. Kelikian H: *Structural alteration in hallux valgus, allied deformities of the forefoot and metatarsalgia,* Philadelphia 1965, WB Saunders, pp 77–83.

36. Kravitz S, Laporta G, Lawton L: KLL progressive staging classification of hallux limitus and hallux rigidus. *In The Lower Extremity,* vol. 1, 1994, pp 56–66.

37. Lamoreux LW: Kinematic measurements in the study of human walking, *Bull Prosthet Res* 10:3–84, 1971.

38. Levens AS, Inman VT, Blosser JA: Transverse rotation of the segments of the lower extremity in locomotion, *J Bone Joint Surg [Am]* 30A:859-874, 1948.

39. Lewis OJ: *Functional morphology of the evolving hand and foot,* Oxford, 1989, Clarendon Press, p 224.

40. Lundberg A, Svensson D, Nemeth G, Selvik G: The axis of rotation of the ankle joint, *J Bone Joint Surg [Br]* 71:94–99, 1989.

41. MacConnaill MA: Some anatomical factors affecting the stabilizing function of muscles, *Ir J Med Sci* 6:160–164, 1946.

42. Mann R: Biomechanics of the foot and ankle. In Mann R, editor: *Surgery of the foot,* ed 5, St Louis, 1986, Mosby–Year Book.

43. Mann RA, Inman VT: Phasic activity of intrinsic muscles of the foot *J Bone Joint Surg [Am]* 46:469, 1964.

44. Mann RA, Moran GT, Dougherty SE: Muscle activity during running, jogging and sprinting, *Am J Sports Med* 14, 1986.

45. Mann R, Nagy J: The function of the toes in walking, jogging and running, *Clin Orthop* 142:24–29, 1979.

46. Manter JT: Movements of the subtalar and transverse tarsal joints, *Anat Rec* 80:397–409, 1941.

47. Michaud T: *Foot orthoses and other forms of conservative foot care,* Baltimore, 1993, William & Wilkins.

48. Morris JM: Biomechanics of the foot and ankle, *Clin Orthop* 22:10–17, 1977.

49. Murray MP, Kory RC, Clarkson BH: Walking patterns in healthy old men, *J Gerontol* 24:169–178, 1969.

50. Oatis CA: Biomechanics of the foot and ankle under static conditions, *Phys Ther* 68:1815–1821, 1982.

51. Oldenbrook LL, Smith CE: Metatarsal head motion secondary to rearfoot pronation and supination, *J Am Podiatr Med Assoc* 69:24, 1979.

52. Perry J: *Gait analysis: normal and pathological function,* New York, 1992, McGraw-Hill, New York.

53. Phillips RD, Phillips RL: Quantitative analysis of the locking position of the midtarsal joint, *J Am Podiatr Med Assoc* 73:518–522, 1983.

54. Root ML, Weed JH, Sgarlato TE: Axis of motion of the subtalar joint, *J Am Podiatr Med Assoc* 56:149, 1966.

55. Root M, Orien W, Weed J: *Normal and abnormal function of the foot,* Los Angeles, 1977, Clinical Biomechanics, pp 10–17.

56. Root ML, et al: Direction and range of motion of the first ray, *J Am Podiatr Med Assoc* 72:600, 1982.

57. Sammarco GJ: Biomechanics of the foot. In Frankel VH, Nordin M, editors: *Basic biomechanics of the skeletal system,* Philadelphia, 1980, Lea & Febiger.

58. Serrafian SK: *Anatomy of the foot and ankle: descriptive, topographic, functional,* ed 2, Philadelphia, 1993, JB Lippincott.

59. Serrafian SK: Functional characteristic of the foot and plantar aponeurosis under tibio talar loading, *Foot & Ankle* 8:14-16, 1987.

60. Sarrafian SK, Topouzian LK: Anatomy and physiology of the extensor apparatus of the toes. *J Bone Joint Surg [Am]* 51:669, 1969.

61. Shereff MJ, Bejani FJ, Kummer FJ: Kinematics of the first metatarsophalangeal joint, *J Bone Joint Surg [Am]* 68:392-398, 1986.

62. Sgarlato TE: *A compendium of podiatric biomechanics*, California College of Podiatric Medicine, 1971, San Francisco.

63. Smith JW: The ligamentous structures in the canalis and sinus tarsi, *J Anat* 92:616, 1958.

64. Stokes AF, Hutton WC, Stotts R: Forces acting on the metatarsals during normal working, *J Anat* 129:579–590, 1979.

65. Winter D: *The biomechanics and motor control of human gait*, Waterloo, Iowa, 1987, University of Waterloo Press.

66. Wright DG, Desai SM, Henderson WH: Action of subtalar and ankle joint complex during the stance phase of walking, *J Bone Joint Surg [Am]* 46:361–382, 1964.

pathomechanics of lower extremity function

Ronald L. Valmassy, DPM

Section I
Basic foot types
Pes planus
Pes cavus
Section II
Functional foot disorders
Frontal plane
Sagittal plane
Transverse plane
Section III
Lower extremity pathology
 1. **Avascular necrosis (osteochondrosis)**
 2. **Calcaneal spur**
 3. **Capsulitis**
 4. **Clawtoe deformity**
 5. **First metatarsal–first cuneiform exostosis**
 6. **Hallux extensus**
 7. **Hallux limitus**
 8. **Hallux valgus**
 9. **Hammer toe deformity**
10. **Interdigital neuroma**
11. **Lateral ankle instability**
12. **Patellofemoral dysfunction**
13. **Plantar fasciitis**
14. **Plantarflexed first-ray deformity**
15. **Retrocalcaneal exostosis**
16. **Sesamoiditis**
17. **Sinus tarsi syndrome**
18. **Stress fractures**
19. **Tailor's bunion**
20. **Tendinitis**
21. **Plantar tylomas**
Summary

Once the practitioner has gained a firm understanding of the basic principles involved in a normally functioning lower extremity, it is possible to fully appreciate how deviation from these norms contributes to the development of lower extremity abnormalities. The biomechanical principles of gait explain how the foot initially functions as a mobile adapter at heel strike, allowing knee flexion, leg rotation, and increased shock absorption, and then converts to a rigid lever to propel us onto our next step. The complex interaction of all the muscles, tendons, ligaments, joints, and bones which make up the lower extremity must function in harmony so that bipedal man can stand, walk, and run in an effective and efficient fashion. When this biomechanical model functions in a faulty fashion, then a host of common lower extremity abnormalities arise. As one proceeds through this chapter, there will be repeated references made to specific types of foot function along with specific types of pathologic conditions. The specific types of pathologic conditions associated with problems occurring in abnormal locomotion were initially described by Steindler as the area of "pathomechanics."[20]

Through the 1960s and 1970s various aspects of normal and abnormal foot function were explored by Inman, Root, Weed, Orien, Sgarlato, and Smith, and culminated in the ability to correlate lower extremity function with specific lower extremity pathologic conditions.[15] Through their application of basic physiologic and anatomic principles to the dynamic process of lower extremity function, we are now able to better understand the mechanism of lower extremity pathomechanical conditions.

Specific types of foot structure and function are responsible for a variety of lower extremity pathomechanical conditions. Section I addresses the specific types of pes planus and pes cavus foot types that may exist. In Section II, specific sagittal, transverse, and frontal plane deformities of the forefoot and rearfoot are presented. A complete understanding of the structural and functional conditions will allow the practitioner to more fully appreciate how various lower extremity pathomechanical conditions arise. The reader is referred to the specific pathologic conditions associated with each foot type. A detailed explanation of each condition is presented in Section III.

SECTION I: BASIC FOOT TYPES

Pes planus

Abnormal pronation is perhaps the most common of all biomechanical problems noted in podiatric prac-
tice. Although pronation through the initial 25% of the stance phase of gait is considered normal, excessive or prolonged pronation is considered pathologic.[19] With pronation, adduction and plantarflexion of the talus, along with eversion of the calcaneus, occur. As the talocalcaneal joint becomes unstable, the midtarsal joint unlocks (see Chapter 1), and pathologic changes occur both proximally and distally. When this type of function is chronic, marked compensatory changes are noted. A variety of lower extremity pathologic conditions such as hallux valgus, contracted digits, neuromas, heel spur syndrome, medial knee pain, and hip and lower back symptoms may be attributed to abnormal pronation.[15] Additionally, it may be noted that most chronic and acute overuse activities of the lower extremity that occur in sports or fitness activities are related to an abnormally functioning foot.[3,5,22] The basic characteristics of a pronated foot include:

1. Excessive calcaneal eversion (beyond 2–3 degrees)
2. Increased flexibility (unless peroneal spasm is present)
3. Uneven weight distribution
4. Hallux valgus, contracted digits, neuroma, heel spur syndrome, etc.
5. Postural symptoms involving the leg, knee, hip, and back

Congenital etiology
1. Gastrocnemius equinus or gastrocnemius-soleus equinus
2. Talipes calcaneovalgus (flexible)
3. Congenital convex pes valgus, vertical talus (rigid)
4. Peroneal spastic flatfoot secondary to tarsal coalition (rigid)
5. Ankle valgus secondary to oblique ankle joint mortise
6. Ligamentous laxity

Functional etiology
1. Compensated forefoot varus
2. Compensation for transverse plane deformities.
   A. Internal femoral torsion or position.
   B. External femoral torsion or position.
   C. Internal tibial torsion or position.
   D. External tibial torsion or position.
   E. Metatarsus adductus.
3. Malinsertion of posterior tibial tendon with or without accessory navicular.

4. Limb length discrepancy. With a significant limb length discrepancy the longer leg functions in a pronated attitude in an attempt to decrease the overall length of the limb. Conversely, if the foot is pronated (unilaterally), then that limb will function as the shorter limb.

Traumatic etiology

1. Posterior Tibial Dysfunction

Complete or partial rupture of the posterior tibial tendon leads to progressive flattening of the arch along with associated abduction of the forefoot relative to the rearfoot. Over time, a unilateral apropulsive type of gait pattern will develop.[7,9,13]

Pes cavus

Although a pronated foot is typically considered the most significant form of abnormal foot function, a highly arched, cavus foot can cause even more significant pathologic changes. The basic characteristics of a cavus foot include[8,9,14]:

1. Limited pronation
2. Rigidity
3. Uneven weight distribution
4. Digital contractures
5. Increased tendency to lateral ankle instability with associated ankle sprains
6. Decreased ankle joint dorsiflexion (osseous block)

The cavus foot type leads to a marked abnormal distribution of stresses through the foot, abnormal weightbearing on contact, and decreased foot mobility. A host of secondary compensatory mechanisms lead to progressively worsening forefoot and rearfoot conditions. The cavus foot may be classified into two types: the anterior pes cavus and the posterior pes cavus.[7,8,14]

Anterior pes cavus

This type of deformity is characterized by sagittal plane plantarflexion of the forefoot relative to the rearfoot. There are four subtypes of this deformity[14]:

1. Metatarsus equinus: plantarflexion of the forefoot relative to the rearfoot at Lisfranc's articulation (tarsometatarsal joint)
2. Lesser tarsus equinus: plantarflexion occurring over the lesser tarsus
3. Forefoot equinus: excessive plantarflexion occurring at Chopart's joint

4. Combined anterior cavus: abnormal plantarflexion occurring at any two or more of the above subtypes.

Posterior pes cavus

This type of deformity is characterized by rearfoot compensation which occurs as a result of a forefoot equinus. This type of equinus is not generally considered a separate type of cavus deformity as it occurs only in response to a forefoot equinus or cavus condition. The deformity actually represents excessive sagittal plane dorsiflexion of the rearfoot relative to the forefoot. This results in an abnormally high calcaneal inclination angle, and is often referred to as pseudoequinus, as there is an apparent clinical lack of ankle joint dorsiflexion.[14,18,28]

Associated conditions

In addition to the classic types of pes cavus, one should be aware of other causes (listed below) of this deformity[1,8,14,15]:

Congenital etiology

1. Congenital plantarflexed first-ray deformity
2. Spasm of peroneus longus
3. Spasm of posterior tibial
4. Weakness of peroneus brevis
5. Weakness of peroneus longus
6. Clubfoot deformity
7. Metatarsus adductus

Functional etiology

1. Uncompensated rearfoot varus
2. Partially compensated rearfoot varus
3. Compensated rigid forefoot valgus
4. Limb length inequality. With a significant limb length inequality, the shorter leg will function in a supinated attitude in an attempt to increase the overall length of the limb. Conversely, if the foot is supinated (unilaterally), then that limb will function as the longer one.

Perhaps the single most important aspect of any cavus foot deformity is to evaluate the patient completely from a neurologic perspective as there are a host of diseases which may result in this apparent mechanical condition. The following represent the most common diseases that may exist as an underlying cause of a pes cavus deformity: Charcot-Marie-Tooth disease, Friedreich's ataxia, poliomyelitis, Roussy-Lévy syndrome, spina bifida and other myelodysplasias, spastic monoplegia or paraplegia, polyneuritis, muscle dysplasia, trauma, angioma of the medulla or other spinal cord tumor,

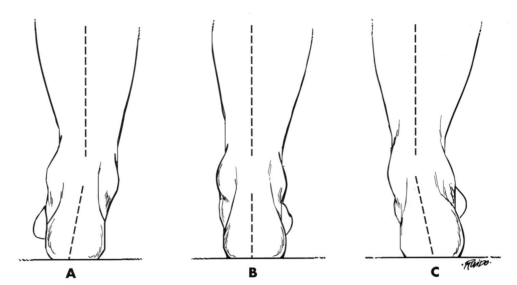

Fig. 2-1. Diagrammatic representations of three basic calcaneal positions: **A,** Inverted calcaneus: This clinical situation is present in the following deformities: uncompensated rearfoot varus, partially compensated rearfoot varus, and rigid forefoot valgus. Additionally, this represents the normally appearing functional position of a rigid cavus-type foot deformity or a rigid, plantarflexed first-ray deformity. A unilateral inverted calcaneus may be demonstrated as compensation for a short limb. **B,** Vertical calcaneus: This clinical situation is generally considered a normal position for the calcaneus in static stance. This position may also be present in the following deformities: compensated rearfoot varus, uncompensated forefoot varus, and flexible forefoot valgus. **C,** Everted calcaneus: This clinical situation is present in the following deformities: rearfoot valgus (rare), partially compensated or compensated forefoot varus, forefoot supinatus, compensated congenital gastrocnemius equinus, and compensated transverse plane condition. This calcaneal position may also be demonstrated in talipes calcaneovalgus, ankle valgus, congenital convex pes valgus (rigid vertical talus), and a peroneal spastic flatfoot. A unilateral everted calcaneus may be demonstrated in a posterior tibial dysfunction or as compensation for a long limb.

arthrogryposis, congenital lymphedema, and congenital syphilis.[4,8–10,14]

SECTION II: FUNCTIONAL FOOT DISORDERS

Frontal plane

Varus

This is a positional or structural deformity that may be present in the forefoot or rearfoot, with each area demonstrating several specific types. A varus position is an inverted position of one part relative to the next. Thus, rearfoot varus deformities represent an inverted position of the foot relative to the leg (Fig. 2-1A). A forefoot varus deformity is an inverted position of the plantar surface of the metatarsals relative to the plantar surface of the calcaneus (Fig. 2-2A).

Rearfoot varus

This is a positional deformity demonstrated as inversion of the rearfoot relative to the ground. This is due to a combination of frontal bowing of the tibia (tibial varum) and the available range of subtalar joint pronation. The greater the degree of tibial varum, the greater the requirement for subtalar joint

pronation (reflected by calcaneal eversion) to allow the heel to reach a vertical position. Rearfoot varus deformities may be categorized as follows:

Uncompensated rearfoot varus. In cases where the degree of tibial varum is greater than the amount of calcaneal eversion available through subtalar joint pronation, the heel will function in an inverted fashion. Specifically, if tibial varum is present without any available subtalar joint pronation (no ability for the calcaneus to evert), then the heel becomes inverted to the same degree as the degree of tibial varum. For example, a patient with 8 degrees of tibial varum with a subtalar joint range of motion of 20 degrees of supination with inversion and 0 degrees of eversion with pronation would stand in an 8-degree inverted position. This relaxed calcaneal stance position reflects the maximally pronated position for this patient's foot.

For associated clinical findings, see Section III, 2, 4, 11, 13, 14, 15, 16, 18B, D, F, 19, 20G, 21A, C, D, F.

Partially compensated rearfoot varus. This type of deformity occurs when the degree of tibial varum is greater than the calcaneal eversion available with subtalar joint pronation. In these cases, the heel will generally function in an inverted fashion, but will

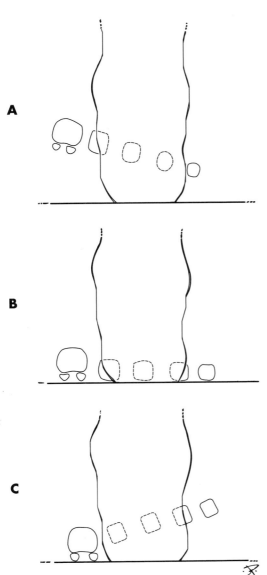

Fig. 2-2. Diagrammatic representations of three basic forefoot positions. **A,** Inverted forefoot: An inverted position of the forefoot relative to the rearfoot may exist when the subtalar joint is placed in its neutral position and the midtarsal joint is locked via a dorsiflexory force placed on the lateral aspect of the forefoot. This reflects a forefoot varus or forefoot supinatus deformity. A structural forefoot varus appears clinically unchanged when a plantarflexory force is placed on the dorsal aspect of the base of the first metatarsal. If the same force were placed on the forefoot in the presence of a forefoot supinatus, the inverted position of the forefoot would completely reduce. **B,** Perpendicular forefoot: A perpendicular position of the forefoot relative to the rearfoot may exist when the subtalar joint is placed in its neutral position, and the midtarsal joint is locked via a dorsiflexory force placed on the lateral aspect of the forefoot. This represents a normal position of the forefoot relative to the rearfoot. **C,** Everted forefoot: An everted position of the forefoot relative to the rearfoot may exist when the subtalar joint is placed in its neutral position and the midtarsal joint is locked via a dorsiflexory force placed on the lateral aspect of the forefoot. This reflects a forefoot valgus or a plantarflexed first-ray deformity. Evaluation of the forefoot-to-rearfoot relationship of this deformity does not reflect whether a forefoot valgus is rigid or flexible.

not be as inverted as the degree of tibial varum that is present. For example, a patient with 8 degrees of tibial varum with a subtalar joint range of motion of 20 degrees of inversion with supination and 5 degrees of eversion with pronation would stand in a 3-degree inverted position. This relaxed calcaneal stance position reflects the maximally pronated position for this patient's foot.

For associated clinical findings, see Section III, 2, 4, 11, 13, 14, 15, 16, 18B, D, F, 19, 20G, 21A, C, D, F.

Compensated rearfoot varus. In cases where the degree of tibial varum is equal to the amount of subtalar joint pronation available, the heel will assume a vertical position relative to the ground. This is considered to be a fully compensated deformity and is the least likely of the three types to develop any significant abnormality. For example, a

patient with 8 degrees of tibial varum with a subtalar joint range of motion of 20 degrees of inversion with supination and 8 degrees of eversion with pronation would stand with a heel-vertical position. This relaxed calcaneal stance position reflects the maximally pronated position for this patient's foot.

For associated clinical findings, see Section III, 15.

Forefoot varus

This is an inverted position of the forefoot relative to the rearfoot at the level of the midtarsal joint. It is due to inadequate frontal plane torsion of the head and neck of the talus occurring during normal development of the foot. Calcaneal eversion is required to fully compensate this deformity and to allow the forefoot to purchase the supporting surface during the midstance and propulsive phases of gait. This typically leads to a pronated foot type with marked calcaneal eversion. This is considered an unstable foot and generally results in a hypermobile first-ray segment. Forefoot varus deformities may be classified as follows:

Uncompensated forefoot varus. If a structural forefoot varus exists and there is no calcaneal eversion beyond the vertical available, then by definition the deformity is considered uncompensated. For example, let us consider a patient with 5 degrees of rigid forefoot varus, with 20 degrees of inversion with supination, 5 degrees of eversion with pronation, and 10 degrees of tibial varum. This patient's resting calcaneal stance position would be 5 degrees inverted. This reflects the maximally pronated position and leaves the forefoot varus deformity uncompensated. From a functional perspective, most patients will have an adequate range of motion within either the oblique axis of the midtarsal joint or within the first ray's range of motion to allow the forefoot to purchase the supporting surface in the midstance and propulsive phases of gait.

Partially compensated forefoot varus. In those cases where the degree of forefoot varus is greater than the available degree of calcaneal eversion, the deformity is considered to be only partially compensated. For example, let us consider a patient with 5 degrees of rigid forefoot varus, 20 degrees of inversion with supination, 5 degrees of eversion with pronation, and 3 degrees of tibial varum. This patient's resting calcaneal stance position would be 2 degrees everted. This reflects the maximally pronated position, and leaves the forefoot varus deformity only partially compensated. Again, additional compensation obtained from both the oblique axis of the midtarsal joint, and within the first ray's range of motion would allow the forefoot to approach the ground during the midstance and propulsive phases of gait.

For associated clinical findings, see Section III, 1A–C, 2, 3–10, 12, 13, 16–18A, C, D, E, 19, 20A–F, H, 21B, C, E.

Compensated forefoot varus. When the degree of forefoot varus is equal to or less than the available degree of calcaneal eversion, the deformity is considered to be compensated. For example, let us consider a patient with 5 degrees of rigid forefoot varus, 20 degrees of inversion with supination, 10 degrees of eversion with pronation, and 3 degrees of tibial varum. Owing to the availability of adequate calcaneal eversion, this deformity would be fully compensated via calcaneal eversion. In cases such as this, the clinical presentation that exists generally reflects a maximally pronated position of the subta-

lar joint. Rather than the calcaneus functioning in a 5-degree everted position as one might expect, the subtalar joint maximally pronates to a 7-degree everted position. This is due to the clinical situation in which a calcaneus that everts beyond several degrees will generally assume its maximally pronated position owing to the force of body weight falling medially to the subtalar joint axis of motion.[15,19]

Forefoot supinatus. The forefoot conditions described above represent osseous abnormalities leading to an inverted position of the forefoot relative to the rearfoot. In cases where excessive compensatory subtalar joint pronation exists, additional motion occurs within the longitudinal axis of the midtarsal joint. For every degree of abnormal calcaneal eversion that occurs throughout the gait cycle, the forefoot must invert a like number of degrees, a situation which occurs within the longitudinal axis of the midtarsal joint. Over a period of time, this results in a soft tissue or positional varus position of the forefoot relative to the rearfoot, which is termed a *forefoot supinatus.* In an off-weightbearing situation, a plantarflexory force placed on the base of the first metatarsal will not alter the forefoot positioning in cases where a congenital osseous forefoot varus exists. However, if a forefoot supinatus deformity exists, plantarflexion of the medial column of the foot will result in an absolute reduction of the forefoot abnormality, such that a perpendicular forefoot-to-rearfoot relationship will be clinically observable.

It should be noted that long-term treatment of a rigid forefoot varus deformity with functional foot orthoses will not produce any effect on the measurable inverted position of that forefoot. However, if a patient with a forefoot supinatus is being treated with functional foot orthoses, the forefoot position will change, as rearfoot motion is controlled and calcaneal eversion is reduced.[15,18]

In these instances, not only will a measurable change in the forefoot-to-rearfoot position be noted but the patient may no longer be capable of tolerating the original orthosis. If this situation arises, the orthosis must be replaced and a new cast fashioned that will more accurately represent the patient's foot. In instances where the practitioner suspects the presence of a forefoot supinatus, the initial casts should be obtained with the medial column maintained in a plantarflexed attitude during the casting. This is accomplished by placing a mild plantarflexory force on the base of the first metatarsal during the casting procedure. This technique is more important when one is prescribing a Root type of functional foot orthosis as opposed to the Blake inverted type, in that the cast correction of the inverted orthosis obliterates any apparent varus attitude of the forefoot. For further information regarding these devices, refer to Chapters 20 and 22.

For associated clinical findings, see Section III, 1A–C, 2–10, 12, 13, 16–18A, C, D, E, 19, 20A–F, H, 21B, C, E.

Valgus

This is a structural or positional deformity that may be present in the forefoot or rearfoot. A valgus position is an everted position of one part relative to the next. Thus, rearfoot valgus deformities represent an everted position of the foot relative to the leg (Fig. 2-1C). A forefoot valgus deformity is an everted position of the plantar surface of the metatarsals relative to the plantar surface of the calcaneus (Fig. 2-2C).

Rearfoot valgus

This condition presents in cases of a marked tibial valgum with an associated excessive degree of subtalar joint eversion with pronation. This is an extremely rare biomechanical presentation. The term must not be confused with, or used to refer to, conditions such as genu valgum, talipes calcaneovalgus, or rigid flatfoot conditions (e.g., peroneal spastic flatfoot, or congenital convex pes valgus).

Forefoot valgus

This is an everted position of the forefoot relative to the rearfoot at the level of the midtarsal joint. It is due to excessive frontal plane torsion of the head and neck of the talus occurring during normal development of the foot. Inversion of the lateral column of the foot must occur to allow the forefoot to purchase the supporting surface during the midstance and propulsive phases of gait. Two forms of compensation may exist for a forefoot valgus deformity, one flexible and the other rigid.

Flexible forefoot valgus. When there is sufficient flexibility within the longitudinal axis of the midtarsal joint to equal the degree of the forefoot valgus, the lateral column of the foot will reach the supporting surface during the stance phase of gait. Although this allows the heel to function perpendicularly during stance, the amount of compensation that occurs leads to a markedly unstable gait with late midstance pronation in propulsion. Lateral instability after heel contact extending into the midstance and propulsive phases of gait may occur.[15,18]

For associated clinical findings, see Section III, 1A–C, 2, 3, 5–10, 12, 13, 16–18A, C, D, E, 19, 20A–H, 21B, C, E.

Rigid forefoot valgus. When range of motion in the longitudinal axis of the midtarsal joint is insufficient to allow the lateral column of the foot to reach the supporting surface, additional compensation via rearfoot supination is noted. This causes the rearfoot to function in an inverted fashion during gait. This allows the lateral column to plantarflex, thereby placing the forefoot on the supporting surface. If this is insufficient to allow the lateral column to fully reach the supporting surface, then additional compensation consisting of adduction and plantarflexion of the oblique axis of the midtarsal joint occurs. Clinically, this appears as a markedly adducted and inverted foot. Lateral instability noted throughout the gait cycle is a hallmark of this type of forefoot valgus deformity.

For associated clinical findings, refer to Section III, 2, 4, 11, 13, 14, 16, 18B, D, F, 19, 20G, 21A, C, D.

Sagittal plane
Compensated congenital gastrocnemius equinus

This deformity occurs when an inadequate amount of ankle joint dorsiflexion is noted in the developing child or adult. A congenital lack of ankle joint dorsiflexion exists when less than 5 degrees of ankle joint motion is noted with the knee extended and the subtalar joint maintained in its neutral position. When this deformity exists, compensation occurs with subtalar joint pronation, which subsequently unlocks the midtarsal joint. This allows independent dorsiflexion of the forefoot relative to the rearfoot, such that 5 to 10 degrees of foot-to-leg motion may occur.[16,17]

The potential for the individual to develop an acquired gastrocnemius equinus due to an abnormally pronated gait pattern must also be considered. If abnormal subtalar joint pronation leads to excessive calcaneal eversion, increased midtarsal joint mobility will occur. From a biomechanical perspective, excessive motion will develop across the oblique axis of the midtarsal joint, which will increase dorsiflexion of the forefoot relative to the rearfoot. Over a period of years, this increasing foot mobility will lead to a limitation of ankle joint movement as the 5 to 10 degrees of foot-to-leg motion required for normal ambulation occurs within the foot rather than at the level of the ankle joint. This ultimately leads to a contracted gastrocnemius. Generally speaking, stretching exercises, functional foot orthoses, and physical therapy will increase ankle mobility if an acquired equinus is present.[5,18,19,23,24,26,27] For a complete discussion regarding partially compensated and uncompensated congenital gastrocnemius equinus conditions, see Chapter 11.

For associated clinical findings, see Section III,

1A–C, 2–10, 12, 13, 16–18A, C, D, E, 19, 20A–F, H, 21B, C, E.

Transverse plane
Compensated transverse plane deformity

Persons with unresolved internal femoral torsion or positional problems, as well as those with an internal tibial torsion, will generally function with their foot in an adducted and pronated attitude.[2,11] Additionally, persons with unresolved external femoral torsion or positional problems, as well as those with an external tibial torsion, will generally also function with their foot in an adducted and pronated attitude.[16,23,24]

Internal femoral torsion represents a lack of external torque or twist within the long axis of the femur during development. The internal femoral position is generally associated with a contracted condition affecting the capsule, ligaments, or muscles of the hip. In both instances the leg will function with the patella in an internally rotated position. Conversely, an external femoral torsion is the result of excessive external torque of the femur during development, while an external femoral position is associated with soft tissue contraction. In both instances, the leg functions with the patella externally rotated. Of note is the possibility of an occult dislocated hip leading to a marked unilateral or bilateral external position of the femur.[23,24,26]

If the position of the tibia relative to the fibula does not advance approximately 13 to 18 degrees in an external direction before the age of 7 or 8 years, then an internal tibial torsion may occur. Conversely, excessive rotation of the tibia relative to the fibula in excess of 18 degrees is consistent with an external tibial torsion.[6,11,12,26]

An additional form of adducted gait may be the result of a metatarsus adductus. This congenital structural anomaly is characterized by adduction of the forefoot relative to the rearfoot. The deformity is characterized by adduction of the metatarsals relative to the tarsals at Lisfranc's joint. This is generally due to an abnormal intrauterine position, an absent medial cuneiform, or malinsertion of the anterior tibial tendon, and is most readily treated in infancy. If allowed to persist, it leads to pain and discomfort at the head of the first metatarsal and the styloid process of the fifth metatarsal.[25,26]

An internal femoral torsion or position, as well as an internal tibial torsion, will lead to internal leg rotation, which ultimately causes the talus to adduct within the ankle joint mortise. This widens the talocalcaneal angle and leads to closed kinetic chain pronation in those persons with a normal amount of calcaneal eversion. Conversely, marked external deviation, as noted with an external femoral torsion or position, or external tibial torsion, will cause the body weight to fall medial to the subtalar joint axis of motion, thereby maintaining the foot in a maximally pronated and abducted attitude. In some instances, compensation for metatarsus adductus leads to abnormal subtalar joint pronation, while in other instances the shoe itself forces the foot into a more pronated attitude.[24,25] Although each of the transverse deformities cited here may cosmetically improve spontaneously over time, the net effect of early compensation, that being an abnormally pronated foot, will persist throughout the person's lifetime.[12,19,26] For a complete discussion of compensated transverse plane deformities, see Chapter 11.

For associated clinical findings, see Section III, 1A–C, 2–10, 12, 13, 16–18A, C, D, E, 19, 20A–F, H, 21B, C, E.

SECTION III: LOWER EXTREMITY PATHOLOGY

In 1977 Root and colleagues[15] provided an in-depth presentation of how abnormal mechanical forces produce lower extremity pathologic conditions. The pathomechanical conditions presented in this section summarize the material initially presented by Root et al.

Most common lower extremity pathologic conditions are the result of an abnormally functioning foot. Although aggravating factors such as footgear, level of activity, weight, and so forth affect various pedal problems, the underlying function of the foot is responsible for the majority of the pathologic conditions that are seen in clinical practice.

In Section II, the various abnormal types of foot function were presented. In this section are outlined the most common lower extremity pathologic conditions attributable to the abnormal functional conditions presented in Section II. By combining the information in these two sections, the practitioner will be able to determine which foot types are responsible for causing specific lower extremity pathologic conditions. Since all of the pathomechanical conditions presented in this section are either precipitated or exacerbated by abnormal foot function, they are all capable of being treated effectively via functional foot orthoses. Although some of the deformities may be more pronounced or chronic, functional foot orthoses are an appropriate and effective method of conservatively managing these various conditions. In cases where the pathomechanical condition has been present for a protracted period of time, surgical intervention may be necessary. However, even in these instances post-

Pathomechanics of lower extremity function

operative use of functional foot orthoses is effective in restoring normal function, increasing postoperative comfort, and decreasing the likelihood of recurrence of the specific pathologic condition.

1. Avascular necrosis (oseteochondrosis)

A. Calcaneal apophysitis (Sever's disease)

This process involves an inflammation of the growth plate of the calcaneus. It is typically found in the 8- to 15-year-old age group (average age, 10–11 years) and generally affects males more than females. Symptoms include generalized pain and discomfort, primarily upon activity (especially running, basketball, baseball); the symptoms progressively worsen and may eventually be noted with all weightbearing activities. Clinical examination reveals medial and lateral calcaneal tenderness on palpation and compression. In extreme cases, the area may appear edematous and slightly erythematous. Although lateral radiographs typically demonstrate an irregular-appearing apophysis, this is generally considered to be a normal appearance for this structure. Extreme cases of involvement demonstrate marked fragmentation of the apophysis with asymmetric findings. The problem is often aggravated by tight posterior musculature associated with a congenital gastrocnemius equinus, or a contracted posterior muscle group. Calcaneal apophysitis is associated with the following mechanical foot types:

1. Partially compensated forefoot varus
2. Compensated forefoot varus
3. Forefoot supinatus
4. Flexible forefoot valgus
5. Compensated equinus
6. Compensated transverse plane deformity

B. Köhler's disease

This is a form of osteochondrosis that affects the navicular. It is generally found in the child aged 3 to 9, affecting males and females in approximately equal numbers. The symptoms affect the dorsal and medial aspect of the foot at the level of the navicular. There may or may not be edema overlying the navicular and the child will generally limp with weightbearing transferred to the lateral aspect of the affected foot. Compression and palpation of the area overlying the navicular will cause discomfort. A comparison of bilateral dorsoplantar radiographs demonstrates thinning or narrowing of the ossification center of the involved navicular. Occasional fragmentation is noted[24]; abnormal pronation generally exacerbates this situation. This condition is associated with the following mechanical foot types:

1. Partially compensated forefoot varus
2. Compensated forefoot varus
3. Forefoot supinatus
4. Flexible forefoot valgus
5. Compensated equinus
6. Compensated transverse plane deformity

C. Freiberg's disease

This form of osteochondrosis affects the lesser metatarsal heads. A loss of vascularity to the metatarsal heads due to a number of possible problems, including mechanical, anatomic, and traumatic etiologies, is responsible for this pathologic condition.[23,24] Freiberg's disease generally affects the second metatarsal head and is most commonly encountered in adolescents aged 13 to 15. Females are affected approximately three times more often than males.

Symptoms include pain over or around the affected metatarsal, while clinical examination reveals localized swelling and thickening of the specific joint area. The joint range of motion is typically limited or guarded in these patients. Typical radiographic findings demonstrated on a dorsoplantar film include a flattened irregularly shaped metatarsal head with a trumpetlike appearance. It should be noted that since the process is gradual, the initial films may not reveal these signs. Osteochondrosis of the metatarsal heads is associated with the following mechanical foot types.

1. Partially compensated forefoot varus
2. Compensated forefoot varus
3. Forefoot supinatus
4. Flexible forefoot varus
5. Compensated congenital gastrocnemius equinus
6. Compensated transverse plane deformity

Orthotic considerations

Control of the abnormal foot function associated with the above osteochondral defects is effective in reducing symptoms and allowing the child to resume his or her normal level of activity. It should be noted that because these conditions are present primarily in the developing child, it is essential that the orthoses be monitored on an annual basis. Normally, the range of effective use for a pair of functional foot orthoses may be from 1 and 1 1/2 years to 3 years, depending on the type of device prescribed and the growth rate of the child.

2. Calcanel spur

This condition is characterized by pain that is present at the plantar-medial aspect of the calcaneus at the level of the medial tubercle. The symptoms are often described as an ache or soreness, and are typically present on arising in the morning or following periods of rest. Symptoms may be present with marked activity or exercise as well. The pain may be associated with inflammation of the plantar fascia at its attachment to the calcaneus or with the proliferative periosteal reaction that occurs as the spur is formed. Excessive tension directed to this area is demonstrated in cases of excessive calcaneal eversion with foot flattening, wherein the plantar fascia becomes chronically stretched. Conversely, a highly arched, supinated cavus foot type in which the plantar fascia is markedly taut and contracted may also lead to this deformity. Lateral radiographs may or may not demonstrate spurring regardless of the level of the symptoms. Minimal periosteal involvement may be noted initially, with more obvious spur formation noted on subsequent films. Although the most common causes of heel spur syndrome are mechanical, the differential diagnosis should include the following: tarsal tunnel syndrome, rheumatoid arthritis, gout, pseudogout, psoriatic arthritis, systemic lupus erythematosus, Reiter's syndrome, peripheral neuropathy, Paget's disease, and ankylosing spondylitis.[1] Aggravating factors include obesity or recent weight gain along with increased athletic activity or a change in footgear.[3,15,22] Calcaneal spurs are associated with the following mechanical foot types:

1. Uncompensated rearfoot varus
2. Partially compensated rearfoot varus
3. Partially compensated forefoot varus
4. Compensated forefoot varus
5. Forefoot supinatus
6. Flexible forefoot valgus
7. Rigid forefoot valgus
8. Compensated congenital gastrocnemius equinus
9. Compensated transverse plane deformity

Orthotic considerations

In most instances, the symptoms associated with mechanical heel spurs may be reduced when functional foot orthoses are worn. As this deformity may be resistant to initial attempts at treatment using standard functional foot orthoses, modifications should be made to the device. These include a deep heel cup (20–24 mm), a plantar fascia accommodation (2–4 mm), the use of an aperture pad within the heel cup, and the addition of shock-absorbing material. If these attempts fail, then a Blake type of functional foot orthosis should be considered. For additional information regarding this device see Chapter 22.

3. Capsulitis

This inflammatory reaction generally affects the second, third, fourth, and fifth metatarsophalangeal joints. Plantar pain at the level of the specific joints involved, with associated erythema and edema, may be noted. Pain is present on direct palpation of the area and increases with active or passive dorsiflexion of the involved joint. In most instances, symptoms are exacerbated by weightbearing and activity, with pain being present primarily in the propulsive phase of gait. The deformity is usually associated with a plantarflexed metatarsal with or without a hammer toe deformity. When the latter is present, it introduces an additional retrograde force into the involved metatarsal head, thereby increasing the deformity as well as the level of symptoms. Capsulitis is associated with the following mechanical foot types:

1. Partially compensated forefoot varus
2. Compensated forefoot varus
3. Forefoot supinatus
4. Flexible forefoot valgus
5. Compensated congenital gastrocnemius equinus
6. Compensated transverse plane deformity

Orthotic considerations

In most cases functional foot orthoses are effective in decreasing the abnormal sagittal and transverse plane forces associated with the development of the capsulitis. In instances where a chronic capsulitis is not completely resolved with functional foot orthoses, application of a metatarsal "cookie" may be helpful. This is fashioned from a firm, resilient material and placed on the superior aspect of the orthosis proximal to the involved joint. This raises the involved metatarsal head, thus decreasing the ability of the plantar soft tissue structures to become stretched.

4. Clawtoe deformity

This condition is synonymous with a hammer toe deformity affecting the proximal and distal interphalangeal joints of the second through fifth digits. Although a hammer toe deformity generally affects one or two digits, the clawtoe deformity affects all the lesser digits fairly equally. When severe, retrograde forces precipitated by sagittal plane displacement of the digits cause pain and lesions may be found beneath the articulating metatarsal heads.[21] This retrograde force is capable of causing a relatively plantarflexed position of each of the involved metatarsals. Causes of a clawtoe deformity include the following: pes cavus, forefoot adductus, forefoot supinatus, congenital plantarflexed first ray, arthritis, spasm or contracture of the short and long flexors, and weakness of the gastrocnemius (primary, post trauma, or post tendon lengthening).[15,21] Clawtoes are associated with the following mechanical foot types[15]:

1. Uncompensated rearfoot varus
2. Partially compensated rearfoot varus
3. Partially compensated forefoot varus
4. Compensated forefoot varus
5. Forefoot supinatus

Orthotic considerations

In instances where the clawtoe deformity is flexible, functional foot orthoses may be able to decrease the contraction of the digits. However, in cases where long-standing contracture has led to adaptive osseous changes, or where the predisposing condition may not be successfully addressed by orthoses (e.g., irreversible weakness of the gastrocnemius), significant reduction of the clawing should not be anticipated.

5. First metatarsal–first cuneiform exostosis

Excessive motion of the first metatarsal during the propulsive phase of gait leads to what has been termed a *hypermobile first ray*. Prolonged dorsiflexion of this segment relative to the more stable first cuneiform leads to the development of a dorsal exostosis at the base of the first metatarsal at its articulation with the distal aspect of the first cuneiform. Pain is generally present with pressure overlying the bumps, and is specifically aggravated by shoe pressure on the involved area. As the exostosis enlarges over time, irritation of the deep peroneal nerve may occur, leading to additional discomfort in the first interspace. The presence as well as the progression of the spurs may be readily documented by a lateral radiograph. A first metatarsal–first cuneiform exostosis is associated with the following mechanical foot types:

1. Partially compensated forefoot varus
2. Compensated forefoot varus
3. Forefoot supinatus
4. Flexible forefoot valgus
5. Compensated congenital gastrocnemius equinus
6. Compensated transverse plane deformity

Orthotic considerations

Although this exostosis may require surgical excision in its later stages, early treatment with functional foot orthoses effectively reduces the hyper-

mobility of the first ray during gait. Ultimately, this decreases the jamming introduced at the dorsal joint margin, thereby relieving symptoms.

6. Hallux extensus

This is a doriflexed attitude of the hallux (greater than 180 degrees) with an increased degree of hallux interphalangeal motion. This generally occurs secondary to a hallux limitus deformity (see Hallux Limitus below) in which a limitation of normal first metatarsophalangeal joint motion leads to excessive sagittal plane movement of the hallux interphalangeal joint. The resultant effect of the dorsiflexion that occurs at this joint level compensates in part for the decreased range of motion of the first metatarsophalangeal joint. Pain may be present on the plantar aspect of the interphalangeal joint and is generally associated with the formation of a plantar keratoma. Distally, a painful subungual exostosis or osteochondroma generally forms, secondary to pressure from the toe box of the patient's shoe, as the hallux is dorsiflexed into the shoe with each step. Additionally, dermatologic conditions affecting the nails, such as paronychia, onychia, or onycholysis may occur secondary to the repeated microtrauma.[15] Hallux extensus is associated with the following mechanical foot types:

1. Partially compensated forefoot varus
2. Compensated forefoot varus
3. Forefoot supinatus
4. Flexible forefoot valgus
5. Compensated congenital gastrocnemius equinus
6. Compensated transverse plane deformity

Orthotic considerations

Functional foot orthoses are generally successful in increasing dorsiflexion of the first metatarsophalangeal joint in functional hallux limitus. If the secondary signs listed previously are not extensive, then they may be reduced as the first-ray range of motion is increased via the orthoses. In other instances, however, the existing abnormality may be so significant as to require surgical intervention.

7. Hallux limitus

This is a restriction of dorsiflexion of the first metatarsophalangeal joint, where there is considerably less than the normal range of 65 to 75 degrees of dorsiflexion.[15] It is found in those patients whose pronated foot type leads to a hypermobile first ray. Additionally, the patient must have a rectus foot type for this deformity to occur, as opposed to an adducted foot type, which will lead to a hallux

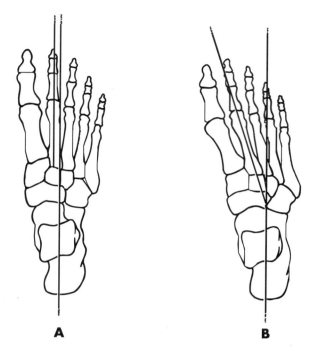

Fig. 2-3. Diagrammatic representations of a forefoot rectus-type foot **(A)** and a forefoot adductus-type foot **(B)**. Abnormal pronation in combination with a forefoot adductus-type foot will generally lead to a hallux valgus deformity.

abducto valgus deformity when a hypermobile first ray is present (Fig. 2-3). Predisposing factors include the following: immobilization of the first ray, which may occur secondary to longstanding abnormal subtalar joint pronation (this leads to adaptive changes at the base of the first ray); osteoarthritis; an excessively long first metatarsal; or a congenital or acquired dorsiflexed first-ray deformity (metatarsus primus elevatus).[15] In some cases, significant trauma affecting the first metatarsophalangeal joint leads to a limitation of first metatarsal joint motion. Often, this develops into a frank hallux rigidus. Generally, a squared or ridge-shaped metatarsal head rather than a round one is present in most cases of hallux limitus. Spurs and other signs of degenerative joint changes are demonstrated on the base of the proximal phalanx of the hallux, as well as on the head of the first metatarsal, which leads to a jamming of the first metatarsophalangeal joint. Pain is generally present over the exostosis, and is typically present in the propulsive phase of gait. It is most marked if the patient is involved in such athletic activity as tennis, racquetball, or running, where great demands are placed on the first metatarsophalangeal joint range of motion.[3,22] Secondary symptoms include hallux extensus, plantar hallux interphalangeal joint lesions, and distal hallux nail symptoms.[15] Hallux limitus is associated with the following mechanical foot types:

1. Partially compensated forefoot varus
2. Compensated forefoot varus
3. Forefoot supinatus
4. Flexible forefoot valgus
5. Compensated congenital gastrocnemius equinus
6. Compensated transverse plane deformity

Orthotic considerations

In instances where a hallux limitus is caused by a hypermobile first-ray segment, functional foot orthoses have been effective in increasing joint motion and decreasing symptoms. The functional foot orthosis allows the midtarsal joint to be locked during the midstance and propulsive phases of gait. This, in turn, restores the normal activity of the peroneus longus, which then becomes capable of maintaining the first ray in a stable position. This degree of stability is provided by its plantarflexory vector of force which, in turn, negates the dorsiflexory ground reactive forces generated during propulsion.

However, in cases where an excessively long metatarsal or structurally elevated first metatarsal is noted, the devices are ineffective in completely relieving the symptoms. In these instances, surgical excision of the spurs, along with shortening of the first metatarsal or a plantarflexory osteotomy of the first ray is required.

8. Hallux valgus

This deformity is associated with an apparent enlargement overlying the medial or dorsomedial aspect of the first metatarsal head. The deformity is caused by increasing adduction of the first metatarsal toward the midline of the body in response to a variety of conditions. The primary factors involved with the development of a hallux abducto valgus deformity include the following[15]:

1. Hypermobility of the first ray in a forefoot adductus foot type. This is the most common cause of hallux abducto valgus. Abnormal pronation leading to a hypermobile first ray in persons with a forefoot adductus foot type go on to develop the classic stages of hallux abducto valgus.
2. Rheumatic inflammatory disease process. Rheumatoid arthritis may cause a hallux abducto valgus, as intraarticular swelling of the involved first metatarsophalangeal joint leads to lateral displacement of the extensor hallucis longus and flexor hallucis longus tendons. Additionally, owing to the associated symptoms present with the lesser

metatarsophalangeal joints, the patient tends to abduct the feet and propel off the medial aspect of the forefoot. The overall effect of this is to increase pronation of the foot during the propulsive phase of gait.

3. Neuromuscular disease. Any neuromuscular disease process that leads to abnormal pronation of the foot may be the cause of a hallux abducto valgus deformity. This includes any disorder that markedly affects the patient's angle of gait, in that either marked adduction or abduction of the foot during gait leads to some degree of foot pronation with a subsequent hypermobile first ray.

4. Surgical intervention. In cases where a fractured tibial sesamoid requires surgical excision, care must be taken to repair the involved capsular structures adequately and to utilize functional foot orthoses post surgery. Because the abductor hallucis brevis and the medial head of the flexor hallucis brevis insert into the tibial sesamoid, disruption of that structure allows a mechanical advantage to be obtained by the transverse and oblique heads of the adductor hallucis brevis, as well as the lateral head of the flexor hallucis brevis. In time, this dynamic imbalance, combined with bowstringing of both the extensor hallucis longus and flexor hallucis longus, leads to a hallux abducto valgus deformity in those patients demonstrating abnormal subtalar joint pronation. Additionally, arthroplasty or arthrodesis of a contracted second digit in the earlier stages of a hallux abducto valgus deformity decreases the buttressing effect of the previously stable digit, thereby allowing the hallux abducto valgus to progress at an increased rate.

In all the above instances, the overall rate of development of a hallux abducto valgus deformity is affected by the following: the extent of abnormal subtalar joint pronation, the extent of subtalar joint and midtarsal joint subluxation, the overall degree of calcaneal eversion, the amount of forefoot adductus present, the extent of inflammation affecting the first metatarsophalangeal joint, the angle and base of gait, stride length, the presence or absence of a propulsive phase of gait, weight, and the type of footgear being worn.[15,19]

The four stages of hallux adducto valgus deformity have been described by Root et al.[15] (Fig. 2-4). The following outlines the progression of the deformity via an abnormally functioning lower extremity with a resultant hypermobile first ray.[15]

Stage 1 is characterized by an apparent abduction or lateral shifting of the base of the proximal phalanx relative to the first metatarsal head. This stage is initiated when the hypermobile first-ray segment dorsiflexes and inverts, thereby creating abnormal transverse and frontal plane movement of the first metatarsal away from the stable proximal phalanx. This is maintained in its normal position by the intrinsic muscles of the foot and does not actually migrate. Therefore, this stage represents movement of the first metatarsal away from the normally positioned proximal phalanx, a situation representative of an unstable first metatarsophalangeal joint. As the deformity progresses, the transverse head of the adductor hallucis, which generally maintains transverse plane stability of the metatarsals during midstance and propulsion, loses its stabilizing ability. This is due to the fact that the first metatarsolphalangeal joint functions in an abnormal and unstable fashion. At this point, the adductor hallucis actually pulls the base of the proximal phalanx away from the first metatarsal head during the propulsive phase of gait.

Stage 1 is characterized by a minor degree of lateral sesamoid displacement. Initial osseous changes involve a slight absorption of subchondral bone medially due to compression of the base of the proximal phalanx against the first metatarsal head. Additionally, deposition of bone occurs laterally. This new bone develops in order to maintain the full articular relationship between the two opposing articular surfaces. Although these changes are easily visualized on a dorsoplantar radiograph, there are no clinical signs evident at this stage. When these findings are noted in the pediatric patient demonstrating abnormal foot function, one may anticipate the eventual formation of a bunion deformity unless treatment with functional foot orthoses is initiated.

Stage 2 in the development of hallux adducto valgus is characterized by actual abduction of the hallux against the second toe. This position is due to a combination of actions precipitated by the extrinsic muscle activity of both the extensor hallucis longus and flexor hallucis longus as each becomes laterally displaced relative to the center of the first metatarsolphalangeal joint. This bowstringing effect initiates an abduction force against the hallux, as well as an adduction force relative to the first metatarsal. Additionally, while the transverse head of the adductor hallucis brevis continues to pull the base of the proximal phalanx away from the first metatarsal, the other intrinsic muscles reinforce the process. The abductor hallucis brevis loses its medial stabilizing force as the first metatarsal moves into slight dorsiflexion during the propulsive phase of gait. As the muscle now approaches the joint with

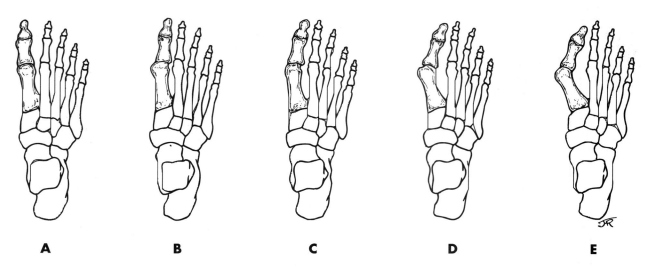

Fig. 2-4. Diagrammatic representation of the stages in the development of hallux abducto valgus as described by Root, Orien, and Weed. **A,** Normal foot. **B,** Stage 1: Lateral displacement. This stage is characterized by lateral deviation of the proximal phalanx relative to the first metatarsal head. **C,** Stage 2: hallux abductus. This stage is characterized by abduction of the hallux against the second digit. **D,** Stage 3: development of metatarsus primus adductus. This stage is characterized by an increase in the intermetatarsal angle between the first and second metatarsals. **E,** Stage 4: dislocation of the first metatarsophalangeal joint. This stage is characterized by marked abduction of the hallux away from the first metatarsal, with loss of joint congruence. (*Redrawn with permission. From Root ML, Orien WP, Weed JH:* Clinical biomechanics: normal and abnormal function of the foot, vol. 2, *Los Angeles, Clinical Biomechanic Corp, 1977.*)

a more plantar vector of force, it is unable to equally address the abductory force of the transverse head of the adductor hallucis brevis. Additionally, the flexor hallucis brevis becomes displaced more laterally relative to the central portion of the first metatarsolphalangeal joint, owing to the lateral displacement of the sesamoids. This, along with the additional pull of the oblique head of the adductor hallucis brevis, adds to the overall effect of abducting the hallux against the second toe.

In this stage, the sesamoids become more unstable and shift laterally, away from the bisection of the first metatarsophalangeal joint. Additional osseous adaptation occurs as the first metatarsal head attempts to maintain its articulation with the base of the proximal phalanx. New bone is added to the distal medial aspect of the first metatarsal head as the joint space becomes wider. Additionally, absorption of bone occurs laterally on the dorsal and distal margin of the first metatarsal head. It is at this point that the first signs of lateral joint deviation may be noted.

As a rule, when the deformity is progressing at a steady rate, bony adaptation maintains symmetric joint margins. However, in cases where a bunion deformity progresses faster than the rate of bony adaptation, unequal joint margins are noted. This is often identified in arthritic or neuromuscular disease processes, where the rate of progression is rapid.

Clinically, stage 2 may be characterized by medial bump pain, lateral hallux nail symptoms, heloma molle formation in the first and fourth interspaces, and a heloma durum overlying the fifth digit. Often, the digital complaints are the patient's chief complaint; the patient may be unaware of the presence of a bunion deformity at this stage of its development.

Stage 3 is characterized by an increased widening of the foot, with a marked increase between the first and second metatarsals noted on a dorsoplantar radiograph. The first metatarsal, along with the first cuneiform, deviates medially owing to the retrograde force generated by the hallux pressing against the stable second digit. This retrograde force is created by the continued bowstringing effect of the extensor hallucis longus and the flexor hallucis longus as they cross the lateral aspect of the first metatarsolphalangeal joint in a more lateral position. Additionally, the intrinsic muscles continue to force the hallux into a more abducted position. Overall, as the distal aspect of the hallux is stabilized against the second digit, the continued pull of the extrinsic and intrinsic muscles places the base of the proximal phalanx of the hallux and the first metatarsal head into a medially displaced position. As the deformity progresses through this stage, the intermetatarsal angle between the first and second metatarsals gradually increases.

At this stage, increased lateral displacement of the sesamoids occurs such that the tibial sesamoid functions in a position lateral to the first metatarsal head. Owing to this lateral displacement, the intrinsic muscles tend to only stabilize the medial aspect of the hallux during propulsion, thereby increasing its frontal plane valgus rotation. Additionally, continued functional bony adaptation occurs which leads to the addition of more new bone on the dorsolateral aspect of the first metatarsal head. This new bone causes the first metatarsal head to become wider, a condition which must occur in order to maintain the functional amount of articulation between the first metatarsal head and the laterally displaced proximal phalanx of the hallux. An aggravation of the clinical abnormality noted in stage 2 may be seen, as well as the presence of frank joint pain.

Stage 4 in the development of the hallux abducto valgus deformity is characterized by a frank subluxation or dislocation of the metatarsolphalangeal joint, and is generally only seen in conjunction with rheumatic inflammatory disease processes such as rheumatoid arthritis. Persons with stage 3 hallux adducto valgus deformity typically alter their gait to the point where they become almost apropulsive. Therefore, it is virtually impossible for stage 4 hallux valgus deformities to occur purely as a result of abnormal biomechanical forces. In cases of stage 4 hallux abducto valgus deformity, the onset of intraarticular swelling causes the extensor hallucis longus and flexor hallucis longus to deviate laterally, initiating a significant bowstringing force across the joint. This, along with continued joint swelling, causes the deformity to progress at a rapid rate. Typically, the second digit is no longer capable of functioning as a stable buttress, as it too becomes unstable because of intraarticular swelling. Subsequently, the hallux will underride the unstable second digit. In instances where a marked metatarsus primus elevatus is present, the hallux may actually override the digit. In both instances, the loss of the stabilizing effect of the second digit allows the first metatarsolphalangeal joint to become dislocated. Hallux abducto valgus deformities are associated with following mechanical foot types:

1. Partially compensated forefoot varus
2. Compensated forefoot varus
3. Forefoot supinatus
4. Flexible forefoot valgus
5. Compensated congenital gastrocnemius equinus
6. Compensated transverse plane deformity

Orthotic considerations

Since functional foot orthoses are capable of restricting abnormal pronation, thereby assisting in restoring normal peroneus longus function, the first-ray hypermobility implicated in the development of a hallux abducto valgus deformity may be controlled. Functional foot orthoses are most effective in treating the early stages of a hallux adducto valgus because they negate the abnormal effect of the extrinsic and intrinsic foot muscles. Not only are they capable of slowing down the progression of the deformity, they are also capable of reducing or eliminating the concomitant clinical symptoms. In cases of stage 3 hallux adducto valgus deformity in which the intermetatarsal angle has progressed beyond 13 degrees, the effectiveness of functional foot orthoses decreases.

Functional foot orthoses may be prescribed preoperatively to diminish a patient's symptoms, as well as to reduce the progression of the deformity prior to surgery. This may avoid a more involved surgical procedure if the patient elects to have the surgery at a later date. The postoperative use of functional foot orthoses is beneficial in restoring whatever element of normal function is not addressed by the surgical procedure itself. If excessive pronation with continued first-ray hypermobility is allowed to continue postoperatively, then one should anticipate prolonged postoperative discomfort, as well as possible recurrence of the initial abnormality.

9. Hammer toe deformity

This deformity is a contracted varus rotated position of any toe, although the fourth and fifth digits are most typically involved. This deformity is in contrast to the clawtoe deformity, which affects all of the lesser digits. Although a significant number of hammer toe deformities are idiopathic, there are a number of mechanical problems that are responsible for precipitating the condition. The pathomechanical and structural problems most likely to precipitate a hammer toe deformity include the following:

1. A plantarflexed metatarsal leads to an isolated hammer toe deformity because the proximal phalanx cannot be adequately stabilized against ground reactive force by the intrinsic muscles. Since the proximal phalanx is fixed dorsally, the activity of the long and short toe flexors during propulsion will buckle the intermediate and distal phalanges.
2. Loss of function of the lumbricale muscle secondary to flaccid paralysis or abnormal insertion leads to a dorsiflexed position of the proximal phalanx.
3. Weakness or flaccid paralysis of the quadratus plantae leads to loss of function of the lumbricales, which in turn leads to multiple hammer toe deformities (clawtoe deformity). The quadratus plantae is the proximal stabilizing force, which must

exist in order to allow the lumbricales to function normally.

4. Imbalance between the medial and lateral interossei leads to an unstable proximal phalanx. Contraction of the long and short toe flexors then results in an isolated hammer toe deformity.

5. Flaccid paralysis or traumatic severing of the long and short toe extensors leads to a hammer toe deformity, as these structures reinforce the action of the lumbricales. Interruption of the normal function of the long and short extensors allows the long and short toe flexors to buckle the intermediate and distal phalanges.

6. A congenital short metatarsal will ultimately function with an increased metatarsal declination angle. This then functions similarly to the previously discussed plantarflexed metatarsal.

7. A forefoot valgus deformity leads to hammer toe deformity of the fourth and fifth digits. This is most likely the result of the combination of a plantarflexed attitude of the respective metatarsals during propulsion and the associated gripping of the digits which are attempting to establish lateral stability in the propulsive phase of gait.

8. Increased pressure from an advancing hallux abducto valgus deformity leads to a hammer toe deformity of the second digit, due to the marked abduction pressure of the hallux. The continued abduction force of the hallux leads to a degree of metatarsophalangeal joint instability, thereby initiating the development of additional hammer toes. It should be noted that surgical intervention directed at reducing a hammer toe deformity of the second digit, in the presence of a hallux abducto valgus deformity, can lead to a rapid progression of the bunion. In most cases, surgical intervention is likely to decrease the overall stability of the digit and allow the hallux abducto valgus deformity to increase rapidly.

9. A pronated and subluxated fifth ray will assume an everted and abducted position. This leads to an unstable metatarsophalangeal joint which ultimately causes the proximal phalanx of the fifth digit to subluxate and develop into a hammer toe.

10. An adducto varus hammer toe of the fourth and fifth digits occurs in cases where forefoot adduction is the result of abnormal subtalar joint pronation. This leads to an increased oblique pull of the long digital flexor. This, associated with an abnormal pull of the quadratus plantae, reduces the effectiveness of the lumbricales, leading to digital contractures. Owing to the fact that the forefoot is abducted, the pull of the long digital flexors also introduces a frontal plane varus element to the deformity. Hammer toe deformities are associated with the following mechanical foot types:

1. Partially compensated forefoot varus
2. Compensated forefoot varus
3. Forefoot supinatus
4. Flexible forefoot valgus
5. Compensated congenital gastrocnemius equinus
6. Compensated transverse plane deformity

Orthotic considerations

When hammer toe deformities of the fourth or fifth digits are noted in the presence of an abnormally pronated foot, functional foot orthoses should be considered. In cases where the hammer toes are the result of a forefoot valgus deformity, the digits contract to grasp the supporting surface to maintain lateral stability. With application of a functional foot orthosis, the contracture reduces and the digits straighten. This generally reduces and eliminates the overlying symptoms associated with a heloma durum. However, if the deformities are associated with a compensated type of forefoot varus deformity, where the hammer toe deformity of the digits is more fixed, functional foot orthoses will generally be ineffective. This is due to the fact that fixed bony adaptation has occurred and the hammered position cannot be reversed. Additionally, the increased pressure placed on the fourth and fifth digits when the inverted forefoot position is corrected with orthoses will generally exacerbate the symptoms. For this reason functional foot orthoses, in cases of varus rotated fourth and fifth digits associated with a compensated forefoot varus deformity, should be prescribed with caution.

10. Interdigital neuroma

This deformity is characterized by pain located in the third interspace. The next most common locations in order are the second, fourth, and first interspaces. A burning paresthesia is present in the interspace which typically radiates to the adjacent digits. Additionally, numbness may be an associated finding. Pain is often relieved by massaging the affected interspace or by removing the shoes. The symptoms increase with athletic activity, increased weightbearing, or tight shoes, and are usually associated with mechanical abnormalities. Specifically, in cases of abnormal subtalar and midtarsal joint pronation, there is excessive transverse plane movement of the metatarsals. From a functional perspective, the first three metatarsals, which articulate with the cuneiforms, act as one functional unit, while the fourth and fifth metatarsals, which articulate with the cuboid, act as another. Excessive movement between these two segments contributes in part to the formation of a neuroma, as well as to exacerbation of the symptoms. Although dorsoplantar radiographs are helpful in delineating abnormal metatarsal head shapes and positioning, the neuroma itself is not visible. Magnetic resonance imaging (MRI) may be useful in cases where multiple neuromas are suspected. Interdigital neuromas are associated with the following mechanical foot types:

1. Partially compensated forefoot varus
2. Compensated forefoot varus
3. Forefoot supinatus
4. Flexible forefoot valgus
5. Compensated congenital gastrocnemius equinus
6. Compensated transverse plane deformity

Orthotic considerations

Control of abnormal transverse plane motion of the forefoot, primarily in the midstance and propulsive phases of gait, is successful in reducing the classic symptoms associated with a neuroma occupying the third interspace. Specifically, in regard to neuromas, orthoses are capable of diminishing excessive transverse plane rotation between the medial and lateral columns of the foot. Neuromas present in additional interspaces may also be successfully addressed, at least in part, when functional foot orthoses are used to control abnormal foot function and abnormal pronation in the propulsive phase of gait. In instances where the symptoms are unresponsive to this initial treatment, a metatarsal "cookie" may be placed on the superior surface of the orthosis proximal to the two involved adjacent metatarsal heads. This modification additionally assists in diminishing transverse plane metatarsal movement and compression.

11. Lateral ankle instability

A sprained ankle is one of the most common problems seen in a podiatric practice. In most instances, this injury or complaint involves the ligamentous structures of the ankle joint. Repeated inversion sprains or generalized ankle instability without trauma is commonly associated with the following:

1. Ligamentous laxity
2. Neurologic deficits
3. Supinated foot types functioning primarily with the heel inverted

Lateral ankle instability is associated with the following mechanical foot types:

1. Uncompensated rearfoot varus
2. Partially compensated rearfoot varus
3. Flexible forefoot valgus
4. Rigid forefoot valgus

Orthotic considerations

Because a significant percentage of chronic lateral ankle problems are associated with either a flexible or rigid forefoot valgus deformity, functional foot orthoses are an effective treatment. When a functional foot orthosis addresses the lateral column instability of the foot (by supporting the everted forefoot position via intrinsic or extrinsic forefoot posting), patients experience dramatic improvement with their lateral stability. This is particularly true in the case of a rigid forefoot valgus deformity, where the foot functions with an inverted rearfoot from heel contact through the propulsive phase of gait.

In instances where a patient with marked lateral instability does not have an inherent everted forefoot deformity, the midtarsal joint may be slightly overloaded when making a cast for an orthosis, so that an artificial everted forefoot position may be introduced into the cast. Although this does not represent the ideal "neutral position," it allows the practitioner to prescribe a device that will markedly increase lateral stability in cases where this condition is the patient's chief complaint.

12. Patellofemoral dysfunction

This condition is characterized by chronic symptoms in the peripatellar area which are usually associated with activity. Symptoms are aggravated by climbing stairs or sitting for prolonged periods of time with a flexed knee position.[3,22] Significant radiographic findings are often absent, while contributing factors often include a weak vastus medialus, a tight vastus lateralis, and anatomic variations of the patella or femoral condyles. Abnormal foot pronation is also implicated. Abnormal calcaneal eversion leading to excessive internal rotation of the tibia relative to the femur produces a transverse plane torque at the level of the knee joint.[22] This twisting motion leads to chronic irritation of the posterior aspect of the patella as it experiences increased compression against the lateral femoral condyle. Patellofemoral dysfunction is associated with the following mechanical foot types:

1. Partially compensated forefoot varus
2. Compensated forefoot varus
3. Forefoot supinatus
4. Flexible forefoot valgus
5. Compensated congenital gastrocnemius equinus
6. Compensated transverse plane deformity

Orthotic considerations

Functional foot orthoses may provide significant relief of symptoms associated with chronic patellofemoral dysfunction. In cases where there is no known significant localized musculoskeletal abnormality, an orthosis may resolve all symptoms. When a localized musculoskeletal problem does exist, an orthosis may be an efficacious adjunctive therapy. When successfully implemented, orthoses can reduce abnormal subtalar joint pronation and the subsequent associated internal rotation of the tibia. This allows the patella to track primarily in the sagittal plane, thereby relieving the symptoms.[3,22,27]

13. Plantar fasciitis

Irritation of the plantar fascia principally involving the medial slip is commonly demonstrated in patients with a pes planus or pes cavus deformity. The discomfort is generally caused by an overstressing of the fascia, and the pain is often localized at the medial calcaneal tubercle. Pain is most often present in the morning upon arising or after sitting for a prolonged period of time. Excessive activity may also exacerbate the problem. Because of its location, as well as its associated symptoms, this condition may be confused with a calcaneal spur. Careful evaluation of the area will allow differentiation. Selective muscle testing of the flexor hallucis longus, flexor digitorum longus, and abductor hallucis brevis should be carried out to determine the specific involvement of these structures. Additionally, care must be taken to carefully palpate the area of involvement to rule out the possibility of plantar fibromatosis or a Dupuytren's contracture. Plantar fasciitis is associated with the following mechanical foot types.

1. Uncompensated rearfoot varus
2. Partially compensated rearfoot varus

3. Partially compensated forefoot varus
4. Compensated forefoot varus
5. Forefoot supinatus
6. Flexible forefoot valgus
7. Rigid forefoot valgus
8. Compensated congenital gastronemius equinus
9. Compensated transverse plane deformity

Orthotic considerations

Functional foot orthoses are efficacious in treating chronic plantar fascial problems. Whenever excessive pronation contributes to this condition, a rigid device, capable of effectively controlling abnormal foot motion, should be used. In the cases of a more rigid, cavus type of deformity without an abnormal pronatory component, a more flexible shock-absorbing material (e.g., Plastazote) may be considered. In both instances the prescription should include the addition of a plantar fascial accommodation (2–4 mm).

14. Plantarflexed first-ray deformity

A plantarflexed first ray may occur as either a structural or positional deformity. In the case of a structural deformity, the first ray is congenitally plantarflexed and is typically found in the cavus foot type. The positional deformity is generally demonstrated as a form of compensation for a supinated foot type. This may occur following Achilles tendon lengthening or rupture, in which the peroneus longus becomes overactive while assisting with heel-off. In other cases, frank spasm of the peroneus longus may cause a plantarflexed first ray. Pain over the entire plantar aspect of the first metatarsal head may develop due to abnormal weightbearing, with specific symptoms involving the tibial sesamoid being most commonly evident. In the congenital type of plantarflexed first ray, the first metatarsal head may not be dorsiflexed to the level of the lesser metatarsals on manual pressure. However, in the positional type of deformity, with application of manual pressure, the first metatarsal may approach the level of the lesser metatarsals. In the case of a congenital plantarflexed first-ray deformity, the range of motion is normal and appears symmetric bilaterally, while it is limited in the positional or accommodative type. A plantarflexed first-ray deformity is associated with the following mechanical foot types:

1. Uncompensated forefoot varus
2. Partially compensated rearfoot varus
3. Rigid forefoot valgus

Orthotic considerations

In cases where functional foot orthoses are used to treat an abnormally inverted rearfoot, a reduction of an accommodative or positional plantarflexed first-ray deformity may occur over time. This results in an eventual decrease of forefoot symptoms, specifically in the area involving the sesamoid apparatus. In the congenital plantarflexed first-ray deformity, eventual resolution of symptoms may be accomplished only by a dorsal wedge osteotomy of the first metatarsal.

15. Retrocalcaneal exostosis

This process involves the presence of an exostosis or bursitis that is generally palpable and symptomatic overlying the posterior or posterior and lateral aspect of the calcaneus. The bursa involved lies between the Achilles tendon and the calcaneus. This is an area of irritation separate from the inflamed superficial Achilles tendon bursa, which is superficial to that tendon. Although this condition is often associated with a congenital anomaly of the posterior surface of the calcaneus, the problem is typically caused and then exacerbated by abnormal shearing forces of the calcaneus relative to the heel counter of the patient's shoes. Specifically, the mechanism involves repetitive rapid eversion of the calcaneus at heel strike against the relatively stable heel counter of the shoes. This process is typically exacerbated by increased activity and stiffer heel counters. A retrocalcaneal exostosis is associated with the following mechanical foot types.

1. Uncompensated rearfoot varus
2. Partially compensated rearfoot varus
3. Compensated rearfoot varus
4. Rigid forefoot valgus

Orthotic considerations

A functional foot orthosis may significantly decrease the abnormal shearing forces noted at heel strike in the mechanical conditions associated with this deformity. Specifically, use of a functional foot orthosis with a rearfoot post will be effective in introducing normal heel contact pronation over the initial 25% of the stance phase of gait. In most instances a 4-degree rearfoot varus post with 4 degrees of motion will be sufficient to introduce normal pronation. In patients with a high-pitched subtalar joint axis of motion with increased transverse plane rotation of the leg, a 2-degree rearfoot varus post with 2 degrees of motion may be more appropriate. On the other hand, patients with a low-pitched subtalar joint axis of motion with restricted transverse plane rotation of the leg func-

tion more efficiently with a 6-degree rearfoot varus post with 6 degrees of motion.

16. Sesamoiditis

This condition is characterized by pain and inflammation plantar to the first metatarsal head, and is associated with excessive pressure on the area. Symptoms are present with active and passive joint motion, as well as upon muscle testing. Increased pressure in this area typically exacerbates the condition. On close inspection, the symptomatic foot generally demonstrates an increased amount of edema compared with the asymptomatic foot. In some instances, avascular necrosis of the involved sesamoid(s) may occur. Predisposing etiologic factors include a plantarflexed first metatarsal, enlarged or multiple sesamoids, acute or repetitive trauma, and inappropriate shoes. In the differential diagnosis one must include the possibility of a fractured sesamoid. In most instances, a fractured sesamoid will result from one traumatic episode, while in others a stress fracture should be suspected in cases of overuse (increased walking or running). Bilateral foot films are useful as an initial screening test. The presence of bilateral bipartite sesamoids is often confusing, as the practitioner may then dismiss the possibility of a fracture. However, one must note that careful evaluation of the plain films may indicate a separation of the fragments on the symptomatic foot, a sign consistent with a fracture of the bipartite sesamoid. In all instances, inconclusive radiographic findings should result in the ordering of a bone scan. Sesamoiditis is associated with the following mechanical foot types.

1. Uncompensated rearfoot varus
2. Partially compensated rearfoot varus
3. Partially compensated forefoot varus
4. Compensated forefoot varus
5. Forefoot supinatus
6. Flexible forefoot valgus
7. Rigid forefoot valgus
8. Compensated congenital gastrocnemius equinus
9. Compensated transverse plane deformity

Orthotic considerations

In cases where abnormal foot function places increased weightbearing on the first metatarsal head during the midstance and propulsive phases of gait, functional foot orthoses will reduce symptoms in that area. In cases where initial treatment with a functional foot orthosis is ineffective, the addition of a flexible forefoot extension with an accommodation fashioned for the area of the symptomatic sesamoid apparatus should prove efficacious.

17. Sinus tarsi syndrome

This condition is associated with compression of the lateral column of the foot secondary to marked abnormal pronation, with resultant calcaneal eversion, and is typically present in younger, active patients. In some instances it may be seen in rheumatologic conditions such as rheumatoid arthritis. Symptoms are localized to the lateral aspect of the foot, primarily lateral to the talar head and at times on the medial side of the canal. The symptoms may be reproduced by direct palpation over the area. Sinus tarsi syndrome is associated with the following mechanical foot types:

1. Partially compensated forefoot varus
2. Compensated forefoot varus
3. Forefoot supinatus
4. Flexible forefoot varus
5. Compensated congenital gastrocnemius equinus
6. Compensated transverse plane deformity

Orthotic considerations

Functional foot orthoses are effective in treating the pain caused by this syndrome. In instances where the patient's symptoms are associated with athletic activity, a Blake inverted orthosis may be useful. In patients with rheumatoid arthritis, an orthosis may be effective in diminishing the symptoms associated with the abnormally functioning foot.

18. Stress fractures

Stress fractures are most often caused by excessive repetitive trauma to a specific area of the foot or lower leg. Faulty foot mechanics often contribute to the development and exacerbation of this condition. Stress fractures are typically characterized by pinpoint pain with associated edema and erythema. In most instances, pain is present that is aggravated by weightbearing. This condition generally involves the neck or shaft of the lesser metatarsals with the second and third metatarsals being most commonly affected. Additionally, stress fractures may often affect the sesamoids, the distal one third of the tibia and fibula, and the proximal aspect of the tibia. Since initial radiographs are often inconclusive in diagnosing the presence of a stress fracture, bone scans will help to establish the diagnosis. The most common sites of stress fractures of the lower extremity are as follows:

A. Second and third metatarsals

Fractures affecting these areas are generally associated with a hypermobile or dorsiflexed first-ray segment, which places increased pressure on the metatarsals, and a pronated foot type. Stress fractures generally involve the neck or midshaft portion of the involved bone. Owing to the stresses placed on the foot while performing ballet en pointe, stress fractures located at the base of the second metatarsal are classically demonstrated with this activity. Stress fractures of the second and third metatarsals are associated with the following mechanical foot types:

1. Partially compensated forefoot varus
2. Compensated forefoot varus
3. Forefoot supinatus
4. Flexible forefoot valgus
5. Compensated congenital gastrocnemius equinus
6. Compensated transverse plane deformity

B. Fourth and fifth metatarsals

Fractures in this area are caused by excessive weightbearing on the lateral column of the foot, seen with a supinated foot type. Stress fractures of these bones typically involve the neck or shaft. An isolated fracture affecting the fourth metatarsal may be present when a dorsiflexed fifth-ray deformity is an additional finding. Stress fractures of the fourth and fifth metatarsals are associated with the following mechanical foot types:

1. Uncompensated rearfoot varus
2. Partially compensated rearfoot varus
3. Rigid forefoot valgus

C. Navicular

Stress fractures in this area may be caused by excessive pronation or following an acute trauma, which is exacerbated by abnormal foot mechanics. Stress fractures of the navicular are associated with the following mechanical foot types:

1. Partially compensated forefoot varus
2. Compensated forefoot varus
3. Forefoot supinatus
4. Flexible forefoot valgus
5. Compensated congenital gastrocnemius equinus
6. Compensated transverse plane deformity

D. Sesamoids

Pain and swelling plantar to the first metatarsal head, especially with palpation of the involved sesamoid, characterize sesamoid fractures. Additionally, symptoms are also present with active and passive movement of the first metatarsophalangeal joint. This condition may be present in either a markedly pronated or supinated foot type. Stress fractures of the sesamoids are associated with the following mechanical foot types:

1. Uncompensated rearfoot varus
2. Partially compensated rearfoot varus
3. Partially compensated forefoot varus
4. Compensated forefoot varus
5. Forefoot supinatus
6. Flexible forefoot valgus
7. Rigid forefoot valgus
8. Compensated congenital gastrocnemius equinus
9. Compensated transverse plane deformity

E. Tibia

Stress fractures in this area generally occur at the anteromedial aspect of the distal one third of the tibia and are characterized by pain, tenderness to percussion, and edema. Pain is present with all weightbearing activities and is typically present with the pronated foot type in athletic patients who demonstrate poor shock absorption. In other instances proximal stress fractures of the tibia may be noted. Clinical signs consistent with the latter include pain, tenderness to palpation and percussion, and edema. Stress fractures of the tibia are associated with the following mechanical foot types:

1. Partially compensated forefoot varus
2. Compensated forefoot varus
3. Forefoot supinatus
4. Flexible forefoot valgus
5. Compensated congenital gastrocnemius equinus
6. Compensated transverse plane deformity

F. Fibula

Stress fractures involving the fibula are usually associated with pain, tenderness to percussion, and edema of the anterolateral aspect of the distal one third of the fibula. Pain is present with all weightbearing activities and is most often noted in patients with a markedly inverted or supinated foot type who do not have adequate shock absorption at heel strike. Stress fractures to the fibula are associated with the following mechanical foot types:

1. Uncompensated rearfoot varus

2. Partially compensated rearfoot varus
3. Rigid forefoot valgus

Orthotic considerations

Functional foot orthoses are effective in preventing additional stress fractures in active persons with abnormal foot function. In the case where one or more stress fractures are noted in a patient with an abnormally pronated or supinated foot, the likelihood of additional fractures developing could be diminished via the use of the orthoses. It should be noted that abnormal foot function may result in either excessive or inadequate motion of the foot and leg during gait. Functional foot orthoses are capable of either reducing abnormal pronation in those patients with a markedly everted rearfoot, or introducing normal pronation in patients with a rigid, inverted rearfoot. In those instances where inadequate shock absorption has precipitated the stress fracture (typically a fifth metatarsal or fibular stress fracture) and the patient does not have subtalar joint motion at heel contact to reach a vertical heel position (uncompensated or partially compensated rearfoot varus), the practitioner should attempt to increase shock absorption through the use of a softer type of orthotic device—for example, Plastazote.

19. Tailor's bunion

A tailor's bunion is a painful enlargement or prominence of the fifth metatarsal head. The pain is generally precipitated by the shearing forces of the shoe, creating an adventitious bursa overlying the fifth metatarsal head. The prominence and the pain may be dorsal, dorsolateral, or plantar-lateral. Generally, a tailor's bunion may be mechanically caused by the following: abnormal subtalar joint pronation, an uncompensated varus deformity, or a congenitally dorsiflexed or plantarflexed fifth-ray segment. In addition to the pain precipitated by the adventitious bursa, a painful hyperkeratotic lesion associated with the head of the fifth metatarsal may be noted.

Radiographic changes demonstrated with this condition are an increased intermetatarsal space along with an apparent increase in the size and lateral deviation of the fifth metatarsal head. This is due to subluxation of the fifth ray. This subluxation places the normal-appearing sagittal plane bowed position of the metatarsal onto the transverse plane, thereby increasing the apparent obliquity of the deformity. Tailor's bunion deformities are associated with the following mechanical foot types:

1. Uncompensated rearfoot varus

2. Partially compensated rearfoot varus
3. Uncompensated forefoot varus
4. Partially compensated forefoot varus
5. Compensated forefoot varus
6. Forefoot supinatus
7. Flexible forefoot valgus
8. Compensated congenital gastrocnemius equinus
9. Compensated transverse plane deformity

Orthotic considerations

Functional foot orthoses are not always capable of reducing progression of symptoms of a tailor's bunion. This is due to the fact that abnormal pronation alone will not cause the condition. This explains why the deformity is not noted in all persons who pronate, even when those persons have other foot abnormalities such as a hallux abducto valgus deformity or hammer toe deformity. In order for a tailor's bunion to occur, abnormal pronation must exist in combination with one of the previously listed etiologic factors. Therefore, depending on the type of abnormal pronation and the extent of the accompanying etiologic factors, an orthosis will be more or less successful on an individual basis.

In most instances, where an uncompensated varus deformity or marked sagittal plane congenital anomaly is present, orthoses do not control the symptoms. In those cases, surgical intervention, generally involving resection of the lateral eminence of the metatarsal head, along with an associated osteotomy, is recommended. On the other hand, if the abnormal pronation is due to compensation for a flexible forefoot valgus, then one may expect that the symptoms can be treated successfully.

20. Tendinitis

This is an inflammation of a tendon which may be caused by overuse or compensation. Similar symptoms also occur as a result of direct injuries, compartmental syndromes, and rheumatologic disorders. In most instances, a tendinitis may be precipitated or exacerbated by abnormal function of the lower extremity.

A. Achilles tendinitis

Insertional Achilles tendinitis may be associated with a retrocalcaneal exostosis or bursitis. In most cases, however, the actual area of involvement is proximal to the insertion into the calcaneus. Inflammation of this area may be caused by a congenitally tight or functionally contracted gastrocnemius, or gastrocnemius-soleus complex, or by strenuous athletic activity.[5,27] It is often exacerbated by a pronated foot type which causes a frontal plane torquing of the tendon. Achilles tendinitis may be associated with the following mechanical foot types:

1. Partially compensated forefoot varus
2. Compensated forefoot varus
3. Forefoot supinatus
4. Flexible forefoot valgus
5. Compensated congenital gastrocnemius equinus
6. Compensated transverse plane deformity

B. Abductor hallucis brevis tendinitis

This is characterized by pain at the origin of the muscle on the medial aspect of the calcaneus, on the medial aspect of the arch, or at its insertion at the medial aspect of the first metatarsophalangeal joint. In most instances, the discomfort is associated with the origin of the muscle. Symptoms are caused or exacerbated by overpronation of the foot, most typically in persons who participate in aerobics and dance-related activities. Abductor hallucis brevis tendinitis is associated with the following mechanical foot types:

1. Partially compensated forefoot varus
2. Compensated forefoot varus
3. Forefoot supinatus
4. Flexible forefoot valgus
5. Compensated congenital gastrocnemius equinus
6. Compensated transverse plane deformity

C. Extensor hallucis longus tendinitis

Pain is present at the dorsum of the first metatarsophalangeal joint often extending proximally onto the dorsum of the foot. Additionally, pain may be present at the level of the ankle joint. Extensor hallucis longus tendinitis may be the result of compensation for overpronation, as the extensor hallucis longus attempts to decelerate abnormal subtalar joint pronation. Additionally, it should be noted that an inflammation of this structure may be caused by an underlying exostosis. Extensor hallucis longus tendinitis may be associated with the following mechanical foot types:

1. Partially compensated forefoot varus
2. Compensated forefoot varus
3. Forefoot supinatus
4. Flexible forefoot valgus
5. Compensated congenital gastrocnemius equinus
6. Compensated transverse plane deformity

D. Flexor hallucis longus tendinitis

Pain is present plantar to the first metatarsophalangeal joint and is usually noted during the propulsive phase of gait. This tendinitis is also associated with compensation for overpronation. Additionally, it may be associated with a hyperextension injury in sports or after increasing speed workouts. It may be caused or aggravated by wearing high-heeled shoes. Flexor hallucis longus tendinitis may be associated with the following mechanical foot types:

1. Partially compensated forefoot varus
2. Compensated forefoot varus
3. Forefoot supinatus
4. Flexible forefoot valgus
5. Compensated congenital gastrocnemius equinus
6. Compensated transverse plane deformity

E. Flexor digitorum longus tendinitis

This is characterized by pain plantar to the lesser metatarsophalangeal joints. Symptoms may also be present in the area of the arch or inferoposterior to the medial malleolus. This condition is associated with abnormal pronation, especially in athletic activity in which the long flexors assist in elevating the heel during propulsion. Flexor digitorum longus tendinitis may be associated with the following mechanical foot types:

1. Partially compensated forefoot varus
2. Compensated forefoot varus
3. Forefoot supinatus
4. Flexible forefoot valgus
5. Compensated congenital gastrocnemius equinus
6. Compensated transverse plane deformity

F. Anterior tibial tendinitis

This condition is characterized by pain in the anterior aspect of the ankle. It is associated with compensation for overpronation as the anterior tibial assists in decreasing abnormal subtalar joint pronation. This condition is often caused by shoe vamp irritation or increased activity in sports. Running up or down hills, which leads to an overuse of the anterior tibial muscle, may cause this classic shin splint injury. The tendon may also become involved when an attempt is made to supinate the foot to avoid weightbearing on the arch or inner ankle. An anterior tibial tendinitis may be associated with the following mechanical foot types:

1. Partially compensated forefoot varus
2. Compensated forefoot varus
3. Forefoot supinatus
4. Flexible forefoot valgus
5. Compensated congenital gastrocnemius equinus
6. Compensated transverse plane deformity

G. Peroneal tendinitis

In this condition pain is present along the inferior or posterior border of the fibular malleolus or on both borders. It typically occurs in persons with a supinated or inverted foot type and a tendency toward lateral ankle instability. It should be noted that involvement of the peroneus longus may be associated with a painful os peroneum, whereas spasm of the peroneus brevis muscle and tendon is generally associated with a symptomatic tarsal coalition. Peroneal tendinitis may be associated with the following mechanical foot types:

1. Uncompensated rearfoot varus
2. Partially compensated rearfoot varus
3. Uncompensated forefoot varus
4. Flexible forefoot valgus
5. Rigid forefoot valgus

H. Posterior tibial tendinitis

This is characterized by pain posterior and inferior to the medial malleolus or at its insertion into the navicular. This generally develops in persons with a pronated foot type. As the foot pronates excessively, the posterior tibial tendon is pulled and strained at its insertion in the navicular. In other instances, it may be secondary to active supination, done to alleviate symptoms of plantar fasciitis or a heel spur. It is commonly associated with an enlarged or accessory navicular tuberosity (os tibiale externum). It should be noted that spontaneous rupture or chronic dysfunction of this tendon leads to a markedly pronated foot. Excessive calcaneal eversion with progressively increasing forefoot abduction is a hallmark of this condition. Posterior tibial tendinitis may be associated with the following mechanical foot types:

1. Partially compensated forefoot varus
2. Compensated forefoot varus
3. Forefoot supinatus
4. Flexible forefoot valgus
5. Compensated congenital gastrocnemius equinus
6. Compensated transverse plane deformity

Orthotic considerations

In cases where abnormal foot function has caused chronic tendinitis, functional foot orthoses have been effective in improving function, specifically, in cases where there has been overuse of the anterior muscles (e.g., anterior tibial and extensor hallucis longus). This is due to the fact that these muscles tend to contract over a longer period of time in attempting to reduce abnormal subtalar and mid-tarsal joint pronation. Additionally, in cases where chronic posterior tibial or Achilles tendinitis is associated with a pronated foot demonstrating excessive calcaneal eversion and forefoot abduction, orthoses dramatically improve function and reduce symptoms. Reduction of forefoot abduction with a functional foot orthosis reduces the workload of the posterior tibial tendon as it attempts to stabilize abnormal oblique axis midtarsal joint abduction. Additionally, in those patients with chronic Achilles tendinitis, maintaining the heel in a vertical position will reduce the frontal plane bowing and torquing. This allows the tendon to function with a more normal sagittal plane vector of force during contraction. Orthoses are also effective in treating recurrent peroneus longus tendinitis with an inverted heel and a rigid forefoot valgus. The orthosis allows the heel to assume a vertical position shortly after heel contact, thereby increasing the overall stability of the foot and alleviating symptoms.

21. Plantar tylomas

These are hyperkeratotic lesions that develop secondary to abnormal shearing forces in association with a bony prominence or with a congenital plantarflexed metatarsal. The hyperkeratotic tissue that accumulates generally becomes symptomatic. In many instances, a nucleated lesion may be found in cases of prolonged or excessive pressure to the affected area.

A. Plantar to first metatarsal

This lesion typically is present in patients with a plantarflexed first-ray deformity (either congenital or acquired). Additionally, this lesion may occur in cases of an enlarged sesamoid or multiple sesamoids. Tylomas plantar to the first metatarsal may be associated with the following mechanical foot types:

1. Uncompensated rearfoot varus
2. Partially compensated rearfoot varus
3. Rigid forefoot valgus

B. Plantar to second and third metatarsal

This lesion typically is present in patients with a hypermobile first ray secondary to a pronated foot type. These lesions are often seen with a hallux abducto valgus deformity. Additionally, the lesions may be associated with a plantarflexed deformity of the respective metatarsal. In some instances the lesion may be noted following surgical correction of an adjacent metatarsal (typically a dorsal wedge osteotomy to raise a plantarflexed metatarsal). A congenital shortening of an adjacent metatarsal may also be responsible for a lesion in this area. Tylomas plantar to the second or third metatarsal may be associated with the following mechanical foot types:

1. Partially compensated forefoot varus
2. Compensated forefoot varus
3. Forefoot supinatus
4. Flexible forefoot valgus
5. Compensated congenital gastrocnemius equinus
6. Compensated transverse plane deformity

C. Plantar to fourth metatarsal

This lesion is common in patients with a hypermobile fifth ray secondary to a pronated foot type. It is often seen with a plantarflexed deformity of the fourth metatarsal or following surgical correction of an adjacent metatarsal (usually a dorsal wedge osteotomy to raise a plantarflexed metatarsal). In some instances, a lesion in this area may develop following surgical correction for a tailor's bunion. Tylomas plantar to the fourth metatarsal may be associated with the following mechanical foot types:

1. Partially compensated forefoot varus
2. Compensated forefoot varus
3. Forefoot supinatus
4. Flexible forefoot valgus
5. Compensated congenital gastrocnemius equinus
6. Compensated transverse plane deformity

D. Plantar to fourth and fifth metatarsal

This lesion typically is present in patients with a supinated foot type and a stable fifth ray. It may be seen plantar to the fifth metatarsal head in association with a rigid cavus foot. Tylomas plantar to the fourth or fifth metatarsal or both, may be associated with the following mechanical foot types:

1. Uncompensated rearfoot varus
2. Partially compensated rearfoot varus
3. Rigid forefoot valgus

E. Plantar to hallux interphalangeal joint

This lesion occurs with a hallux extensus secondary to a hallux limitus deformity. Additionally, it may be seen when an accessory interphalangeal joint ossicle is present. Tylomas plantar to the hallux interphalangeal joint may be associated with the following mechanical foot types:

1. Partially compensated forefoot varus
2. Compensated forefoot varus
3. Forefoot supinatus
4. Flexible forefoot valgus
5. Compensated congenital gastrocnemius equinus
6. Compensated transverse plane deformity

F. Plantar and lateral to styloid prominence

This lesion is typically found in patients with a supinated foot type and a hypermobile fifth ray. It may additionally be noted in patients with an accessory ossicle in this location (os peroneum or vesalianum). Tylomas plantar or lateral or plantar and lateral to the styloid prominence may be associated with the following mechanical foot types:

1. Uncompensated rearfoot varus
2. Partially compensated rearfoot varus
3. Rigid forefoot valgus

G. Dispersive lesions plantar to the lesser metatarsals

These lesions develop in patients with a supinated foot type in which all the lesser metatarsals function on the same plane. Dispersive tylomas plantar to the lesser metatarsals may be associated with the following mechanical foot types:

1. Uncompensated rearfoot varus
2. Partially compensated rearfoot varus
3. Rigid forefoot valgus

Orthotic considerations

Since most plantar tylomas are caused or exacerbated by abnormal biomechanical shearing forces occurring during gait, functional foot orthoses are effective in decreasing the rate of formation as well as the extent of the symptoms. Orthoses are most effective in dealing with lesions plantar to the second or third metatarsal in instances where a hypermobile first ray is the only pathologic condition evident. Once normal function is restored to the peroneus longus, and the first ray is capable of accepting weight in propulsion, lesions plantar to the lesser metatarsals become less evident.

In cases where a lesion is located plantar to the fourth or fifth metatarsal in patients functioning with a rigid forefoot valgus, support of the lateral column of the foot with a functional foot orthosis (in patients with adequate range of motion to assume a vertical heel position) will reduce shearing forces to that area. The use of a forefoot extension with additional protection of the involved area via aperture accommodation is often an effective adjunctive modification in more severe cases.

In patients with a longstanding abnormality, and a nucleated tyloma, or in patients with a congenitally plantarflexed metatarsal, orthoses will not fully reverse the pathologic condition. Although the patient may be made more comfortable with an orthosis, surgical shortening or elevation of the involved metatarsal via a dorsal wedge osteotomy may be necessary for complete resolution.

Summary

This chapter has presented the common types of foot function and compensation present in persons functioning in a biomechanically unsound or unstable fashion. Additionally, the pathologic conditions caused by specific types of foot malfunction have been presented. By correlating specific foot types with resultant abnormalities, the practitioner will be more aware of the abnormal mechanical forces acting on the lower extremity. On acquiring a more complete understanding of this process, the practitioner will be able to provide effective and efficient treatment.

References

1. Barenfeld PA, Wesley MS, Shea JM: The congenital cavus foot, *Clin Orthop* 79:119-126, 1971.
2. Blount, P: *Fractures in children,* Baltimore, Williams & Wilkins, 1955
3. Brody, DM: Running injuries, prevention and management, Clin Symp 32:4, 1980.
4. Crenshaw AH: *Campbell's operative orthopaedics,* St Louis, Mosby–Year Book, 1971.
5. Dirix A, Knuttgen HG, Tittel KT: *Olympic book of sports medicine,* Oxford, England, Blackwell, 1988.
6. Elftman H: Torsion of the lower extremity, *Am J Physiol Anthropol* 3:255, 1945.
7. Giannestras NJ: *Foot disorders: medical and surgical management,* London, Henry Kimpton, 1967
8. Green DR, Ruch JA, McGlamry ED: Correction of equinus related forefoot deformities. *J Am Podiatry Assoc* 66:768–780, 1976.
9. Jahss MH: *Disorders of the foot and ankle: medical and surgical management,* Philadelphia, WB Saunders, 1991.
10. Kominsky SJ: 1991 *Yearbook of podiatric medicine and surgery,* St. Louis, Mosby–Year Book, 1992.
11. Hutter CG, Jr, Scott W: Tibial torsion. *J Bone Joint Surg* [Am] 31:511, 1949.
12. LaPorta G: Torsional abnormalities, *Arch Podiatr Med Foot Surg* 1:47–61, 1973.
13. Mann RA: *Surgery of the foot and ankle,* St. Louis, Mosby–Year Book, 1992.
14. McGlamry E, Dalton, editor: *Comprehensive textbook of foot surgery,* Baltimore, Williams & Wilkins, 1987.
15. Root, ML, Orien, WP, Weed JH: Clinical Biomechanics: Normal and Abnormal Function of the Foot, vol 2. Los Angeles, Clinical Biomechanics Corp, 1977.

16. Root ML: A discussion of biomechanical considerations for treatment of the infant foot, *Arch Podiatric Med Foot Surg* 1:41–46, 1973.

17. Scherer, P: Heel spur syndrome: pathomechanics and nonsurgical treatment *Am Podiatr Med Assoc* 87:68–72, 1991.

18. Sgarlato TE: A Compendium of Podiatric Biomechanics. San Francisco, California College of Podiatric Medicine, 1971.

19. Sgarlato TE: Tendon Achilles lengthening and its effect on foot disorders, *J Am Podiatry Assoc*, 65:849, 1975

20. Steindler A: Kinesiology. Springfield, Ill, Thomas, 1955.

21. Stuart F: Clawfoot—its treatment, *J Bone Joint Surg*, 6:360–367, 1924.

22. Subotnick S: *Sports medicine of the lower extremity.* New York, Churchill Livingstone, 1989.

23. Tachdjian MD: *Pediatric orthopedics,* Philadelphia, WB Saunders, 1972.

24. Tax H: *Podopediatrics,* Baltimore, Williams & Wilkins, 1980.

25. Valmassy RL: Conservative Treatment of Metatarsus Adductus, Podiatry Arts Laboratory, Pekin, IL 1981.

26. Valmassy RL: Biomechanical evaluation of the child, *Clin Podiatry* 1:563–579, 1984.

27. Valmassy RL: Conservative Versus Surgical Management of Foot Pathology, Perspectives in Podiatry, Podiatry Arts Laboratory, Pekin, IL 1987.

28. Yale AC, Hugar DW: Pes cavus: the deformity and its etiology. *J Foot Surg* 20:159-162, 1981.

the classification of human foot types, abnormal foot function, and pathology

Paul R. Scherer, DPM
Jack L. Morris, DPM

The literature
The method
Foot type pathology
  Set 1
  Set 2
  Set 3
Summary

The amazing and infinite variety of the human foot has often stimulated attempts to develop a method of classifying foot types. Further impetus for classification has emerged from a desire to define the "normal foot," from which we could then better define the abnormal and the possible sources of pathologic change and deformity. In this chapter we present the reasons why a foot classification system is necessary. We then review previous attempts at classification and their failings. Finally, we present a new method that seems to satisfy clinicians' needs and, we hope, will improve the effectiveness of various treatments.

The need for a classification of foot types is apparent to anyone treating feet. Several questions prevail with each group of patients. Why do some feet develop abnormalities and others not? Why are some feet more susceptible to injury while seemingly similar feet are not? Why do some surgical procedures work on some feet while the same procedures fail on other feet? Why do some abnormalities respond to simple conservative therapy while other feet require extraordinary invasive therapy? Do these aberrations occur because there are distinct variations in the human foot? Do the variations respond to disease, deformity, trauma, and treatment differently?

Our primary objective is to establish an orderly method of approach to diagnosing and treating foot ailments. The first step therefore is to understand the variations that occur, and the second is to recognize the abnormal conditions that may be found in the various types.[6] Unfortunately, most descriptions of surgical and nonsurgical therapy disregard the obvious variations of feet. Yet authors and practitioners consistently question why their therapies are not universally successful!

A classification system must do more than just pigeonhole feet. The classification must account for appearance so that each type is consistently recognizable by all healthcare providers. A consistent and universal terminology must therefore also be used. The classification should account for the incidence and prevalence of pathologic changes and deformities in each foot type. The classification must be complete so that all feet will fit into the system and be identifiable in relationship to the other foot types. There must be a "normal," and this "normal" means that no pathologic changes are present and that foot function is efficient. Finally, the classification system must be without regard to sex, race, or age in a manner that allows for the identification of a research model. If all these criteria are met, investigators will be able to demonstrate the effectiveness of their tests and treatments far more accurately.

The literature

The first classification of foot types was probably done for the purpose of fitting shoes. This continues today, with many more technologic advances, but still only accounts for size and shape and rarely function and abnormalities. For this reason, our historical review of foot classification methods is restricted to the medical literature.

A literature search reveals that anatomists first attempted classification in the eighteenth century by describing the foot characteristics of various races and cultures.[7] In the nineteenth century a great deal of attention was placed on the obvious flatfoot[3] and, curiously, the length of the second toe.[4] The significance of the latter was probably related to the overwhelming predominance of English male anatomists performing the investigations.

In the twentieth century cultural and ethnic classification systems were introduced and foot types subdivided by country of birth and even religion.[5] An attempt was also made during this period to classify foot types by occupation.[8] Cultural classification continues today with contemporary authors in the 1980s investigating "pure" cultures for the incidence of high or low arches in whites, nonwhites, and Asians without regard to relevant criteria.[1,9]

In 1949 the first intelligent, clear, logical, and honest attempt at classification appeared—J.M. Hiss's *Functional Foot Disorders.*"[6] Hiss recognized that valid diagnosis and treatment improved with a recognition of the normal variations of the human foot. Further, fundamental mechanical and pathologic changes in feet create symptoms and are related to disturbances in function. The thought that structure affects function and malfunction creates symptoms was revolutionary. The Hiss classification further described foot types such as highly arched, low-arched, functional eversion, rigid feet, flexible feet, and even some arthritic feet as actual variations of "normal." The foundation of our classification is based on these concepts.

Additional past classifications have included metatarsal length patterns,[12] foot shape and contour,[10] forefoot weight distribution patterns,[11] walking patterns,[14] and footprints,[15] and have served more to confuse than to clarify. The plethora of additional references to foot classification in the literature, aside from those cited above, indicates that a valid and universal classification has yet to be described.

The method

The contemporary description of forefoot-to-rearfoot measurement[13] allowed consideration of mid-

REARFOOT \ FOREFOOT	Everted	Perpendicular	Inverted
Inverted	1	2	3
Perpendicular	4	5	6
Everted	7	8	9

Fig. 3-1. The forefoot-rearfoot position matrix used to differentiate foot types. The horizontal axis represents the forefoot-to-rearfoot position of each foot, and the vertical axis represents the rearfoot-to-ground axis.

tarsal joint position and motion and resulted in dividing the foot into three forefoot-to-rearfoot general categories: (1) everted forefoot (valgus), (2) perpendicular forefoot, and (3) inverted forefoot (varus).[13] We incorporated the forefoot observation into the new method of classification but rejected the rearfoot position because of historical problems with understanding the confusing influence of tibial varum. Further, the lack of weightbearing examinations led the authors to adopt the standing calcaneal position interrelated to the forefoot-to-rearfoot position.

Rather than using degrees of varus or valgus angulation of the forefoot or calcaneal position we simply accepted the three observations of everted, perpendicular, and inverted. These are simple observations that are easily repeatable and universally understood. Ordering the three choices of forefoot position and the three choices of rearfoot-to-the ground position in a matrix gives nine foot types, as demonstrated in Figure 3-1. The horizontal axis describes the forefoot position, and the vertical axis describes the rearfoot position. The top row of the matrix describes all feet that have an inverted calcaneus, but allows for perpendicular forefoot in the center, an everted (valgus) forefoot on the left, and an inverted (varus) forefoot on the right-hand side of the matrix. The lower row allows for all everted calcaneal feet, but with the same forefoot-to-rearfoot differentiation. The matrix also allows for our normal model foot in the center of the matrix which has both a perpendicular forefoot-to-rearfoot relationship as well as a perpendicular calcaneus-to-ground relationship.

As we started to place feet into our matrix we found that many of the previous classification systems started to pattern themselves within the system (Fig. 3-2). Rigid highly arched and cavus feet fell within the upper left of the matrix (lower numbers) and flexible flatfeet toward the lower right (higher numbers). This patterning satisfied our goal to create a classification method that would group foot types and their abnormalities.

As the classification was applied to the clinical reality of feet, a grouping of external appearance, x-ray findings, gait patterns, and various deformities was noted. The most dramatic was the grouping of hallux abducto valgus deformities by severity and formation. The upper row of the matrix demonstrated little or no hallux abducto valgus and

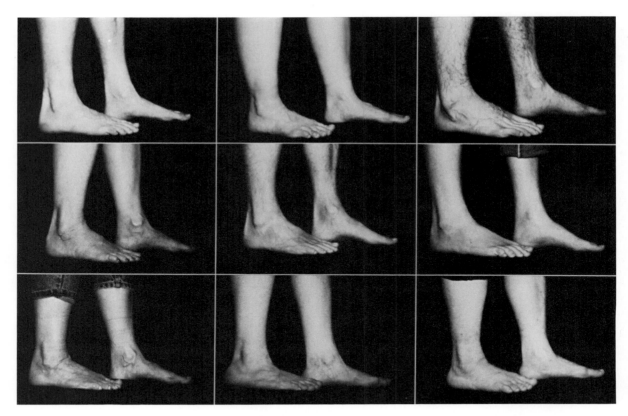

Fig. 3-2. The appearance of each foot type as classified in the matrix of Figure 3-1. Type 5, the center of the matrix, is the "normal foot."

only an occasional hallux limitus, whereas the lower row demonstrated a significant incidence of hallux abducto valgus with the severity of deformity increasing from left to right. Speculation suggests that this is related to the hypermobility of the foot, which increased concurrently with foot type numbers and is related to the heel position. The system allowed the deformity to group itself in a recognizable pattern and it also surrounded foot type 5, which was the normal model.

This method of classification requires a disclaimer relative to neuromuscular and congenital diseases. These categories deserve their own classification because of their unique ability to deform both structure and function during the development of the lower extremity. The addition of the deformed foot that results from neuromuscular and congenital disease would only confuse classification.

General observations by appearance created a familiarity that most foot care providers can recognize (Fig. 3-2). The familiar terms of rigid valgus or Shaffer foot fall only in type 1; calcaneal valgus in type 3; global cavus in type 4; and the narrow flatfoot in type 7. The intent of this system is to provide a universal classification that will allow

other authors and researchers to more accurately describe the type of human feet they are studying.

Foot type pathology

Now that the foot types and their characteristics have been presented, we will proceed with the unique pathologic changes associated with each foot type. Similarities can be seen in each foot type with regard to calcaneal position and the stability or instability of the midtarsal joint. The midtarsal joint position and response to loading are the keys to describing pathologic changes encountered in the foot types. To clarify the discussion of pathology, a reference to tissue type and disease entity is essential. The lower extremity structures are divided into five tissue types, and each tissue type has five disease categories that include most lower extremity disorders. The five tissue types are (1) skin, (2) muscle, fascia, and tendon, (3) vascular, (4) neurologic, and (5) osseous. The five disease categories are (1) tumors, (2) infections, (3) congenital, (4) mechanical, and (5) metabolic.

If we follow this grouping and address each foot type in accordance with the tissue type, the patho-

Forefoot

Type 1
Inverted calcaneus
Forefoot valgus

Type 2
Inverted calcaneus
Perpendicular forefoot

Type 3
Inverted calcaneus
Forefoot varus

Type 4
Perpendicular calcaneus
Forefoot valgus

Type 5
Perpendicular calcaneus
Perpendicular forefoot

Type 6
Perpendicular calcaneus
Forefoot varus

Type 7
Everted calcaneus
Forefoot valgus

Type 8
Everted calcaneus
Perpendicular forefoot

Type 9
Everted calcaneus
Forefoot varus

logic classification becomes more organized. The mechanical problems encountered with these classifications will be the primary focus. The forefoot categories are shown in the box above.

Before the presentation of each foot type, the function of each foot and what motions occur to place the foot on the floor are discussed. The foot is described from heel contact to forefoot loading together with the compensation that occurs.

Set 1

Type 1: inverted calcaneus– everted forefoot (valgus)

The calcaneus contacts the floor inverted in this foot and then everts to a fully pronated position that leaves the calcaneus inverted to the floor. The forefoot loads medially and with the forefoot everted three resulting possibilities exist. When the forefoot valgus is equal to the rearfoot varus the foot is compensated. If the forefoot valgus is greater than the rearfoot varus the longitudinal midtarsal joint axis supinates the medial column. If the forefoot valgus is greater than the rearfoot varus by more than 5 degrees the rearfoot will invert at the subtalar joint after the longitudinal midtarsal joint axis is fully supinated. This foot is usually stable at the midtarsal joint and presents as a rigid cavus-type foot. The clinical findings are as follows:

Skin

- Intractable plantar keratosis, valgus <5 degrees—none
- Intractable plantar keratosis, valgus >5 degrees—1–5

Nerve

- Neuroma, third interspace

Muscle-fascia

- Haglund deformity
- Functional equinus
- Fasciitis when long midtarsal joint axis supinates

Osseous

- Heel spur syndrome due to inadequate shock absorption
- Retrocalcaneal exostosis
- Ankle instability
- Bunion <5 degrees of valgus—none
- Bunion >5 degrees of valgus—hallux limitus or rigidus
- Tailor's bunion <5 degrees—none
- Tailor's bunion >5 degrees—plantar

Gait

- Adducted
- Laterally unstable
- Subtalar joint inverted >5 degrees

Type 2: inverted calcaneus– perpendicular rearfoot to forefoot

The calcaneus contacts the floor inverted and everts to a fully pronated position that is still inverted. The forefoot is perpendicular and therefore not in contact with the floor medially, thus creating severe lateral loading. The medial column must plantarflex to get to the floor or the subject must abduct the foot. The clinical findings are as follows:

Skin

- Intractable plantar keratosis—4–5

Nerve

- None

Muscle-fascia

- Haglund deformity

Osseous

- Retrocalcaneal exostosis
- Heel spur syndrome due to inadequate shock absorption
- Bunion—none
- Tailor's bunion—plantar
- Tailor's bunion dorsal with subluxed fifth ray

Gait

- Abducted and medial side roll-off
- Adducted with short lever push-off

Type 3: inverted calcaneus–inverted forefoot (varus)

The calcaneus contacts the floor and everts to a fully pronated position that is still inverted. The forefoot is off the floor in an inverted position. The lateral column is severely loaded. The foot abducts to place the forefoot down to the floor, and the knee bends to compensate for the abduction. This foot still demonstrates a stable rearfoot and midtarsal joint. The clinical findings are as follows:

Skin

- Intractable plantar keratosis—4–5 and hallux
- Hammer toe due to weightbearing—2

Nerve

- None

Muscle-fascia

- Equinus, functional

Osseous

- Retocalcaneal exostosis
- Heel spur syndrome
- Sinus tarsi syndrome
- Ankle valgus
- Genu valgum—knee pain
- Bunion—none
- Tailor's bunion—plantar
- Subluxed dorsal tailor's bunion—5
- Hammer toe—2

Gait

- Very abducted to place foot on floor
- Apropulsive
- Genu valgum with waddling-type progression

The first set of types 1, 2, and 3 demonstrate a stable foot. They all have this in common because the calcaneus is fully pronated in an inverted position. This maintains the midtarsal joint in a stable position with the forefoot fairly rigid. This set of feet are the highly arched cavus-type foot, with a gradual decline in arch height in type 2 and 3, but still in the cavus category. Bunions are of the hallux rigidus type due to the stability and limited first-ray motion. Tailor's bunions have plantar lesions unless the fifth ray subluxes causing a dorsal-type bunion to form. The inverted rearfoot in this set is prone to a retrocalcaneal exostosis deformity because of the inverted fully pronated calcaneal position.

Set 2

Type 4: perpendicular rearfoot–everted forefoot (valgus)

The calcaneus contacts the floor inverted and everts to a perpendicular and fully pronated position. The forefoot is everted and the longitudinal midtarsal joint axis (medial column) supinates to place the forefoot horizontal to the floor. If the forefoot valgus angulation is 5 to 7 degrees, the longitudinal midtarsal joint axis absorbs the range of motion. If it is greater than 7 degrees, the subtalar joint will require additional supination in order to place the lateral column on the floor. This set of foot types 4, 5, and 6 are also characterized by a stable rearfoot and midtarsal joint, as described for set 1. The clinical findings are as follows:

Skin

- Lateral heel callus
- Intractable plantar keratosis <5 degrees—none
- Hammer toe and heloma dura—4–5
- Intractable plantar keratosis >5 degrees—1–5

Nerve

- Neuroma—2nd interspace

Muscle-fascia

- Plantar fasciitis
- Achilles tendonitis
- Functional equinus

Osseous

- First metatarsal cuneiform exostosis
- Bunion—dorsal limitus or rigidus
- Tailor's bunion—>5 degrees—plantar
- Tailor's bunion <5 degrees—none
- Increased shock in gait
- Retrocalcaneal exostosis
- Heel spur syndrome

Gait

- Normal progression
- With high valgus, resupination of the forefoot is present at midstance

Type 5: perpendicular rearfoot–perpendicular forefoot

The calcaneus contacts the floor inverted and everts to a perpendicular, fully pronated position. The forefoot is perpendicular and is therefore on the floor and void of any abnormally directed ground reactive forces. This foot type is the normal foot and does not exhibit any abnormalities. Although this foot is considered to be the normal foot type, external forces (femoral or tibial torsion and equinus) may still create late midstance pronation and develop minor pathologic changes. For all intents and purposes this classification of type 5 is considered normal.

Type 6: perpendicular rearfoot– inverted forefoot (varus)

The calcaneus contacts the ground inverted and everts to a perpendicular and fully pronated position. The forefoot is elevated from the floor so the foot abducts and the knees bend to place the forefoot down. The rearfoot is stable and the medial forefoot has minor pressure and ground reactive force. The subject will abduct and roll off the medial side of the foot and be moderately apropulsive in gait. The clinical findings are as follows:

Skin
- Callus—1 and hallux
- Intractable plantar keratosis—1, 2, 4, 5
- Hammer toe due to weightbearing—2

Nerve
- Joplin neuroma
- Neuroma—2nd interspace

Muscle-fascia
- Posterior tibial syndrome
- Anterior tibial syndrome
- Extensor substitution

Osseous
- Genu valgum
- Tailor's bunion—plantar
- Subluxed fifth ray—dorsal tailor's bunion
- Bunion—none

Gait
- Apropulsive gait—full-foot plant–type gait

The common characteristics of set 2, comprising types 4, 5, and 6, are a stable rearfoot and midtarsal joint. When the calcaneus is perpendicular or inverted, as seen in set 1, the midtarsal joint is stable and the abnormality in the forefoot is that seen with a stable foot. Bunions, as seen in type 4, are of the hallux limitus or rigidus type seen with supination of the long midtarsal joint axis. Type 4 is prone to retrocalcaneal exostosis. The normal foot is in this set is presented by type 5.

Set 3

Type 7: everted rearfoot– everted forefoot (valgus)

The calcaneus contacts inverted, then everts to the floor. The midtarsal joint collapses and the longitudinal midtarsal joint axis supinates owing to pronation of the rearfoot. The rearfoot everts until no more motion is available in the subtalar joint. This is the most significant foot for pathologic disorders. The foot is hypermobile with the midtarsal joint responding to eversion of the rearfoot. The abnormality in this set is that seen with a hypermobile foot. When the valgus exceeds the motion available in the longitudinal midtarsal joint axis (5–7 degrees), the rearfoot may resupinate, but generally the body weight is too forceful on the subtalar joint axis to allow the foot to be resupinated. If this occurs, subluxation of joints must take place.

Skin
- Medial heel callus
- Intractable plantar keratosis <5 degrees—2
- Intractable plantar keratosis >5 degrees—1–5
- Heloma durum and hammer toe 5—2, 4, 5

Nerve
- Calcaneal neuroma
- Neuroma—2nd-3rd interspace
- Tarsal tunnel syndrome
- Sinus tarsi syndrome

Muscle-fascia
- Posterior tibial syndrome
- Plantar fasciitis
- Vascular
- Complicates all problems

Osseous
- Sinus tarsi syndrome
- Cuboid syndrome
- First metatarsal–cuneiform exostosis
- Bunion—medial
- Tailor's bunion—lateral
- Stress fracture—2, 3
- Mechanical heel spur syndrome

Gait
- Calcaneus everted
- Moderately propulsive
- Abductory twist
- Late midstance pronation

Type 8: everted rearfoot–perpendicular forefoot

The calcaneus contacts the floor inverted and everts past perpendicular to the floor. The forefoot is perpendicular so the longitudinal midtarsal joint axis supinates and the midtarsal joint collapses with respect to eversion of the calcaneus. This foot is also classified as hypermobile because the midtarsal joint collapses and the forefoot becomes hypermobile. The abnormality is that seen in a hypermobile-type foot.

Skin
- Medial calcaneal callus
- Intractable plantar keratosis—2, 3
- Heloma durum and hammer toe—2, 4, 5

Nerve
- Calcaneal neuroma
- Infracalcaneal neuritis
- Neuroma—2nd-3rd interspace
- Tarsal tunnel syndrome

Muscle-fascia
- Plantar fasciitis
- Posterior tibial syndrome

Osseous
- Heel spur syndrome—mechanical
- Sinus tarsi syndrome
- Cuboid syndrome
- Stress fracture—2nd, 3rd metatarsals
- Bunion—medial

Gait
- Progression normal
- Calcaneus everted
- Collapse of arch at forefoot loading
- Late midstance pronation
- Foot appears to peel off floor at midtarsal joint collapse

Type 9: everted rearfoot–inverted forefoot (varus)

The calcaneus contacts the floor inverted, everts to perpendicular, and continues to evert until the forefoot is on the ground. When more than 4 degrees of forefoot varus is present, the subtalar joint everts to its full range of available motion. The gait is abducted, and the subject tends to roll off the medial side of the foot with a very apropulsive gait.

Skin
- Medial calcaneal callus
- First midtarsal joint and medial callus
- Intractable plantar keratosis—2
- Heloma durum and hammer toe—2, 4, 5

Nerve
- Calcaneal neuroma
- Tarsal tunnel syndrome
- Neuroma—3rd interspace

Muscle-fascia
- Plantar fasciitis
- Posterior tibial syndrome
- Extensor substitution

Osseous
- Heel spur syndrome
- Sinus tarsi syndrome
- Bunion, mild—medial
- Stress fracture—none

Gait
- Very apropulsive
- Abducted if varus is greater than subtalar joint pronation
- Whole foot on floor with severe flatfoot
- Whole-foot contact leaving floor at same time

The third set, types 7, 8, and 9, have in common an everted calcaneal position. These feet are also characterized by an unstable midtarsal joint and hypermobile forefoot. This set has medial bunions when present and lateral tailor's bunions because of splaying and hypermobility. There are also more rearfoot abnormalities owing to arch collapse and jamming of the midtarsal and subtalar joints. These types are the flatfoot-type feet seen clinically.

Summary

A new classification for human foot types has been presented. The different foot types are grouped into three sets. The sets range from a highly arched cavus foot type in the first set to a moderate arch in the second. These two sets demonstrate a stable rearfoot and midtarsal joint–type foot. The third set is the hypermobile, everted rearfoot with collapse of the midtarsal joint which develops the flatfoot type. The abnormalities associated with all nine foot types were presented. The sets were developed to simplify the classification of foot function and the incidence of abnormalities noted in each group.

References

1. Braun S, Basquin L, Mery C: The contour of the normal foot, *Rev Rhum Mal Osteoartic* 2:127-133, 1980.
2. Cavanagh PR, Rodger S, MM: The arch index: a useful measure from foot prints, *J Biomech* 20:547, 1987.
3. Flower WH: *Fashions in Deformity*, London, Macmillan, 1881.
4. Harrison JP: On the length of the second toe of the human foot. London, *British Association Report* 606, 1882.
5. Hawkes OA: On the relative lengths of the first and second toes of the human foot from the point of view of anatomy and heredity, *Genetics* 3:249, 1914.
6. Hiss JM: *Functional Foot Disorders*, ed 3. Los Angeles, Oxford University Press, 1949.
7. Jones FW: *Structure and Function as Seen in the Foot*, Baltimore, Williams & Wilkins, 1944.
8. Lambrinudi C: The feet of industrial workers, *Lancet* 2, 24:1980, 1938.

9. Lee HI: Anatomical studies on the structure of joints of the foot in South Kyushu Japanese, *Acta Med Okayama* 48:57, 1978.

10. Lorimer DL: *Neale's Common Foot Disorders,* ed 4, Edinburgh, Churchill Livingstone, 1993.

11. Martorell JM: Hallux disorder and metatarsal alignment, *Clin Orthop* 157:14, 1981.

12. Regnauld B: *The Foot* New York, Springer-Verlag, 1986.

13. Root M, Weed J, Orien W: The Normal and Abnormal Function of the Foot, Los Angeles, California Clinical Biomechanics Corporation, 1977.

14. Schwartz RP, Heath AL, Morgan DW, et al: A quantitative analysis of recorded variables in the walking pattern of "normal" adults, *J Bone Joint Surg* [Am]46:324, 1964.

15. Weissenburg R: The shape of the hand and the feet, *Z Ethnologie* 27:82, 1885.

the spine, an integral part of the lower extremity

Irene Minkowsky, MD
Robert Minkowsky, MD

Selected anatomy
Screening test
Muscle imbalance
Lifting
Leg length inequality: the pelvic tilt
   syndrome

Pes planovalgus (foot pronation)
Pes cavus
Functional foot orthoses
Spine biomechanics
Gait
Functional pathology

Selected anatomy

Low back pain is a very common problem which affects 60% to 80% of the population at some point in their lives.[22,25] However, in only 20% to 30% of cases is a specific anatomic diagnosis made such as disk herniation, spinal stenosis, spondyloarthrosis, or spondylolisthesis. In the remaining 70% to 80% the cause is termed idiopathic.[14,19] The etiology in this group becomes clearer, however, if focus is placed on spinal biomechanics or the effect on the spinal axis of lower extremity problems such as muscle imbalance, leg length difference, or abnormal foot function.[1,12,14]

The back, a complex mechanical and neurologic structure, extends from the skull to the pelvis, and connects to the lower extremity primarily through muscles and fascia. The foot and lower extremity are the base of support for this human scaffold, the spine. The true vertebrae are: 7 cervical, 12 thoracic, and 5 lumbar. The pseudovertebrae or fused vertebrae are: 5 sacral and 4 coccygeal. The bodies of the true vertebrae are separated by disks except at C1–C2.

Vertebral size increases from the top to the bottom of the column to better sustain the compressive load of the body weight and the load due to physical effort.[5]

Spinal curves

The neutral spine with its level pelvis is composed of three curves that contribute to energy conservation in standing, walking, and during mechanical stresses. There is an anterior convex curve or lordosis in the cervical and lumbar spine, and an anterior concave curve or kyphosis in the thoracic spine (Fig. 4-1). Any exaggeration or reduction of these normal curves modifies the inherent mechanics of the spine from neutral mechanics to non-neutral ones.

Facet joints

The zygoapophyseal (facet) joints or small synovial posterior joints control spinal motion, and in the lumbar spine bear 10% to 40% of the total load[10] (Fig. 4-2). Because of the lumbar lordosis, there is a constant anterior shearing force, especially at the lumbosacral (L5–S1) joint, the most stressed spinal joint. This force is resisted by the opposing sacral facets below and by the posterior ligaments attaching to the posterior spinous ligaments.

The normal lumbar lordosis of 30 to 40 degrees is defined by the *sacral* or *lumbosacral angle* formed by a line drawn between the L5–S1 space and the horizontal (Fig. 4-3). The *facet angle,* drawn on an oblique erect x-ray film between the facet and the horizontal, determines the congruence of the facet as well as the degree of friction. Abnormal facet shape

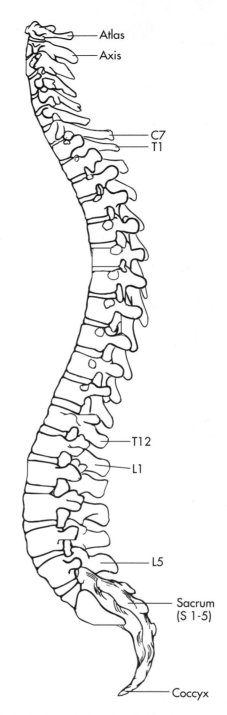

Fig. 4-1. Lateral view of the spine demonstrating cervical and lumbar lordosis and thoracic kyphosis.

or an asymmetric angle such as that seen with leg length inequality leads to increased interfacet stress and eventually degenerative changes.

Sacrum and sacroiliac joint

The sacrum, a triangular fused bone, is inserted between the two innominates which comprise the

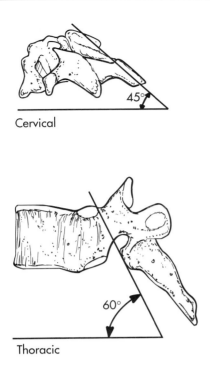

Cervical

Thoracic

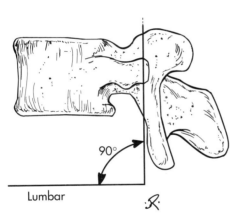

Lumbar

Fig. 4-2. Facet plane angulation.

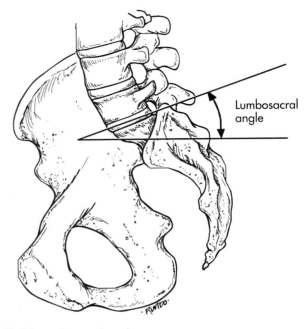

Fig. 4-3. Lumbosacral angle.

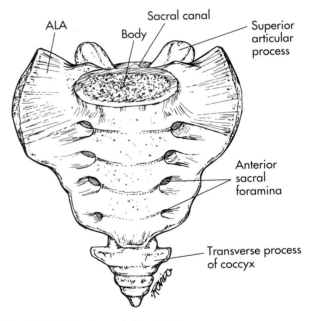

Fig. 4-4. Anterior view of the sacrum.

ilium, ischium, and pubis. This forms a mechanical interlinked ring with the lumbosacral and the two sacroiliac joints in the back and the pubis in the front (Fig. 4-4).[5]

The sacroiliac joint, which connects the sacrum to the ilium, is an amphiarthrodial, or only slightly movable, joint.[1,14] Its stability depends on:

1. Sacroiliac joint configuration, which is L-shaped with a short upper limb and a longer lower limb connecting at the level of S2. Each limb has a bevel in opposite directions which produces an interlocking mechanism. In addition, the ilium is convex and the sacrum concave, which creates an articular mechanism.

2. Extensive ligamentous support, which includes the sacroiliac ligaments (interosseous, posterior sacroiliac), as well as the accessory sacroiliac ligaments (iliolumbar, sacrotuberous, sacrospinous) (Fig. 4-5).

The symphysis pubis is also an amphiarthrodial joint stabilized by the superior, arcuate, and interpubic ligaments.

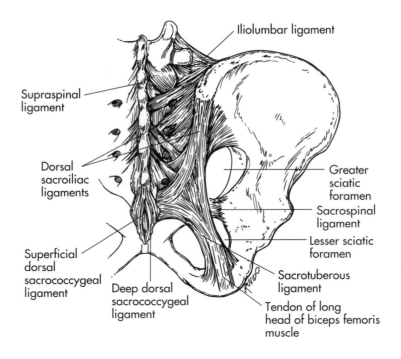

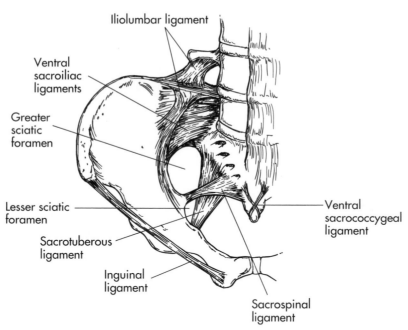

Fig. 4-5. Anterior and posterior views of the ligaments of the sacrum.

Musculoskeletal connections

Owing to its anatomic position between the feet and the head, the lumbopelvic unit influences and is very much influenced by the lower extremity below (especially during weightbearing activities) and the trunk, upper extremities, and craniocervical junction above through myofascial, neurologic, and vascular connections.

The origin and insertion of the muscles of the lower trunk, back, and hip extend over large areas, which explains how pain can radiate along any part of the functional muscle unit, far from the immediate area of injury, and influence distant osseous and joint structures (Fig. 4-6).

1. The abdominal muscles and the adductors of the thigh attach to the pubis from above

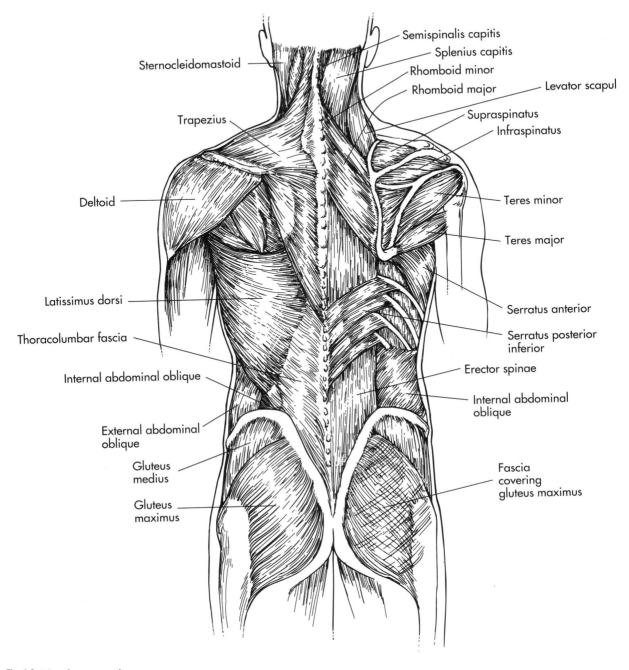

Fig. 4-6. Muscle connections.

Labels on figure:
Sternocleidomastoid
Trapezius
Deltoid
Latissimus dorsi
Thoracolumbar fascia
Internal abdominal oblique
External abdominal oblique
Gluteus medius
Gluteus maximus
Semispinalis capitis
Splenius capitis
Rhomboid minor
Rhomboid major
Levator scapul
Supraspinatus
Infraspinatus
Teres minor
Teres major
Serratus anterior
Serratus posterior inferior
Erector spinae
Internal abdominal oblique
Fascia covering gluteus maximus

and below, respectively; they influence pubic mechanics, and therefore gait.

2. The quadratus lumborum connects the rib cage (12th rib) to the iliac crest; tightness of this muscle may be responsible for recurrent ilial imbalance by cephalad pull on the ilium (Fig. 4-7).

3. The psoas links the thoracolumbar junction to the lesser trochanter of the femur, in effect connecting the midspine to the leg (see Fig. 4-7).

4. The piriformis, the only sacroiliac muscle, connects the anterior surface of the sacrum to the greater trochanter of the femur and participates in sacral torsion and hip tightness (Fig. 4-8).

5. The diaphragm, the primary respiratory muscle, has extensive musculoskeletal attachments to the upper lumbar vertebrae, lower six ribs, xiphoid process, and lower extremity through the psoas. In addition,

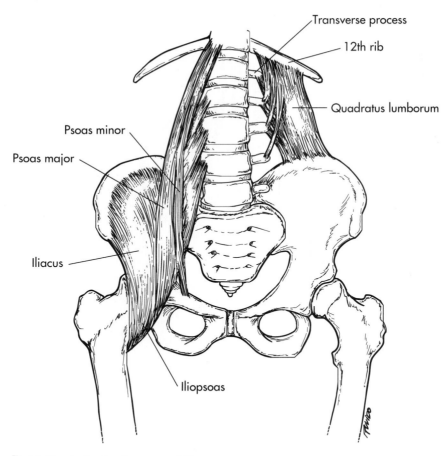

Fig. 4-7. Quadratus lumborum and iliopsoas.

its innervation is through the phrenic nerve, which originates from the cervical plexus. Thus the cervical, thoracic, and lumbar spinal segments are linked to the rib cage and to the lower extremity through this muscle. If the function of the diaphragm is altered, all of the above structures will be affected as well as the intrathoracic pressure, influencing venous and lymphatic return.[16]

Screening test

Because of these connections it is essential to look not only at a symptomatic area but also to screen the complete musculoskeletal system, as dysfunction in one region may affect a distant area. Included in this screening evaluation are gait and posture, trunk and rib cage motion, upper and lower extremity range of motion, and lumbar and sacroiliac mechanics.[13] Any lower extremity abnormality resulting from muscle tightness, ligament sprain, or joint degeneration will affect the pelvic girdle.

The integrity of the hip, knee, and ankle mecha-

nism in the lower extremity may be assessed as follows:

1. Taking the hip, knee, and ankle joints through their full range of motion in the squat test (Fig. 4-9).
2. Ascertaining the length of the lower extremity muscles including hamstrings, quadriceps, iliopsoas, and tensor fascia lata (Fig. 4-10).
3. Measuring the hip range of motion.
4. Scanning for cutaneous hypersensitivity through a skin rolling test (Fig. 4-11) which may reflect underlying areas of segmental dysfunction.

In performing the screening test we are looking for evidence of somatic dysfunction—that is, any alteration in the somatic system or body framework, including joints, muscles, fasciae, nerves, and vascular structures.[13] The elements that define dysfunction are remembered by the mnemonic ART (Asymmetry of form or function, e.g., scoliosis, drooping of a shoulder, gait abnormality; Range of motion,

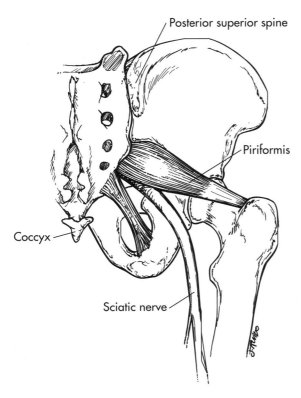

Fig. 4-8. Piriformis.

including both quantity and quality of motion; Tissue texture abnormality, which in the spinal axis is hypertonicity detected by palpation in the deep fourth-layer muscles of the spine, the multifidi, and the rotatores).

The foot is connected to the lumbosacral region via the hip, knee, and ankle joints. The muscles crossing the hip joint and attaching to the innominate make this bone functionally part of the lower extremity. The sacrum, on the other hand, should be viewed as a component of the vertebral axis.

Muscle imbalance

Muscle imbalance is a term used to describe asymmetry in the length of a muscle during passive range of motion. This evaluation is performed bilaterally and notes the presence of asymmetric distribution of stress along the osseous structures with resulting dysfunction and coordination problems. This may be present with a pronated foot, short heel cord, or hamstring and tensor fascia lata tightness.[1,13,19]

Commonly tight and inhibiting muscles in the lower back and leg are:

- Quadratus lumborum
- Erector spinae and gluteus maximus
- Iliopsoas
- Piriformis
- Tensor fascia lata
- Hamstrings and quadriceps
- Adductors
- Gastrocnemius

Commonly weak and inhibited muscles are

- Gluteus medius—affecting pelvic stability
- Abdominals—affecting spinal bracing and pubic function

The goal of treatment is functional restoration of the musculoskeletal system. An attempt to achieve muscle balance is one aspect of this goal.[13,17,19] One means of treatment of tight muscles involves a 3 to 5-second isometric contraction followed by a total physiologic relaxation which allows passive stretching of the tight muscles for 10 to 20 seconds.

A home program also emphasizes proper sequencing with stretching of the tight muscles before any attempt at strengthening the weak muscles can freely occur.

Lifting

The vertebral body and the annulus column are natural shock absorbers, and the annulus derives this property from its capacity to tighten and become strong and rigid. On the other hand, the end plate of the vertebral body is a weak structure that often fails and breaks.[27]

Lifting occurs by contraction of multiple muscles: the erector spinae (spine extensor), the gluteus maximus and hamstrings (hip extensors), and the abdominals. The hip extensors are the strongest muscles and are helped by the posterior ligaments, which tense up when abdominal pressure increases[2] (Fig. 4-12). These are the supra- and interspinous ligaments, the facet joint capsule, the ligament flavum, the posterior longitudinal ligament, and the lumbar fascia. If the range of motion of hip extension is reduced, back problems can occur as the strong hip extensors fail to perform through a full range and are substituted for by weaker, rapidly overused structures such as the abdominal muscles.[22] The farther the line of gravity is shifted forward, the more active the muscles of the back need to become.[20,21]

Leg length inequality: the pelvic tilt syndrome

Podiatrists, osteopaths, chiropractors, and nontraditional healers pay more attention to leg length disparity than do most physicians.

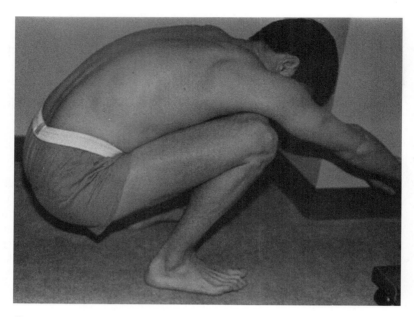

Fig. 4-9. Squat test.

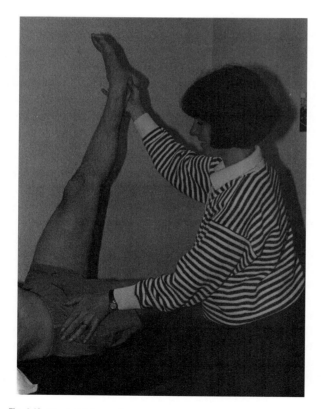

Fig. 4-10. Straight leg raise.

Subotnik differentiates between an anatomic and a functionally short leg.[15]

1. An anatomic short leg tilts the pelvis down, producing a functional scoliosis with convex-ity to the short side.[15] Balance is restored by lateral bending of the spine toward the longer leg. Axial rotation coupled with lateral bending twists the lowest intervertebral joint and its musculoskeletal ligamentous structures, resulting in inflammation and pain.[25] This is also the most damaging combination of motion for the intervertebral disk.[8] This flexible scoliosis corrects in the sitting or lying position. With time though, the scoliosis can become more rigid[25] (Fig. 4-13).

2. A similar tilting of the pelvis with functional shortening of the leg can occur as a result of sacroiliac or iliosacral torsions. These are, respectively, dysfunction between the sacrum and the ilium or between the ilium and the sacrum. This problem requires correction of the sacroiliac dysfunction before leveling of the pelvis can take place (Fig. 4-14).

3. Structural congenital scoliosis is not accompanied by leg length inequality or low back pain, and remains rigid or unchanged through changes of position.

Etiology

There are multiple causes of inequality of leg length varying from congenital to acquired problems such as epiphyseal growth dysfunction, fractures, poliomyelitis, juvenile rheumatoid arthritis, foot pronation, arthrodesis of the knee, and arthroplasty of the hip.[25]

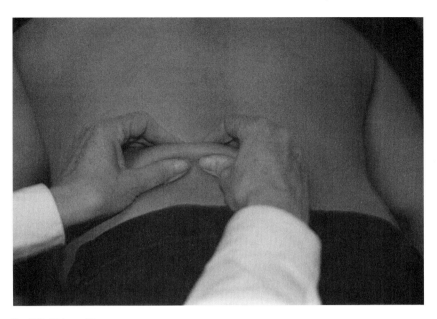

Fig. 4-11. Skin rolling.

Symptoms

Symptoms occur from asymmetric tensions in the functional scoliotic curves or sacroiliac strain imposed by the tilted pelvis. Symptoms can also involve the neck region through compensatory cervical scoliosis.[1,25] Symptoms generally occur within 30 minutes of standing, and are relieved by sitting. Bending and straight leg raising tests are not helpful in making the diagnosis. This represents a very different clinical picture from that of a disk herniation.

In most studies, the prevalence of leg length inequality in the low back pain population is increased compared with asymptomatic controls. A discrepancy greater than 5 mm is seen in 75% of the low back pain group, and in 44% of the asymptomatic controls.[8,11,25] A 4-mm difference is considered significant.[12]

Although there is still controversy regarding the role of leg length difference and low back pain, a strong association is recognized.[8,11,12,25] Differences of less than 9 mm (3/8 in.) are difficult to see and measure clinically, and can remain asymptomatic, whereas an inequality of 12.5 mm is easier to detect, and imposes a lateral shift of the upper border of the sacral plane by 4 degrees, compensated for by the lower spinal ligaments and muscles.[11] Electromyography shows an increase in the activity of several muscles, even with a difference of 10 mm.[8]

Clinical and radiographic measurements

Clinical measurements of leg length inequality remain in general unreliable and may be influenced by landmark palpation difficulties in obese patients, hypoplastic iliac crests, and pronation of the feet or concomitant sacroiliac torsion. Thirty percent of clinical measurements differ from radiographic measurements, the clinical findings indicating greater differences.[25]

To date, the best radiographic technique, with accuracy to within 1.5 mm, is an erect lumbosacral anteroposterior (AP)-lateral film, the feet 6 in. apart with the beam perpendicular to the iliac crest, visualizing the femoral heads[12] (Fig. 4-15).

1. The leg length difference is measured by dropping a perpendicular to a horizontal line joining the most superior points of the femoral heads.

2. The sacral base plane inclination is measured by dropping a perpendicular through the top center of the femoral heads and intersecting it with a line joining the most posterior part of the promontory of the sacrum and comparing the right and the left sides. X-ray films should not be done until pelvic mechanics are corrected.

Self-correction

An attempt is made by the body to self-correct the leg length inequality by posteriorly rotating the

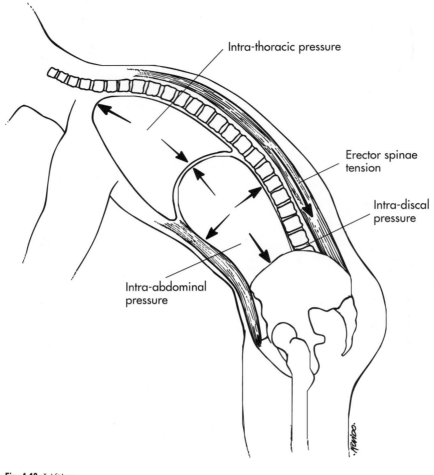

Intra-thoracic pressure

Erector spinae
tension

Intra-discal
pressure

Intra-abdominal
pressure

Fig. 4-12. Lifting.

innominate and pronating the foot on the long side. This leads to a functionally shorter leg. The innominate rotation contributes to correcting the difference by 6 mm (1/4 inch).[1] Similarly, the innominate can also be rotated anteriorly to lengthen the short side.

Lift therapy

Sacral base unleveling in response to leg length difference is one of the most common findings, and probably the only one worth correcting.

Lift therapy should be directed toward leveling the sacral base even if the leg length difference dictates a different conclusion; for example, in the presence of a right sacral tilt with a short left leg, a lift should be placed on the right side to level the sacral base as long as the sacral base inclination is not secondary to a sacroiliac torsion.[12]

Differences in the sacral base of up to 8 mm can be corrected by a lift inside the shoe. Beyond 8 mm, 50% is corrected outside the shoe on the short side, and 50% is accomplished by deepening the bottom of the shoe on the long side.

A heel lift is not as physiologic as a full-length shoe lift. Definitely, lift therapy in the presence of metatarsalgia should only be done with a full lift to reduce any increase in metatarsal stress.[25]

Lifting in the presence of spondylarthrosis or severe degenerative changes of the spine should be more progressive, starting at 50% of the measured difference, to allow for adaptation of the soft tissue and the paraspinals.[12] A lift may also encourage further hip and knee joint contracture, which are associated with arthritis.[25] If the lift aggravates the symptoms a review of the postural film and consideration of concurrent abnormalities are indicated.

In general, lift therapy provides good results.[8,10-12] In particular, patients with spondylolysis or spondylolisthesis demonstrate a good response because the leg length inequality may be a major aggravating factor in their conditions. One patient with a refractory plantar wart healed with sacral base leveling.[11]

The pelvic tilt syndrome is accompanied by other objective clinical findings. They include the side of

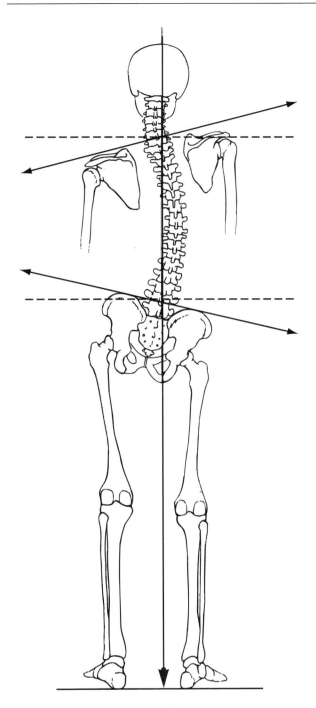

Fig. 4-13. Pelvic tilt short leg syndrome.

the low back pain; facet and sacral angles; muscle and ligament tightness; bursitis; hip, knee, and ankle changes; and foot adaptations.[1,8,10,25,26]

The short leg is characterized by the following:

- Usually on the right side
- Lateralization of the chronic low back pain
- Anterior rotation of the innominate (can lengthen the leg by 6 mm)
- Reduced facet angle (produces degenerative joint changes)

- Tensor fascia lata tightness and myofascial tightness
- Trochanteric bursitis
- Lateral knee joint degeneration
- Foot supination
- Pes cavus

The long leg is characterized by the following:

- Usually on the left side
- Drooping of the shoulder with elevation of the iliac crest on the long side
- Piriformis tightness with sciatic impingement
- Iliopsoas tightness
- Inguinal ligament tightness
- Decreased sacral angle and increased lordosis
- Posterior innominate torsion (can shorten the leg by 6 mm)
- Superolateral hip joint degeneration resulting in 5-mm shortening*
- Medial knee joint degenerative changes
- Pes planus

Pes planovalgus (foot pronation)

Foot pronation is a combination of subtalar eversion, forefoot abduction and dorsiflexion, and flattening of the plantar vault comprising the anterior, medial, and lateral arch. In the normal gait pattern, pronation of the foot occurs after heel strike, terminates prior to midstance, and lasts no more than 25% of the gait cycle until the foot and leg externally rotate in preparation for push-off. Abnormal pronation continues through toe-off and results in strain of the sacroiliac and lumbosacral joints, eventually leading to instability and abnormal thickening of the inguinal ligament.[1]

Flattening of the medial longitudinal arch produces postural symptoms as a result of fascia and muscle tension and functionally shortens the extremity. It internally rotates the hip, tightens the iliopsoas, and tilts the pelvis forward. This increases the sacral angle or lumbar lordosis. There is a downward rotation of the sacroiliac joint impinging the sciatic nerve between the piriformis or, because of an anatomic variation, between the piriformis and the sacrospinous ligament. At the knee, it creates a valgus stress with pubic dysfunction.

* Osteoarthritis of the hip: with varus angulation or adduction of the thigh on the longer side under a tilted pelvis there is a reduced weightbearing area of the femoral head, and this produces higher stress per square centimeter of the weightbearing area. This contributes to the formation of degenerative joint disease.

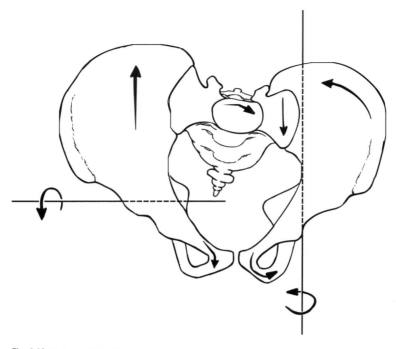

Fig. 4-14. Pelvic distortion.

Abnormal foot pronation is associated with a short Achilles tendon and gastrocnemius-soleus group, and tightness of the hamstrings, tensor fascia lata, and erector spinae. This produces low back pain through the short leg, pelvic tilt, scoliosis, and the effect on sacroiliac structures.

There are a host of causes for an abnormally pronated foot. They include ligamentous laxity, weak muscles, deviation of the joint axes of the subtalar and midtarsal joints, compensation for a short Achilles tendon, and compensation for transverse plane deformities of the femur and tibia.

Functional instability of the foot after trauma is due to muscle incoordination rather than to weak ligaments, scarring of sprained structures, or talus instability.[6]

Pes cavus

Pes cavus, a combination of subtalar inversion, forefoot adduction, and plantarflexion with elevation of the longitudinal arch, stresses the lateral knee joint, tightens the tensor fascia lata with sciatica-like pain, and clinically shortens the Achilles tendon. In combination with low back pain this is called the Ober syndrome.[1]

Functional foot orthoses

Custom-made orthoses have a corrective value affecting stress distribution up the lower extremity and the spinal axis. Orthoses may be to the foot what

a shoe lift is to sacral base unleveling in the presence of lower limb discrepancy.

The role of functional foot orthoses in the overall management of low back disorders cannot be overemphasized. There are three types of abnormal foot function that are capable of precipitating or exacerbating low back problems. In the first instance the foot will undergo a large range of abnormal subtalar joint pronation with excessive midtarsal joint subluxation and calcaneal eversion. This may be seen in cases of compensated forefoot varus, flexible forefoot valgus, ligamentous laxity, or posterior tibial dysfunction. In these cases, marked internal leg rotation occurs from heel contact through the propulsive phase of gait, which leads to excessive internal hip rotation and sacroiliac ligament tightness. In the other two instances, the problem is due to the inability of the foot to properly attenuate the normal amount of shock precipitated with each heel strike. The two foot types responsible for this situation include the foot that is maximally pronated at heel contact and remains in that attitude through the stance period of gait, and the rigid, supinated pes cavus foot. The maximally pronated foot is generally associated with a compensated gastrocnemius equinus, a compensated transverse plane deformity, or possibly with a peroneal spastic flatfoot. The rigid, supinated cavus foot may be associated with a rigid forefoot valgus, a plantarflexed first ray, an uncompensated or partially compensated rearfoot varus, or possibly one of a host of neurologic disturbances (e.g., Charcot-

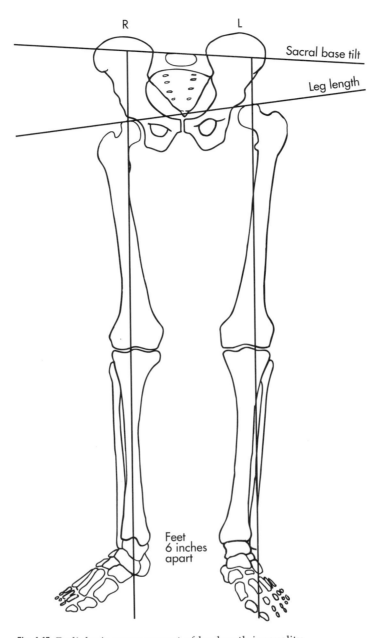

Fig. 4-15. Radiologic measurement of leg length inequality.

Marie-Tooth disease or Friedreich's ataxia). In patients that function with this foot type, normal shock absorption cannot occur, and the jarring shock of each step is transmitted directly to the paravertebral area.

In patients in whom excessive pronation is evidenced, the functional foot orthoses can decrease the overall degree of motion while allowing normal heel contact pronation to occur (pronated or pronating foot type). In patients whose foot functions in a more rigid fashion, the devices may be critical in initiating normal motion with increased shock absorption (supinated, cavus foot type). By so doing, the orthoses introduce normal heel contact

shock absorption, thereby decreasing the stress to the lower back.

Spine biomechanics

The zygoapophyseal or facet joints are part of the motion segment of the vertebral axis. Their orientation, which varies between spinal regions, determines the type of movement that will predominate in a particular region.

The lumbar facets are oriented sagittally and medially and permit flexion-extension and side bending, but not rotation, whereas the thoracic facets with a more coronal orientation favor side

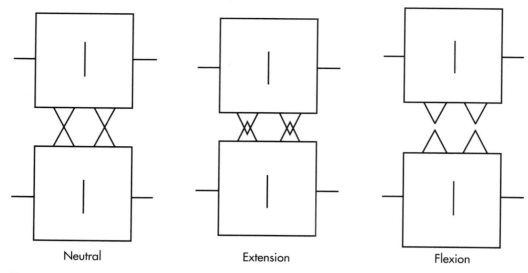

Neutral   Extension   Flexion

Fig. 4-16. Facet movement: flexion and extension.

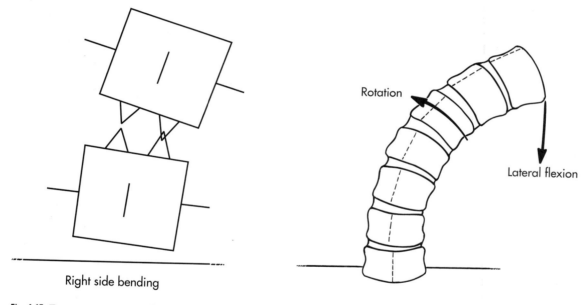

Right side bending

Fig. 4-17. Facet movement: side bending and rotation.

bending and rotation.[24,27,28] In the thoracic spine limitation of movement also results from the attachment of the ribs to the demifacets found on the vertebral bodies.[4]

Movement in an individual facet joint resembles the movement of an accordion.[13] With flexion, the facets gap open; with extension, they close (Fig. 4-16). With side bending the ipsilateral facet joint closes and the contralateral one opens (Fig. 4-17). For example, with right side bending the right facet closes and the left facet opens. With left side bending, the left facet closes and the right facet opens.[20]

Neutral spine mechanics is defined by the presence of the normal cervical and lumbar lordoses and

dorsal kyphosis. Fryette[9] and later Greenman[13] described neutral mechanics as that in which the facet joints are not engaged or are "idling." In this condition, introduction of side bending in a spinal segment will produce rotation to the opposite side. This is known as *type 1 mechanics* and is operative in the thoracic and lumbar spine.

If flexion or extension is introduced in these areas, the facets are "engaged" and they control vertebral motion. Under these circumstances, side bending and rotation are to the same side. This is known as *type 2 mechanics* or *non-neutral mechanics* and is operative in the thoracic and lumbar spine whenever a segment is flexed or extended.

Because of the anatomy of the cervical spine, type 2 mechanics is always operative from C2 to C7. The available motion at C2 is simply rotational and the occipito-atlantoid joint 1 follows type 1 mechanics.[4]

Lumbosacral joint

The sacrum is suspended by ligamentous structures between the ilia. Although still controversial, it is generally accepted that there is a small amount of movement permitted in the sacroiliac joints.[3,26,28]

At the sacral base there is an opposite coupling movement with the last lumbar vertebra, L5.[13] With forward bending of the spine, the sacral base moves posteriorly and the apex anteriorly into what is termed *counternutation*. With backward bending of the spine, the sacral base moves anteriorly and the apex posteriorly into *nutation*. This anteroposterior movement of the sacrum occurs around a theoretical axis at S2.

Greenman[14] has logically defined the oscillatory movement of the sacrum that occurs during the walking cycle as occurring about theoretical oblique axes drawn from each sacral base to the opposite inferolateral angle (ILA) of the sacrum. The axes are designated according to their point of origin. The right oblique axis extends from the right sacral base to the left ILA of the sacrum; the left oblique axis extends from the left sacral base to the right ILA.

During the normal walking cycle from left heel strike to right heel strike, the sacrum faces right on the right axis, returns to neutral, and then faces left on the left axis. In this movement cycle of the sacrum, side bending and rotation occur to opposite sides. This is termed *neutral sacral mechanics.*

With forward bending of the trunk, the sacrum counternutates. If one then turns to one side, the sacrum rotates to the opposite side, producing a backward torsion about an oblique axis. This is termed *non-neutral sacral mechanics*. The lumbar spine is flexed and rotated to that side, and is using type 2 non-neutral mechanics. If one attempts to straighten up from this position without returning to neutral, the articular mechanism of the lumbosacral joint may jam as the lumbar spine attempts to change from a situation using type 2 mechanics to one that uses type 1 mechanics. This type of joint behavior is responsible for the saying, "well man bent over, cripple stood up."

Pubis

The pubis, which forms the axis of rotation for the innominates during gait, has an oscillatory movement pattern.[14] With one-legged standing, the ipsilateral pubis may shear upward. This is most pronounced during the ligamentous laxity of pregnancy as are any dysfunctions in the pelvis.

Innominates

The innominates behave functionally as part of the lower extremity.[14] During gait there is a rotatory movement in an anteroposterior direction.

If the concave-convex relationship between the sacrum and innominate is reversed so that the innominate is concave, there is a tendency for the innominate to rotate medially or laterally in what is termed an *inflare-outflare*. With reduction of the bevel, forces driving it cephalad or caudad may shear the innominate *upward* or *downward.*

The theoretical construct developed by Greenman to explain functional and structural changes in the pelvis is logical and based on clinical observation, but needs further investigatory confirmation.

Gait

The complex relationship between the different parts of the pelvis is most apparent during gait (Fig. 4-18). At *right heel strike*, the right innominate rotates posteriorly, the left anteriorly.[14] The sacrum is rotated left and the spine is straight, but rotated left. At *right leg midstance*, the right leg is straight, and the right innominate is beginning to rotate anteriorly. The sacrum has rotated right, side-bent left, and L5 has rotated left and is side-bent right. At *left heel strike*, the left innominate is posterior and begins to rotate anteriorly. After right toe-off, the right innominate rotates posteriorly. The sacrum is level, but rotated right, as is the spine. At *left leg midstance*, the left leg is straight, the sacrum is rotated left, side-bent right, and the lumbar spine is rotated right, side-bent left. Should any dysfunction be present altering the normal mechanics of the innominates, sacrum, lumbar spine, or pubis, the normal gait pattern will be affected.

A simple way to screen for normal pelvic mechanics is to first observe gait, looking specifically for rotation of the lumbar spine to the contralateral side at midstance. The curve should be smooth and rounded; a flat section is indicative of a spinal segment that is not behaving normally or is dysfunctional.

The forward flexion test[13] can be used to assess normal iliosacral and sacroiliac mechanics when performed standing and sitting (Fig. 4-19). With one's thumbs resting on the inferior surface of the posteroinferior iliac spine, there is cephalad excursion of the thumb with trunk flexion. If there is locking of the sacroiliac mechanism with trunk forward bending, asymmetric motion occurs, with an early and excessive motion on the locked side as the whole sacroiliac mechanism shifts forward as one unit.

By utilizing these screening measures one may

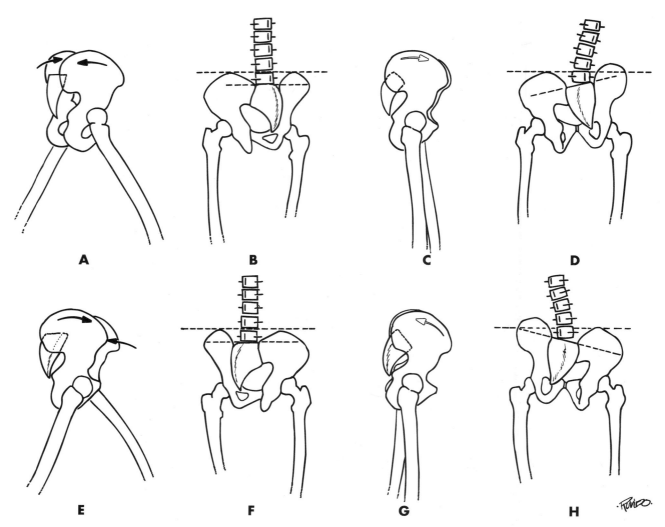

Fig. 4-18. A and **B,** At right heel strike, the right innominate rotates posteriorly, the left anteriorly. The sacral base is level and faces left. The lumbar spine is straight and rotates left. **C** and **D,** At right midstance, the right innominate rotates anteriorly. The sacrum rotates right and side bends left. The lumbar spine rotates left and side-bends right. **E** and **F,** At left heel strike, the left innominate is posterior and begins to rotate anteriorly. The sacrum is level but rotated right, as is the lumbar spine. **G** and **H,** At left midstance, the left innominate rotates anteriorly. The sacrum rotates left and side-bends right; the lumbar spine rotates right and side-bends left. (*From Greenman, PE: Clinical aspects of sacroiliac function in walking. J Manual Med 5:125–130, 1990. Used with permission.*)

develop a clinical impression regarding what role abnormal mechanical behavior in the lumbar spine or pelvis may be contributing to problems with gait.

Functional pathology

Janda[17] and Lewitt[23] have focused attention on the functional pathology of the neuromuscular system, for in the majority of patients, pain and altered function are not adequately explained by anatomic pathology. Rather, there is an imbalance between muscles with mainly a postural role and muscles that are more phasic or dynamic. The former are frequently tight and short, whereas the latter are weak and inhibited by the tight muscles.[18] It is this

imbalance that creates a functional alteration of movement patterns and frequently results in pain.

In the thighs and pelvis Janda has termed this imbalance the *pelvic crossed syndrome*.[19] It is characterized by tight hip flexors, hamstrings, lumbar erector spinae, and weak and inhibited gluteal muscles and abdominals. This imbalance has an important effect on posture with a forward pelvic tilt, increased lumbar lordosis, and flexed hip. The weak gluteals affect gait. In this syndrome the normal muscle activation sequence for hip extension of the hamstrings, gluteals, and lumbar and thoracolumbar paraspinals is frequently altered, with increased stress on the thoracolumbar junction that can result in dysfunction and altered compen-

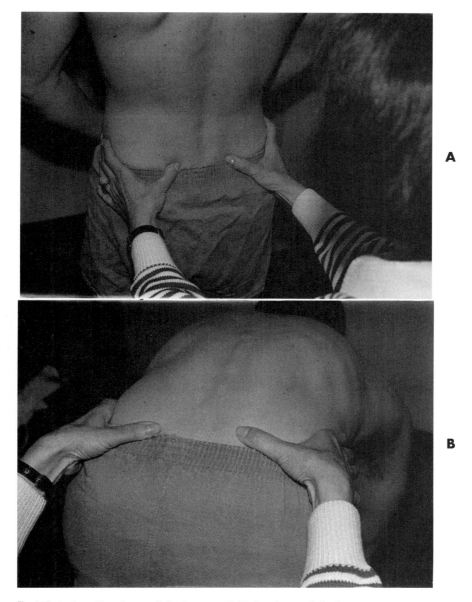

Fig. 4-19. A, Standing forward flexion test. **B** Sitting forward flexion test.

sation farther cephalad, even with activation of the scapular muscles.

In the ankle, functional alterations were found to be responsible for chronic ankle instability following a sprain, resulting from altered afferent impulses coming from the injured joint affecting muscle coordination.[6,7] This concept may apply anywhere in the body. Joint injury affects proprioceptive impulses from injured nerve endings in the surrounding ligaments. Through spinal reflex, muscle function changes, affecting movement patterns, which in turn affect joint function. A vicious cycle is created. Altered movement patterns spread both vertically and horizontally, and what begins as a local phenomenon may ramify throughout the musculoskeletal system.

According to Sherrington's law of reciprocal innervation, tight muscles have an inhibitory effect on their antagonists. Trying to strengthen weak muscles may thus be ineffective. In fact, in attempting to strengthen weak muscles, one can paradoxicallystrengthen antagonists, creating a further imbalance.[17] By first stretching the tight muscle, the weakened antagonist may spontaneously improve in strength.

To understand low back pain it is essential to look not only at the back and its biomechanics but to carefully screen and examine the whole body.

Particular emphasis should be placed on structural and functional problems in the lower extremity and foot, as they are frequently important contributing factors to spinal dysfunction.

Acknowledgment

We thank and acknowledge our mentor, Dr. Philip Greenman, for inspiring us to learn the art of segmental evaluation and treatment.

References

1. Botte RR: An interpretation of the pronation syndrome and foot types of patients with low back pain, *J Am Podiatry Assoc* 71:243–253, 1981.

2. Cailliet R: *Low back pain syndrome,* Philadelphia, FA Davis, 1981.

3. Colachis S, Worden RE, Bechtol CO, Strohm BR: Movement of the sacroiliac joint in the adult male: a preliminary report, *Arch Phys Med Rehabil* 44:490–498, 1963.

4. Dvorak J, Dvorak V: *Manual medicine,* New York, Springer-Verlag, 1984.

5. Finneson BE: *Low back pain,* ed 2., Philadelphia, JB Lippincott, 1980.

6. Freeman MAR: Instability of the foot after injuries to the lateral ligament of the ankle, *J Bone Joint Surg* 47:669–677, 1965.

7. Freeman MAR, Dean MRE, et al: The etiology and prevention of functional instability of the foot, *J Bone Joint Surg* [Br] 47:678–685, 1965.

8. Friberg O: Clinical symptoms and biomechanics of lumbar spine and hip joint in leg length inequality, *Spine* 8:643–651, 1983.

9. Fryette HH: Principles of Osteopathic Technic. Carmel, Calif, Academy of Applied Osteopathy, 1954.

10. Giles LGF: Lumbosacral facetal joint angles associated with leg length inequality, *Rheumatol Rehabil,* 20:233–238, 1981.

11. Gofton JP: Persistent low back pain and leg length disparity, *J Rheumatol* 12:747–750, 1985.

12. Greenman PE: Lift therapy: use and abuse, *J Am Osteopath Assoc* 79:238–250, 1979.

13. Greenman PE: *Principles of manual medicine,* Baltimore, Williams & Wilkins, 1989.

14. Greenman PE: Clinical aspects of sacroiliac function in walking, *J Manual Med* 5:125–130, 1990.

15. Grundy PF, Roberts CJ: Does unequal leg length cause back pain? *Lancet* 2:256–258, 1984.

16. Hollinshead WH: *Functional anatomy of the limbs and back,* Philadelphia, WB Saunders, 1976.

17. Janda V: *Muscles, central nervous motor regulation and back problems.* In Korr I, editor: *The neurobiologic mechanisms in Manipulative Therapy.* New York, Plenum Press, 1978.

18. Janda V: *Muscle weakness and inhibition (pseudoparesis) in back pain syndromes.* In Grieve GP, editor: *Modern manual therapy of the vertebral column.* New York, Churchill Livingstone, 1986.

19. Janda V: Muscle and back pain: assessment and treatment of impaired movement patterns and motor recruitment. Presented at Physical Medicine Research Foundation meeting, Las Vegas, 1983.

20. Kapandji IA: *The physiology of the joints,* ed 2, vol 3, New York, Churchill Livingstone, 1974.

21. Kapandji IA: *The physiology of the joints,* ed 5, vol 2, New York, Churchill Livingstone, 1982.

22. Kirkaldy-Willis WH, editor: Managing low back, ed 2, New York, Churchill Livingstone, 1988.

23. Lewit K: *Manipulative therapy in rehabilitation of the locomotor system,* ed 2. Oxford, England, Butterworth-Heinemann, 1991.

24. Netter FH: *Nervous system in the Ciba collection of medical illustrations,* West Caldwell, NJ, Ciba Foundation.

25. Rothenberg RJ: Rheumatic disease aspects of leg length inequality, *Semin Arthritis Rheum* 17:196–205, 1988.

26. Vleeming A, editor: First Interdisciplinary Congress on low back pain and its relation to the sacroiliac joint. San Diego, 1992.

27. White AA, Panjabi MH: *Clinical biomechanics of the spine,* ed 2. Philadelphia, JB Lippincott, 1990.

28. Williams PL, Warwick R, Dyson M, Bannister LH: *Gray's Anatomy,* ed 37. New York, Churchill Livingstone, 1989.

biomechanical principles of running injuries

Richard J. Bogdan, DPM

Office techniques
Clinic-based techniques
Hospital-based techniques
Low back injuries
Hip injuries

Iliotibial tract irritation
Knee injuries
Leg injuries
Foot injuries

Treatment of the athlete and his or her injury starts with the basic premise that the history and physical examination are specific for the sport and for the individual. The practitioner should question the athlete thoroughly until the cause of the injury has been determined. The diagnosis is confirmed by the physical examination.

Commonly, the athlete is evaluated in the office setting. The following outline of evaluation techniques will be helpful in the determination of the cause of many common athletic injuries. Specifically, the guidelines for the evaluation of running injuries within an office, clinic, or in a hospital-based practice are explored in this chapter.

Office techniques

Once the patient's history of the injury has been taken (Fig. 5-1) and the possible causes of the injury have been identified, the practitioner is in a position to choose the most appropriate examination techniques.

As with all physical examinations, the practitioner should observe the affected area, noting any swelling or change in color. This is then followed by palpation of the site and surrounding areas. The patient's response to the pressure applied is often a valuable indicator of the extent of injury. Palpation of the area should also provide information on the type of swelling that is present, if it is indurated or fluctuant for example. Any temperature change in the area should be noted at this time.

Next, the quality of the joint range of motion should be tested on both the affected and nonaffected side. As the findings so far are subjective, it is important to quantify the range of motion. The objective findings of the arthrometric examination should include examination from the hips to the toes. (For a complete discussion regarding this examination see Chapter 6.)

In order to reduce the subjective errors of these evaluation techniques, it is suggested that the arthrometric examination be performed utilizing two different instruments and repeating each measurement three times.[4]

The next step in the physical examination is muscle evaluation. This examination includes evaluation of both muscle strength and flexibility. (For a complete discussion regarding this examination, see Chapter 9.) This examination provides information necessary for the evaluation of the balance or symmetry of movement. This should be considered relative to the overall body movement patterns and as it pertains to specific joints. The range of motion is influenced by: (1) muscle strength, (2) flexibility, and

(3) positional influences that may alter structural positions during functional activity.

The first observation of the functional positions of an athlete will include weightbearing stance and gait. When treating athletes, it is preferable that they be observed performing their specific athletic activity. In the case of the runner, observation of him or her running is of immense value in making a diagnosis.

Clinic-based techniques

Clinic-based techniques are usually more sophisticated than office techniques and may be more expensive. Although these tests may be carried out in some private offices, they are typically done in a large clinic or university setting. Examples of these tests include the following:

1. Stress plate or barograph for evaluation of impact load to foot and limb
2. Accelerometers for evaluation of vertical and shear acceleration and deceleration
3. Video (digital) and goniometric evaluation of motion
4. Electromyography (EMG) evaluation of the neuromuscular sequence of the movement of the joints
5. Isokinetic muscle testing for dynamic muscle imbalance

Hospital-based techniques

The hospital-based evaluation includes the following:

1. Radiographs (more extensive than plain films)
2. Bone scans
3. Computed tomography (CT)
4. Compartmental pressure readings of the leg
5. Sonography
6. Magnetic resonance imaging (MRI)
7. Biochemical tests

Low back injuries

The painful back complaint is common among athletes, particularly runners. It affects runners of all ages. Often the problem arises from faulty mechanics of the foot or leg, or both. The effect on the back may be so limiting that it affects all aspects of the runner's life. The most common reasons for back pain in the runner are the following:

1. How many years have you been running? _____
   _____
2. How many miles/day do you average? _____
3. How many times do you run per week? _____ per day? _____
4. How many miles is your longest run during the week? _____
5. What pace (min/mile) do you average in your workouts? _____
6. How do you train? (circle)   long slow distance   long fast distance   fartlek
   intervals   sprint training   other _____
7. What type of terrain do you usually run on? (circle)
   grass   dirt   concrete   asphalt   sand   artificial track   hilly   flat   other
8. Do you regularly run on any canted surfaces (e.g., beach)? _____
9. At what time of day do you normally run? (circle)   morning   afternoon   night
10. What type of runner do you consider yourself? (circle)
    beginning   intermediate   advanced   competitive
11. What goals have you set for yourself in running? _____
    _____
12. How often do you race? _____
13. What distances do you normally race at? _____
14. What model of running shoes do you wear?
    For training _____
    For racing _____
15. What is the most important feature you look for in your running shoe? (circle)
    comfort   styling   recommendation from friends   sports shop recommendation
    running magazine rating   cheapest in price   other _____
16. How long have you been running in your present pair of shoes? _____
17. Do you wear any of the following in your running shoes? (circle)
    Spenco insole   varus wedge   orthotics   arch supports   other _____
18. Do any of your pairs of shoes make your injury/pain better or worse? (please describe)
    _____
19. Do you "build up" your running shoes to keep the outsole from wearing out too quickly? (If yes, what do you
    use?) _____
20. How do your shoes fit? (circle)   too short   long   narrow   wide   just right
21. How many pairs of socks do you wear when you run? _____
22. Do you stretch before you run? _____ How long? _____
23. Do you stretch after you run? _____ How long? _____
24. Do you warm up before you run? _____ How long? _____
25. Do you warm down after you run? _____ How long? _____
26. Do you supplement your running program with muscle-strengthening exercises? _____
    Please describe the goals of this program. _____
27. Do you participate in any other sports or any other types of exercise program? _____
    (please describe) _____
28. Are you on a special diet? _____ What type is it? (circle)
    vegetarian   macrobiotic   high protein   low salt   low fat   other _____
29. Are you presently feeling (circle)   completely healthy   fatigued   injured?
30. Did you modify your training/racing schedule prior to your injury? (please describe) _____
    _____
31. Did you run a particularly hard race or hard workout immediately prior to your injury? (please describe) __
    _____
32. Did you switch to another pair of running shoes prior to your injury? (please describe) _____
    _____
33. Did you modify your footgear in any way prior to your injury? (please describe) _____
    _____
34. Was there any direct trauma associated with your injury? (please describe) _____
    _____
35. Did you have another injury or any discomfort in your feet or legs prior to your injury that you tried to train
    through? (please describe) _____
36. How did you treat yourself or modify your training following your injury? _____
    _____ Did it help? _____
37. Have you ever been treated by a sports medicine specialist? _____
    By whom? _____ For what problem? _____

Fig. 5-1. A runner's history questionnaire.

- Functional short leg
- Anatomic short leg
- Bilateral excessive pronation of feet
- Muscle imbalance (previous injuries)
- Muscle spasm (acute injury)
- Medical (ankylosing spondylitis, spondylolisthesis, spondylolysis)

Since the evaluation is somewhat the same for all of the conditions in the above list, the following is typical of a runner's injury and subsequent complaint.

Consider a runner in his or her mid-thirties who complains of pain across the lower back. The runner points to the central portion of the lumbar area. This person has been running for several years and occasionally runs in road races. The runner trains at a 7:30-min/mile pace on rolling hills and streets. The low back pain begins as a stiffness that develops into an ache at the end of the run. The runner is currently training to run a half-marathon 6 months hence and would like to be more comfortable by that date. Investigation of the complaint requires a thorough history of the patient's running activity and its relationship to the back complaint. The detailed examination technique is as follows:

Evaluation

The initial physical evaluation begins with the athlete standing. The athlete should be clad in shorts and singlet for ease of observation. The athlete should be viewed from the back, the front, and the side. This allows observation of the overall posture.

Note the specific position of the head (tilted forward or to the side), shoulders (tilted to one side or positioned anteriorly), arms (one lower than the other), back (kyphotic or lordotic), hips (tilted to one side), knees (flexed), rearfoot (everted or inverted), and forefoot (abducted or adducted). Check for symmetry of these positions.

When the athlete is standing, observe the level of the posterosuperior iliac spines and iliac crests, (Fig. 5-2), observing the patellae and the positions of the lower legs for any asymmetry.

When the athlete lies down, observe the curvature in the back, the position of the hips, and the position of the knees (Fig. 5-3). This position provides an impression of the spine in the off-loaded position. Examine the area of complaint. Look for any signs of primary vertebral disorder or discogenic disease. Note the level of the anterosuperior spines. If necessary, a detailed neurologic examination is performed (Table 5-1).

If the lateral or oblique spinal films of the lumbar area or Lasègue's maneuver (straight leg lift which places tension on the sciatic nerve and spinal

Table 5-1
Neurologic examination

Test	Area
Power	Hip flexors (L2) Quadriceps (L3) Anterior tibial (L4) Extensor hallucis longus (L5) Flexor hallucis longus (S1) Hamstrings (S2)
Dermatome sensation	Medial midthigh (L2) Superior aspect of knee (L3) Medial arch (L4) Dorsum of foot (L5) Lateral aspect of foot (S1) Popliteal fossa (S2)
Muscle tenderness	Quadriceps (L4) Anterior tibial (L5) Calf (S1)
Reflexes	Patella (L4) Achilles tendon (S1) Plantar (Babinski's sign) (S1)
Sciatic nerve	Straight leg and Lasègue's sign Bowstring test

nerves) (Fig. 5-4) are questionable, referral to a consultant for evaluation is necessary.

A biomechanical examination of the entire lower extremity should then be performed and documented.

The office examination must now concentrate on observation of the functional positions of the runner's limbs. What should be elicited from the functional examinations is the status of the body's functional symmetry. The use of bathroom scales is an easy way to observe overloading of one extremity relative to the other. Although this does not indicate the cause or level of the inequality, scales are capable of quantifying the imbalance. This represents a static measurement.

Next, the practitioner should evaluate motion from one side to the other for any asymmetric movement. This asymmetric movement is the main means of recognizing the influence of leg length differences on the body.

Motion analysis and functional symmetry

The relaxed calcaneal stance position (RCSP) and its relationship to limb asymmetry must be assessed. The practitioner must compare the RCSP of one side with the other. This is done by observing the heel bisection during the stance phase of gait (Fig. 5-5), comparing it with the RCSP and the neutral calcaneal stance position (NCSP). If the RCSP measurement indicates that one heel is everted more than the other (>3 degrees), one should note the existence of a functional or positional asymmetry at the level of

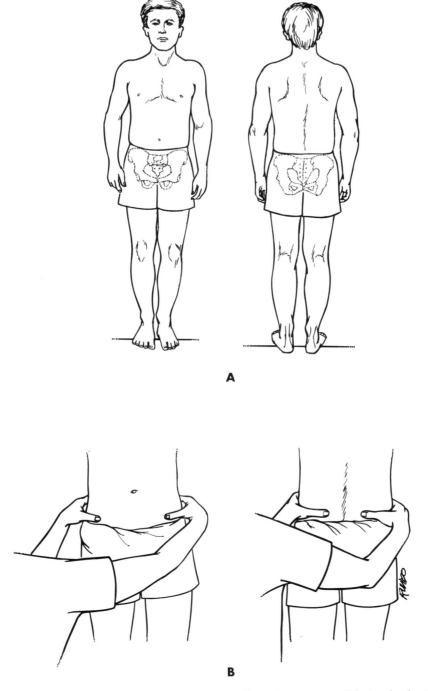

Fig. 5-2. A, Anterior and posterior views of the pelvis. **B,** Clinical assessment of the levels of anterior and posterior iliac spines.

the hip, either in the transverse plane or the frontal plane. If symmetry of the RCSP is noted, then there is an equal maximally pronated functional position for the subtalar joints. The clinician should observe the possibility of an anterior pelvic instability (anterior pelvic tilt), which may be a more

likely cause of the back complaint than a limb length inequality of the functional or structural type.

In determining the functional limb asymmetry, the clinician will need to consider other causes:

1. Evaluation of the running environment may

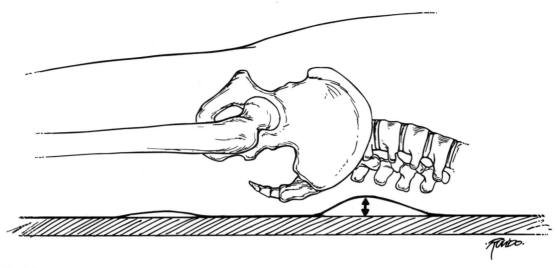

Fig. 5-3. Curvature of the lower back with the patient supine.

reveal that the runner is running on a canted (tilted) surface, downhill, on a beach, or on an unstable surface.

2. Evaluation of the patient's shoe may demonstrate a structural deviation of the midsole or heel from the reference vertical line (Fig. 5-6). This could be a sign that the foot strike or the construction of the shoe may be disturbing the functional position of the limb.

Limb measurement

There are a variety of techniques that may be utilized to assess the presence of a limb length inequality. The following is used to evaluate the anatomic or structural limb length difference. The clinician should start the measurement from a proximal position at the level of the hips. The anterior iliac spines represent a relatively reliable bony landmark in the pelvis. A measuring tape is stretched to the prominence of the medial malleolus (the distalmost aspect of the tibia) or the medial aspect of the ankle joint. A measurement is then recorded and compared with the measurement of the contralateral side. As with all measurements, it should be repeated. This technique is the most commonly used method to measure limb length. Several other techniques are commonly used and are noted elsewhere in this book (Fig. 5-7). These can be correlated in both a non-weightbearing position or a weightbearing position with the subtalar joint in a neutral position.

Hip injuries

A runner complains of a vague, aching pain deep in her hip. She points to the deep portion of her right hip. This runner has been running on a golf course near her home, as well as on the roads. She has not experienced any problem with her back for several weeks. She has been participating in occasional road races with no pain until last week.

This runner trains at an 8:00-min/mile pace on rolling hills and a 7:45- to 7:30-min/mile pace on the streets. Her hip pain begins as a stiffness that develops into an aching type of pain following a run. The runner is training to run a half-marathon 2 months later, and would like to be more comfortable so that she may do some speed workouts. She also has been playing some recreational basketball. The patient should be evaluated by a thorough history and examination.

The practitioner should be aware that an initial evaluation must include examination for a malfunction of the foot or leg. Any malalignment of the foot or leg can create an overuse or acute load on the osseous or soft tissue structures of the hip.

A leg length inequality, anatomic or functional, may affect the hip-supporting structures similarly to its effect on the low back. It may cause a biomechanical imbalance that will stress the muscles, ligaments, and joint cartilage about the hip joint. These stresses are due to the compensation the body must perform in order to equalize its function from one side to the other.

Could this possibly represent a low back abnormality with referred pain to the hip? The clinician must perform a detailed examination of the hip and evaluate the biomechanical structure in conjunction with the runner's function. The clinician should refer back to the neurologic examination shown in Table 5-1.

Muscle imbalances may be present in many hip complaints, resulting from either overtraining or structural imbalances. The following specific muscle

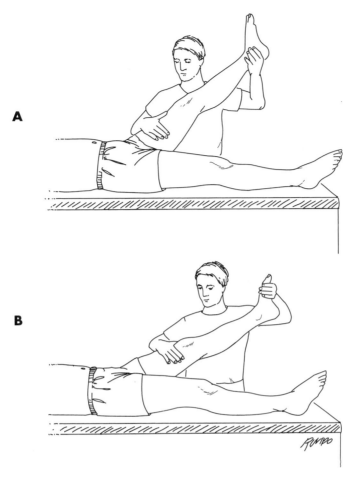

Fig. 5-4. Lasèque's sign: This test is performed by raising the straight leg to the point where the patient experiences pain radiating down the leg **(A).** At this point, the leg is lowered slightly until no discomfort is noted. The foot is then dorsiflexed **(B).** If this produces radiating pain down the leg, the test is positive for sciatic nerve stretch or irritation.

testing should be included in a general muscle test examination of this area.

Evaluate the hip abductor (external rotator) vs. the hip adductor (internal rotator) muscles. Evaluation of the balance of strength and flexibility between the extensors and flexors of the thigh should be performed next. This is usually performed manually in the office. The practitioner should grade the muscles by the following standard "5 over 5" reporting method (For a complete discussion regarding this examination, see Chapter 9). Data are collected and compared with the unaffected side. Next, flexibility is evaluated by comparing the unaffected side with the affected side (Fig. 5-8).

More extensive functional muscle evaluation via an isokinetic device (e.g., Cybex*) may be needed to confirm any subtle findings of the clinical evaluation.

For example, when weakness of the quadriceps musculature occurs during a 12-mile run, a Cybex examination may be done to compare one side with the other. The Cybex reproduces the level at which the difference occurs because it tests the athlete at the speeds that they obtain during the athletic event.

Analysis of the structure of the lower extremity may determine a higher degree of varus angulation in the thigh or knee complex (genu varum), the tibia, or the subtalar joint. Compensation for these deformities creates an internal limb position that produces a moderate shock wave affecting the hip, back, and thigh. It also creates a higher degree of the limb varus phenomenon during running. The muscular control of this functioning limb type may produce fatigue of the lateral and extensor muscle groups of the thigh and hip regions, because this musculature attempts to stop internal rotation of the limb.

* Lumex Inc., Cybex Division, Ronkonkoma, NY 11779.

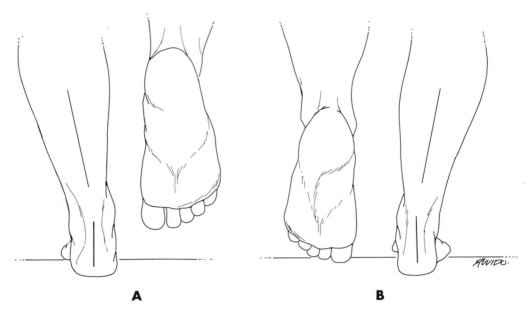

Fig. 5-5. Observation of the heel bisection during the stance phase of running. **A,** A normal heel position in midstance. **B,** Excessive pronation at midstance.

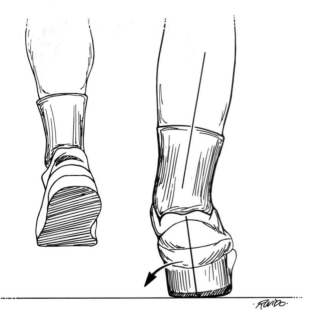

Fig. 5-6. Structural deviation of running shoes.

The cavus foot type (a forefoot valgus that compensates by inverting the rearfoot, or in combination with a compensated rearfoot varus or a partially compensated rearfoot varus) contributes to the lack of shock absorption. The pes planus (forefoot varus) foot type contributes to overuse and fatigue from an excessive amount of pronation.

The differential diagnosis includes a number of

syndromes. The following are some of the common causes of mechanically induced hip pain:

1. Illiotibial tract irritation
2. Strain of a muscle about the hip
3. Greater trochanteric bursitis
4. Stress fracture of the femoral neck
5. Piriformis syndrome
6. Pubic rami stress fractures
7. Illiac crest fracture
8. Slipped capital femoral epiphysis (10:12 male/female)
9. Congental hip dysplasia

Clinical palpation of the region may help to identify an anatomic cause. To distinguish between a structural lesion and an osseous lesion, the following is performed.

The patient is placed on an examination table and the hips are extended. A rotation test of the thigh placed through the full range of motion is performed (Fig. 5-9). This should stress the hip and localize any complaint of pain, possibly from a lesion involving the cartilaginous surface or the ligamentous structures of the hip joint. These positions are reproduced when evaluating the strength of the muscles and tendons that govern the joint's movement.

Further inspection of the painful site may be necessary using regional x-ray films, bone scans, CT scans, or MRI. As the practitioner evaluates the

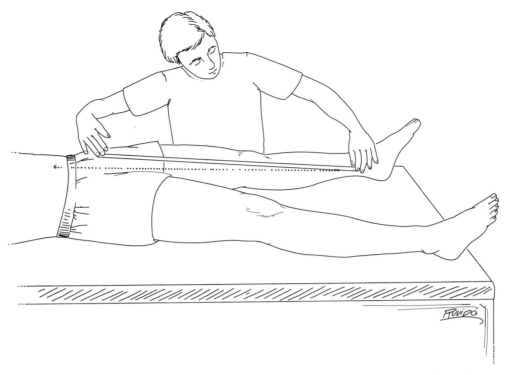

Fig. 5-7. Measurment of limb length. This method demonstrates measurement of the distance between the anterior iliac spine and the medial malleolus. When assessing limb length inequality, a combination of clinical and radiographic assessments are most accurate.

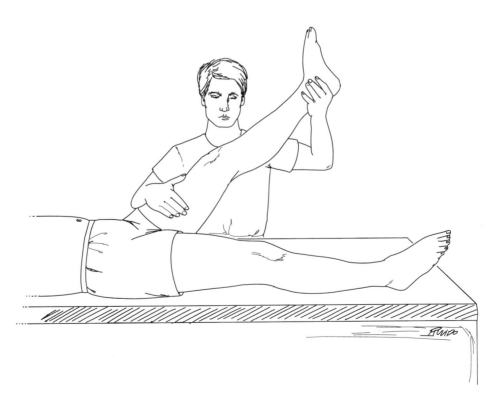

Fig. 5-8. Testing hip flexibility. Each hip is extended to determine the flexibility of one limb relative to the other.

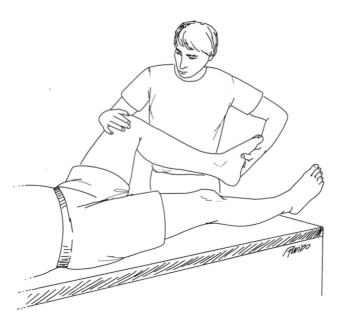

Fig. 5-9. Hip rotation test. Pain elicited via this maneuver is consistent with cartilaginous or ligamentous involvement.

information obtained, a more specific determination regarding the cause of the pain may be attained.

Iliotibial tract irritation

This syndrome is usually precipitated when a runner trains extensively on a downhill terrain. The problem occurs as a result of a constant need to control the bent knee. Along with this flexed knee position, the lateral compartmental muscles of the thigh are continuously attempting to stabilize the knee from buckling laterally (Fig. 5-10). The practitioner should observe the functional position of the knee while the runner is running. The best way to do this is via a slow-motion video camera. This allows the practitioner to observe the position of the limb at heel strike, then at midstance, and finally, in the propulsive phase of gait. The practitioner can evaluate the degrees of angulation of flexion of the knee in the sagittal plane and the degree of valgus or varus angulation in the frontal plane.

The type of running described here tends to tighten the iliotibial tract as the thigh musculature repeatedly contracts when an athlete runs downhill. The iliotibial tract also responds to tightening because the lower extremity demonstrates a limited ability to properly attenuate the shock while the athlete is running downhill. Another factor in this scenario is that many athletes do not stretch this area of their thighs before or after running.

An intrinsic or anatomic limb malalignment may intensify while running downhill resulting from the fatiguing of the foot or the inequality of one limb's function relative to the function of the other limb.

The overactivity of the thigh muscles in this runner may create an overload of a muscle group or a single muscle, which will then become strained. Any one of the following muscles may develop a weakness: iliopsoas, rectus femoris, sartorius, gluteus medius, and piriformis.[5,6]

Another problem in the area of the hip that the practitioner must consider with iliotibial band irritation is either a greater trochanter friction bursitis or a stress fracture involving the femoral neck. The friction bursitis is located directly under the iliotibial tract and may be palpable when inflamed. As the muscular structures about the lateral compartment of the hip and thigh fatigue, an imbalance develops where one muscle group maintains a contracted position. This creates a tissue that is not resilient to the firm structures rubbing beneath. There is a clicking of the bursa that can be felt when the leg is flexed or rotated inward (the common position of the pronated foot and limb complex).

A stress fracture involving the femoral neck is a more deeply positioned complaint.[7] It is generally located in the vicinity of the groin and may refer pain to the periphery. It may present in a similar fashion to the types of pain seen with a pubic rami or iliac crest stress fracture.[9,10] The former is located toward the midline and in line with the pelvis, while the latter is located more proximally, toward the origin of the tensor fascia lata.[2]

The moderate stress of running downhill may be responsible for the stress of the osseous structures about the hip. This stress may cause fatigue fractures of the osseous structures about the hip.[16]

Further evaluation may be necessary via regional x-ray films, bone scans, CT scans, or MRI.

Knee injuries

A runner complains of pain around the inside and front of his knee. He points to the central portion and medial aspect of the knee. This runner has been running for several weeks trying to increase his training schedule. He has occasionally raced on roads. The runner trains at a 7:30-min/mile pace on rolling hills and on streets. The pain is described as a stiffness that develops into an ache at the end of the run. The runner is training to run a half-marathon a few months hence and would like to be more comfortable by that date. The complaint is explored by a thorough history and examination of the following areas of the knee:

Patellar region

Since the knee functions in the sagittal plane, any significant deviation from this position results in a change of both the femorotibial joint and the

A

B

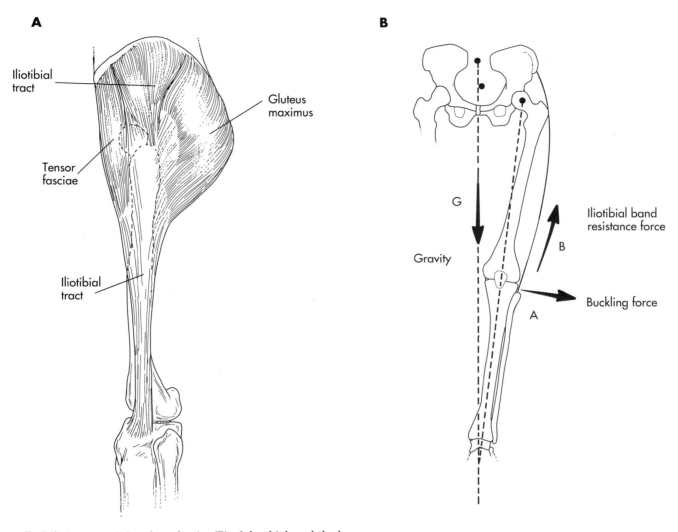

Iliotibial tract

Gluteus maximus

Tensor fasciae

Iliotibial tract

G

Gravity

Iliotibial band resistance force

B

Buckling force

A

Fig. 5-10. Anatomy (**A**) and mechanics (**B**) of the thigh and the knee.

anterior patellofemoral joint. These joints respond to the terrain the runner runs on (shock absorption) and the functional position that the feet have owing to their structure or the footgear-surface interface.

This runner has a history of running on the very uneven surface of a golf course. He also plays recreational basketball. He has a moderate Q angle (>10 degrees) (Fig. 5-11) and a forefoot varus of moderate degree (7 degrees with full compensation via eversion of the subtalar joint upon stance and during gait). Therefore, he is considered a moderate pronator during function.

The common condition that develops is classically reported as the "runner's knee syndrome" where the patella is malaligned to its origin and insertion points on the femur and tibia. The cartilage of the patella and the retinacular and ligamentous structures become strained and inflamed. The site of the pain is usually on the medial side of the patellofemoral joint.

Stress testing of the patellofemoral joint with movement of the knee from flexion to extension may help rule out a synovial plicae or tendinitis (Fig. 5-12).

Medial joint line

Knee symptoms affecting this site may be associated with the patellofemoral complaint.[1] It may be that the collateral ligament is strained or that a small tear of the the medial meniscus is present. Use of meniscal testing maneuvers, McMurray's (Fig. 5-13) and Apley's compression tests (Fig. 5-14), may provide the diagnosis.

Central deep joint

Symptoms affecting this site generally involve a tendinitis of the patellar ligament that is painful on pressure or during a fall. If the knee is functioning in a markedly flexed position, the pain is located deeper and involves an internal structure such as

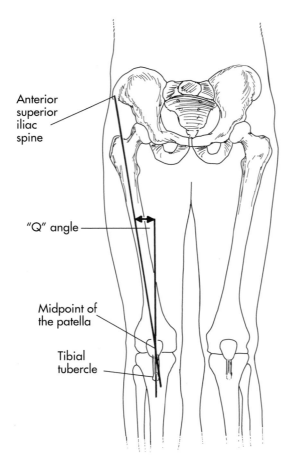

Fig. 5-11. Measurement of the Q angle. A high Q angle may predispose the athlete to patellar problems as the structure assumes a more laterally deviated functional position during gait.

the fat pad, or the anterior or posterior cruciate ligaments. These conditions may appear with the extreme pronator who has a functional flexed knee position associated with a tight hamstring or heel cord syndromes.

Lateral joint line

Lateral knee symptoms may be associated with a strained lateral collateral ligament.[11] Additionally, they may be associated with the illiotibial band causing a bursitis, a popliteus tendon tendinitis, or a small tear of the lateral meniscus. (Fig. 5-15). These conditions are associated with athletes who demonstrate significant pronation or poor shock absorption related to a structural genu varum and a supinated foot type.

Posterior joint line

The posterior knee is rarely symptomatic. However, the strain of the popliteus muscle, inflammation of the hamstring tendons, or herniation of the posterior capsule into a popiteal cyst may cause symptoms

(see Fig. 5-15). These problems may be associated with training on uneven terrain or found in the athlete who is performing other sporting activities that require side-to-side movements such as basketball and contact sports.

Leg injuries

We now consider the runner who develops a complaint of pain across the front of the shin. The runner points to the central portion of the shin area. This runner has been training at a 7:10-min/mile pace on rolling hills and on streets. His shin pain develops after he runs on a hard paved surface. The pain begins with a stiffness that develops into an ache by the end of a run. He has some numbness or tingling between the second and great toes.

The runner is planning to run a half-marathon 2 months hence and would like to be more comfortable by that date. Let us explore his complaint by a thorough history and examination.

The examination of the part by palpation elicits a painful area in the midportion of the shin. Pain seems to progress from anterior to lateral along the muscle belly rather than from the anterior medial ridge of the tibia. This site suggests a differential diagnosis that includes the following[14]:

1. Compartmental syndrome, anterior vs. lateral or posterior
2. Extensor tenosynovitis
3. Stress fracture, tibial or fibular
4. Medial stress syndrome
5. Deep thrombophlebitis

The cause and diagnosis are determined when the following is considered:

Diagnosis of compartmental syndrome requires that the runner complain of tightness while running and an ache after the rest phase begins. The runner complains that his foot gets heavier during the run. He also experiences a tightness in the midportion of the leg. While testing the extensor muscle group, the patient complains of pain and a "full" feeling in the front portion of the leg.[12,17]

At this point in the examination, the practitioner should observe the runner's gait, and the mechanical makeup of the lower extremities.[15,21] A treadmill evaluation will provide insight into the dynamic movements of the foot relative to the leg. The clinician may evaluate the extent of pronation or supination that occurs during running. Reproduction of the activity may precipitate the problem and allow the patient to be more specific in regard to the location and nature of the symptoms.

A wick or slit catheter (Fig. 5-16) pressure analysis

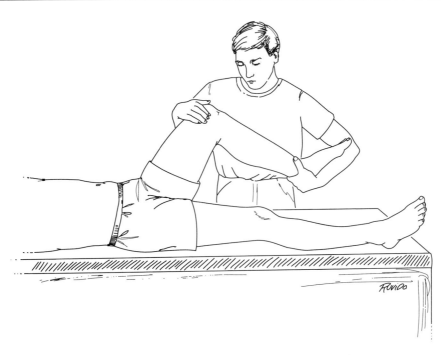

Fig. 5-12. Stress testing of the patellofemoral joint. This maneuver attempts to elicit pain with movement of the knee from a flexed to an extended position.

of the leg's compartments[3] is performed to evaluate the variance of the compartmental pressure from the norm of 40 mm Hg and radiographs or a triphasic bone scan is done to rule out osseous involvement.[18]

The osseous causes are generally found in either the proximal, midportion, or distal part of the tibia. They usually present as an area that is sensitive to palpation. A tuning fork test may be positive. The athlete is placed on an examining table and a stethoscope is placed on the opposite side of the suspected fracture. The clinician attempts to hear the vibrating tuning fork. If a vibrating hum is heard, the bone is not fractured. These areas of pain may not represent true fractures but partial stress reaction or stress fractures. Bone scans are helpful in the diagnosis of this type of stress fracture as no other means of evaluation can detect them in the early stages.

It is essential to evaluate the function of the foot in these cases,[15,21] because stress fractures are usually associated with a foot structure that does not provide adequate shock absorption in the initial contact phase of gait. This abnormal structure and function includes a fully compensated forefoot varus (fixed pronated foot), a forefoot valgus compensated by a supinated subtalar varus (pes cavus) and a rearfoot varus (uncompensated, partially compensated, or compensated). These foot types function at the end of range of motion of pronation, which allows for the shock to overload and fracture the tibia or fibula.

Treatment will generally include rest or modified activity, reduction of inflammation (ice, electrical therapy, nonsteroidal anti-inflammatory drugs), and the establishment of appropriate ranges of motion for the subtalar and midtalar joints of the foot using functional foot orthoses.

Foot injuries

A runner complains of pain in both her rearfoot and forefoot. She points to the central portion of the left heel, posterior and plantar-medial. The runner has been running for a month in road races and on a track. She is training at a 7:00-min/mile pace on rolling hills and on the track at a 6:00 min/mile pace.

The forefoot pain is described as a soreness that develops into an ache at the end of a run or after standing for any period of time. The ache usually radiates from the midfoot to the forefoot. The rearfoot complaints have been present for several weeks. Initially the pain was tolerable, and it waxed and waned depending on the terrain and the number of miles she ran during the week. She is still planning to run a half-marathon a few months hence and would like to be more comfortable by that date. The complaints are explored by a thorough history and examination.

Rearfoot

After inspection, the complaints in the rearfoot appear to be separate entities relative to the forefoot

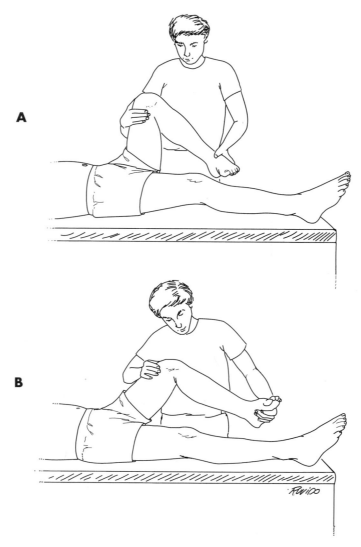

Fig. 5-13. McMurray's test. **(A)** To test for a torn meniscus the knee is fully flexed, rotated, and extended. The fingers are placed on the joint line, and a click or a grinding sensation is palpated for within the joint. **(B)** By extending the knee while applying a varus force to the foot and internally rotating the tibia, a torn medial meniscus may be compressed. This causes pain or produces a click. Following this, the same procedure may be performed with the leg in an external position. First, the knee is flexed and the tibia is externally rotated. By extending the knee while applying a valgus force to the foot and externally rotating the tibia, a torn lateral meniscus may be compressed. This causes pain or produces a click.

and midfoot. A portion of the rearfoot pain is located behind and about the Achilles tendon. Palpation elicits the following differential diagnosis (Fig. 5-17).

1. Partial tendon rupture
2. Tendinitis
3. Bursitis (associated retrocalcaneal exostosis)
4. Os trigonum syndrome

Although mechanical causes of rearfoot pain are numerous, a rearfoot that is inverted throughout the early contact phase of gait creates a significant stress on the posterior lateral aspect of the heel, which is a likely cause of the above conditions. These stresses are due to an uncompensated or partially compensated rearfoot varus, or an inverted rearfoot associated with a rigid functioning forefoot valgus. This rearfoot varus may additionally overload the Achilles attachment or the tendon itself. Also, limited ankle dorsiflexion can compound the abnormal effects and exacerbate the symptoms, or be the sole cause of the symptoms.

The pronated foot type associated with excessive eversion of the heel may also be a significant contributor to these symptoms. This foot type creates significant twists within the tendon, and

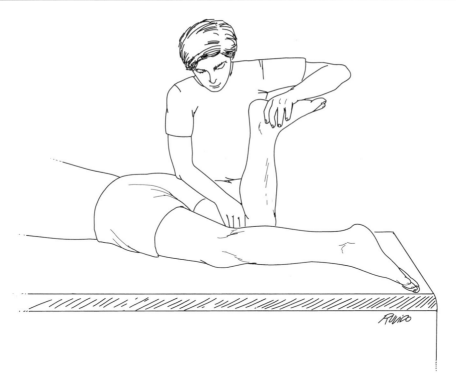

Fig. 5-14. Apley's compression test. The examiner pushes the tibia downward and simultaneously rotates it. If this produces pain, then one should suspect a posterior horn tear of the medial meniscus. This pain should not be present if the tibia is distracted from the femur and simultaneously rotated.

associated excessive torques at the level of its insertion into the calcaneus.[3] The everted heel foot types may be found with a limb length asymmetry causing excessive pronation of one side, as compensation for limited ankle dorsiflexion, for a severe (>7 degrees) forefoot varus, and a moderately flexible forefoot valgus deformity. Additionally the practitioner should consider that the patient's training is excessive and contributes to the overuse syndrome. The clinical judgment may be reinforced by appropriate adjunctive tests such as x-ray films, tomograms, bone scans, or MRI. Arthrography of the ankle or subtalar joint may be necessary.

Following evaluation of the posterior calcaneal symptoms, the complaint in the area of the plantar heel should be examined. The following are the most likely diagnoses:

1. Plantar fasciitis or enthesitis
2. Bursitis
3. Nerve entrapment
4. Stress fracture

The athlete's response to palpation will narrow the differential diagnosis. The above diagnoses are generally associated with overuse syndromes due to elongation of the longitudinal arch in the transverse

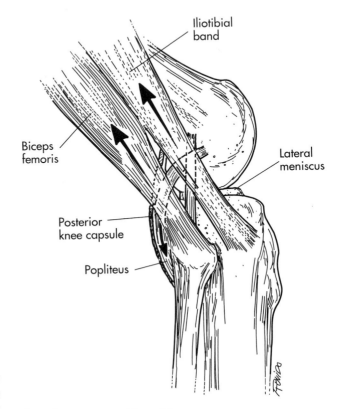

Fig. 5-15. Posterior and lateral knee anatomy.

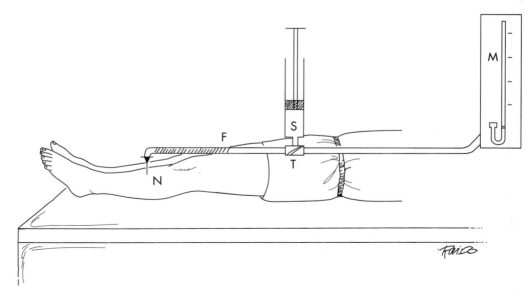

Fig. 5-16. The wick or slit catheter compartmental pressure analysis system. *N,* 18-gauge needle; *F,* fluid meniscus; *S,* syringe; *T,* three-way trap; *M,* mercury manometer.

and sagittal plane.[20] Several foot types can create the arch elongation which occurs for an inappropriate or prolonged period of time. During the gait cycle, the elongation of the foot may be too abrupt for the elastic modulus of the plantar fascial tissue. The pes cavus foot type (inverted rearfoot compensation from the rigid forefoot valgus) is generally the cause of the abrupt elongation in the sagittal plane direction and the pronated foot types (forefoot valgus compensated in the longitudinal axis, rearfoot varus, and forefoot varus) are responsible for elongation in the sagittal and transverse direction.

Radiographs (stress fractures, calcaneal spurs, bursitis), EMG or nerve conduction studies (nerve entrapment), bone scans (stress fracture, enthesitis), CT scans, or MRI may be necessary to arrive at the appropriate diagnosis.

Midfoot

We now consider the pain described as an ache in the midfoot that migrates to the forefoot. The complaint is explored by a thorough history and examination. Pressure palpation of the midfoot produces pain circumferentially about the midfoot and at the proximal aspect of the metatarsals. Movement with and without muscular activity generates continuous pain. The differential diagnosis includes

1. Navicular stress fracture or reaction
2. Spring ligament strain
3. Os tibiale externum syndrome
4. Stress fracture of a metatarsal
5. Calcaneal navicular coalition

A navicular stress fracture is the most significant injury in this group and should be ruled out. Early evaluation with a bone scan is essential. A CT scan may determine the level and extent of the fracture if the bone scan is positive.

Specific foot types associated with the above include

1. Limited ankle dorsiflexion
2. Pes cavus foot type (bony block type or soft tissue limited type)
3. Pronated foot type with eversion of the heel of the foot

These foot types undergo compensation, then create a large torque to the attachments of the navicular and midtarsal joint. The everted heel foot types are found with a limb length asymmetry causing excessive pronation of one foot over the other, a limited ankle dorsiflexion foot type, severe (>7 degrees) forefoot varus and a moderately flexible forefoot valgus. Additionally, excessive training will contribute to functional overuse and fatigue. In all instances, clinical judgment must be reinforced by appropriate adjunctive tests such as x-ray films, tomograms, bone scans, or MRI.[19]

Forefoot

The runner now complains of pain in her forefoot. She points to the central portion of the ball of the left foot. The forefoot pain is described as a soreness that develops into an ache at the end of a run or after standing for any period of time. The ache usually radiates to the midfoot. Initially the pain was tolerable and it waxed and waned depending on the

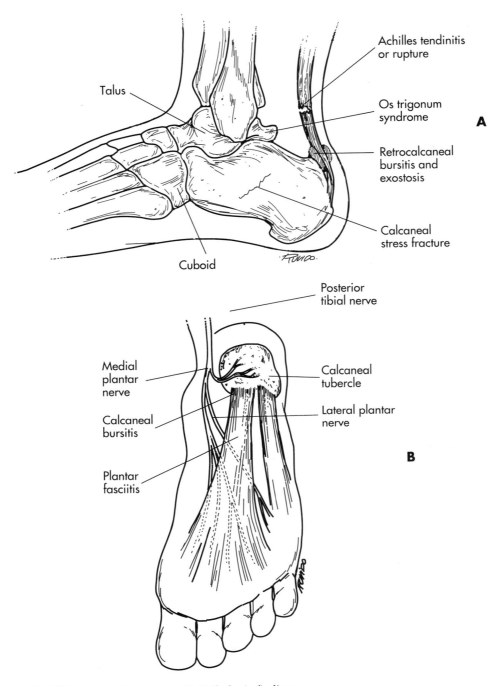

Fig. 5-17. Rearfoot **A,** Anatomy. **B,** Pathologic findings.

terrain and the number of miles she ran during the week. She is still planning to run a half-marathon a few months hence and would like to be more comfortable by that date.

With palpation of the involved area of the forefoot, the painful site is localized to the third and fourth metatarsal shafts and heads. The differential diagnosis includes

1. Disorders associated with metatarsalgia

2. Stress fracture or fractures

3. Morton's neuroma

Because of the occasional radiation of pain that the runner describes, one may need to perform tests that rule out nerve entrapment. Ultrasound[8] or MRI have been utilized clinically to investigate the forefoot interspaces for masses. The differential diagnosis of a stress fracture or stress reaction is demonstrated through the use of multiple radiographic views or bone scans. Clincally, the tuning fork test, as well as the history, may be definitive.

The differential diagnosis of disorders associated with metatarsalgia usually includes clinical findings located in the area of the metatarsophalangeal joints. These findings include swelling in this region or pain upon distraction of the digits. The plain film may be helpful in demonstrating patterns of the metatarsals, metatarsus primus elevatus, or signs of a functional hallux limitus.

There are specific foot types that may be implicated. A flexible forefoot valgus in association with a moderate rearfoot varus will create a significant imbalance of the forefoot within the transverse plane. The imbalance exists between the stabilizing points of the medial and lateral column. If they are in an elevatus position, the middle segments will become overloaded. Any activity that involves fore-and-aft movements of the leg and foot may increase stresses to the metatarsal region.

The aim of this chapter has been to develop the clinician's [2] awareness of the individual biomechanical aberrations of the lower extremity and how they relate to overuse and acute injuries.

References

1. Carson WG Jr: Diagnosis of extensor mechanical disorders; *Clin Sports Med* 4:231, 1985.
2. Clancey WG, Folty AS: Illiac apophysitis and stress fractures in adolescent runners, *Am J Sports Med* 4:214, 1972.
3. Clement DB, Taunton JE, Smart GW: Achilles tendinitis and peritendinitis: etiology and treatment, *Am J Sports Med* 12:179–184, 1984.
4. Elveru RA, Rothstein JM, Lamb RL: Goniometric reliability in a clinical setting: subtalar and ankle measurements, *Phys Ther* 68:672–677.
5. Garrett WE, Safran MR, Seaker AV, et al. Biomechanical comparison of stimulated and non stimulated muscle pulled to failure, *Am J Sports Med* 15: 448, 1987.
6. Grace TG: Muscle imbalance and extremity injury. *Sports Med* 2:77, 1985.
7. Hajek MR, Noble HB: Stress fractures of the femoral neck in runners, *Am J Sports Med* 10:112, 1982.
8. Harichaux P, Viel E: *Application de l'ultrasonographie à l'effet Doppler à la physiologie et médicine du sport.* In Commandre FA, Bence YR (eds): *Explorations fontionnelles neuromusculaires.* Paris, Masson, 1982, pp 96–108.
9. Harris WH, Murray RO. Lesions of the symphysis in athletes, *Br Med J* 4:211, 1974.
10. Koch R, Jackson D: Pubic symphysitis in runners, *Am J Sports Med* 9:62, 1981.
11. Lutter LD: Cavus foot in runners, *Foot Ankle* 1:225, 1981.
12. Martens M, Backaert M, Vermant G, et al: Chronic leg pain in athletes due to a recurrent compartment syndrome, *Am J Sports Med* 12:148–151, 1984.
13. Matsen F, Mayo K, Sheridan G, et al: Monitoring of the intramuscular pressure, *Surgery* 79: 702–709, 1976.
14. Matsen F, Winquist R, Krugmire R: Diagnosis and management of compartment syndromes, *J Bone Joint Surg* [Am] 62:286–291, 1980.
15. Meisser SP, Pittala KA: Etiologic factors associated with selected running injuries, *Med Sci Sports Exerc* 20: 501–505, 1988.
16. Noakes TD, Smith JA, Lindberg G: Pelvic stress fractures in long distance runners, *Am J Sports Med* 13:120, 1985.
17. Rorabeck C. *A practical approach to compartmental syndromes.* Part 3. Inst Course Lect 32:102–113, 1983.
18. Rupani H, Holde L, Espinola R. et al. Three phase radionuclide imaging bone imaging in sports medicine. *Radiology* 156:187–196, 1985.
19. Stafford SA, Rosenthal DI, Gebhardt MC, et al: MRI in stress fracture, AJR, *Am J Roentgenol* 147:553, 1986.
20. Torg JS, Pavlov E: Overuse injuries in sport: the foot, *Clin Sports Med* 11:125–130, 1983.
21. Vitasolo JT, Kvist M: Some biomechanical aspects of the foot and ankle in athletes with and without shin splints, *Am J Sports Med* 11:125–130, 1980.

biomechanical examination of the foot and lower extremity

Bart W. Gastwirth, DPM

Physical setting and layout
The biomechanical examination

The musculoskeletal examination of the lower extremity is divided into several parts: the arthrometric examination, muscular strength and tone assessment, postural assessment, and dynamic assessment. It is imperative that the clinician create a clinical environment that is comfortable for the patient and that appropriate time is allotted to do all that is necessary to perform a complete and detailed examination. When performing the examination the clinician should strive to minimize patient movement; that is, the patient is first examined supine, then prone, then standing, then walking.

Physical setting and layout

To perform a biomechanical examination the following instruments should be available: a tractograph, a gravity gonionmeter, a tape measure, a protractor, and a felt-tip pen (with water-soluble ink) (Fig. 6-1). The ideal examination table is a padded flattop examination table with adjustments for height. A well-lighted walkway about 30 feet long is needed for gait assessment. The patient should be dressed appropriately for the examination. The clinician will need to record the measurements, and a suitable form should be available (see Appendix).

The biomechanical examination
Hip joint measurement

The hip joint is a ball-and-socket joint whose range of motion is measured in all three planes. The patient is placed supine on the examination table.

The anterior superior iliac spines are placed in the same plane as the table (Fig. 6-2). The examiner palpates the medial and lateral femoral epicondyles just proximal to the knee joint.

Internal and external hip range of motion

The calipers of a gravity goniometer are placed on the medial and lateral epicondyles. The leg is then internally rotated to the end range of motion (Fig. 6-3). Any motion beyond this point causes trunk rotation. The normal amount of internal motion is 45 degrees. The same procedure is

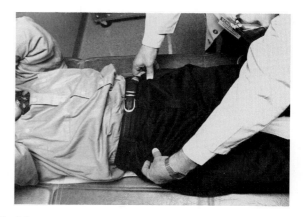

Fig. 6-2. The hips are placed in the frontal plane.

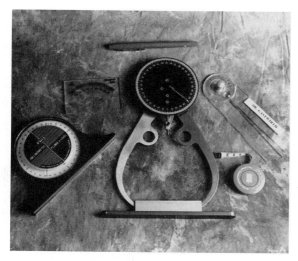

Fig. 6-1. Biomechanical instruments include an inclinometer, gravity goniometer, tractograph, tape measure, protractor, and felt-tip pen.

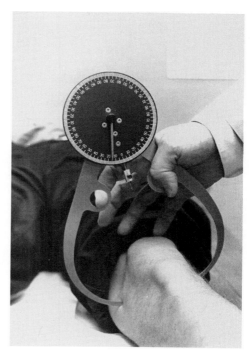

Fig. 6-3. The arms of the gravity goniometer are placed on the medial and lateral femoral epicondyles, and the leg is internally rotated.

repeated with the leg moved in the direction of external rotation (Fig. 6-4). The normal amount of external motion is 45 degrees. Since hip motion is influenced by the muscles and ligaments that originate and insert around it, the procedure for measurement is repeated with the patient in an upright sitting position. The neutral position of the hip is midway point between the maximal internal and maximal external rotation points.

Hip flexion

With the patient supine the tractograph is placed with one arm following the lateral border of the upper leg from a point from the greater trochanter to the lateral epicondyle of the femur with the other arm along the lateral surface of the trunk of the body (usually parallel to the superior surface of the flat examination table). The center of the goniometer is at the hip joint. With the knee extended, the leg is raised (Fig. 6-5) The usual range of hip flexion with the knee extended is 70 degrees or greater. The same procedure is repeated with the knee flexed (Fig. 6-6). Knee flexion allows for greater motion since the hamstrings are relaxed. The usual range of motion is 100 degrees or greater with the knee flexed. A gravity goniometer may also be used.

Hip extension

The patient is placed in a prone position. The same reference sites as used for hip flexion are identified. With the knee both flexed and extended, the range of motion of hip extension is determined (Figs. 6-7 and 6-8). The normal range of hip extension is 20 degrees with the knee extended and 30 degrees with the knee flexed.

Hip abduction and adduction

A tractograph is placed with one arm following the line connecting the anterior superior iliac spines and the other arm bisecting the upper leg. The leg is then adducted and abducted and the measurements are recorded (Figs. 6-9 and 6-10). Normal hip abduction is 45 degrees and adduction is at least 20 degrees.

Knee position

The knee joint is a highly complex joint and a common site of sports-related injuries. The motion of the knee is measured primarily in the sagittal plane (flexion and extension). Deviations from the frontal plane often predispose the knee joint to additional pathomechanical faults and therefore

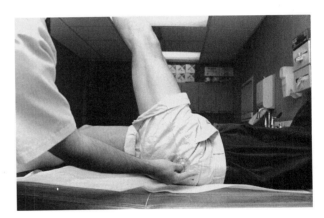

Fig. 6-5. The arms of the tractograph are lined up with the bisection of the trunk and the lateral bisection of the leg, and the leg is flexed.

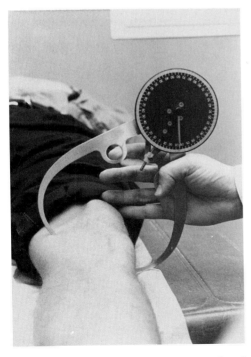

Fig. 6-4. The arms of the gravity goniometer are placed on the medial and lateral femoral epicondyles, and the leg is externally rotated.

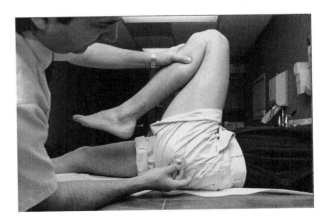

Fig. 6-6. Hip flexion is measured with the knee flexed.

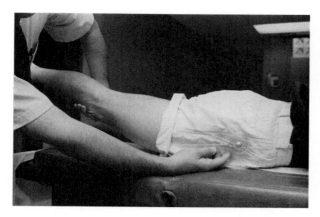

Fig. 6-7. Hip extension is measured with one arm of the tractograph bisecting the trunk and the other arm bisecting the lateral aspect of the upper leg.

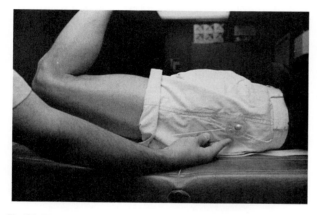

Fig. 6-8. Hip extension is measured with the knee flexed.

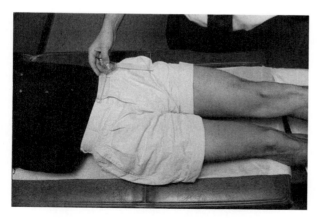

Fig. 6-9. Hip adduction is measured with one arm of the tractograph lined up with the anterior superior iliac spines and the other arm bisecting the femur while the leg is moved to its end range of adduction.

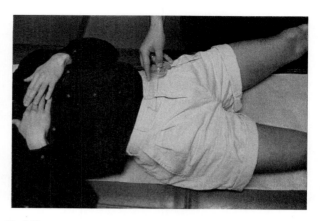

Fig. 6-10. Hip abduction is measured.

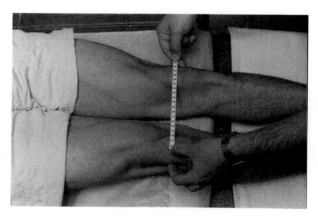

Fig. 6-11. The examiner notes and measures any frontal plane knee deformities.

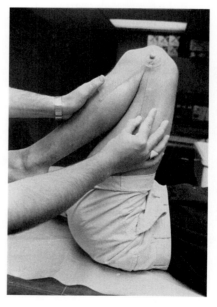

Fig. 6-12. Knee flexion is measured with one arm of the tractograph placed on the lateral bisection of the upper leg and the other arm bisecting the lower leg. The center of the tractograph is placed at the knee joint axis.

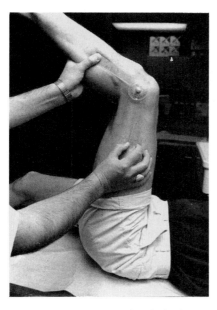

Fig. 6-13. Knee extension is measured with the knee moved into its end range of extension.

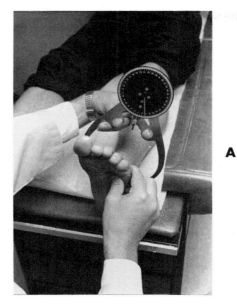

A

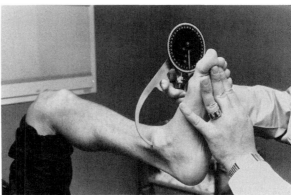

B

Fig. 6-15. A and B, The arms of a gravity goniometer are placed on the malleolar bisections, and the measurement of malleolar position is determined.

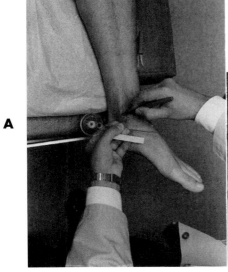

A

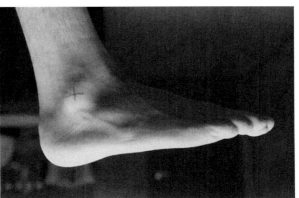

B

Fig. 6-14. The bisections of the medial (A) and lateral (B) malleoli are determined and marked.

require inspection (Fig. 6-11). Knee flexion is measured with one arm of the tractograph placed along a line bisecting the lateral border of the femur and the second arm along a line bisecting the lower leg. The center of the tractograph is placed at the knee joint axis (Fig. 6-12). Knee flexion is measured with the hip extended and the hip flexed. The normal

range of motion equals 140 to 160 degrees of knee flexion with the hip flexed and 120 degrees of flexion with the hip extended. Knee extension is also measured with the hip flexed and extended (Fig. 6-13). With the hip flexed at 90 degrees the normal amount of knee extension equals 160 degrees, or 20 degrees of flexion. With the hip extended, knee extension equals 180 degrees, or 0 degrees of flexion. Inability of the knee to flex or extend normally is generally consistent with quadriceps or hamstring tightness. The position of the knee in the frontal plane is determined by having the patient lie in a supine position with the pelvis in the frontal plane. The lower legs are gently brought together. Should the knees meet prematurely with the position of the feet being separated, a valgus deformity, genu valgum, is present. The examiner quantifies the extent of the deformity by measuring the distance between the opposing medial malleolar bisections. Conversely, should the feet touch first with a separation being noted between the knee joints, a genu varum is the most likely cause. The varus deformity of the knee is quantified by measuring the distance between the opposing medial condylar surfaces of the knee.

Malleolar position

Malleolar position is a reflection of true tibial torsion, which cannot be measured clinically. The examiner should palpate and then mark the bisection of the medial and lateral malleoli (Fig. 6-14). This is not always represented by the high point of the malleolus. The knee is then placed with the

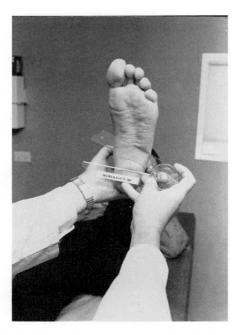

Fig. 6-16. An alternative measurement of malleolar position using a tractograph.

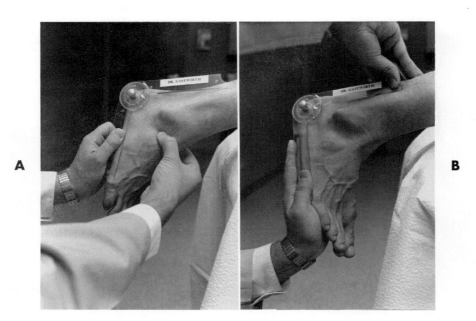

Fig. 6-17. A and **B,** The proper position of tractograph placement is demonstrated for ankle joint range of motion.

transcondylar axis in the frontal plane. The arms of a gravity goniometer are placed at each of the malleolar bisections, and the angle is measured (Fig. 6-15). A tractograph can also be used (Fig. 6-16). The normal malleolar position is 13 to 18 degrees external. Care must be taken to neither pronate nor supinate the subtalar joint when obtaining this measurement. When the examiner touches the foot during this measurement, a closed kinetic chain situation is created. Therefore, inadvertent supination of the foot while obtaining this measurement will increase the degree of malleolar position. Conversely, inadvertent pronation of the foot while obtaining this measurement will decrease the degree of malleolar position.

Ankle joint measurements

The ankle joint is a pronatory-supinatory joint. Its movement has been described as a coning-type movement, primarily in the sagittal plane. To measure ankle joint range of motion, the subtalar joint is placed in its neutral position. A tractograph is placed at the level of the ankle joint with one arm of the tractograph along the lateral leg bisection and the other arm along the lateral margin of the foot (Fig. 6-17A). The transcondylar axis of the knee should be in the frontal plane and the knee should be fully extended. The examiner then applies a loading force to the forefoot to allow the ankle joint to dorsiflex to its end range of motion (Fig. 6-17B). The normal range of ankle dorsiflexion gradually

decreases with time. After the age of 15 years, normal ankle joint dorsiflexion is 5 to 10 degrees with the knee extended. Inadvertent pronation of the subtalar joint while recording this measurement will unlock the midtarsal joint, thereby allowing its oblique axis to dorsiflex. If this occurs, the examiner may incorrectly assess a normal range of motion when in fact a true limitation might exist. The examiner repeats the same procedure with the knee flexed in order to record the range of motion of the ankle joint, eliminating the influence of the gastrocnemius muscle (Fig. 6-18). Ankle joint dorsiflexion with the knee flexed should approach 15 degrees. If limitation of ankle joint motion is noted in both knee extension and flexion, then a gastrocnemius-soleus equinus may exist. Because a bony ankle block may be responsible for the same clinical picture, stress lateral radiographs should be obtained. To complete the evaluation of the ankle the examiner moves the foot in the direction of plantarflexion (Fig. 6-19). The normal amount of plantarflexion of the ankle joint is 40 to 70 degrees. The range of motion is then recorded.

First-ray position

The first ray has its own independent axis of motion. It is a pronatory-supinatory joint, although first-ray position and excursion are determined in the sagittal plane. With the subtalar joint placed in its neutral position the examiner grasps the second through fifth metatarsal heads between the thumb and index finger of one hand. The nail plate of the thumb is placed parallel to the plane of the metatarsals. The other hand holds the first metatarsal head in a similar fashion (Fig. 6-20A). With the foot evenly loaded the examiner moves the first metatarsal dorsally and plantarly and records its motion (Figs.

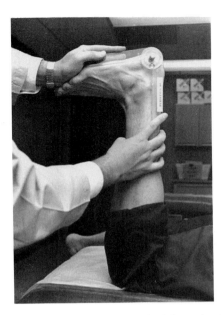

Fig. 6-18. The ankle joint is dorsiflexed while maintaining the subtalar joint in its neutral position.

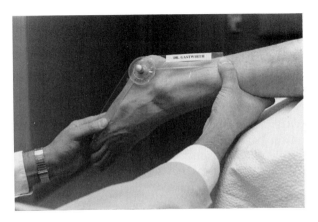

Fig. 6-19. The ankle joint is plantarflexed.

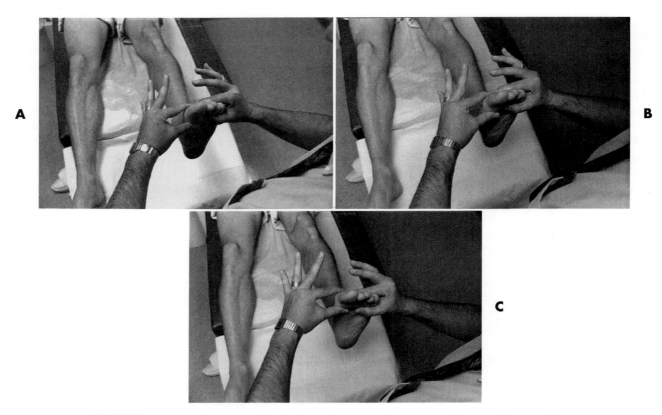

Fig. 6-20. The proper placement of the hands to determine first metatarsal range of motion, from neutral **(A)**, to plantarflexion **(B)**, to dorsiflexion **(C)**.

6-20**B** and **C**). The normal range of motion is 10 to 12 mm, with dorsal excursion equaling plantar excursion. The examiner records its full range of motion as well as the position of the first metatarsal relative to the second metatarsal. In this fashion, a dorsiflexed or plantarflexed first-ray deformity may be diagnosed. Asymmetric first-ray positions are common in the same individual, and are associated with asymmetric foot function.

First metatarsophalangeal joint measurements

First metatarsolphalangeal joint range of motion may be measured in two ways. The medial aspect of the proximal phalanx is identified. The dorsal excursion of the hallux is measured against the medial bisection of the first metatarsal, allowing the first metatarsal to plantarflex. The dorsal range of motion is 65 to 75 degrees (Fig. 6-21). If the proximal point of reference is the plantar surface of the foot,

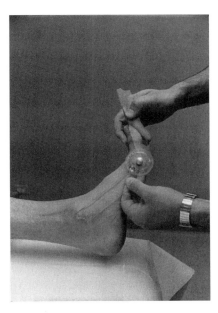

Fig. 6-21. First metatarsophalangeal dorsiflexion is measured by placing one arm of the tractograph against the medial bisection of the proximal phalanx and the other arm against the medial bisection of the first metatarsal while the hallux is maximally dorsiflexed.

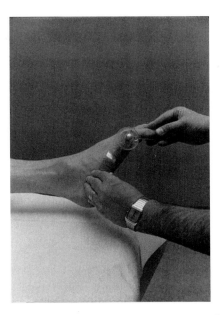

Fig. 6-23. First metatarsophalangeal joint plantarflexion is determined.

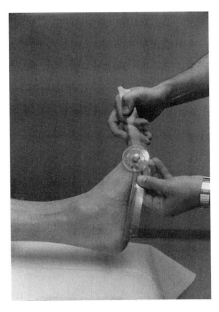

Fig. 6-22. First metatarsophalangeal joint dorsiflexion is measured with the proximal arm of the tractograph placed along the planter surface of the foot.

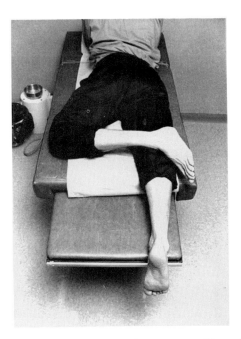

Fig. 6-24. The patient is placed in the supine position with the transcondylar axis of the knee in the frontal plane.

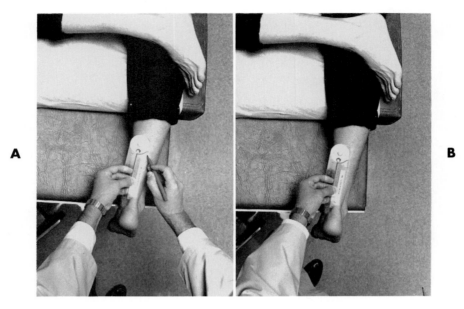

Fig. 6-25. A and **B,** Bisection of the lower one third of the leg is performed.

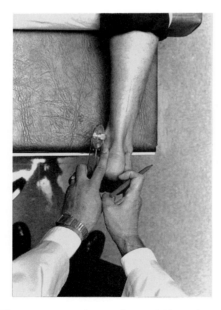

Fig. 6-26. The examiner palpates the medial and lateral aspect of the heel.

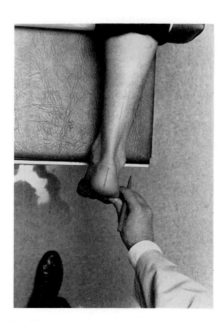

Fig. 6-27. A heel bisection line is drawn.

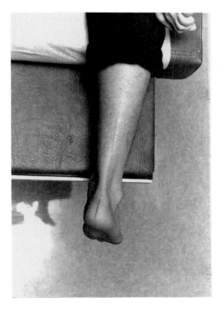

Fig. 6-28. The bisection lines of the heel and leg.

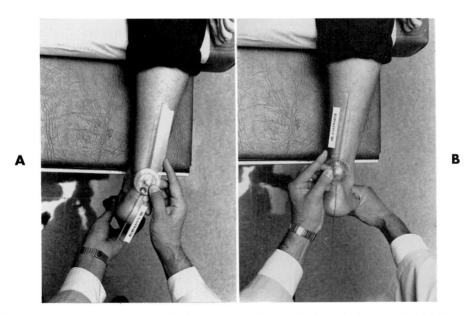

Fig. 6-29. The subtalar joint is moved to its end range of inversion **(A)** and eversion. **(B)** Motion and excursion values are recorded.

the range of dorsal excursion will be closer to 20 degrees (Fig. 6-22). Plantarflexion of the first metatarsolphalangeal joint is normally 45 degrees, the reference point being the plantar surface of the foot (Fig. 6-23).

Subtalar joint measurements

The subtalar joint is a pronatory-supinatory joint whose main component of motion is in the frontal plane. It is the frontal plane motion that is used as the standard to define the subtalar joint neutral position. The average range of motion of the subtalar joint is 30 degrees: 20 degrees of inversion motion and 10 degrees of eversion motion. To measure the subtalar joint, anatomic landmarks are established. The patient lies prone on a flat examination table and the knee is placed in the frontal plane (Fig. 6-24). The lower one third of the leg is marked on its posterior aspect. This is done by determining and marking the medial and lateral margins of the leg with a felt-tip pen, bisecting the marks and connecting them with a line (Fig. 6-25). Three sites are used for greater accuracy. Next, the posterior aspect of the heel is marked. The examiner palpates the calcaneus on its superior, middle, and inferior levels and bisects each location (Fig. 6-26). A felt-tip pen is used to mark the location and connect the points of reference (Figs. 6-27 and 6-28). Continuing the line onto the plantar aspect of the foot is useful because it allows the examiner to evaluate the forefoot-to-rearfoot measurement more accurately. A goniometer is placed with its central point at the level of the subtalar joint. One arm of the tracto-

graph is placed on the superior line of the leg and the other arm is placed at the heel bisection line. The examiner then passively moves the subtalar joint into its end range of inversion and eversion motions and records its excursion values (Fig. 6-29). Care must be taken to place the foot at a right angle to the leg. Inadvertent plantarflexion of the foot during, this measurement introduces additional frontal plane motion to the ankle, thereby inaccurately increasing the total range of subtalar joint motion.

Subtalar neutral position

The subtalar joint neutral position is determined in the following manner: the clinician palpates the medial and lateral aspect of the talar head as the

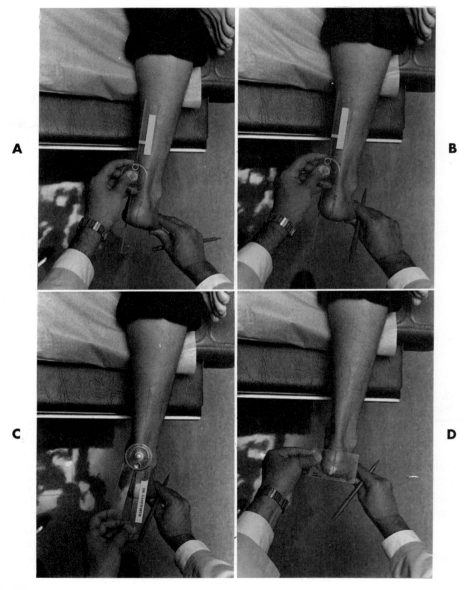

Fig. 6-30. A–D, The subtalar joint neutral position is determined and recorded.

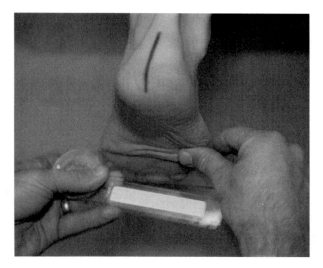

Fig. 6-31. The examiner compares the position of the plane of the forefoot to the rearfoot bisection with the subtalar joint in its neutral position and with the midtarsal joint maximally pronated to determine the forefoot neutral position.

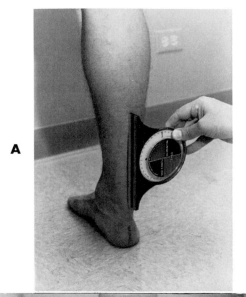

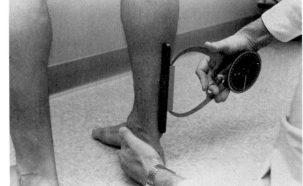

Fig. 6-32. A and **B,** With the patient standing in the angle and base of gait and the subtalar joint held in its neutral position, the angle of the bisection of the lower leg relative to the ground determines the tibial position.

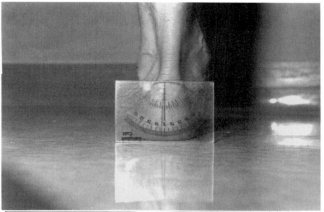

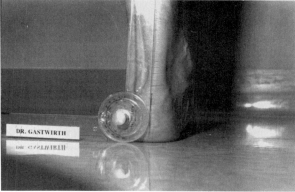

Fig. 6-33. A and **B,** The resting calcaneal stance position is determined by measuring the posterior bisection line of the heel to the ground with the foot relaxed.

subtalar joint is moved from an everted to an inverted position. When the talar head is felt to be the same on its medial and lateral sides, the examiner adds a loading force to the forefoot and the ankle joint is dorsiflexed to 90 degrees or to its end motion if less than 90 degrees. The position of the heel bisection is then compared with the leg bisection. The clinician may draw a line from the leg to connect to the heel for ease of measurement (Fig. 6-30**A** and **B**). The numeric value can be measured by using a tractograph or protractor (Fig. 6-30**C** and **D**).

Forefoot position

The forefoot position is measured in the following manner. With the subtalar joint maintained in its neutral position, the examiner applies a dorsiflexion loading force to the forefoot, with thumb and index finger holding the foot in the toe sulcus across the lesser toes. Care is taken not to dorsiflex or plantarflex the metatarsophalangeal joints. Utilizing a tractograph held with the other hand, the practitioner views and records the plane of the metatarsal heads as compared to the rearfoot bisection (Fig. 6-31). This is accomplished by lightly placing the tractograph arm across the plane of the metatarsal heads.

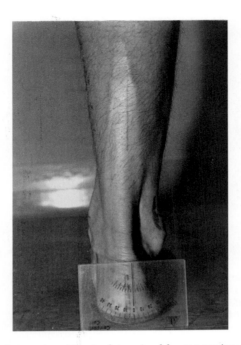

Fig. 6-34. Neutral calcaneal stance position is determined by measuring the heel position to the ground with the subtalar joint held in its neutral position.

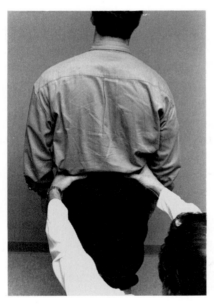

Fig. 6-35. The posterior superior iliac spines are palpated and checked for symmetry.

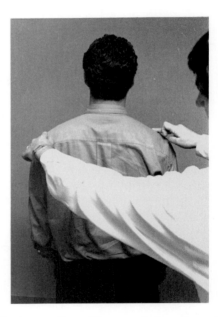

Fig. 6-36. The top portion of the scapula is compared with its contralateral side.

The angular relationship of the plane of the first through fifth metatarsals and the plane of the second through fifth metatarsals is recorded. The normal forefoot position should be perpendicular to the heel bisection with the subtalar joint in its neutral position and the midtarsal joint fully pronated or locked.

Stance measurements

Tibial position

The patient is asked to stand and is placed in the angle and base of gait as determined from gait assessment. The examiner places the foot in its neutral position and places the arm of a goniometer or inclinometer along the posterior leg bisection line

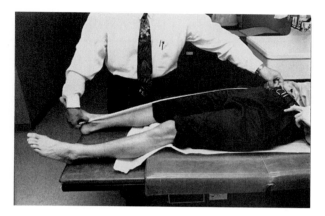

Fig. 6-37. With the patient placed in the supine position the leg lengths are measured from the anterior superior iliac spine to the bisection of the medial malleolus.

(Fig. 6-32). The normal relationship of the lower portion of the leg to the ground is 0 to 4 degrees of varus angulation.

Resting calcaneal stance position

With the patient standing in the angle and base of gait, the posterior surface of the calcaneus is measured (Fig. 6-33). The examiner should check the heel bisection line relative to the osseous structure to ensure that skin stretching has not altered the accuracy of the heel bisection. If there is any doubt that the original line has shifted, then the heel should be bisected again in the standing position.

Neutral calcaneal stance position

The posterior heel bisection is measured with the subtalar joint in its neutral position (Fig. 6-34).

Postural considerations

With the patient in the angle and base of gait, the posterior superior iliac spines are palpated and checked for symmetry (Fig. 6-35). The top portion of the scapula is compared with the contralateral side (Fig. 6-36). Variations of height may be due to limb length inequalities or aberrant spinal curvatures.

Limb length measurements

The patient is placed in the supine position with care taken to place the anterior superior iliac spines in the frontal plane. Using a tape measure, the distance from the anterior superior iliac spine to the medial malleolar bisection is determined and compared with the adjacent limb (Fig. 6-37). An additional method of determining limb length inequality is to have the patient stand in the angle and base of gait. Palpation of the anterior superior iliac crests, as well as the greater trochanters of the femur and the pelvic brim may indicate a limb length inequality. This evaluation should be carried out in both the relaxed and neutral calcaneal stance positions. An asymmetric limb length that improves with both feet maintained in their neutral positions suggests a functional limb length inequality. If a discernible difference exists with the patients in both the relaxed and neutral positions, then a structural limb length difference may be responsible. Building up the apparent shortened limb with sheets of plastic (e.g., 3 or 4 mm of polypropylene) until there is no clinically observable asymmetry will provide the examiner with an approximation of the shortage. A standing pelvic radiograph may also be utilized to more specifically determine the extent of the limb length inequalities.

References

1. Blake RL, Ross AS, Valmassy RL: Biomechanics gait evaluation, *J Am Podiatr Med Assoc*, 71:341–343, 1981.
2. Blake RL, Valmassy RL. Runner's knee examination form, *J Am Podiatry Assoc* 71:397–403, 1981.
3. Finkelstein HB, et al: *Basic Concepts of Physical Therapy for the Lower Extremity*, Chicago, Scholl College of Podiatric Medicine, 1983.
4. Frankel VH, Nordin M: *Basic Biomechanics of the Skeletal System*, Philadelphia, Lea & Febiger, 1980.
5. Gould JA, Davies GJ: *Orthopaedic and Sports Physical Therapy vol 2.* St Louis, Mosby–Year Book, 1975.
6. Green DR, Sgarlato TE, Wittenberg M: Clinical biomechanical evaluation of the foot: a preliminary radiocinematographic study, *J Am Podiatry Assoc* 65:732–755, 1975.
7. Hoppenfeld S: *Physical Examination of the Spine and Extremities*, New York, Appleton-Century-Crofts, 1976.
8. Kapandji IA. *The Physiology of the Joints, 3 vols.* New York, Churchill-Livingstone, 1970.
9. LaPorta GA, Scarlet J: Radiographic changes in the pronated and supinated foot: a statistical analysis, *J Am Podiatry Assoc*, 67:334–338, 1977.
10. MacConaill MA, Basmajian JV: *Muscles and Movements: Basis for Human Kinesiology*, ed 2, Huntington, NY, RC Krieger, 1977.
11. Orien WP, et al, *The National Orthopedics/Biomechanics Curriculum*, 1991.
12. Root ML, Orien WP, Weed JH, et al, *Biomechanical Examination of the Foot, vol 1.* Calif, Los Angeles Clinical Biomechanics, 1971.
13. Root ML, Orien WP, Weed JH: *Normal and Abnormal Function of the Foot, ed 1*, Calif, Los Angeles Clinical Biomechanics, 1977.
14. Sgarlato TE: *A Compendium of Podiatric Biomechanics*, San Francisco, California College of Podiatric Medicine, 1971.
15. Valmassy RL: Biomechanical evaluation of the child, *Clin Podiatry* 1:563–579, 1984.
16. Valmassy RL, Stanton B: Tibial torsion: normal values in children, *J Am Podiatr Med Assoc* 79:432–435, 1989.

Appendix: evaluation of lower extremity capability and performance

NAME: _____ #: _____ DOB: __/__/__ DATE: __/__/__

CHIEF COMPLAINT: ___ EXAMINING PHYSICIAN: _____

I. RELEVANT HISTORY
   A. All congenital and hereditary deformities and disorders and all lower extremity trauma:
   _____

   B. Current footgear: _____

   C. Current vocational activities: _____

   D. Current recreational activities: _____

   E. Pertinent past activities: _____

   F. Previous lower extremity treatment: _____

   G. Plantar lesions: _____
      Right _____ Left _____
   H. Dorsal lesions: _____
      Right _____ Left _____

II. EVALUATION OF ANGLE AND BASE OF GAIT
    WEIGHTBEARING X-RAY STUDIES

III. KINETIC STANCE (GAIT): Record all abnormal variations and asymmetries
     A. Angle of gait: R)   (L)
     B. Base of gait: _____ inches.
     C. Contact period: _____

     D. Midstance period: _____

     E. Proplusive period: _____
     F. Postural considerations: _____

	Right	**Left**
IV. STATIC STANCE		
A. Relaxed calcaneal stance position:	INV/EV	INV/EV
B. Neutral calcaneal stance position:	INV/EV	INV/EV
C. Frontal plane tibial position:	INV/EV	INV/EV
(measured with subtalar joint in neutral)		

V. EVALUATION OF MOTION AND POSITION—SUPINE
   Record all axis variations and abnormal quality of motion under Comments

A. Hip joint:	EXTENDED	INT/EXT	INT/EXT
	FLEXED	INT/EXT	INT/EXT
	NEUTRAL	INT/EXT	INT/EXT

   Comments: _____

B. Knee joint: Record only abnormalities

	Right	Left
C. Malleolar relationship:	INT/EXT	INT/EXT

D. Comparative morphologic and length
   variations of the lower extremities: _____

VI. EVALUATION OF MOTION AND POSITION—PRONE
Record all axis variations and abnormal quality of motion under Comments

	Right	Left
A. Subtalar joint:	SUP/PRO	SUP/PRO
Neutral position (foot to leg):	INV/EV	INV/EV

Comments: _____

_____

B. Midtarsal joint:	VAR/VAL	VAR/VAL

Comments:

C. Ankle joint:

Knee extended:	DOR/PLN	DOR/PLN
Knee flexed:	DOR/PLN	DOR/PLN

Comments: _____

_____

D. First ray:	DOR/PLN	DOR/PLN

Comments: _____

_____

	Right	Left
E. First Metatarsophalangeal joint	DOR/PLN	DOR/PLN

Comments: _____

_____

F. Lesser metatarsophalangeal joints:
   Comments: _____

_____

VII. MANUAL MUSCLE TESTING FOR STRENGTH:
Record only abnormal findings

VIII. MANUAL MUSCLE TESTING FOR LENGTH:
Record only abnormal findings

IX. DIAGNOSTIC IMPRESSIONS:
1.
2.
3.
4.
5.

X. TREATMENT RECOMMENDATIONS:
1.
2.
3.
4.

Reprinted from O'Brien WP, editor, *A curriculum for podiatric orthopedics and biomechanics.* 1991 Edition. N.O./B.F.C.

gait evaluation in clinical biomechanics

Charles C. Southerland, Jr., DPM

Introduction

Gait analysis
Plantar lesion patterns

Dynamic examination
A review of basics
Site location for gait analysis and TBFR
   sequence
Line of progression
Phasic observations
Crosschecking and verifying

Neurologic and acquired gait abnormalities
Myopathies
Neuromuscular junction
Lower motor neuron dysfunction
Upper motor neuron dysfunction

Summary

Introduction

Podiatric medicine is unique among healthcare disciplines for the amount of time spent training its students in the principles of biomechanics. Curricula in medicine and surgery, which must necessarily occupy a considerable portion of podiatric medical school agendas, do not serve to make the podiatrist stand apart from other primary healthcare professionals. All medical students must learn essential details of medicine and surgery. No other group of healthcare professionals in the world spends as much time in their professional education learning "the application of mechanical laws to living structures, specifically to the locomotor systems of the human body"[8] as do podiatrists. Clinical *gait evaluation* must be a fundamental skill for podiatric physicians. While all seven schools of podiatric medicine have developed courses on gait evaluation, nomenclature, method, and outcome have yet to become standardized within the practicing community. Often, practitioners trained in the east must wrestle with shorthand script from those trained in the west, and vice versa. Simple terms such as "antalgia," "compensation," and "festination" are used to describe complex details of bipedal ambulation that may require different forms of intervention and therapy. Many practitioners have expressed a need for some reproducible model which can be used to express the finer details of dynamic gait on a static image such as a piece of paper.

In quest of a logical, easily interpreted, consistent, and reproducible model for gait evaluation, it is perhaps best to survey those instruments which are in use in the academic and practicing community. Surprisingly, there are very few. The California form is used by the California College of Podiatric Medicine as a patient evaluation form (Fig. 7-1). It incorporates features which include range-of-motion (ROM) testing along with observed gait evaluation to record the most relevant features of a biomechanical evaluation. This type of evaluation sheet has been used for nearly 15 years in a variety of forms, and has worked reasonably well as a clinical tool and teaching instrument. The form relies on checked boxes or written commentary.

Langer Biomechanics has a gait evaluation form which goes with its EDG electronic gait evaluation system[10] (Fig. 7-2). The form uses a program interface to display data and, ultimately, so-called data analysis statements (DASs). The DASs draw conclusions from intrinsic data noted on EDG sensor leads to determine abnormalities. Language is used on a DAS that is common to all podiatrists, and easily understood regardless of their training.

The graphs and summaries that precede these DAS commentaries are not always well understood by clinicians, nor is the correlation between the graphs and summaries and the DAS conclusions. The EDG text *A Practical Manual of Clinical Electrodynography*[13] explains the correlations, but requires considerable study. Most clinicians do not correlate data with much more than the DAS in drawing clinical conclusions on which to base treatment algorithms. Also, EDG instrumentation, while sophisticated, does not offer information on all factors that may affect gait, and which may be either observed or treatable. Other electrodiagnostic modalities, such as EMED, F-Scan, and Gait Track, offer sophisticated information about some subset of gait analysis which, while quite detailed, do not take into account the most pertinent aspects of "the big picture" of clinical pathomechanics in gait.

In an effort to standardize orthopedic and biomechanics nomenclature, the National Orthopedics/Biomechanics Faculties Committee (NO/BFC) has developed a text, *A Curriculum for Podiatric Orthopedics and Biomechanics.*[7] Within the text is a biomechanical clinical examination form called "Evaluation of Lower Extremity Capability and Performance." While an excellent review form for teaching detailed examination steps, the form is long and cumbersome to work with. In addition, the gait evaluation component of the evaluation form is basically blank, leaving it up to the user to fill in observations, which may be extensive or brief. Given the length of the form, the gait portion typically tends to be brief, and again, the vocabulary used on this national form may tend to reflect regional training.

Various commercial laboratories leave space on their prescription forms for clinical evaluation observations and measurements as an aid in helping technicians to develop orthoses. However, none of the laboratories have developed a standard format for recording clinical values and assessments.

In quest of a valid format for gait evaluation, research began in 1987 to experiment with various formats in conveying the concept of gait analysis to students of podiatric medicine. Several existing forms from various sources were used among different cohorts of junior- and senior-level students. The best features from each form were then combined into a single form and used as a testing vehicle. The essentials of successful interaction with any form rely on a personality profile that demonstrates motivation, receptivity, critical objectivity, and reliable comparative model distribution.[21] A scale of reproducibility was developed to determine the efficacy of forms used by various populations of clinical practitioners. Predictably, among those us-

EVALUATION OF LOWER EXTREMITY
CAPABILITY AND PERFORMANCE

Name:_____ #_____ DOB:___/___/___ Date of Exam:___/___/___

Chief Complaint: Examining Physician:

I. Relevant History

Plantar Lesions   Dorsal Lesions
Right   Left   Right   Left

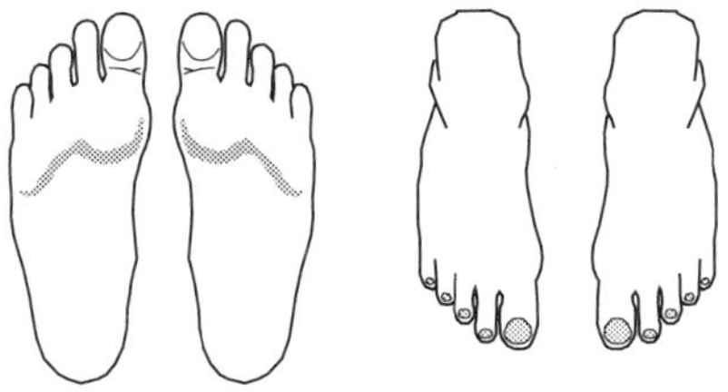

II. Kinetic Stance (Gait) (Record abnormal variations and asymmetries)

    A. Angle of gait: (R)   [ADD/ABD] (L)* [ADD/ABD]   B. Base of gait: inches.

           [Right]   [Left]

    C. Contact period:

    D. Midstance period:

    E. Propulsive period:

    F. Postural considerations (limb length/asymmetry):

III. Evaluation of Motion and Position – Supine (record axis variations and abnormal quality of motion)

		[Right]	[Left]	
A. Hip joint:	Extended.	INT./EXT.	INT./EXT.	
	Flexed.	INT./EXT.	INT./EXT.	
	Neutral.	INT./EXT.	INT./EXT.	

Comments:

    B. Knee joint: (record only abnormalities)

    C. Malleolar relationship: [Right]   INT./EXT. [Left]   INT./EXT.

A

Fig. 7-1. The California form. **A,** Front of form.   *Continued.*

ing the form in the beginning, we found a wide range of variance in data recorded when examinations were performed on the same subject or patient. Typically, researchers expect an increasing reliability to be reflected on measurable parameters when examining an abstract instrument such as a clinical evaluation form. Indeed, we find that reproducibil-ity does increase with experience in using the form referred to in this chapter. Generally, by about the fourth or fifth patient evaluation, the level of reproducibility in comparative studies of different examiners on the same patient was quite high. The balance of this chapter discusses the instrument that has evolved for documenting gait evaluation. For

IV. Evaluation of Motion and Position: Prone (record axis variations and abnormal quality of motion)

		[Right]	[Left]
A. Subtalar joint:		SUP./PRO.	SUP./PRO.
	Neutral position: (foot to leg)	INV./EV.	INV./EV.
	Comments:		
B. Midtarsal joint:		INV./EV.	INV./EV.
	Comments:		
C. Ankle joint:	Knee extended:	DOR./PLN.	DOR./PLN.
	Knee flexed:	DOR./PLN.	DOR./PLN.
	Comments:		
D. First Ray:		DOR./PLN.	DOR./PLN.
	Comments:		
E. First metatarsal-phalangeal joint:		DOR./PLN.	DOR./PLN.
	Comments:		
F. Lessor metatarsal-phalangeal joints:			
	Comments:		

V. Static Stance

	[Right]	[Left]
A. Relaxed calcaneal position:	INV./EV.	INV./EV.
B. Neutral calcaneal position:	INV./EV.	INV./EV.
C. Frontal plane tibial position:	INV./EV.	INV./EV.
(Measured with STJ in neutral)		

VI. Manual Muscle Testing (record only abnormal findings)

VII. Evaluation of Weight-Bearing X-rays (taken in angle and base of gait)

VIII. Diagnostic Impressions: IX. Treatment Recommendations:

1.   1.

2.   2.

3.   3.

4.   Student

5.   Clinician

Fig. 7-1, cont'd. The California form. **B,** Back of form.

purposes of accuracy in gait evaluation, the form has been found to be reliable, reproducible, and highly interpretable.

Gait analysis

Gait analysis is divided into two major segments: static and dynamic. In the static portion, available ROMs are measured from hip to toe. In the interest of consistency, sequencing should always be the same. Therefore, the form attempts to evaluate according to a "top-to-bottom, front-to-rear" (TBFR, pronounced "TeeBFuR") sequencing. This static portion of the gait evaluation process attempts to reproducibly *quantify* motions in the lower extremity, whereas the dynamic evaluation section at-

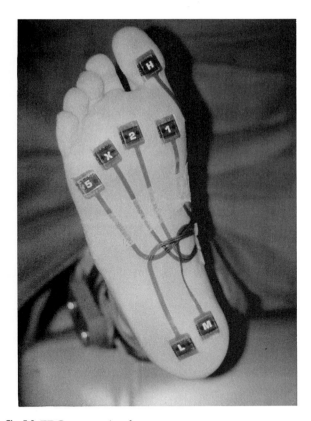

Fig. 7-2. EDG sensors in place.

tempts only to reproducibly *qualify* observations. Quantification and qualification are mechanisms which have long been considered essential standards in scientific analysis.[12]

Within static portions of the evaluation form, examination data are further broken down into open and closed kinetic chain. The sequence of evaluation following a TBFR format is as follows (Fig. 7-3):

I. Static examination
  A. Open kinetic chain (OKC)
    1. Patient supine (semi-Fowler's position)
      a. Hip ROM
      b. Knee position (qualified)
      c. Tibial torsion
      d. Ankle joint dorsiflexion—knee extended
      e. First-ray ROM
    2. Patient prone
      a. Ankle joint dorsiflexion—knee flexed
      b. Subtalar joint (STJ) maximum inversion
      c. STJ maximum eversion
      d. *Calculated* STJ neutral position
      e. Forefoot-to-rearfoot position
      f. Plantar lesion patterns
  B. Closed kinetic chain (CKC)

1. Angle and base of gait
2. Limb length (from anterior superior iliac spine to medial malleolus)
3. Tibial position
4. Neutral calcaneal stance position (NCSP)
5. Relaxed calcaneal stance position (RCSP)

The second half of the evaluation form deals with dynamic examination, and is the focus of this chapter. Dynamic activity is intrinsically more difficult to capture on a sheet of paper, which is itself in essence a static image. It must be the aim of the form, therefore, to capture that moment of evaluation in which the anatomy is physiologically most deviated from an accepted ideal norm. Again, following the TBFR format, points of evaluation include:

II. Dynamic examination
  A. Head tilt
  B. Facial symmetry
  C. Shoulder drop
  D. Spinal linearity
  E. Hip tilt
  F. Q angle
  G. Patellar position
  H. Tibial position
  I. STJ
    1. ROM
    2. Neutral position
    3. Rearfoot position
    4. STJ compensated position
  J. Forefoot-to-Rearfoot position
  K. Angle and base of gait relative to line of progression (LOP)
  L. STJ dynamic graph
  M. Phasic observations
    1. Stance
      a. Contact
      b. Midstance
      c. Propulsive
    2. Swing

Given the above data criteria, it should be possible to draw conclusions about almost any abnormality that is expressed through gait. Figure 7-4 shows the complete evaluation form. The sheet of paper, printed on one side, contains all the information listed above, and offers considerable space for marginal notations. In addition to the above-noted parameters, there are several shorthand notation systems on the form which we will review as they pertain to gait analysis. Most of the first half of the form (see Static Examination) is part of a biomechanical examination process which

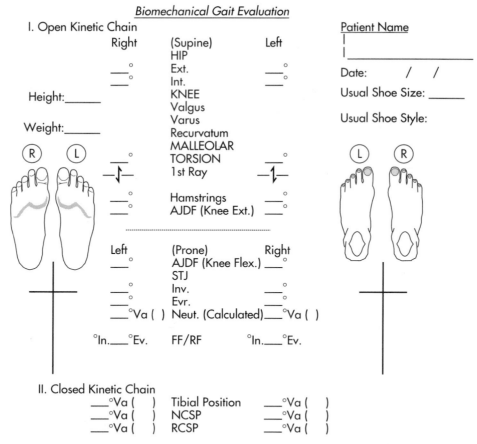

Fig. 7-3. Static portion of the gait evaluation form.

should be familiar to most clinicians. It is discussed in depth elsewhere in this text. Our principle focus for the balance of this chapter is on the dynamic portion of the evaluation form, which is the essence of clinical gait analysis.

Although clinical biomechanical evaluation is covered elsewhere in this text, there is one feature of the static examination which we must refer to in order to understand one essential feature of gait analysis, that is, subtalar joint range of motion (STJ ROM). While the total range of motion of the subtalar joint may not be apparent during dynamic gait analysis, it is most important that the clinician understand the limits of this motion, as well as the reference neutral positions in both the open (STJ neutral position) and closed (neutral calcaneal stance position, NCSP) kinetic chains. STJ ROM occurs from forces directed to an angular momentum driven around the axis of the STJ from a primary moment located on the anterior and medial talar dome. Because this force is directed toward eversion, the range of eversion is normally limited in comparison to the range of inversion, which is not driven by distribution forces of gravity. The most

common formula used to express this relationship is a 2:1 ratio of inversion to eversion. Determining the midpoint of this total 2:1 ROM is done both mathematically and clinically. The STJ neutral position (STJ Neut) is calculated as follows:

Method A
STJ Neut = (maximum eversion of STJ from distal 1/3rd of leg)° − (total STJ ROM/3)°
that is, if the calcaneus *inverts* 22 degrees from the distal one third of the leg, and the calcaneus *everts* 8 degrees from the distal one third of the leg:
$$STJ\ Neut = 8° − (8° + 22°/3)$$
$$STJ\ Neut = 8° − (30°/3)$$
$$STJ\ Neut = 8° − 10°$$
$$STJ\ Neut = −2°$$
Note: By convention, a minus sign implies varus angulation, while a plus sign implies valgus angulation.

Method B
STJ Neut = [(total STJ ROM/3) × 2] − maximum inversion of STJ from distal 1/3rd of leg
Using the same measured indices from above:
$$STJ\ Neut = [(30°/3) × 2] − 22°$$

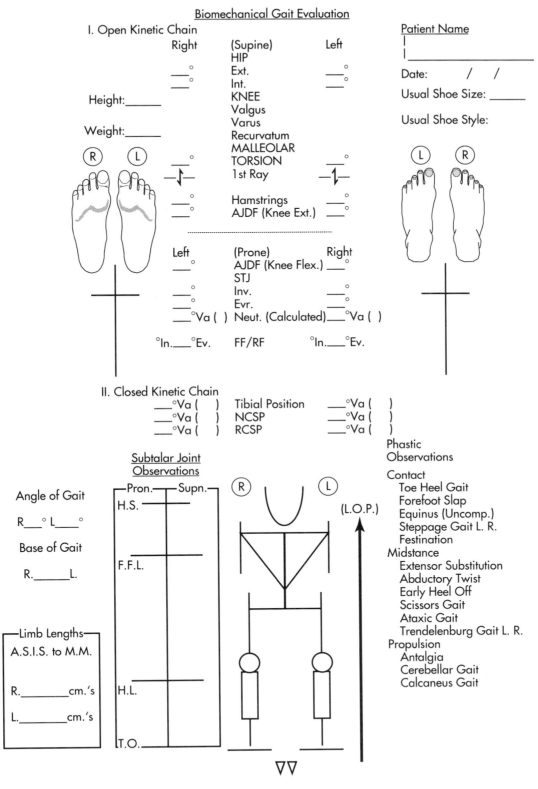

Biomechanical Gait Evaluation

I. Open Kinetic Chain

Right	(Supine)	Left
	HIP	
___°	Ext.	___°
___°	Int.	___°
	KNEE	
	Valgus	
	Varus	
	Recurvatum	
___°	MALLEOLAR TORSION	___°
	1st Ray	
___°	Hamstrings	___°
___°	AJDF (Knee Ext.)	___°

Height:_____

Weight:_____

Left	(Prone)	Right
___°	AJDF (Knee Flex.)	___°
	STJ	
___°	Inv.	___°
___°	Evr.	___°
___°Va ( )	Neut. (Calculated)	___°Va ( )
°In.___°Ev.	FF/RF	°In.___°Ev.

Patient Name
| _____

Date: /   /

Usual Shoe Size: _____

Usual Shoe Style:

II. Closed Kinetic Chain

___°Va ( )	Tibial Position	___°Va ( )
___°Va ( )	NCSP	___°Va ( )
___°Va ( )	RCSP	___°Va ( )

Subtalar Joint Observations

Pron.——Supn.—
H.S.

F.F.L.

H.L.

T.O.

Angle of Gait

R___° L___°

Base of Gait

R._____L.

┌─Limb Lengths─┐
A.S.I.S. to M.M.

R._____cm.'s

L._____cm.'s

(L.O.P.)

Phastic Observations

Contact
  Toe Heel Gait
  Forefoot Slap
  Equinus (Uncomp.)
  Steppage Gait L. R.
  Festination
Midstance
  Extensor Substitution
  Abductory Twist
  Early Heel Off
  Scissors Gait
  Ataxic Gait
  Trendelenburg Gait L. R.
Propulsion
  Antalgia
  Cerebellar Gait
  Calcaneus Gait

Fig. 7-4. Gait evaluation form.

$$STJ\ Neut = [10° \times 2] - 22°$$
$$STJ\ Neut = -2°$$

There is a shorthand method of recording STJ ROM which bears mentioning at this point. Conventional physics has long since assigned standards to most concepts of linear and angular motion.[5] When conveying concepts related to angular motion, physicists recognize that angular motion in two dimensions may occur. In a two-dimensional universe, it is relatively simple to assign titles to these motions such as the universally understood direction of a clock. Therefore, in describing angular motion in only two dimensions, the terms *clockwise* and *counterclockwise* are used. While various combinations of momentum, force, acceleration, and moments of inertia may be applied, generally, a plus value is ascribed to counterclockwise rotation, while a minus value is most often ascribed to clockwise rotations. This convention cannot be adopted without the caveat that rotation does not in reality occur within a two-dimensional universe. While concepts of "clockwise" and "counterclockwise" apply very effectively to a clock with a one-sided face, the roles are reversed when one views rotation from the opposite perspective. Movements that appear clockwise on one side of the circle appear counterclockwise on the other side. Unfortunately, in an enantiomeric universe, it is difficult to describe rotational motion in three dimensions other than to refer to it as "fixed angular motion." Therefore, it is often helpful to represent angular motion on paper from a two-dimensional perspective (i.e., as if there were no other side, no mirror image, no left or right hemisphere). When referring to varus rotations, we attempt to represent them as (−) counterclockwise. When referring to valgus rotations, we attempt to describe them as (+) clockwise. Understanding this, it is possible to use an intersectional diagram to describe in simple terms information that is most relative to STJ function. A cross-shaped diagram is inscribed as the template or basic illustration onto which additional data can be recorded. The lower, longer arm of the cross represents a ray that is continuous with the distal third of the tibia. The upper shorter arm of the vertical segment of the cross represents a perpendicular plane to the ground relative to the leg. A horizontal crossbeam represents a transverse plane intersection of the STJ (Fig. 7-5).

Varus movement of the calcaneus in a frontal plane around the STJ axis (relative to the distal third of the tibia) occurs in a clockwise (−) direction. Rotational vectors drawn above the horizontal line in a clockwise direction imply tibial varus angulation. Rotational vectors drawn below the horizontal line in a counterclockwise (+) direction imply tibial

valgus angulation. An additional line with an **N** drawn onto its distal point represents the neutral position of the STJ. This shorthand method of recording measured and calculated data becomes very useful in identifying limits of compensation during active gait.

Plantar lesion patterns

Just prior to starting a dynamic evaluation, the last point of examination in OKC should be to record lesion patterns. On the evaluation form are line drawings of feet which provide a place to record areas of hyperkeratosis (Fig. 7-6). The examiner runs his or her thumb or finger along the entire plantar surface and records, in traced shades, areas of greater or lessor callus formation. Both dorsal and plantar surfaces are represented. Hard and soft corns, intractable plantar keratomas, nucleated keratomas, and tylomas of any observable description (whether or not symptomatic) should be traced onto representative areas of the illustration. It is well established that shearing forces acting on plantar surfaces caused by compensatory mechanisms will form nontender, but clearly discernible tyloma patterns with great predictability.[18]

These patterns are important in recording, and later in contrasting, separately measured parameters with pathomechanical evidence of compensation deformities. It is also useful at this point to detail other soft tissue abnormalities such as the Haglund deformity, plantar fascial bowing and masses, hallux abducto valgus (HAV), hammer toes, clavi, and tailor's bunions. In tracing lesions onto line drawings of the foot, an effort should be made in gray-scale tracing to make denser lesions appear darker, and mild lesions appear lighter (Fig. 7-7).

Dynamic examination

In developing a method for recording dynamic gait cycle observations, attempts were made at various methods of detailing information. Many generations of ergonomic studies have demonstrated that shorthand systems such as the Fischer projections of organic molecules[16] tend to become a preferred method for representing and compressing data. In quest of a shorthand system for demonstrating dynamic gait analysis, a homunculus has been developed that provides a framework diagram for recording details of gait analysis that are observable during gait. In an effort to refer to this homunculus through a simple nomenclature, the acronym **GHORT** (**g**ait **h**omunculus **o**bserved **r**elational **t**abular, pronounced "GORT," rhymes with "short") is used (Fig. 7-8).

Shorthand Template for STJ Observations

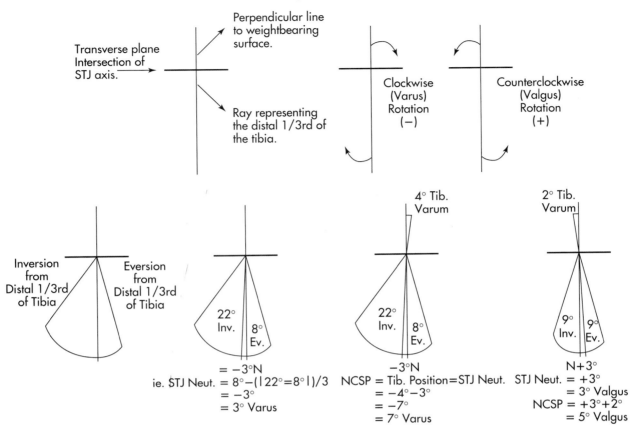

Fig. 7-5. Subtalar joint shorthand template.

We use GHORT to express features of pathomechanical gait that are observable, interpretable, and reproducible. In developing this system over about 5 years, we have found that, with some practice, various observations from different examiners evaluating the same patient tend to come together and after about four or five evaluations, clinicians are independently recording the same details on a given patient. Also, most persons using this system are able to read evaluations recorded by other clinicians and draw the same conclusions about what another recorder has observed.

A review of basics

Before going into detail on the GHORT system, it is necessary to first review some basic concepts which all practitioners have become well-acquainted with through education, clinical training, and experience. *Gait* is defined as "the manner or style of walking."[8] Gait is made up of repetitive steps and strides. A *step* is that distance covered from a given point on the foot to the same point on the other foot during one half of a complete bipedal gait cycle. A *stride* is that distance covered by a given point on the foot during

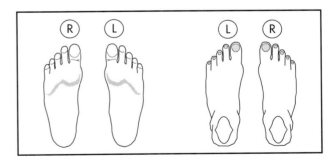

Fig. 7-6. Blank feet templates.

one complete cycle of gait. *Cadence* is a quantitative term which defines the number of steps per minute in a measured movement of constant velocity. Normal walking cadence is about 100 to 120 steps per minute.[9,11,14] Speed walking and sprinting cadences cannot be quantified owing to the wide variations that exist in terms of forward velocity. Walking and running are separate functions. They are, perhaps, more accurately defined as "double stance phasic gait" (walking) and "double float phasic gait" (running).[15]

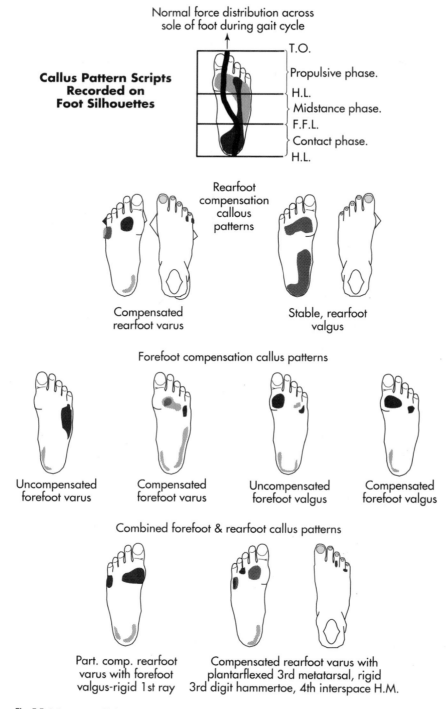

Normal force distribution across
sole of foot during gait cycle

**Callus Pattern Scripts
Recorded on
Foot Silhouettes**

T.O.
Propulsive phase.
H.L.
Midstance phase.
F.F.L.
Contact phase.
H.L.

Rearfoot
compensation
callous
patterns

Compensated
rearfoot varus

Stable, rearfoot
valgus

Forefoot compensation callus patterns

Uncompensated
forefoot varus

Compensated
forefoot varus

Uncompensated
forefoot valgus

Compensated
forefoot valgus

Combined forefoot & rearfoot callus patterns

Part. comp. rearfoot
varus with forefoot
valgus-rigid 1st ray

Compensated rearfoot varus with
plantarflexed 3rd metatarsal, rigid
3rd digit hammertoe, 4th interspace H.M.

Fig. 7-7. Many small feet templates with lesion patterns.

The two functions are separated by a transition in repetitive patterns. A walking form describes both feet on the ground at the same time during some part of the cycle. A running form describes both feet off the ground at the same time during some part of the cycle. Both cycles have in common a weight-bearing *stance phase* and a nonweightbearing *swing phase*. In any method of interpretive analysis it is best to go from the best known to the less certain or unknown. The known reference plane in gait, the so-called normal walking gait, is more correctly defined: double stance phasic gait. Root et al.[18] have refined original work done by Inman et al. to a familiar graph for the biphasic gait cycle consisting of stance and swing phases. Stance phase is further broken down into *periods,* namely contact, mid-

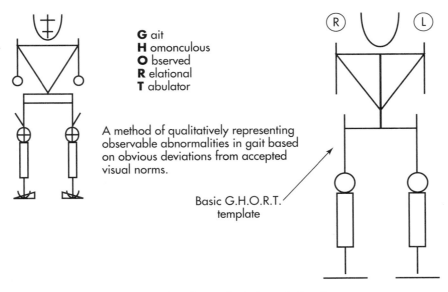

G ait
H omonculous
O bserved
R elational
T abulator

A method of qualitatively representing observable abnormalities in gait based on obvious deviations from accepted visual norms.

Basic G.H.O.R.T. template

Fig. 7-8. GHORT (*g*ait *h*omunculus *o*bserved *r*elation *t*abulator).

stance, and propulsive periods. Some authors[6] subdivide the propulsive period into subperiods of push-off and balance assist. Other authors attempt to describe two periods of swing phase.[17] Because the classification of gait remains largely debatable, we have adopted the familiar Rootian cycle, which contains the most accepted essentials of observed gait (Fig. 7-9).

By referring to this graph, one can categorize events which take place during gait relative to some period or phase of activity. Keeping in mind that this cycle is repetitive, a reference starting point is usually the beginning of stance phase. Stance phase initiates with heel-strike (HS), sometimes called heel contact. This also begins the contact period. Contact period lasts from HS through forefoot loading (FFL) and occupies about 27% of the stance phase or 16% of the total gait cycle. The next period occupies most of stance phase and is called midstance. Midstance begins with FFL and ends with heel-lift (HL). It is during midstance that the majority of energies from ground reactive force (GRF) are absorbed by the body. The most "pathologic" moments of the cycle usually occur during midstance. Midstance occupies about 40% of stance phase or 25% of the total gait cycle. A great deal has been written about shear forces acting on the foot during the first two periods of stance. It is beyond the scope of this chapter to go into great detail on the finer points of shear, stress, and strain, so I will attempt to limit this discussion to those aspects that are most directly observable in gait analysis. The final period of midstance is propulsion. Propulsive period begins with HL and ends with toe-off (TO). Propulsion occupies the last 33% of stance phase or about 20% of the total gait

cycle. As previously mentioned, the propulsive period is subdivided by some into two subperiods. These subperiods tend to be quite subtle, and contribute little to differentiating etiologies in pathomechanics. For this reason, we deal with propulsion as a single period and do not attempt to assign events to subperiods of push-off or balance assist.

After TO, the foot passes into an OKC event, swing phase. Swing phase begins with TO and ends with HS. It occupies 40% of the total (normal) gait cycle. While sometimes subdivided into early and late swing periods, for our purposes, swing phase is best detailed as a single phase during which only a few things occur in the OKC foot that bear on pathomechanics.

Having identified points of reference for one complete stride, it remains to relate our single cycle event to the true bipedal activities which gait entails. In correlating the events of one hemisphere with the other, we discover the following relationship occurring during a normal double stance phasic gait cycle as contrasted with double float phasic gait (Fig. 7-10). It is useful at this point to take essential points of evaluation which should have been previously measured in the static portion of the biomechanical evaluation, and determine how each point is affected by various transitions in the gait cycle. For example, the observed position of maximum pathomechanical effect on the STJ during gait is RCSP during middle and late midstance. Knowing something about the limits of motion of the STJ, and compensation theorems of the foot, one can relate what is happening to the invisible STJ by observing the rearfoot position. It is possible to have an in-

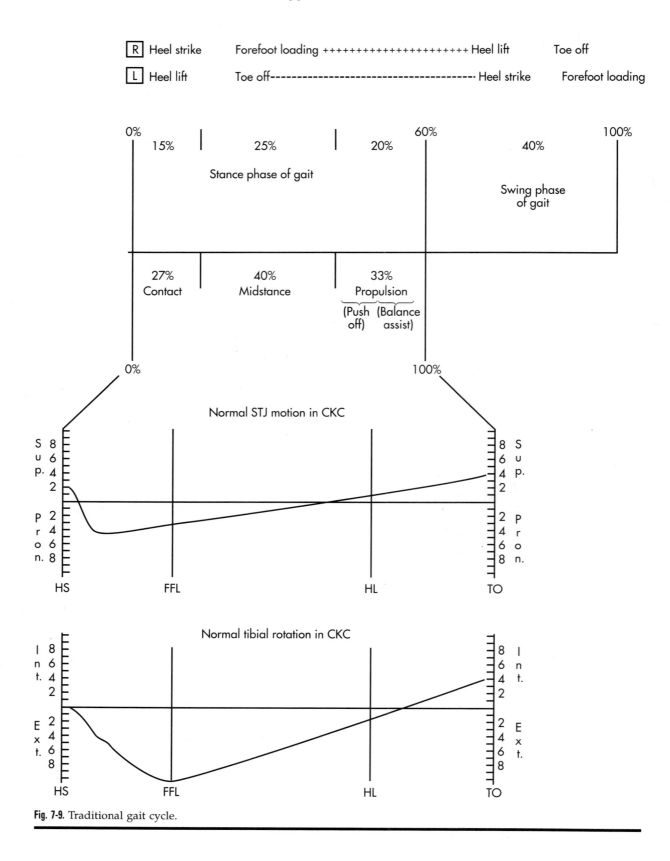

Fig. 7-9. Traditional gait cycle.

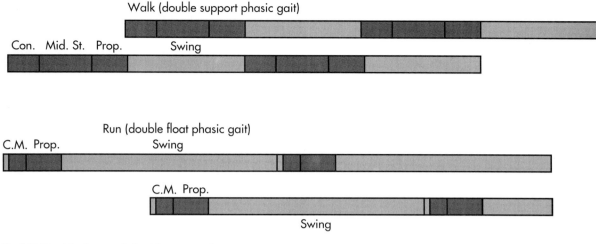

Fig. 7-10. Double float and double stance phasic gait.

verted rearfoot that is either pronated or supinated. This observation can only be truly perceived by relating back to static examination data. For this reason, true gait analysis is both a static and a dynamic process.

It is also useful at this point to review the so-called theorems of compensation of the foot. Adopted by the NO/BFC, there are seven currently accepted theorems of foot compensation. *Compensation* is defined as those mechanisms which exist within the foot to balance variations in ranges of motion between the ground, the forefoot, the rearfoot, and the leg. The theorems are as follows:

1. The heel and forefoot will always attempt to purchase the ground unless prevented by limitation of motion *(purchase)*.

2. The rearfoot will always attempt to compensate to a perpendicular with the weight-bearing surface unless influenced by some proximal or distal force *(rearfoot perpendicularity)*.

3. If driven to valgus more than 2 degrees beyond perpendicular by some proximal or distal force, the rearfoot will "fall through" to its end ROM in the direction of eversion *(rearfoot fallthrough)*.

4. If the rearfoot is unable to purchase with normal dorsiflexion of the ankle joint, the midtarsal joints (MTJs) will offer additional dorsiflexion to the foot by unlocking and maximally pronating against a maximally everted rearfoot. Therefore, equinus results in pronation of the entire foot *if the heel contacts the ground*. If an equinus deformity is so severe that the heel does not contact

the ground at all during stance phase, supination of the foot will occur *(equinus)*.

5. The forefoot loads under the lateral column and compensates under the medial column. Therefore, the forefoot compensates primarily in the direction of inversion from its fully loaded neutral position *(forefoot loading)*.

6. The order of compensation of the forefoot is: (1) MTJ longitudinal axis supination to end ROM, (2) early STJ mobilization, (3) MTJ oblique axis supination, and (4) late STJ supination *(forefoot sequencing)*. Remember the mnemonic LA-SOS (*l*ong *a*xis, *s*ubtalar joint early; *o*blique axis, *s*ubtalar joint late).

7. The metatarsal parabola will generally splay in a predictable direction as the foot goes through the motions of supination to pronation. In the "normal" foot, the fourth metatarsal remains fixed in supination or pronation *(metatarsal splay)* (Fig. 7-11).

Again, the best way to understand an infinite domain of abnormals is in relation to a given norm and to understand trends that progress with pathologic processes that tend to occur as opposites away from the reference normal position.

Site location for gait analysis and TBFR sequence

Selection of a location for gait analysis is important. There should be a straight, level walkway, such as a long corridor, sufficient to permit the patient acceleration to and deceleration from normal cadence. A gravity level should be used to ascertain that the walkway is level, especially relative to the frontal plane of the patient. An unlevel surface may give the impression of shoulder tilt or limb length discrep-

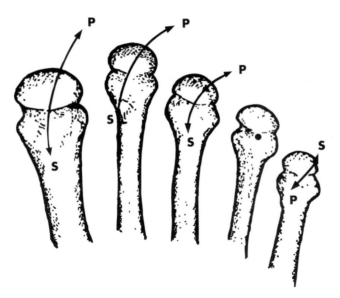

Fig. 7-11. Metatarsal splay. *(From Root ML, Orien WD, Weed JH: Clinical biomechanics: normal and abnormal function of the foot. Clin Biomech, 1971.)*

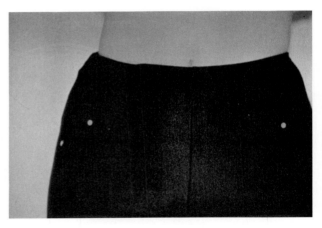

Fig. 7-12. Demonstrating landmarks (anterior superior iliac spine) through clothing.

ancy. Ideally, there will be a tile line or some straight line running down the center of the walkway to represent a line of progression. The area should be well lighted and free of traffic which may interfere with an unobstructed view of the patient. When presenting for gait evaluation, the patient should wear clothes that will make observations easy and reliable. Leotards or shorts and a T-shirt are best. Beware of shoulder pads, now commonly seen in many T-shirt fashions, and belt lines, which may often not represent a true transverse line across the midsection. Anatomical landmarks, such as the anterior superior iliac spine, or kneecap, are the only truly reliable references to use in gait, and a patient should wear clothing that will allow visualization of these features (Fig. 7-12).

Long hair should be tucked or rolled so as not to affect facial position or shoulder visibility. It is best to have the patient walk back and forth several times prior to recording impressions. This permits the examiner to develop an impression regarding normal cadence and posture. The patient will typically be self-conscious for the first few steps. Ask him or her to not look down at the ground, but straight ahead and to let the arms swing comfortably. When evaluating a child, ask the child to walk back and forth between two familiar people rather than have a parent hold the child's hand while walking as this will significantly alter a normal gait pattern. Observe each point in the TBFR sequence as much as possible both going and coming, and record points which seem consistent.

Eyes

Start with the eyes. The eyes should be level to the horizon, or in this case, level to the ground (Fig. 7-13**A**). The acquisition of a level horizon is one of three systems for balance and stability which the sensory side of the central nervous system (CNS) uses to determine the spatial relationship of the body to its environment. Other systems are the inner vestibular cochlear apparatus of the middle ear and proprioception from relative muscle groups transmitted via the dorsal column medial lemniscus.[3] Seasickness, for example, is caused by, among other sensory disturbances, loss of acquisition of a level horizon. Unless limited by some cervical constraint, the eyes will always seek a level horizon. This is a good starting point to begin the evaluation. Record the eyes as a level horizontal line that is subtended by a midsection dividing the face into two equal sagittal hemispheres. Next, look at the mouth. In a neutral facial expression, the mouth should be more or less parallel with the eyes. Collectively, mouth and eyes form a cephalic reference plane for recording observations of tilt in other parts of the upper body (Fig. 7-13**B**). From here, we can begin to detail points of gait by observing the following features (Fig. 7-14):

Head
Shoulders
Arm length and swing
Back midline
Hips
Q angle
Knees
Tibial position
STJ motion
Rearfoot position
Forefoot-to-rearfoot position

Shoulders

Having established a reference plane from the eyes and mouth, the next point of reference is the shoulders. The major point of observation here is tilt. Does one shoulder droop more than the other when ambulating routinely? To fully appreciate shoulder drop, imagine the plane of the shoulders as a seesaw resting on either the top of a hill, or just off to one side of a hill. On the top of the hill, one side of the seesaw will rise to a height equal with the other. If the seesaw is placed slightly off the top of this hill, the downhill side of the seesaw will not rise to the same height as the uphill side. In the case of shoulder drop, while both shoulders rise and fall with the counterbalancing effect of arm swing, rising and falling occur relative to a level or inclined plane. If the level is inclined to the patient's right side, the drop of the right shoulder will be greater than the drop of the left shoulder, like a seesaw on the side of a hill (Fig. 7-15**A** and **B** on p. 165). This should be recorded as a diagonal line drawn between the two shoulder posts on GHORT. Together with shoulder drop, arm length and swing should be recorded. If the shoulder is truly dropping to one side, the arm on that side will seem longer than the arm on the opposite hemisphere. A dropped shoulder will cause the hand to extend down further in the resting posture and arm swing. The longer distance will cause the hand also to seem to swing farther forward than the opposite extremity. To record this, extend the line of the arm on the longer side, and draw a circle at the bottom of the arm line that is bigger than another circle drawn at the bottom of the side of the shorter arm. Arm swing occurs in a sagittal plane that does not exist as a third dimension on a flat piece of paper. The larger circle is intended to convey the concept of appearing to swing farther forward than the smaller circle on the opposite extremity. This records that one arm seems longer than the other, and swings farther forward than the other. For obvious reasons, these features, along with head tilt, are best recorded as the patient is ambulating at normal cadence, walking toward the observer.

In the otherwise normal adult, shoulder drop, along with arm extension and forward swing, tends to occur on the same side as the structurally longer extremity.[1] The reason for this goes back to head tilt and level gaze. Over the course of a lifetime, as eyes seek a level horizon, the body gradually compensates by dropping the shoulder that is higher as a result of the limb length discrepancy. This can be demonstrated by placing the foot of a blindfolded, normal, healthy adult on a plane that is slightly elevated (e.g., with a textbook placed under the foot). A normal CNS causes the shoulder on the side of the elevated extremity to drop down as the eyes seek a level horizon, even behind a blindfold. Over several years of compensation with adolescent development, the spine develops a subtle scoliosis to compensate for the phenomena of eye balance and leveling.[2] If there is a visible scoliosis, this should be recorded along the midline of the upper torso on GHORT; more often, however, it will be too subtle to appreciate in a normal gait analysis (Fig. 7-16**A-C** on p. 166).

In the event of a very obvious lordosis or kyphosis, a curved line should be placed next to the midline and the recorder should mark an *L* or *K* next to the line to indicate *k*yphosis or *l*ordosis. Once again, the limits of a two-dimensional piece of paper prevent recording details of the z-axis which occur in a truly sagittal plane. Children, unlike adults, may not have fully developed this structural compensation. For that reason, in prepubescent children, it is usual to recognize a shoulder drop to the side of the short limb.

Hips

Prior to beginning, the examiner should have palpated the anterior and posterior superior iliac spines. Relate the positions of these constant structural features to the belt line. Beware of using the beltline as a constant plane of reference. This may give a false impression of tilt. In viewing gait for evaluation of hip tilt, one should observe the patient both going and coming. Again, apply the concept of a seesaw on a plane which may be either level or tilted. Hips, like shoulders, tend to seesaw with ambulation. Most often, the reference plane about which this seesaw effect takes place will demonstrate a tilt with the high side to the longer limb. Therefore, in the normal adult, one would expect to see a shoulder drop to the same side as the hip rise. Draw a level or diagonal line between the two posts on the hip area of GHORT to represent this (Fig. 7-17 on p. 167). Do not impose expectations on observations. Over the course of many evaluations, the careful clinical observer encounters many habitus that do not fall within the norm (e.g., hip drop on the same side as shoulder drop in an adult, or structural variations imposed by injury, disease, age, etc.).

Q angle

The Q angle is not easily measured with a great degree of accuracy. However, the concept of Q angle is one that may be observed qualitatively and recorded as a line that intersects the thigh line on GHORT at the knee. This also should be observed with the patient coming and going. If the observer perceives a considerable amount of Q angle, this should be expressed as illustrated in Figure 7-18 on p. 167. Often, a high Q angle is associated with genu

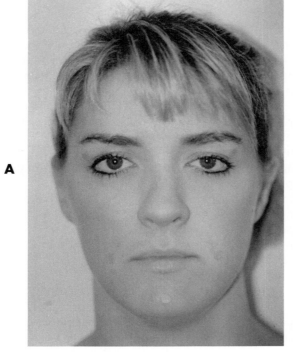

A

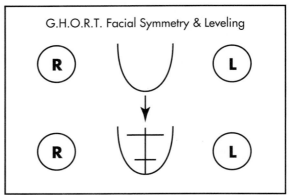

B

Fig. 7-13. Observation of facial landmarks.

Recorded Points of Evaluation on G.H.O.R.T.

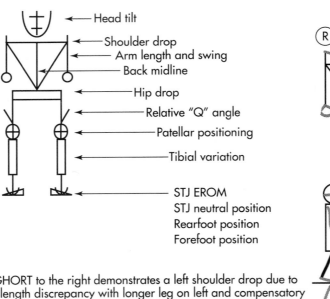

— Head tilt

— Shoulder drop
— Arm length and swing
— Back midline

— Hip drop

— Relative "Q" angle

— Patellar positioning

— Tibial variation

— STJ EROM
STJ neutral position
Rearfoot position
Forefoot position

Example: The GHORT to the right demonstrates a left shoulder drop due to
limb length discrepancy with longer leg on left and compensatory
scoliosis. There is bilateral compensated STJ varus with EROM
compensation on right due to forefoot varus.

Fig. 7-14. Top-to-bottom, front-to-rear sequence on GHORT.

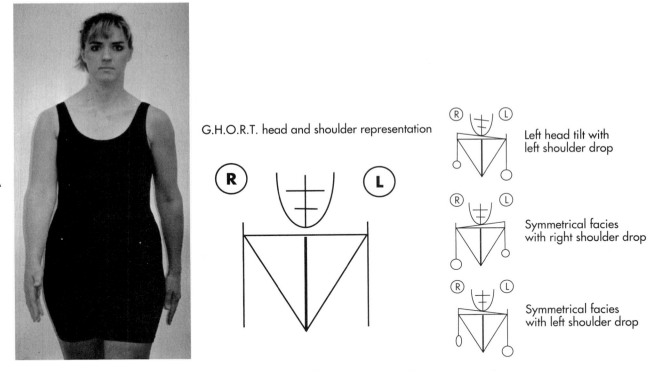

G.H.O.R.T. head and shoulder representation

Left head tilt with
left shoulder drop

B

Symmetrical facies
with right shoulder drop

Symmetrical facies
with left shoulder drop

A

Fig. 7-15. A, Observation of shoulder level and arm swing. **B,** Head, shoulder, and arm recording form.

valgum and coxa vara. This may have some bearing in orthotic therapy and should be recorded if it appears dramatic to the examiner. The fine line between normalcy and abnormality here is purely subjective, but we have noted in form evaluations that most clinicians who perceive enough Q angle to record the feature make the notation on patients demonstrating measured Q angles in excess of about 25 degrees.

Knee position

Moving down from hips to thighs to knee, the next point of notation is knee position. This is recorded relative to the patella. The patella may take one of nine gross positions on the anterior aspect of the knee. It may be centered on both the transverse and long axis of the knee joint. The patella may be located proximal and medial, proximal and central, proximal and lateral, distal and medial, distal and central, or distal and lateral. This offers some insight into femoral torsion as the patellae will be inevitably oriented along a line that is formed by the bowstringing of the patellar and quadriceps tendons, and also, to a lesser degree, to the relationship of the convex lateral patellar facet with the patellar groove formed between the medial and lateral distal femoral condyles. Although the patellar position is primarily observed with the patient walking toward the observer, the orientation of the knee joint may also be somewhat discernible from the orientation of

the popliteal fossae as the patient walks away. Patellar position should be recorded as the intersection of cruciform lines drawn in circles representing knee portions of GHORT (Fig. 7-19 on p. 168).

Tibial position

Although recorded quantitatively in CKC, part of the static examination, tibial variations of varus or valgus angulation should again be noted qualitatively here. The examiner should draw either a straight line or a bowed line to demonstrate that the tibia is oriented in either a linear direction from knee to ankle, or curves as it progresses distally from knee to ankle. Most often, one tends to observe a "bowing varus" and a "linear valgus" in tibial positioning. It is rare for the tibia to bow in the valgus direction. More often, valgus angulation will occur with a concurrent genu valgum, whereas tibial varum may often exist without any apparent coronal plane, genu deflection, or even with a slight amount of apparent genu valgum. This particular observation is made with the patient both coming and going, but greater credence should be placed on observation of the *shin line* with the patient ambulating toward the examiner (Fig. 7-20 on p. 168).

Subtalar joint

The STJ is recorded as both a neutral position relative to STJ ROM and a rearfoot position. The two are differentiated by the terms *subtalar joint position*

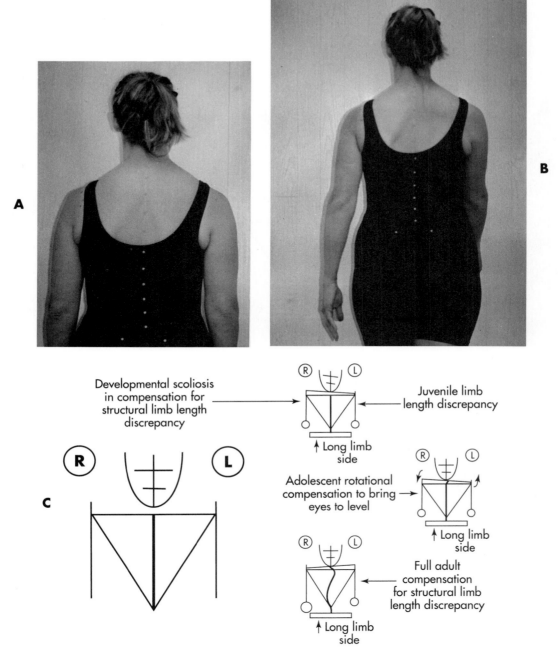

Fig. 7-16. **A,** Scoliosis is apparent with patient standing. **B,** Scoliosis is not apparent during gait. **C,** Development of scoliosis.

and *rearfoot position.* Because the entire STJ ROM may not be observable in normal ambulation, the examiner should begin this portion of the evaluation by taking the total STJ ROM as recorded from the OKC static portions of the evaluation form, and draw in an approximate arc of motion that relates angles of eversion and inversion relative to the distal third of the tibia. This distal tibial third is represented by a line that appears below the tibial

position box on the inferior portions of GHORT. After drawing in arcs to represent motions of inversion and eversion from the tibia, a long line should be drawn in to express STJ Neut relative to the line that represents the distal third of the tibia. This line should have an *N* at the bottom to differentiate it from the line of maximum inversion, the line of maximum eversion, and the distal third of the tibia. As mentioned before, enantiomers are

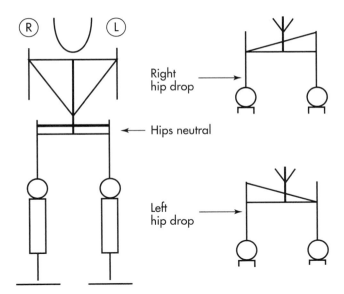

Fig. 7-17. Hip drop to right and left on GHORT.

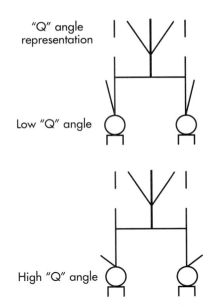

Fig. 7-18. Q angle on GHORT.

difficult to express on paper. *Viewing GHORT as if it were a figure walking toward the observer,* the *left* STJ complex fits in the STJ template standard discussed previously (i.e., clockwise to varus angulation). To demonstrate the chirality of this shorthand notation, the *right* STJ complex should have a mirror-image or backward *N* to show that this is an enantiomeric representation of the template standard. Prior to recording the observed STJ positions, the examiner should have traced in a 2:1 arc at the bottom of the leg lines or on the distal third of the tibia. This arc should be taken from the biomechanical evaluation portion which measures STJ ROM. With this nonobserved template already traced onto the homunculus, the observer should now observe the rearfoot during gait.

The rearfoot may take up any one of several positions. It may be perpendicular to the weight-bearing surface, everted to end range of motion, or forced into varus angulation by limitation of motion. The apparent rearfoot position should be drawn in below a horizontal perpendicular line that is located at the bottom of the distal third tibial line. Keep in mind that the rearfoot position appears relative to the ground. It may be inverted, everted, or perpendicular. This inverted, everted, or perpendicular position of the rearfoot *does not* accurately express the true position of the STJ. In virtually any rearfoot position, the STJ may be either neutral, pronated, or (rarely) supinated. The observer should attempt to record the STJ position after compensation has occurred by a highlighted, heavy, or colored line somewhere along the STJ arc of motion. As mentioned earlier, the total STJ arc of motion cannot be actually observed. Therefore, the

RCSP, the position the calcaneus takes when the rearfoot is fully compensated in midstance, must be deduced by realizing the relationship between rearfoot position, the calculated STJ position, and the tenets of compensation which dictate (1) that the rearfoot will always attempt to come to perpendicular unless driven beyond perpendicular by some proximal or distal force; and (2) that when the rearfoot is driven beyond perpendicular in the direction of eversion by more than 2 degrees, it will fall through to its end ROM. Summing these two tenets, an astute observer can detail by a highlighted or thickened line drawn above the arc of STJ motion, the STJ position when maximum loading occurs, and then, by a solid line *below the ground reference plane,* the rearfoot position when maximum loading occurs. Maximum loading represents that point, usually from about the middle to the last half of midstance, in which there is maximum vertical load on the STJ induced by GRF. This is the moment in which the kinetic chain must distribute maximum forces and therefore is most subject to the deleterious effect of pathomechanics. It is this moment, therefore, that should be captured on paper to represent the observer's impression of gait as represented by GHORT (Fig. 7-21 on p. 169).

The ability to detail the entire motion of the STJ from HS to TO is also important information. A foot that remains pronated longer than normal must distribute forces over a longer curve, and has less of an opportunity to balance propulsive loading forces against the structural adaptation of supination. The so-called propulsive phase of gait has relatively little to do with actual propulsion. Forward motion

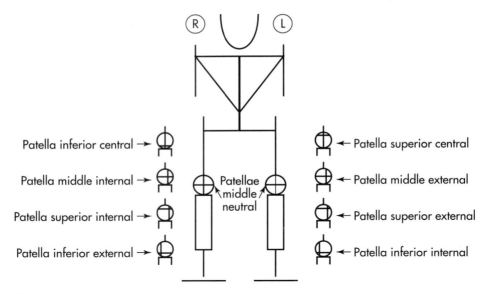

Fig. 7-19. Knee positions on GHORT.

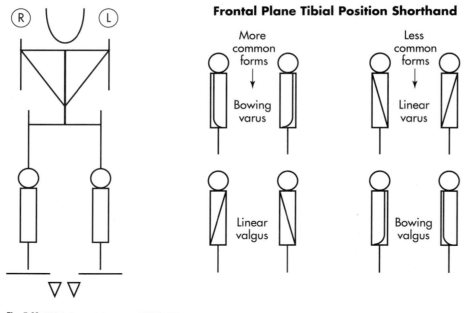

Fig. 7-20. Tibial position on GHORT.

occurs primarily because of "falling forward." This occurs as a result of the pendulous transfer of body weight over a fulcral foot plant in midstance. Further insight into the position of the STJ throughout the entire gait cycle is, however, very important from the perspective of what can be done biomechanically to improve energy distribution up the kinetic chain. Once again, given the limits of a static impression on a piece of paper, the only way to do this is to chart the progressive positions of the STJ on a graph that details the coordinates of time and STJ position and motion. Referring now to the graph that is located to the right side of GHORT (see Fig.

7-8), begin by identifying the position of the STJ at the moment of HS. In an ideal foot, this is about 2 degrees inverted. Then trace a line along the graph to represent the position of the STJ as it passes through the stance phase. By graphing the position, one can also detail motion, as every single point on the graph line demonstrates a slope. Examples of the effect of different forms of forefoot-to-rearfoot pathomechanics are illustrated in Fig. 7-22 on p. 170.

Forefoot
The relationship of the forefoot to the rearfoot is significant for a number of reasons. Inverted and

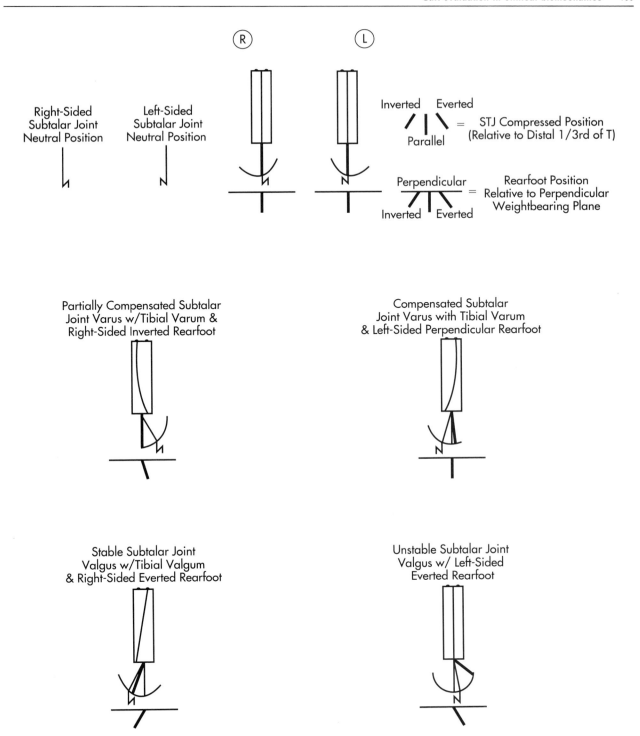

Fig. 7-21. Subtalar joint rearfoot positions on GHORT. Subtalar joint shorthand representations.

everted forefoot deformities bear considerable influence in foot function. The patient should be observed while advancing toward the examiner. Looking at the ball of the foot, directly under the first metatarsophalangeal joint just prior to FFL, one can appreciate the position of the forefoot as it begins to load. On GHORT, in between the STJ complex are two triangular-shaped structures on

which the observation of OKC forefoot orientation may be recorded (Fig. 7-23 on p. 171). If the forefoot is exactly neutral to the rearfoot, a horizontal line should proceed out from the apex of the triangle to describe the lateral column of the foot. This is then joined through a perpendicular triangular structure to the superior base of the first metatarsophalangeal joint triangle. If the observation is one of forefoot

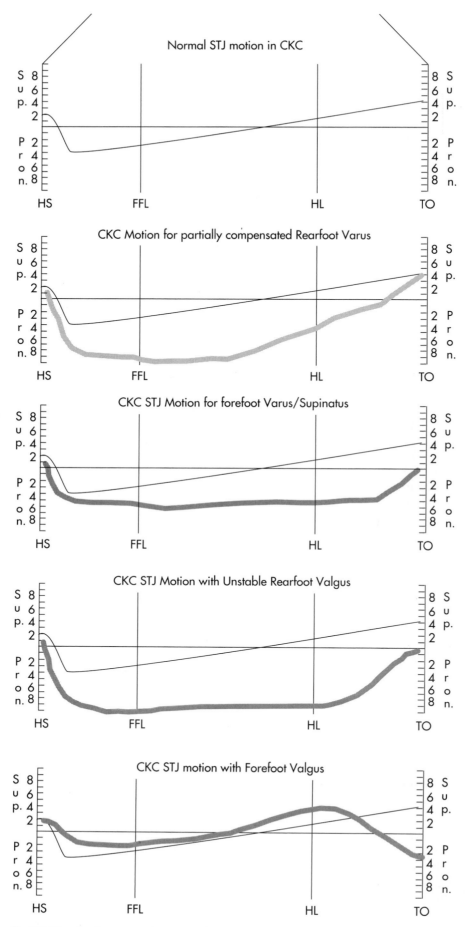

Fig. 7-22. Graphs demonstrating normal, compensated rearfoot varus, unstable rearfoot valgus, forefoot varus, and forefoot valgus angulation.

Forefoot Template Shorthand Illustrations

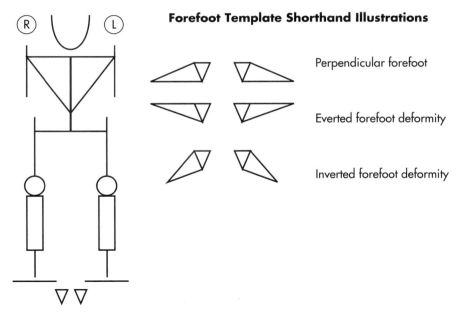

Perpendicular forefoot

Everted forefoot deformity

Inverted forefoot deformity

Fig. 7-23. Forefoot template and example of valgus, varus, and perpendicular forefoot positions.

varus angulation, the line proceeding out from the inferior apex of the first metatarsophalangeal joint triangle should be inclined downward, then back upward to give the impression of inversion. Conversely, if a forefoot valgus angulation is observed, the line should be inclined upward with a level, horizontal line directed back to the superior base of the first metatarsophalangeal joint triangle.

Line of progression

At this point, it is useful to record several steps by tracing blocked footprints relative to the LOP. This should give an impression of the relative angle and base of gait while actually ambulating. While these are not quantitative angles of gait, as were those recorded during the static phases of this examination, qualitative impressions of gait can be very valuable in crosschecking and verifying the accuracy of data recorded on static portions of the evaluation form. For example, in the absence of more proximal torsional forces (i.e., femoral ante- or retrotorsion or inversion or eversion or tibial torsion) acting on the foot, one would expect feet with higher STJ axes (i.e., increased transverse plane component axis deviation) to demonstrate a narrower angle of gait and, probably, a slightly wider base of gait (Fig. 7-24).

Phasic observations

During various phases and periods of gait, there are phenomena which can be noted by careful observation. Between HS and FFL, there may be excessive

shock load or poor shock absorption. There may be instability of the ankle joint due to lateral ligamentous instability. Between FFL and HL, a phenomenon called "abductory twist" may be observed. This represents an unlocking of the MTJ which occurs during the last half of midstance should resupination of the STJ fail to occur. The MTJ unlocks and causes the rearfoot to abduct on the forefoot, making for a less propulsive or less springy propulsive phase. Another event occurring during the late midstance and propulsive periods is antalgia, or guarding, which occurs when the patient prevents a painful foot from going through extremes of motion via reciprocal muscle group recruitment. This also results in an apropulsive, less efficient induction into swing phase. Early heel-off, caused by compensated equinus, may be observed in late midstance with effects seen into the propulsive period as well. Steppage gait is observed primarily throughout swing phase and is noted by a failure of recruitment of anterior muscle groups. Both steppage gait and equinus may produce toe-to-heel instead of heel-to-toe gait during the contact period. There are a host of neurologic abnormalities which are not easily related to the normal gait cycle. These are detailed later, but notations regarding some of these abnormalities are best made in the areas of phasic observations on the evaluation form (Fig. 7-25).

Crosschecking and verifying

The validity of gait evaluation is only as strong as the integrity of the examiner. It is sometimes

Line of Progression Relative to Angle and Base of Gait

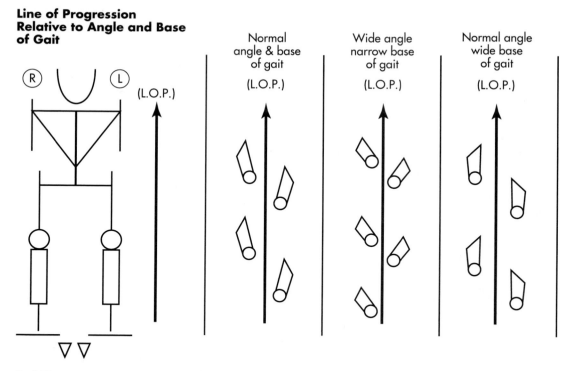

Fig. 7-24. Line of progression and angles of gait.

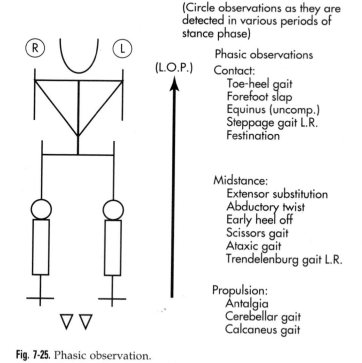

(Circle observations as they are detected in various periods of stance phase)

Phasic observations

Contact:
Toe-heel gait
Forefoot slap
Equinus (uncomp.)
Steppage gait L.R.
Festination

Midstance:
Extensor substitution
Abductory twist
Early heel off
Scissors gait
Ataxic gait
Trendelenburg gait L.R.

Propulsion:
Antalgia
Cerebellar gait
Calcaneus gait

Fig. 7-25. Phasic observation.

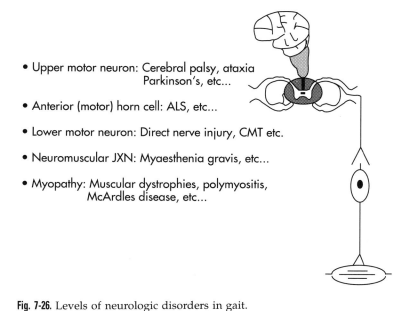

- Upper motor neuron: Cerebral palsy, ataxia Parkinson's, etc...

- Anterior (motor) horn cell: ALS, etc...

- Lower motor neuron: Direct nerve injury, CMT etc.

- Neuromuscular JXN: Myaesthenia gravis, etc...

- Myopathy: Muscular dystrophies, polymyositis, McArdles disease, etc...

Fig. 7-26. Levels of neurologic disorders in gait.

difficult not to impose preconceived notions onto the evaluation form. Even the most sincere recorder may be influenced by his or her expectations of findings. For this reason, it is essential that the clinician review the evaluation form at this point and crosscheck data in an attempt to verify the credibility of the recorded instrument. Compare callus patterns and phasic observations with points of observation. For example, compensated rearfoot varus anguation on a perpendicular forefoot should produce callus patterns that demonstrate a shearing tyloma below the second, fourth, and fifth metatarsals. Lack of external rotation at the hip should produce in-toeing in the absence of compensating torsional deformity in the tibia. A limb length discrepancy is often compensated functionally by pronation of the STJ on the long side, and supination of the STJ on the short side. There are a host of similar relationships which should be obvious to a well-trained clinician who takes the time to go back, crosscheck, and verify. Accuracy of data lends greatly to correctly perscribing orthotic devices.

Neurologic and acquired gait abnormalities

There are abnormalities of gait associated with neurologic lesions or that are acquired through injury or progressive disease states and which bear recording of details that do not relate well with normal gait. GHORT was constructed in template form to relate most directly with typical musculoskeletal variances from normal gait. When extreme variances exist, GHORT may still be used to construct a simple, shorthand method of detailing observations, but the template may require modification. Neurologic gait abnormalities are best catalogued by the level at which they occur in gait (Fig. 7-26).

Myopathies

For purposes of this discussion, we classify neurologic disorders beginning at the level of muscle impulse conduction, and start by identifying disorders of gait caused by myopathies. This includes proximal myopathies (nemaline myopathy, muscular dystrophy, etc.), distal myopathies (infant onset, late onset, distal muscular dystrophy, etc.), centronuclear myopathy, and alcoholic myopathy. While the word *myopathy* refers to any disease affecting muscle, it refers here to forms of the disease that cause proximal muscle weakness. The effect is that of a so-called dystrophic or atrophic gait, which results in exaggerated alternation of lateral trunk movements with an exaggerated elevation of the hip suggestive of the gait of a duck or penguin.[20] It is frequently associated with Gowers' sign or requires manual assistance in rising from a seated position by pushing down on the thighs (Fig. 7-27).

Neuromuscular junction

The next level of gait disturbance is at the neuromuscular junction. The most common disorder seen at this level is myasthenia gravis. This disease is very difficult to capture as a static image because the

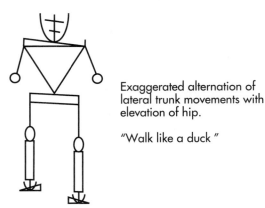

Exaggerated alternation of lateral trunk movements with elevation of hip.

"Walk like a duck "

Fig. 7-27. Dystrophic gait.

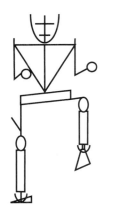

Loss of peroneal innervations with exaggerated hip flexion to compensate for foot drop

Fig. 7-29. Steppage gait.

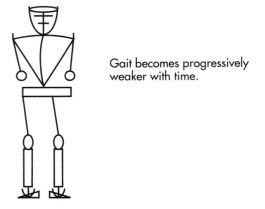

Gait becomes progressively weaker with time.

Fig. 7-28. Myasthenia gravis.

patient starts out walking normally but fatigues easily and loses good posture with difficulty in maintaining even an erect position of the head and neck. The most drastic moment of the disease may be illustrated by GHORT (Fig. 7-28).

Lower motor neuron dysfunction

Progressing proximally along the peripheral nervous system, pathologic changes of the lower motor neuron (LMN) are next in line. The most common LMN abnormality is loss of efferent function distal to some point of interrupted impulse transmission. A commonly affected LMN nerve to demonstrate abnormality in gait is the common peroneal nerve. Owing to its vulnerable position about the head and neck of the fibula, along with other traumatic changes affecting its course (e.g., the anterior compartmental syndrome), common peroneal nerve paralysis has acquired a definition of its own in terms of altered gait cycles, the so-called steppage gait[19] (Fig. 7-29). LMN injury or dysfunction may, of course, occur at any point along the circuits innervating the lower extremity. Sciatic nerve injury may result in a functionless, insensate lower extremity, or

lesser degrees of dysfunction such as guarding, antalgia and dragging of the limb, or isolated footdrop.[4] Injury to the popliteal nerve may affect both the common peroneal and posterior tibial muscles, resulting in a more flaccid, exaggerated form of steppage gait with no structural loading possible. While steppage gait may not detail the exact point of disruption in an LMN circuit, it fairly well represents the concept of LMN dysfunction, with the exception of femoral nerve cessation. In this case, the entire limb is circumducted to the advantage of muscle groups innervated by the sciatic and obturator nerves. Understanding LMN dysfunction requires a conceptual review of nervous circuitry in the lower extremity. Innervations below the knee are relatively well understood, and generally satisfy the sequencing chart shown in Figure 7-30.

Calcaneus gait refers to a gait cycle that results when the gastrocnemius-soleus muscles are paralyzed with lack of push-off and a shift of the tibia posteriorly over the talus at the end of stance phase. Above-the-knee sequencing of muscle firing has been well studied but not well correlated. There remain a number of varying opinions about mean electromyographic activity in "normal" gait above the knee. For this reason, it is perhaps best to classify general trends of recruited muscle activity during phasic gait by muscle groupings above the knee. We attempt to do this by conceptualizing all muscles within a muscle group as firing together. While this certainly *does not* happen in reality, the perception aids greatly in relating an LMN neurologic disorder to normal gait cycle activity. Figure 7-31 roughly demonstrates sequencing of muscle activity above the knee by groupings and associates these groups with respective innervations. Disruption of nerve routes by injury, development, disease, or metabolism will affect the gait cycle accordingly.

A common form of LMN dysfunction affecting

**Below the Knee
Neuromuscular Sequencing**

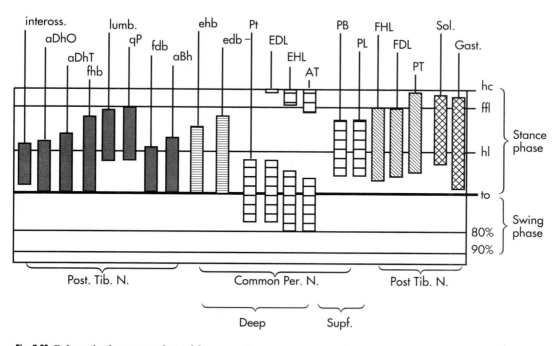

Fig. 7-30. Below-the-knee muscle and lower motor neuron sequencing.

**Neuromuscular Sequencing
(By muscle Groups)
Above the Knee**

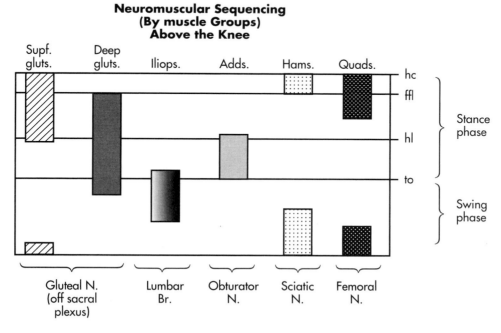

Fig. 7-31. Above-the-knee lower motor neuron and muscle sequencing.

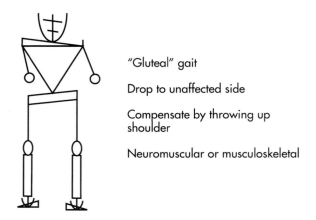

"Gluteal" gait

Drop to unaffected side

Compensate by throwing up shoulder

Neuromuscular or musculoskeletal

Fig. 7-32. Trendelenburg's gait without dystrophy.

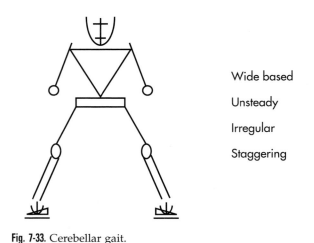

Wide based

Unsteady

Irregular

Staggering

Fig. 7-33. Cerebellar gait.

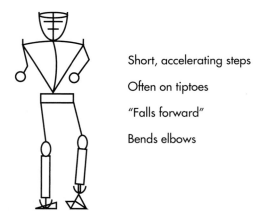

Short, accelerating steps

Often on tiptoes

"Falls forward"

Bends elbows

Fig. 7-34. Festinating gait.

the gluteal muscle groups is expressed in gluteal, or Trendelenburg, gait. This is characterized by paralysis of the gluteal muscles with a listing of the trunk *toward the affected side.* As the patient ambulates, the weightbearing hip cannot be fixed by the gluteal muscles. As a result, the opposite hip tends to drop

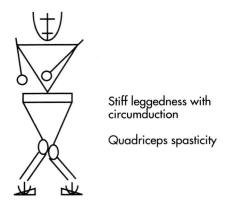

Stiff leggedness with circumduction

Quadriceps spasticity

Fig. 7-35. Scissors gait.

and the trunk inclines to that side. Frequently, the patient attempts to compensate by throwing the shoulder of the drooping hip side upward to assist in raising the swinging leg, and compensating for ipsilateral hip abductor weakness. While some authors consider dystrophic and Trendelenburg gait to be synonymous, there are visible differences that differentiate the two. Trendelenburg gait is more often seen in non-neurologic, "waddling" disorders, such as congenital hip dislocations, than as a result of isolated hemispheric neurologic disorders. Trendelenburg gait is routinely seen after Achilles tendon lengthening procedures. It will remain as long as posterior leg muscle weakness persists (Fig. 7-32).

Prior to discussion of upper motor neuron (UMN) dysfunction and following in sequence from caudal to cephalad levels of neurologic effect on gait, it is worth mentioning that there are a host of disorders that affect the interface between the LMN and the UMN. These are characterized by lesions of the anterior motor horn cells or diseases like amyotrophic lateral sclerosis (ALS). ALS results in progressive degeneration of neurons that give rise to the corticospinal tract and of motor cells of the brainstem and spinal cord resulting in deficit of UMNs and LMNs. It is characterized by fasciculations and progressive loss of muscle capacity with wasting. Such neurologic disorders do not have a specific effect on gait, but tend to have a cumulative effect, as in myasthenia gravis.

Upper motor neuron dysfunction

Moving up the CNS into the cerebrum, we encounter lesions of cerebellar dysfunction caused by cerebral tumors, abscesses, injuries, syphilis (tabetic), multiple sclerosis, and so forth. This level of disorder results in cerebellar or "ataxic" gait. The pattern is typified by wide-based lurching, an unsteady gait with a tendency to fall toward the affected side of the CNS lesion. Gait is often uncoordinated, with an abrupt HS, followed by a double forefoot loading sequence or "double toe tap" (Fig. 7-33).

At the extrapyramidal system nucleus, paralysis agitans, or Parkinson's disease, demonstrates a very characteristic "festinating gait." This is a gait disorder in which the patient initiates voluntary gait by "falling forward" or leaning far enough forward to stimulate the CNS to develop repetitive gait commands. The patient moves involuntarily with short, accelerating steps, often on tiptoe and with elbows bent (Fig. 7-34).

Perhaps the most common form of UMN disorder seen in clinical gait evaluation is that due to cerebral palsy. This results most often in a spastic type of gait in which the legs are adducted to the point that circumduction is necessary in order to produce forward motion. This type of gait is commonly nicknamed "scissors" gait because the sliding back and forth of one leg upon the other appears scissorslike in the frontal plane (Fig. 7-35).[22]

Other forms of gait have been described. As previously mentioned, *antalgic gait* is a compensating gait induced by voluntary guarding of a painful extremity. *Charcot's gait* is the term used to describe the ataxic type of gait seen in Friedreich's ataxia. Terms like *drag-toe* and *footdrop gait* are self-explanatory. *Heel-toe gait* is a term often used to describe the normal sequencing from HS to TO. *Helicopod gait* occurs when the feet describe half-circles as they shuffle along during contact and early midstance phase. This is seen frequently in hysterical disorder. *Intermittent double step gait* is a hemiplegic gait in which there is a pause after the short step of the normal foot or after the step of the hemiplegic side. *Oppenheim's gait*, seen in rare cases of multiple sclerosis, represents an atypical form of ataxia in which there is dramatic oscillation of head, limbs, and body.[8]

Summary

While it behooves the biomechanical clinician to recognize and represent all the above forms of neurologic gaits described, the vast majority of patients seen in the clinic will demonstrate some more subtle form of musculoskeletal disorder which fits well in the GHORT template previously described for gait analysis. While seemingly complex at first glance, one will find that the form is quite logical and therefore easy to follow. In familiarization studies, after about the fifth evaluation, most clinicians seem to have easily mastered the form. Gait evaluation must be a scientific process. It should involve the assimilation of quantitative and

qualitative data that are reproducible and verifiable. It should be within the grasp of every podiatrist to understand and interpret visual variations from a normal gait cycle and to represent these variations on a simple recording medium such as paper. Using the instrument described above, along with a bit of practice and review, competent gait analysis can be a unique, powerful biomechanical tool in the armamentarium of the clinical practitioner concerned with gait.

References

1. Bailey HW, Beckwith CG: Short leg and spinal anomalies—their incidence and effects on spinal mechanisms, *J Am Osteopath Assoc* 36:319, 1937.
2. Balis WJ, Rzonca EC: Functional and structural limb length discrepancies: evaluation and treatment, *Clin Podiatr Med Surg* 5:509–519, 1988.
3. Bannister R, editor: *Brains clinical neurology*, ed 5, Oxford, 1978, Oxford University Press.
4. Bigos SJ, Coleman SS: Foot deformities secondary to gluteal injection in infancy, *J Pediatr Orthop* 4:560–563, 1984.
5. Beuche FJ: *Schaums outline of theory and problems of college physics*, ed 7, New York, 1979, McGraw-Hill.
6. Burns MJ, McGlamry ED: *Fundamental principles of foot surgery*, Baltimore, 1987, Williams & Wilkins.
7. *Curriculum for podiatric orthopedics and biomechanics*, 1991, National Orthopedics/Biomechanics Faculties Committee.
8. *Dorlands Illustrated Medical Dictionary*, ed 27, Philadelphia, 1988, WB Saunders.
9. Drillis RJ: The influence of aging on kinematics of gait. In *The geriatric amputee*, report of conference sponsored by Committee on Prosthetic Research and Development of the Division of Engineering and Industrial Research. Washington, DC, April 13–14, 1961. Publication 919, 1961. National Academy of Sciences–National Research Council, Washington, DC.
10. *EDG evaluation form*, EDG software documentation version 4.8, Langer Biomechanics, Deer Park, NY.
11. Finley FR, Cody KA: Locomotive characteristics of urban pedestrians. *Arch Phys Med Rehabil* 51:423, 1970.
12. King LS: *Medical thinking: a historical preface*, Princeton, NJ, Princeton University Press, 1982.
13. Langer, et al: *A practical manual of clinical electrodynography*, ed 2, Langer Foundation for Biomechanics and Sports Medicine Research, Deer Park, NY, 1989.
14. Molen NH, Rozendal RH. Some factors of human gait, *Proc Kon Ned Akad Wet Ser C* 69:522, 1966.
15. Molen NH, Rozendal RH, Boon W: Graphic representation of the relationship between oxygen consumption and characteristics of normal gait in the human male, *Proc Kon Ned Akad Wet Ser C* 75:305, 1972.
16. Morrison RT, Boyd RN: *Organic chemistry*, ed 3, Boston, 1976, Allyn & Bacon.
17. Perry J: The mechanics of walking. A clinical interpretation, *Phys Ther* 47:778, 1967.
18. Root ML, Orien WP, Weed JH: *Normal and abnormal function of the foot clinical biomechanics*, Vol 2, Los Angeles, 1977, Clinical Biomechanics 319.
19. Sutherland DH: *Gait disorders in childhood and adolescence*, Baltimore, 1984, Williams & Wilkins.
20. Sutherland DH, et al: The pathomechanics of gait in Duchenne muscular dystrophy, *Dev Med Child Neuro* 23:3–22, 1981.
21. Swift EH, Eliot AB: *Quantitative measurements and chemical equilibria*, San Francisco, WH Freeman.

computerized gait evaluation

Eric Arthur Fuller, DPM

Theoretical uses
    Diagnosis
    Normal values
    Prediction of high-risk patients
    Determination of need for treatment
    Evaluation and documentation of progress
Approaches to computerized gait analysis
Technical aspects
**The difference between reality and
    instrument measurement**
Statistical aspects
Types of measurement
Summary

This chapter is intended to assist readers who are interested in computerized gait analysis. It will help them to choose the right device for their needs and to understand the limitations of the technology, which is essential if they are to interpret test results effectively. It will also help readers to understand the research literature of computerized gait analysis.

This chapter initially examines the theoretical approaches to the use of gait analysis, then the technical and statistical problems encountered when using such analysis. Next, various methods of measuring gait are compared, with particular emphasis placed on the differences between force measurements and motion measurements, and the additional information that can be attained from the combination of the two.

Theoretical uses

There are several possible and distinct uses of computerized gait analysis systems. If a practitioner is considering acquiring one of the systems he or she should consider the specific use of the measuring device. Computerized gait analysis cannot be substituted for sound clinical judgment and common sense.

Diagnosis

Programming a computer to make a diagnosis is extremely difficult even if the computer could take into account the complete history and physical examination. The data obtained from gait analysis is only a small portion of the information needed to make a diagnosis. For most disorders the computer would have to be programmed with data from a series of normal and abnormal patients. A clinician would then have to decide who is abnormal and who is not. If a clinician is able to determine this on his or her own, a computer is not necessary. A similar situation occurs when the measurements of a group of subjects with a known abnormality are programmed into the computer. It must be determined beforehand who is normal and who is not. The subjects used for the measurement would have to demonstrate obvious disorders or else normal people would be included with the patients demonstrating abnormalities. The analysis system then may not be able to distinguish the borderline subject because that individual would not demonstrate adequate abnormal findings.

Normal values

The establishment of normal values is another potential use of computerized gait analysis. The problem of establishing normal values is similar to that of having the computer make a diagnosis. The establishment of normal values implies that there are no significant differences among normal subjects. In other words, the assumption is that all normal people walk exactly the same. When the measurements of a "normal" population are measured and averaged, the individual differences among them are lost. This was shown to happen with electromyographic (EMG) measurements during gait when the averaging of all the subjects produced a profile that did not resemble any of the subjects.[4] For more discussion on the establishment of a range of normal values, see Statistical Aspects below.

Prediction of high-risk patients

One of the most promising areas of gait analysis is the use of pressure distribution measurement for prediction of ulceration in people with insensate feet.[20] A simple measure could be used to predict patients that need immediate treatment and those whose treatment could be delayed.

Gait analysis instrumentation can be used to evaluate clinical judgment as to which patients belong in high-risk populations. For example, arch height has been used as a clinical indicator of foot function. However, arch height does not correlate with shock absorption or the amount of flattening during gait.[66] Another common belief is that there is a correlation between body weight and foot pressure. Body weight does not correlate with peak pressure under the foot.[42] In Morton's foot (short first metatarsal) there are higher pressures under the second metatarsal head compared with the non-Morton's foot, but there are high second metatarsal head pressures in the non-Morton's foot as well.[77]

Determination of need for treatment

This subject is related to the prediction of high-risk populations. If a patient is in an identifiable high-risk population the analysis equipment could then document that the patient requires treatment. In addition, if the need for treatment is clinically obvious, the analysis equipment can be used to select the best option from several different treatment protocols. For example, in patients that underwent a proximal tibial osteotomy for knee pain secondary to a varus knee position, those patients that had a lower adduction moment on their lower leg had better clinical results than patients with a higher adduction moment.[96] It has also been suggested that gait assessment could be used to help determine the need for total knee replacement, because patients who have a worse preoperative evaluation show the greatest improvement postoperatively.[52]

Beyond determining the need for treatment, gait

analysis may help determine the type of treatment, especially if specific measurements are found to correlate with pathologic findings. For example, it has been found that when the flexion moment at the first metatarsophalangeal joint increases, bunion deformities tend to increase.[80] Treatment plans could be evaluated on their ability to reduce flexion moments. Computerized gait analysis has been suggested for determining which style of leg orthosis is best for paraplegic patients.[45] This study was a preliminary study in which paraplegic patients were given several styles of orthoses and a period of time to learn how to use the devices, following which gait measurements were done. The subjects were asked which device they liked best. The values that they exhibited with this device were chosen to represent the ideal situation. For computerized gait analysis to be useful in determination of the best orthosis, the analysis should predict which device the patient would like best. This study appropriately required that all of the subjects become accustomed to the device before measurement. After trying all of the orthoses, it is the patient, not the computer, who should decide which device he or she liked best. The data from the analysis are never used to make this decision and it may not be possible for computer analysis to accurately predict the correct orthosis for a paraplegic patient before the patient wears it.

Evaluation and documentation of progress

Gait analysis instrumentation can provide an objective evaluation of the progress of a patient from one visit to the next. It is difficult for a practitioner to remember a gait pattern from a previous visit. A few words in a chart may help the practitioner recall to some degree what the gait was like a week before, but the full documentation that computerized analysis can provide is more complete. However, in a study in which foot switches, EMG, and goniometers were used to measure gait, it was noted there were no changes in the pattern following treatment, even though the patient and the observers believed that there was improvement.[52] This result can be explained in two ways. Either the patient and observers were overly optimistic and there were no changes in gait, or there were changes in gait that were not detected by the methods used. Goniometers and foot switches measure only the position of the foot and leg; they do not measure the moments that cause the motions of the foot and leg. It has been noted that there are changes in joint moments over time when there has not been much change in the position and motion of the leg.[96]

Gait analysis instrumentation can be used to evaluate the efficacy of a specific treatment. Such evaluation is critical in comparing the costs of various treatments. For example, removal of a callus can reduce plantar pressure under the foot of a diabetic.[112] In rheumatoid feet with high plantar pressure there is a marked decrease in plantar pressure after a forefoot arthroplasty.[9] Insole materials differ in regard to their reduction of peak plantar pressure.[81] Different immobilization devices display great variability in reducing plantar pressures.[85] Placement of cast rockers more posteriorly decreased pressures on the forefoot.[71,85] It should be remembered when comparing one treatment with another that all patients do not respond the same to similar treatments. Altering midsole density reduced the force on the foot more on some feet than on others.[37] One must note that averaging all these patients may obscure the positive effects of treatment in the individual patient.

Approaches to computerized gait analysis

The several approaches to the clinical use of computerized gait analysis vary in complexity. The first approach to be discussed is theoretical modeling of the foot. In this approach the foot is examined the way an engineer would examine a building. The second approach, the empirical approach, is somewhat less sophisticated. A measurement corresponding with a certain abnormality is used as an indicator of that abnormality. The indicator is used without necessarily understanding the relationship between the measurement and the abnormality. The final approach is the "before-and-after" approach, which is to see if there is a change in gait measurement after treatment intervention. These are not necessarily completely distinct approaches. A basic understanding of the nature of the measuring approach will help the clinician in assessing the value of the data obtained.

It is also important to understand the type of injury that is to be treated or prevented. Traumatic injuries are usually related to single identifiable events and they may have identifiable risk factors. Whether or not a traumatic injury occurs is a random event, but the risk factors may help in predicting the chances of the injury. The other type of injury is an overuse or repetitive injury. This injury is the result of repeated stress which eventually causes tissue damage. Hopefully, through the use of computerized gait analysis, this type of stress can be easily identified and reduced before injury occurs.

Modeling

The perfect gait analysis system would be capable of measuring stress in anatomical structures and then determining whether the structure could handle this stress without being damaged. Mechanically caused pain is the result of an anatomical structure being stressed beyond its limit. It is very difficult to measure directly the forces acting on structures. An example of direct measurement is the placing of a strain gauge on the Achilles tendon[47] or tibia.[51] Even direct measurement of the tibia strain may have some inaccuracies due to the placement location on the tibia. Additionally, the axial compressive forces can affect the output of the strain gauge.[83] Overall, direct implantation of measurement devices is not practical clinically.

However, stress on anatomical structures can be estimated by the use of anatomical models.[83] A computerized model may be used to calculate the internal forces from the motions and external forces that are measured by gait analysis devices. An example of an internal force is the compressive force at the talotibial joint. The peak external force acting at the ankle joint is approximately 2.7 times body weight and occurs at 0.09 second after heel contact during a slow jog. However, the peak force calculated with a model at the talotibial joint is 11 times body weight and occurs at 0.11 second.[83] The compression force at the ankle joint is equal to ground reactive force plus the compression force from the Achilles tendon. At the time of peak force at the ankle joint, 82% of the force comes from muscle.[83] The Achilles tendon forces for the model[83] were very similar to the values obtained with a strain gauge.[47]

The steps that are required for using anatomical models to predict injury are to: (1) identify the structure that is injured, (2) determine the stress limits of the structure, (3) determine the stress placed on the structure, and (4) identify the factors that influence the stress.[70] Each step involves uncertainties. It is often difficult to determine the exact anatomical structure that is injured. One author has questioned the assumption that shin splints are related to the posterior tibial muscle.[59] This study found that the pain and increased radiotracer uptake in the tibia was located at the insertion of the medial head of the soleus, which is anatomically distinct from the insertion of the posterior tibial muscle. Determining the stress limits of a structure is difficult because the limit is related to the cross-sectional area of the structure.[70] In other words, if the quality of the collagen is equal, then a thicker tendon is stronger than a thinner tendon. Anatomical structures may vary in size by 100% from person to person.[70] Determining the stress placed on a structure can also be difficult owing to the problem of redundancy. If it is assumed that the only structure that prevents the arch of the foot from collapsing is the plantar fascia, then the estimated

stress in the plantar fascia will be too high because the stress in the intrinsic muscles will have been ignored.[83] Finally, determination of the factors that influence stress is probably the easiest and most important step in the process. Motions or positions of parts of the body that cause stress in a particular anatomical structure can be determined through cadaver studies. The purpose of modeling is to determine the stress on an anatomical structure. To determine the stress on a structure that cannot be measured directly the model must be used to calculate the forces acting on the structure from the forces and motions that can be measured. To calculate the internal forces many measurements or assumptions have to be made. For example, it was reported that a change in the Achilles tendon lever arm from 4.5 to 5.0 cm resulted in a peak stress reduction from 62 to 56 MPa.[83]

The variables that must be measured are the position, velocity, and acceleration of each of the segments of the lower extremities and the location and direction of ground reactive force on the foot. The values that have to be obtained or assumed are the location of the center of mass and the moment of inertia of each of the segments of the body.[104] These values are necessary because the joint moments and joint reactive forces are calculated from the angular and linear accelerations and the ground reactive force. The ankle force and moment can be determined from the accelerations of the foot. After the ankle force is known, it can be used to calculate the force at the knee if the leg accelerations are known.[104] The calculations continue for the rest of the body. The important point is that the stress on a structure cannot be known from its position alone. For example, the subtalar joint may be maximally pronated with a 50-N-m moment from the ground reactive force holding it in that position or it may have only a 5-N-m moment holding it pronated. Both feet are maximally pronated, but the stress on the structure that is stopping pronation is markedly different between the two feet.

Empirical approach

The empirical approach is different from the modeling approach in that the stress on an anatomical structure is assumed to be related to a measurable quantity. This stress on a particular structure is not measured or even calculated, but it is assumed that when there is pain, the structure has had excessive stress. If a particular gait analysis measurement can be found to have a correlation with the pain, then that measurement can be used as an indicator of the effectiveness of a preventive treatment or the probability of injury in a particular patient. With this approach the mechanism of injury does not have to be known. In the previously mentioned example of posterior shin splints, calcaneal eversion was found to be related to the symptoms and it was assumed that the pathologic finding was related to the posterior tibial muscle attachment. The pain resolved with varus wedges[94] placed in the shoes and the calcaneal eversion decreased even though the actual abnormality was located at the head of the soleus muscle.[59] There are two major steps in the empirical approach: (1) a measurement must be found that is related to the pathologic finding, and (2) when that measurement is altered by treatment the pain decreases.

The empirical approach requires well-designed prospective studies that measure the gait of subjects who later develop injuries. The reason for prospective studies is that a patient may alter his or her gait in response to the pathologic change,[9] and it can never be known, after the injury, whether the gait changes observed after the injury were the cause or the result of the injury.[70] For further assessment of approaches used with gait analysis instrumentation, see the reviews by Nigg and Bobbert[70] and Winter and Bishop.[106]

An example of the use of the empirical approach is the study of the relationship between pronation and the patellofemoral syndrome. The first part of the empirical model is satisfied because it has been demonstrated that pronation does correlate with the problem.[5] It was also demonstrated that wedges placed in the shoes can alter pronation.[68] Finally, it has been demonstrated that a 20-degree valgus wedge causes the patella to move by 1.6 mm.[49] To measure this small amount of motion steel pins had to be placed in the patella and the femur, because in video analysis the motion of markers placed on the skin is greater than the motion of the patella.[15] The pins and the large wedge are not routinely used in a clinical setting, but they were required to demonstrate a difference in the position of the patella. If pain can be alleviated by wedging, the empirical approach can be used, because the amount of patellar movement does not need to be known.

In the above example, gait analysis would be used only to assess the treatment. Diagnosis would be extremely difficult, because the amount of pronation needed to cause pain differs from one person to another. The difficulty in establishing normal values is discussed under Statistical Aspects below.

Discussion

The two approaches are not mutually exclusive. The modeling approach can help in choosing the proper measurements for assessment of injuries or treatments, and will prevent random searches for the best indicator of a particular abnormality. The modeling approach can be used to pick the most likely indicators of an abnormality, and these can be further investigated using the empirical approach. It should again be emphasized that computerized gait analysis should provide information beyond what the practitioner can obtain on his or her own. Gait analysis should be able to predict, with reasonable accuracy, whether or not a patient is likely to incur an injury and whether a particular therapy will lead to relief of symptoms. All too often practitioners concentrate on the process of measurement and forget that a device must have some predictive value to be truly useful in prevention of injuries.

Technical aspects
Data acquisition and storage

It is important that the clinician understand the technical aspects of computerized analysis. All of the devices discussed here have limits to their ability to produce accurate measurements. Understanding the causes of these limits will enable the clinician to make better decisions regarding the use and acquisition of the instrumentation. Often, the device that is on the cutting edge of current technology is not the one that the clinician has in the office. Understanding the trade-off between cost and performance is important in deciding on which technology to use. Some of the following concepts are related to the technical abilities of gait analysis instrumentation to produce reliable data. There are several steps in the production of data: (1) choice of data gathering device; (2) performance by the subject; (3) attaining the raw data signal; (4) processing the data; (5) storage of data and (6) production of output to the clinician. At each of these steps, information can be lost or altered in such a way as to make the measurement less meaningful. However, some of these limitations are related to decisions made at the time of acquisition of the instrument and thus can be disregarded for general clinical use.

The output signal from a measurement device will have some noise present when it is used. Noise is an unwanted variation in the signal. An example of noise is the television set that is tuned to a station where there is no signal. What is seen is static, which must be removed to produce a good picture. Sources of noise for kinematic analysis include electronic noise, spatial inaccuracies of the digitizing system, and human error if the digitizing is done by hand.[104] Another source of noise is the movement of markers placed on the skin relative to the bones they are supposed to represent.[10] For further information on processing of raw data the reader is referred to Winter's text.[104] One method of eliminating noise

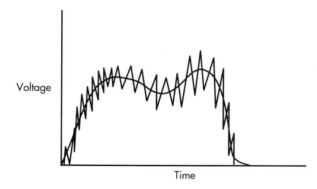

Fig. 8-1. The jagged line represents the actual values measured from the device. The other line is the result after data smoothing.

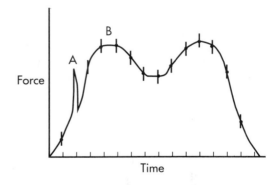

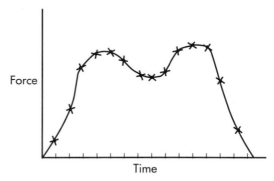

Fig. 8-2. The effects of sampling rate and frequency of signal. The top curve is the continuous force applied to the sensor. The marks on the curve indicate when the data for the bottom curve are sampled. The sampling frequency was not high enough to measure peak A, but it was high enough to measure peak B.

when a force sensor is used to measure the time of contact is to set a threshold at which the reading commences. If the threshold is set too low, random noise may trigger the switch, creating an artificially long contact period. To prevent this the contact switch can be set at 50 N instead of 1 N. This difference in threshold may explain differences in length of contact reported by different investigators for a similar experiment.[29]

Data smoothing

Data smoothing is a mathematical process by which noise is removed. This can also be called fitting a curve to the data.[104] For example, the output of a measuring instrument that produces a very jagged curve when all the points are connected will produce a smoother curve after data fitting (Fig. 8-1). The smoothing reduces error caused by noise.[109] One of the methods for producing a smoother curve is called a low pass filter. Oscillations in the raw data above a certain frequency are removed and oscillations of a lower frequency are allowed to pass through. Bobbert et al.[10] have shown that different cutoff frequencies may be necessary for measurements of the head, hip, and leg to produce an accurate representation of what is occurring. However, data smoothing may reduce peak values that actually exist, thus producing inaccuracies.[10] An example of this is the single, short duration force peak that sometimes occurs at heel contact (Fig. 8-2). The tradeoff in data smoothing is between producing generally more accurate data and a loss of some peak values. For further information on data smoothing the reader is referred to Winter's text.[104]

Data sampling

It is believed that one of the biggest advantages of computers is the ability to convert analog data from the continuous output from a sensor to digital

data.[16] For example, a single force sensor will create a continuous but variable voltage over time that correlates with varying force values. Digitization of the voltage signal requires measuring the voltage at a particular instant in time and assigning a numeric value to the voltage. In a given time period there are an infinite number of instants at which the voltage may be sampled. The upper limit of sampling may be determined by cost, data storage capacity, or the physical properties of the sensor. The lower limit of the frequency is determined by the signal itself. The sampling theorem states that "the process signal must be sampled at a frequency at least twice as high as the highest frequency present in the signal itself."[104] The process signal is the signal that is sampled at a particular instant in time. A variable whose value oscillates in 5.0 ms must be sampled at a minimum every 2.5 ms. An example of a high-frequency signal that must be sampled at a high rate is peak pressure on the heel during contact. The peak pressure may last for less than 0.04 second, so the signal should be sampled at least every 0.02 second.[60] The sampling theorem is critical in the digitization process.

The simple answer to the requirement of the

sampling theorem is to sample more often. There is, however, a limit to the amount of data that can be collected at one time, and there is a limit to the number of calculations that can be made from those data before the processing time increases significantly. Furthermore, the speed and storage capacity of computers are rapidly improving, so that ever-increasing amounts of data collection and processing can be done in a reasonable time. Understanding how computers manipulate data will help the clinician determine which piece of hardware needs to be upgraded to improve the performance of the analysis instrument.

The speed of the incoming data must match the computer's ability to record these data. There are two kinds of basic memory in computers, random access memory (RAM) and read-only memory (ROM). These memories are in different parts of the hardware. For the computer to use information it has to be in RAM. When the RAM memory becomes full, part of the data has to be stored in ROM. It takes time for the computer to write this information to the ROM hard drive. This is one reason why personal computers are faster when additional RAM is added. When a large amount of data is gathered in real time it has to be stored in RAM because the computer cannot write it into ROM fast enough. After the data gathering has finished the computer can then write the information into ROM. One of the major distinctions between RAM and ROM is that when the power to the computer is turned off the data in RAM is lost.

The term *read-only memory* is a little confusing. In the past ROM for computers has primarily represented magnetically encoded data on disks. The data could not only be read but could be written and erased by the computer. This is important for data that are changing from day to day (e.g., patient files). More recently, compact disk ROM (CD-ROM) has been developed, which at this time cannot be modified by personal computers. The information on CD-ROM is encoded by the disk manufacturer. The advantage of CD-ROM is that large amounts of data can be stored in a small amount of space, and the information is more durable than that encoded on magnetic disks. Recommendations on the amount of RAM and ROM that should be acquired are useless because the technology is changing rapidly. To say that retrieval of information from ROM is slow is a relative statement. It is only slow when compared with RAM. Retrieval of ROM data is much faster than retrieval of data on magnetic tape. The reason for this is that the computer can go directly to the location on the disk where the information is stored. To access information on a tape, the tape must be wound to the location of the data.

Calibration

The electronic output from a sensor must be calibrated with real life to make the data useful. When the sensor has an output of 5 mV the absolute value of force on the sensor must be known or measurable. In fact, this is how calibration is done. Several known forces are applied to the sensor and the output is measured. Linearity is the desired property of the sensor that describes the relation between the force applied and the electrical output. A particular sensor could have an output of 5 mV when the force applied is 5 N, and the output could be 10.3 mV when the force applied is 10 N. This is an example of nonlinearity. If the calibration is done well and over small enough intervals, the computer can take nonlinearity into account. Devices that apply force uniformly over a large area have been developed so that many small sensors can be calibrated at the same time.[62] Optical force measuring systems cannot be calibrated in this manner, because the total force on the device would cause it to break.[62] However, small areas of optical devices can be calibrated at a time.[8,9] The total force from optical devices can be calibrated with another type of sensor that measures the same data at the same time.[9]

There may be loads for which the sensor cannot be calibrated. The sensor can "max out" at a certain level, and an added force will not produce any higher output from the sensor. Manufacturers should publish the effective range of their sensors. If the sensor reaches its maximum at a value that is obviously going to cause tissue damage, its ability to distinguish different amounts of stress at lower levels may still be useful. The range of measurement must be greater than the range of possible nonpathologic values. Another difficulty in calibration and the use of force-sensing devices is the response rate of the device. For example, one noncommercial force sensor was observed to achieve 95% of its voltage output in 0.05 second.[85] If the force under the sensor rose and fell in 0.02 second, the sensor would be unable to detect the peak value. This difficulty also points to the need for calibration under the conditions in which the device will be used.

A problem similar to slow response rate is drift. Drift is a change in electrical output that sometimes occurs when there is no change in the force applied to the sensor. A decision must be made at the time of calibration about the time the calibration is made relative to when the known load is applied. If the measurement is to be after the person has been standing on the sensor for 2 minutes, then the calibration should be made after the load is applied for this amount of time as well. If rapid loading and unloading is of interest, then for maximum precision the device should be calibrated shortly after the load is applied. However, if a 5% error and the loss of some peak values are acceptable, then the timing of calibration is not that important. The amount of acceptable error must be determined for the specific use and compared with the precision required for the use for each type of device.

When using three-dimensional video or film analysis, this must be calibrated as well. The computer does not know the location of one camera relative to another, so this has to be determined before the positions of body parts can be established. One method of calibration is to set a series of markers at known locations, take readings of the markers with all the cameras, and then correlate the positions of the markers recorded from each camera with the computer.[90]

EMG signals can also be calibrated. This is done by having the subject perform a maximum voluntary contraction and recording the level of EMG output. Smaller outputs can be graded against the maximum to give a relative level. This value can be compared across subjects. The problem of nonlinearity also occurs with EMG measurements. This difficulty can be solved by having the subject produce several different moments at varying joints and measuring the EMG output.[3] However, muscle length and speed of contraction may make accurate calibration difficult.[3]

A concern with the use of any device is how often it requires recalibration. If any component of the device wears out over time, the output of the sensor could be affected. The difficulty of recalibration is a concern as well, especially if the device has to be sent back to the manufacturer for recalibration. Manufacturers of analytical devices should be able to tell the user how often the device will require recalibration.

Data presentation

There are many steps between the collection and processing of raw data and the presentation of data to the interested clinician. Many of these steps are never seen by the clinician who is using the gait analysis device, because the computer has been programmed to do them automatically. The software must digitize, calibrate, smooth, store, and present the data. The programming and electrical engineering required to do this often makes this the most expensive part of the gait analysis device. The ease with which information can be extracted from a gait analysis device depends on the presentation of the data by the software. Examples of types of presentation include pressure mountains (Fig. 8-3) or color plots for pressure distribution or stick figures for the representation of motion. Of course,

the graphing of numeric data over time is an easy way to visualize changes in gait. Comparison of one graph with another requires some special statistical manipulations, and this is discussed below.

The choice of data presentation is often determined by the manufacturer of the analysis device. Once the basics of how computers store and retrieve data are mastered, then most commercially available analysis systems have software that is relatively easy to use. As with any new application, adequate time should be allowed for learning how to use the software. The data presentation should include all the information that the clinician is interested in and should be easy to use and learn. If an important parameter is excluded from the software, the user will either have to write his or her own software or pay someone else to write it. Prior to acquisition of a gait analysis system the literature should be carefully reviewed to determine what values are useful.

Durability

When selecting a gait analysis device an important concern is the short- and long-term durability of the device and its components. For example, the sensor should last at least as long as the measurement that is to be performed. In an early version of a pressure distribution sensing device it was noted that after 12 measurements the total force dropped by 20%.[79] If the measurement protocol required 12 measurements, then this particular device could not reliably appraise any difference smaller than 20%. A way to circumvent this problem is to use new identical sensors for subsequent trials. This procedure was attempted and it was noted that these factory-calibrated sensors had different force values for their first use in identical situations. This difference between sensors is a problem because the comparison then must be made with the same sensor. This turned out to be ineffective as well because of the drop in total force over time. (The manufacturer has since changed the calibration procedure because temperature and method of application of the sensor affected the output.)

Long-term durability is important in the choice of a gait analysis device. There is a distinctive tradeoff between a force-measuring device with disposable sensors that cost less than $40 and one with a sensor that may need to be repaired once every 5 years at a cost of $4,000. A problem with assessing the durability of gait-measuring devices is that most are so new that they do not have a valid frequency-of-repair record.

Subject-test interaction

One of the major problems in gait analysis is that the test itself may alter gait. Just as the blood pressure

N/cm²
59

N/cm²
59

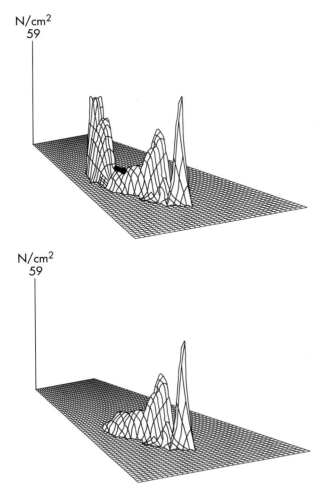

Fig. 8-3. Representation of pressure: the height of the mountain represents the amount of pressure under that particular location. *Above,* A maximum pressure plot in which the maximum pressure at each sensor is displayed. This does not represent any specific moment in time. *Below,* The pressure at a particular moment in time after the heel has left the ground.

analysis is to measure the effects of treatment or to distinguish between the normal and the pathologic and not the changes in gait caused by the measurement.

Assessment is further complicated by the fact that velocity of gait affects many variables. In fact, the subject's chosen velocity of gait may vary with treatment. It has been shown that vertical ground reactive force[48,65,69] and the anteroposterior component of ground reactive force[65] vary with running speed. Therefore, it is critical when measuring ground reactive force to hold the velocity of the subject constant. Other variables that have been shown to vary with velocity are joint power[101] and peak pressure.[17] This variation illustrates the important interrelationship among variables. For example, a treatment directed toward reducing force on the foot could be falsely determined to be ineffective if the subject had a faster gait as a result of the treatment.

Another interaction between the subject and the test is the effect of the subject's pain on his or her gait. A study done on the effects of a proximal tibial osteotomy that was used to treat excessive tibial varum[96] compared clinical results with static and dynamic values preoperatively and postoperatively. The clinical results were more closely related to the adduction moment on the knee during gait than to the amount of the static varus deformity. (Adduction moment is a measurement of how much ground reactive force will increase the varus deformity.) The study also found that patients who walked more "normally" tended to have a higher adduction moment. Subjects who had a lower adduction moment tended to walk with their leg more externally rotated. The authors concluded that some people alter their gait in such a way as to reduce the pain from the deformity.[96]

The same question of pain and gait has been raised in relation to hallux abducto valgus. Sanders and co-workers[80] note that with hallux abducto valgus there is a tendency to decrease weightbearing on the first ray,[35,43] but they also showed that flexion forces on the hallux increase the deformity. Perhaps an attempt is made by the patient to reduce flexion forces by shifting weight to the lateral side of the foot.

Another confounding interaction could result from the added weight of, or hindrance from, the data collection instruments. Instruments that need to be attached to the body include in-shoe force sensors and EMG leads. There are three basic methods of transferring information from data collection devices attached to the body to the computer, where they can be processed. Telemetry uses a mini–radio transmitter with a receiver and

may go up when the patient's arm is compressed by the cuff, gait may be altered because the patient is conscious of being tested. One experimenter attributed an increase in double support time to the fact that the subjects were afraid of walking on a treadmill.[91] Another study noted that elderly subjects had an increased heart rate while walking on a treadmill compared to walking in a hallway, but younger subjects exhibited no change.[34] If the change were consistent it might not be a problem, but there is often a learning effect. In a study of novice treadmill users compared with persons experienced on the treadmill, the novices had higher heart rates, blood pressures, and perceived exertion.[26] Whether the effect is from fear or simply getting used to the test, these studies show that the test has some effect on the subject. The goal of

then transfers the data to the computer. The second method is to store the information in a pack attached to the body and download the data at a later time. The third method is to have wires leading from the sensors on the patient directly to the free-standing computer. There are tradeoffs between cost, convenience, and interference with the patient for each of these methods.

The effect of added weight from instrumentation depends on what is being measured. When additional load is applied to limbs the kinematic pattern does not change, but moment, joint forces, and metabolic demand are increased.[56] Therefore, if measurement of motion is desired, added mass may not be a problem. The effects of added mass are greater when the mass is placed more distally.[56] Therefore, the transmitter or data collection storage device should be snugly attached to the trunk.

One method to reduce the interference of wires connected to a patient is to have the patient use a treadmill. Treadmills are also convenient for visual analysis because many steps can be analyzed consecutively. With over-ground running, only the step that the camera has in focus can be analyzed. However, the treadmill itself can affect the measurement of gait. The amount of training needed to reduce the treadmill effects on gait is currently under debate.[3,91] This debate is important enough to explore in some detail as gait analysis would be much more convenient with a treadmill in a clinical setting where space is limited. In a study by Arsenault and co-workers, treadmill walking and over-ground walking were compared using segmental energy analysis and EMG activation.[3] There were no significant segmental energy changes, and only one of the muscles measured showed a significant difference. The authors concluded that treadmills are satisfactory for gait analysis. However, in this study they held the cadence of gait constant and noted a shortening of stride length of 4%.[3] The authors suggest that if a treadmill with a longer surface were used, this shortened stride might be prevented. Also, stride length tends to increase with time of practice on the treadmill.[82] The reason for the shortened stride may be that the subject is afraid of falling off the end of the moving surface.

One of the major problems associated with treadmills involves changes in the variability of gait. A decrease in vertical and horizontal velocity while on the treadmill has been observed,[25] but most other studies note an increase in the variability of gait. This variability is reduced as the subject becomes more accustomed to the treadmill over time. The time needed to adapt is currently under study. One study says that several practice sessions totaling 1 hour of treadmill time are required for consistent gait.[95] The authors also observed that some subjects adjust more quickly than others.[95] Other investigators noted that gait had stabilized halfway through the second 15-minute training session.[82] Both of these studies noted that the first 2 minutes of any session were more variable than any time later in the session. Finally, Cavanagh and Henley[16] report that they found one 15-minute training session to be adequate for analysis.

There has been some debate over whether the treadmill is capable of adding energy to the stance leg by pushing it backward. Theoretically, there is no difference between over-ground walking and treadmill walking.[91] Walking on a treadmill is like walking in an airplane. The motion of the subject with respect to the surface that he is walking on is the same, but the motion with respect to the earth is different. The measurements of the subject must be made relative to the belt of the treadmill and not to the floor underneath the treadmill. The surface of the treadmill should not bounce when it is landed on, because this bounce would make the treadmill act as a shock absorber and thus alter the measurements. A 10% change in the instantaneous velocity of the treadmill belt has been noted.[75] This change probably occurs because the load on the treadmill is much less before heel contact than after heel contact, especially in running. The variation in velocity may be reduced by using treadmills with large flywheels that provide greater inertia. This problem may also be remedied to a lesser extent by more powerful motors driving the treadmill.

In summary, when treadmills are used for gait analysis they should ideally have (1) a surface significantly longer than the subject's stride length; (2) a surface that does not bounce; (3) a belt that does not change velocity; and (4) a system that measures movement relative to the treadmill belt and not to the floor.

The difference between reality and instrument measurement

After the technical problems mentioned above have been solved the computer is able to produce large amounts of data from the measurements. The question is whether these data represent useful information. Whether or not this information is useful depends on the precision and validity of the data. Precision can be determined by measuring the same motion several times and observing how much the data change from one measurement to the next. Validity is related to whether what is being measured is actually related to what it is thought is being measured.

Precision

One of the major difficulties in assessing precision is the variability of human walking. When the position of a marker on the subject varies, is this attributable to random error in the measuring device or is one stride actually different from the next? In video analysis, where the position is determined by the computer, the computer may make the same "random" error every time. For example, if the actual measurement of an angle is 5.5 degrees, the computer may always round this up to 6.0 degrees. In a study on three-dimensional video analysis it was found that the stride-to-stride variability was much greater than the variability caused by recalibrating the system.[2] This implies that the measurement system was precise enough. Another source of error in video analysis is marker placement. A study of hip motion, in which markers were removed and reapplied, found that there were systematic changes in the measurements.[92] The investigators also found that range of motion and the time when the motion reversed direction did not change. This concept may be important for measurement of calcaneal motion, because maximal eversion relative to the ground is dependent on marker placement. Although the above examples were related to video analysis, the concept of precision is important for all measurement devices. A problem with each device is determining what level of precision is accurate enough to be useful.

Validity

There are two important factors to consider in assessing the validity of the measurement. First, the user must ensure that what is being measured is really what is thought is being measured. Second, it must be determined whether the measurement is related to the abnormality. Subtalar joint pronation, ground reactive force, and motion measurement in general will be discussed in relation to these concepts.

One of the major assumptions in the measurement of subtalar joint motion is that the shoe moves with the heel when the subtalar joint pronates or supinates. In a study where holes were cut into the heel counter of the shoe it was found that in a side-to-side movement the shoe motion does not correlate with heel motion.[76] The investigators also found that the correlation between shoe and heel motion was worse when larger holes were cut into the shoe. This result implies that stiffness of the heel counter is important when measuring shoe motion relative to heel motion. The same authors found that in running, as compared to side-to-side motion, the difference between shoe markers and heel markers was less.[89] Another question, not addressed by these studies, is whether the skin markers accurately represent the motion of the calcaneus for all people. It is not known how much the skin over the calcaneus moves relative to the bone.

Two assumptions are made when defining subtalar joint pronation as motion between the calcaneal bisection and the leg. The first is that this motion represents only talocalcaneal motion and not any ankle joint motion. The second assumption is that all of the subtalar joint axis motion is in the frontal plane. If the ankle joint is at an angle to the plane of measurement, there will be some contribution from ankle joint motion to the measured inversion and eversion of the calcaneus to the leg. Subtalar joint motion is not entirely in the frontal plane, and motion measured only in the frontal plane will underestimate the true motion of the subtalar joint. Scott and Winter[84] have developed a mathematical model for this motion that requires three-dimensional measurement and assessment of the location of the subtalar joint axis. This mathematical model can differentiate ankle joint motion from subtalar joint motion. The authors found that two-dimensional model assumptions caused an error between 6% and 22% in calculation of joint moment compared to the three-dimensional model's position of the axes. The error increased with larger deviations of the axes away from the cardinal body planes.[84]

One of the most difficult problems in correlating subtalar joint pronation with abnormalities is deciding which aspect of motion is important. Hamill and co-workers[39] noted that some researchers believe that the total amount of pronation is important while others believe the speed of pronation is important. Both speed and total pronation may be important, but perhaps for different disorders. It has been speculated that the internal rotation of the leg associated with pronation may be responsible for pathologic changes.[14,32] The foot that appeared the most "pronated" was the foot that showed the most internal leg rotation.[32]

The value for subtalar joint motion depends on how that value was obtained. One of the earliest papers on subtalar joint motion used a goniometer that was attached to the leg and the shoe to measure the motion.[111] The authors found that the normal subtalar joint moves between 4 and 6 degrees in the stance phase of gait. The authors mentioned that they treated subtalar and midtarsal joints as the same. However, later authors have treated these results as a function of the subtalar joint only.[78] Researchers using three-dimensional video analysis have found averages of approximately 15 degrees of subtalar joint motion.[2,84] The norms established with one measuring device should not be compared with the values obtained with another.

Subtalar joint motion cannot be determined from the position of the ground reactive force. A simple example can be used to explain this. Visualize two feet striking the ground at the same time, one with its forefoot at an angle of 3 degrees to the ground and the other at an angle of 6 degrees. If the medial forefoot of each foot were to hit the ground at the same time, the timing of ground reactive force would be identical, but the feet would have different velocities and amounts of pronation. Now, imagine those same two feet hitting the ground, but this time have the medial forefoot of the 6-degree inverted foot hit in twice the time it takes compared to the other foot. The more inverted foot had to evert farther to reach the ground, but it cannot be known from force plate data if it started more inverted or pronated slower (Fig. 8-4).

One of the major assumptions of ground reactive force measurement is that the magnitude of ground reactive force is related to pathologic changes.[69] This sounds plausible, but the results of reducing force have been difficult to measure. Materials used to reduce the magnitude of ground reactive force in running shoes[69] and on sports surfaces[67] have not demonstrated a correlation between material tests and a reduction of force. An example of a material test is the measurement of the deceleration of an instrument, of a known mass, when it is dropped onto a shoe or an insole material. Force is equal to mass times acceleration. Different materials exhibit different rates of deceleration and hence there will be differing amounts of peak force on the instrument. The force reduction with material tests is not seen with people wearing shoes made from these materials while running.[69] However, when subjects land after dropping from a height there was a reduction of the magnitude of ground reactive force when the the midsole material in their shoes had been altered.[37] Although ground reactive force did not change much in running there were changes in the motions of the lower extremity.[69] Materials can alter ground reactive force in some situations, and they cause alteration of body mechanics in others.

Ground reactive force per se does not represent all of the available sources of compressive force when measuring stress on the joints. Ground reactive force in running can range from 1.6 to 2.3 times body weight during heel contact, but it has been calculated that the compression force at the talocrural joint can reach 11 times body weight during the stance period while jogging slowly.[83] This compression force comes from the triceps surae pulling the tibia down and the calcaneus up. Ground reactive force represents only a small portion of the total force acting at this time. It is not clear whether the rapid onset of ground reactive force or the high magnitude of joint compressive force is more likely to be related to pathologic changes. More research is needed to determine which, if any, abnormalities are related to ground reactive force.

The measurement and description of motion can produce a host of data. Motion by itself does not tell us anything regarding the forces that cause the motion. It has been demonstrated that the moments at the joints do not correlate well with motion exhibited at the joints.[101] This may occur because hip extension can also produce knee extension and vice versa. Therefore, using motion to infer which muscles are acting is not a valid method of analysis.

Statistical aspects

In using any test to differentiate normal from abnormal populations, some basic understanding of statistics is required. This is especially true for computerized gait analysis. Some of the statistical problems occur when deciding whether a measurement is different enough to change the treatment or to judge if the treatment is successful.

Confidence limits

One of the most frequently used methods of determining normal from abnormal populations is the use of confidence limits. Confidence limits are set by first measuring a "normal" or "asymptomatic" population and establishing a distribution of values for this population. Then a confidence limit is chosen for this range of values.[9] The limit could be 1[99] or 2 SD[18] from the mean, or it could be set by excluding the 5% of measures that are farthest from the mean; this is a 95% confidence limit. Usually this means that values lower than the value at the 2.5th percentile and values higher than the 97.5th percentile are termed abnormal. This method is better than using a percentage change. For example, a change of 50% for one measurement could represent a clearly abnormal value, whereas a 50% change in another would be less than 1 SD from the mean.[41] One problem in using percentage occurs when the value is near zero. A small change in the value will produce a large percentage change without this being meaningful.[41] The percentile cutoffs do not have this problem. However, when using 95th percentile cutoffs, 5% of normal feet will be termed abnormal.[20] Also, the use of cutoff values may not be sensitive enough to demonstrate an abnormality. When measuring plantar pressures the 2-SD cutoff allows a large amount of overlap when comparing insensate feet with normal feet.[18] Many feet that would be at risk would fall into the normal range.

A   **B**

Time 1

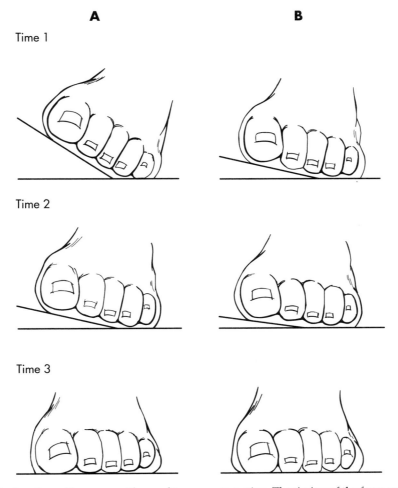

Time 2

Time 3

Fig. 8-4. The location of force cannot be used to measure motion. The timing of the force on the first metatarsal head would be the same for both of the feet above, but the left one would have pronated faster because it started more inverted. Force measurement devices cannot measure the angle of the foot to the ground.

Normal variation

Every step is not the same. The body has to compensate for changes in the terrain, making turns and errors in placement of the foot. Balance control requires constant variability because each step during gait is a controlled fall. In gait the foot is never under the center of mass but the body is always accelerating toward the midline.[55] Because of the requirements of balance for each step, it is logical that the motions of each step are different. This step-to-step variation is demonstrated with subtalar joint motion,[23,111] medial-to-lateral component of ground reactive force,[65] EMG,[58] hip and knee moments,[110] and foot placement.[55,102] Even though an individual demonstrates variation, his or her pattern may be distinguishable from the patterns of other people.[23] In running economy, the single standard deviation in variation is 1.32% and

the 95% confidence limit is 2.64% from the mean when treadmill experience, time of day, footwear, training, and performance are controlled. Therefore, in evaluating treatment the change in economy should be greater than this to state that it is effective.[61]

Normal variability may make it difficult to obtain a "true value" for the average of a single subject. The number of measurements required to get this true value depends on the variability of the measurement. For example, if a measurement varies by 50% from stride to stride, to establish a reliable average value it has to be measured more times than if it varies by 5% from stride to stride. For measurements of pressure distribution it is recommended that five samples be taken to establish an average step.[20] In a study in which running economy was measured by mechanical analysis, it was found that when establishing normal values for a group, a single stride analysis is sufficient, but multiple trials are necessary for the establishment of averages for individuals.[61] Therefore, a single subject should be measured multiple times before and after treatment so that an average can be obtained.

Often, it is assumed that the body should be symmetric, that is, that the left foot should behave the same way as the right. If there is a difference between right and left it is assumed to be abnormal. This has been found to be a poor assumption because some variables that are relatively stable will demonstrate up to 4% asymmetry.[41] There are other problems in the measurement of asymmetry. It was found that when subjects walked in one direction on a walkway, one leg was found to be dominant, but when they walked in the opposite direction, the other leg was dominant.[41] The authors' concluded that the walkway being near a wall had some influence on how the subject walked. A study that compared the effects of spinal manipulation and back exercises on back pain and symmetry of gait noted that the pain reduced more with exercise, while the symmetry reduced more with manipulation.[40] It is still questionable whether the more symmetric gait is better.

Across-subject

When determining an average or "normal" pattern the combination of several individual patterns may produce a norm for the population that does not resemble any of the individual patterns.[3,6,30] This fact is important for determining the effectiveness of a treatment. The entire population may not demonstrate a benefit, but some individuals in the population may benefit. The treatment should not be discarded because it did not help everyone in the population.

Error types

Four interpretations are possible when a measurement is taken. The measurement can correctly say that a person is abnormal or normal. There are, however, two categories of statistical error, commonly called Type I and Type II. Type I error occurs when the test says that the subject is normal when in fact the subject is abnormal. Type II error is the error that says the subject is abnormal when in fact the subject is normal. Understanding that these errors can occur is critical in computer gait analysis.

An example of a Type II error is defining a pressure reading for the foot that would be termed abnormal. A study found that all feet that ulcerated in neuropathic patients had pressures greater than 1.07 MPa. However, a large number of non-neuropathic diabetic patients and 7% of normal subjects had pressures higher than this figure.[7] This pressure level has some significance as an indicator, but many normal people are in this high range.

An example of the second kind of statistical error is a study that demonstrated that 70% of rheumatoid patients had high plantar pressures and pain, but 30% had pain without high plantar pressures.[9] In this case 30% of the patients would not be treated if the sole criterion was the value of the plantar pressure distribution.

Comparison of waveforms

Often data are plotted as a value over time. Several points of information can easily be seen when figures are plotted as a waveform. The peak value and the time at which the peak value occurred are two easily obtainable pieces of data. However, some procedure is needed to compare the shape of one curve relative to another curve over time. One procedure is to divide the curve into discrete time periods and calculate the average value for each time period. The variation for each time period can then be averaged for many total measurements. For an example of the mathematics involved, see Kadaba and co-workers.[46]

The process of converting the waveform into discrete time periods is similar to digitizing analog data. The time periods should not be made too large or data could be lost (see Data Sampling above). One of the difficulties of comparing analog data from one stride to the next is that one stride may be a few milliseconds longer than the next. Numeric data can be manipulated so that the time can correspond to a percentage of the gait cycle. As an example Winter has calculated the EMG value at intervals of 2% of stride length.[99] There is a tradeoff between the possibility of losing information and the number of calculations that are necessary. If the value is calculated at every 1% of the stride, then twice as many calculations must be done. These additional calculations may not provide any more information if the original signal does not oscillate significantly within 2% of the stride.

Comparison of force values across subjects is difficult because people who are heavier will have higher force outputs, but not necessarily pressures.[20] It is possible to compare output of force devices between subjects of different mass by dividing the force output by the person's body weight.

Types of measurement

There are several types of gait analysis measurement, including force measurement, motion measurement, electrical activity, and oxygen consumption. Oxygen consumption cannot be appropriately used for the prevention and treatment of injuries. Its proper setting is in a human performance laboratory where the economy of gait is being refined rather than being assessed for the extent of abnormality. Each of the other types of gait measurement will be discussed.

Force and pressure measurement

There are many devices that are available to measure force and pressure. Devices can vary quite significantly in how they measure the force, and how the force is measured can affect the output of a device. The differences in the technology of devices can affect the results of the measurements. In deciding whether a particular device is useful for the measurement in question it is important to know something about how the device works.

It is important to understand the distinction between force and pressure. Pressure is equal to force divided by area. The total force acting on the calcaneus represents its total load. The pressure under the calcaneus may not be a measure of the total load on the calcaneus.[75] This is because pressure is measured by using very small sensors that can measure force, and pressure is the force on the sensor divided by the area of the sensor. A foot whose highest pressure is noted under the second metatarsal head may also have the highest load under the first, as the second has approximately half the area of the first.[29] Pressure cannot be accurately determined by dividing the force acting on the entire foot by the area of the entire foot.[19] Discrete locations may have much higher pressures than other parts of the foot.[17,56]

The output of a pressure sensor can depend on the sensor itself. Two factors that affect the output of the sensor are the size and compliance of the sensor. The pressure reading can also depend on how the data are processed after they leave the sensor.[53] Larger rigid sensors can concentrate pressure, whereas transducers that are compliant can actually reduce the true pressures by accommodating to an existing deformity.[20] Since the force on a sensor is divided by the area of the sensor, the size of the sensor is critical in giving the final value. Different devices provide different results on the same foot owing to a different sensor-effective area.[21] For example, a single metatarsal could apply its force to a sensor that is either 0.75 or 1.0 cm^2. The force applied is the same but the measured pressure reading is different. This example demonstrates the importance of resolution of the pressure distribution device. The resolution that is needed depends on the area and shape of the structure that is to be measured.[62] Heel pressure decreases and metatarsal

pressure increases with sensor size.[60,62] It should be reiterated that pressure measurements are gauged by individual, small-force sensors.

Force measurement

This discussion of force sensors is divided into two parts. The first part is an examination of the advantages and drawbacks of the different electronic methods for gathering data. Each method produces an electrical signal that is compared to a calibrated value to produce a value of force for the particular sensor. The second part is a discussion of how the force data are presented to the clinician. An electrical method for gathering data can be used in several different ways to present data.

The original force measurement sensor was a rubber mat impregnated with ink. The more pressure applied to the mat, the more ink left on a piece of paper. Ink mats are inexpensive and may provide some information on static stance and the maximum pressure achieved during gait. Ink mats are limited in their ability to differentiate between pressure levels and their ability to give a value of pressure over time.[20]

There are five types of electronic sensors for measurement of force. These are (1) strain gauge, (2) piezoelectric, (3) optical, (4) resistive, and (5) capacitance sensors.[62,104] Strain gauges are time-independent, that is, they have little drift.[62] The disadvantages of strain gauges are that they require a large amount of deformation and have a limited range of measurement and a limited response time. Piezoelectric devices are very linear,[36,62] but they are temperature-dependent, not easily bent, and exhibit drift.[9] Resistive sensors can be made very thin, but they are temperature-sensitive, exhibit drift, and one type of resistive sensor is susceptible to breakage, necessitating that the sensors be disposable. The quality of capacitance sensors is determined by the material that separates the metal plates that are charged. Capacitance sensors are easily calibrated, but their output changes when they are bent.

Optical sensors work by placing a plastic film over a sheet of glass. Differing amounts of pressure cause different amounts of light to be refracted. The glass is filmed with a video camera and the pressure is correlated with a gray scale.[8,9] The resolution and the frequency of measurement are determined by the video camera.[9] Optical systems are very good at providing spatial resolution, but they are not appropriate for measuring high pressures that have a short duration.[9] Optical systems can only measure the pressure of the bottom of the shoe or a bare foot in contact with the floor.

There are three basic devices that utilize the different types of sensors. The first device is a solid plate under which either piezoelectric or strain gauge sensors are placed and the vertical and horizontal components of force applied to the plate are measured. From these data the center of pressure can be calculated.[104] However, the location of the foot relative to the force plate has to be input manually. One method is to attach an ink-soaked string to the shoe or foot, measure the location of the foot contact, and compare this with the center-of-pressure data.[101] Although this method cannot provide specific locations of high localized force, it can provide mediolateral and anteroposterior components of ground reactive force. These components, along with the center of pressure, are important for calculating the moment about joint axes.

The second type of device is the discrete sensor. Either a single sensor or a group of sensors that are usually the size of a metatarsal head are applied directly to the foot. Discrete sensors provide data about a specific location on the foot that solid plate sensors cannot,[37] but they cannot give the location of the center of pressure. Because these sensors have to be reapplied with each use there is a day-to-day repeatability error of 9.9% across all locations, with some locations exhibiting an even higher error.[38] All of the electrical devices except the optical have been utilized as discrete sensors. These sensors can be and usually are used inside shoes. Brodsky et al.[12] have stated that one commercially available discrete sensor in common use is neither reliable nor accurate.

Another device that falls loosely into the force measurement category as a discrete sensor is the foot switch. A foot switch is a force sensor that tells only whether force is present or not. Several switches are placed on various locations of the foot and the timing of the force on these locations is recorded. Foot switches are excellent for recording cadence and time of contact for the various locations on the foot. They cannot measure motion; they can only give the location of the foot when it is on the ground.

The third type of device is a matrix of small-force sensors. The combined output of these sensors, called a pressure distribution, provides information on specific locations on the foot. At this time there is no commercially available device that can measure horizontal (shear) as well as vertical forces at discrete locations on the foot. Pressure distribution devices can either be embedded in a walkway or they can be made to fit inside a shoe. The devices embedded in a walkway can give the vertical forces at a specific location for a single step on a bare foot. However, the walkway devices cannot provide information on the location of the pressure inside the shoe. The in-shoe devices may be used to record

many consecutive steps. One disadvantage of the in-shoe device is that the sensor has to be connected directly to the computer or to a temporary data storage device that is attached to the body. For further discussion of this problem see Technical Aspects above. These pressure distribution devices can provide the location of the center of pressure without the manual input of the location of the foot that is needed for solid-plate force sensors. This occurs because the outline of the foot relative to the center of pressure is already available.

A final and dramatically different method of measuring force is the use of accelerometers. Accelerometers work on the principle of Newton's second law: force is equal to mass times acceleration. A small mass is placed on a force transducer and when there is an acceleration of the mass the transducer will have an electrical output proportional to the acceleration. If the acceleration and the mass of the body part are known, the force acting on the body part can be calculated. A single accelerometer is able only to measure force perpendicular to the surface of the minitransducer and therefore only the acceleration in this direction can be measured. For obtaining the complete direction and magnitude of the force, three accelerometers are used. They are arranged so that one measures anteroposterior acceleration, another measures mediolateral acceleration, and a third measures vertical acceleration. One problem with accelerometers is that they not only respond to landing shock but also to rotations of the body part to which they are attached.[50] When measuring accelerations of the tibia it is suggested that the accelerometer be placed near the ankle, where the rotation is less, rather than near the knee.[50] Accelerometers have also been considered for measurement of motion, because if accelerations are known, the position may be calculated. The problem to be overcome is separating the acceleration due to shock from the acceleration resulting from motion, without having to measure ground reactive force or motion at the same time. This separation is advantageous because accelerometers are inexpensive compared with the force- and motion-measuring devices. But the problem of separating shock from motion forces is a formidable one.

One common way to present force data is in the form of a center-of-pressure curve, sometimes called the gait line. The center of pressure is a mathematically derived point that represents the average point of force acting on the foot at a single moment in time. The center-of-pressure curve is a representation of the change in the center of pressure over time. A common misconception is that the center of pressure represents an actual location of where force is on the

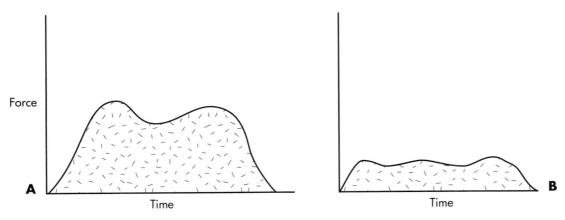

Fig. 8-5. Force time integrals, also called impulses, are represented by the shaded areas. Essentially the value of the impulse is the average force times the time that it is applied. The time of contact for each curve is the same, but the integral is higher for **A.**

foot. To illustrate why this idea is erroneous, consider a foot that has equal weight on the heel and forefoot and no weight on the midfoot; the center of pressure would be on the midfoot region even though the foot does not contact the ground in this location. The center of pressure may be utilized to calculate the moment from ground reactive force about the joints of the foot.[72,88] For example, a foot with a center of pressure that is more lateral from the subtalar joint axis than an average foot will have a greater pronation moment about the axis, and in this foot the subtalar joint will tend to pronate faster than the average foot. There are specialized mathematical methods available for comparing center-of-pressure paths from one subject to another.[63] Further study in this area may lead to center of pressure being a useful measure of the progress of treatment.

Another way to analyze pressure data is to integrate the pressure time curve. This value provides a quantity that represents how much time the pressure is high. An integral is measurement of the area under the curve (Fig. 8-5) and is essentially the average force multiplied by the time the force is applied. The time factor may be important in determining whether tissue damage will occur. It has been shown in animals that very high pressure for a short amount of time can cause skin ulceration, and a smaller amount of pressure can cause an ulcer if applied for a longer amount of time.[64] It is unknown, at this time, whether peak pressure or the pressure time integral correlates more closely with tissue damage.[20] The load on a particular structure may also be integrated over time, and this quantity has been given the name "impulse." The difference between the two integrals may be illustrated by looking at the different measures on the heel and on a metatarsal head. The pressure time integral and the force time integral for a single sensor is propor-

tional because the pressure is equal to the force on the sensor divided by the area of the sensor. The total force on the heel comes from adding values from several sensors together, and the integral of this force value may not be proportional to the average pressure time integral from all the sensors. The pressure time integral is more important for assessment of skin ulceration, and the force time integral is more valuable for evaluating the effects of fatigue on a bone. An error in the use of time integrals can come from noise from the sensors. Noise may give the sensor a positive value when it should equal zero, thus causing the value for the integral to increase by the magnitude of the noise times the time that it is present. This error can be prevented by integrating only the values above a threshold (Fig. 8-6). The threshold should be set so that the amount of noise that is eliminated does not reduce the value of the integral significantly.

An example of the usefulness of pressure time integrals is in quantifying the effect of rheumatoid arthritis on the forefoot. In rheumatoid arthritis, "when abnormally high pressures were reached, the length of time that these levels remained high was often a substantial percentage of the foot ground contact time."[9] Unfortunately, pain does not necessarily correlate with pressure. It was found that 70% of rheumatoid patients had high plantar pressures and pain, and 30% had pain without high plantar pressures.[9]

It should again be noted that the velocity of gait has an important effect on force and pressure. If comparison between treatments is to be attempted, the velocity of gait should be held constant. Gait velocity will also have an effect on the time the foot is in contact with the floor. This factor could dramatically affect time integrals, because the force may remain the same at different speeds, but the

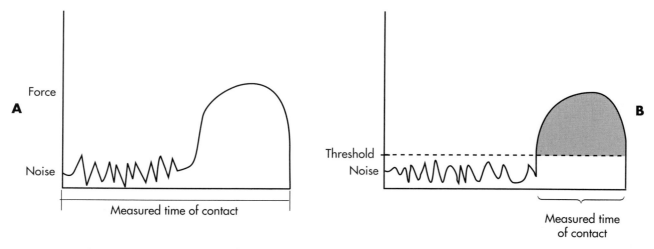

Fig. 8-6. Force time integral above a threshold value. The noise in **A** leads to an artificial increase in the value of the integral. This can be eliminated by integrating only the force above the threshold, **B.**

time it is applied would increase. Even when steps are taken at the same velocity, the difference in time at a specific location may be enough to alter the time integral. More research is needed on the effects that force, pressure, and time have on tissue damage. If it were found that the time a force was applied to a location was useful in predicting or evaluating an injury, then a foot switch could be used to evaluate the injury instead of a more expensive force sensor.

Measurement of motion

There are several methods by which motion can be measured, and they vary in their complexity and accuracy. The methods include projection angles, Euler angles, and screw displacement axes. Projection angles and Euler angles assume there is a fixed anatomical axis relative to the two bones that determine the joint. Projection angles are the angles measured when the line that defines each bone is projected onto a single plane. This occurs when a picture is taken and the position of the markers on the bones is projected onto the focal plane of the camera (Fig. 8-7). This method is called two-dimensional analysis because the distance of the markers from the focal plane of the camera is not known, and therefore projection angles do not fully determine the position of the bone. Projection angles are accurate when the axis of motion of the joint is pointed at the camera, and they become increasingly less accurate the more the axis is angled to the camera.[2]

Euler angles are angles that are determined from the position and orientation of the bones. Strictly speaking, Euler angles measure the angle between a fixed segment and a moving segment.[1] This is difficult to employ for the lower leg because neither the calcaneus nor the leg is fixed. This can be compensated for by measuring the three-dimensional position and orientation of each bone relative to the ground and then measuring the change in position of the bones relative to one another.[2] Three-dimensional position measurement is best done with two cameras that are perpendicular to one another. Additional cameras may be helpful because markers may not be visible to two cameras all of the time. Euler angles can be used to measure the motion relative to the three cardinal planes or around a specific axis of motion. Determination of motion around a specific joint axis is more clinically relevant but it requires knowledge of the location of the axis.[2] The axis location can be estimated and this estimation has given between 6% and 22% improvement of measurement of the absolute motion about the subtalar joint.[84] Measurement about the three cardinal body planes assumes that the axis lies in one of those planes. In either case the use of Euler angles assumes that the axis of rotation remains fixed relative to the bones and therefore the degrees of freedom of the joint are limited. It has been noted that the axis can change relative to bones as motion occurs.[31,93] However, the change in the axis of motion is not significant enough to make the assumption of a single axis invalid when making clinical measurements.[84]

Measurement of motion with screw displacement axes is not limited to joints that are constrained to move around a single axis. Screw displacement axes allow measurement of 6 degrees of freedom (1 degree of freedom for linear motion and 1 degree of freedom for angular motion in each of the cardinal planes). In this method an instantaneous center of rotation is determined; then the angular motion

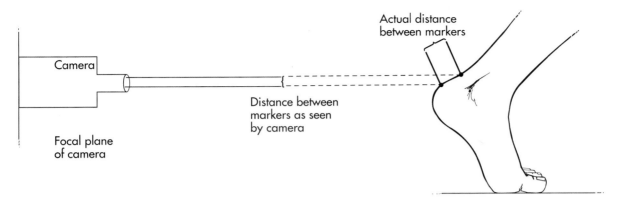

Fig. 8-7. The projection of the position of markers onto the plane of the film. A single camera cannot measure the distance between two points. There is also a distortion in the measurement of angles.

about the axis and any linear displacement along this axis is measured.[1] The difference between Euler angles and screw displacement axes can be seen if the ankle joint is used as an example. The Euler angle method assumes that the ankle joint has only 1 degree of freedom, which is plantar- and dorsiflexion within the sagittal plane. The ankle joint, in pathologic conditions, can show inversion and eversion in the form of talar tilt. The ankle joint can also show displacement when there is a positive anterior drawer sign. Neither of these motions is measured with the use of Euler angles. If both anterior drawer and talar tilt motions are insignificant, the motion measured at the ankle joint should be the same for both Euler angles and screw displacement axes. Scott and Winter[84] found that the ankle and subtalar joints could be treated as monocentric single–degree of freedom joints during the stance phase of walking for the subjects that they measured.

The choice of method of measurement is dependent on the accuracy that is needed for the specific analysis. It has been demonstrated that projection angle measurement of calcaneal eversion is sufficiently sensitive to demonstrate a correlation between the amount of eversion and the likelihood of injury.[5,54] However, two-dimensional analysis is highly sensitive to the angle of gait relative to the camera.[2] It remains to be seen if three-dimensional measurement can improve the prediction of injury. If a modeling approach is to be used, then the screw displacement axis may be employed as an indicator of injury. It has to be determined if the motion that is related to pain is large enough to be detected by video analysis. Pain may not even be related to motion at all; it may be related to force.

There are three tools that are generally used to measure motion: (1) goniometers, (2) video cameras, and (3) accelerometers. Each tool may fit into one or more of the methods of measuring motion. Electronic goniometers usually consist of a hinge and two arms that are applied to different body parts which vary their voltage output depending on the angle between the two arms. These devices are relatively inexpensive, easy to calibrate, and can be very accurate.[44] Since these devices are attached to body parts and they have hinges, they require the assumption that the joints are single–degree of freedom hinge joints. The goniometer can lose accuracy if its hinge is not precisely aligned with the joint axis.[1] The goniometer can also quickly become cumbersome if more than one joint at a time is measured. Each goniometer needs a wire or a radio signal to communicate with the recording device. A difficulty can occur if the bone on either side of the joint is not readily accessible. For example, goniometric studies of the subtalar joint have to contend with the fact that the talus is inaccessible for goniometer arm attachment. Goniometric studies using one attachment on the leg and one on the forefoot have attempted to improve the situation by using a dual goniometer with one axis lined up with the ankle joint and one axis lined up with the subtalar joint.[58,111] With this approach, however, midtarsal joint motion makes the measurement of the other two joints less accurate. Another disadvantage of goniometers is that the angle of the body part relative to the ground cannot be known. This makes it difficult to perform kinetic analysis.[1]

The most commonly used tool for measuring motion is stereometry. Stereometry refers to the use of two or more cameras to establish the position of an object in space. Film, television, or direct digitizer cameras can be used. For film and television, an image is captured and the positions of the markers are then digitized from the image so that the computer can process the information. This process is called direct linear transformation. When this

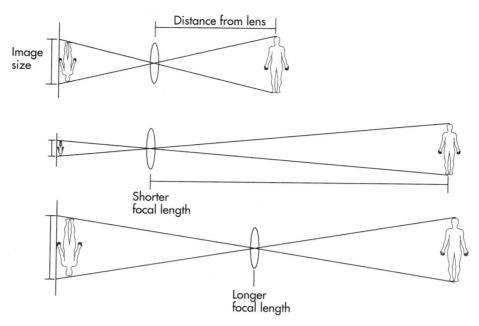

Fig. 8-8. The effects of the distance from the lens and the focal length of the lens. The farther the object is from the lens, the smaller the image. A longer focal length lens can increase image size. For measurement from images the largest image is best.

method was first used with film cameras, each frame was projected and a person was required to manually record the position of each marker in each frame. This is very time-consuming, but it is as precise as automatic digitization. Film is impractical for clinical use because there is a long turnaround time for processing. The difference between television and automatic digitization is that the automatic digitizers automatically record the position of the markers without making a video picture, whereas in television analysis the video picture is taken and then analyzed. For automatic digitization of the position of markers, the device has to distinguish the markers from the background. This requires highly reflective markers.

There are several factors that determine the accuracy of stereometric analysis, including image size, marker motion, and the number of markers used. Image size is determined by the distance from the camera and the focal length of the lens. Ideally, image size should be as large as possible so that measurement error is minimized[104] (Fig. 8-8).

Marker motion can occur between the marker and the skin or between the skin and the shoe. If markers are placed on the shoe there can be motion between the bone and the shoe.[76,89] At least three non-colinear markers are required to define a segment for three-dimensional motion. Using more markers will improve the accuracy of position and orientation measurements. More markers reduce the error caused by the motion of a single marker. This assumes that all the markers do not move the

same amount and that the average position of each marker accurately represents the position of the bone underneath it. One strategy for decreasing marker motion is to attach the markers to hinged sticks. In this study[10] it was found that the impact force peak could be predicted by measuring motion and velocity at heel contact. (This was a prediction of the force at impact and not of the ground reactive force throughout gait.) The impact force could be predicted even though the running style was changed by the subject.[10] Without the sticks, marker motion made the force prediction inaccurate. This measurement appears to be similar to that using goniometers, but a goniometer could not be used because the velocity of the segments relative to the ground is required to make the prediction of ground reactive force.

The final instrument for analyzing motion is the accelerometer. The principle of how an accelerometer works was described above under Force Measurement. In order to measure motion of a body part, two triplane accelerometers are positioned on the body part as far apart as possible. If one end of the body part rotates faster than the other the accelerations at each accelerometer will be different.[13] Angular motion can be calculated from the difference between accelerations at the two ends of the body part. These calculations are complex[1] and the complexity increases as more body parts are measured. In addition, the calculations have to take into account the accelerations from ground reactive force. Accelerometers also suffer the same problem as goniometers in that their position relative to the ground is difficult to determine.[104] The problem could theoretically be solved if the position of the body relative to the ground could be programmed at the start of the measurement. It remains to be seen if these problems can be overcome to make accelerometers a clinically useful measurement tool.

Electrical measurement

There are two electrical measurements that are commonly made in the diagnosis of patients: nerve conduction studies and EMG. Nerve conduction studies are important, but are not necessarily involved in gait analysis, so they will not be discussed here. EMG, however, is an important tool in gait analysis because it gives some insight into the functioning of muscle during gait. Essentially, EMG is the measurement of the voltage changes that occur with depolarization of a muscle. The measurement can be done with either surface electrodes or electrodes that penetrate into the muscle belly. Surface electrodes require more amplification of the signal and may have more interference from other muscles. For an excellent review of the physics of EMG measurement and processing, see Winter's text.[104] EMG can be used as an on/off signal to tell that the muscle is active, or it can be quantified relative to the force produced by the muscle. When used as an on/off signal there must be a threshold designated for when one begins, because noise can make the signal appear to be on longer than it should. This threshold is difficult to determine because it may be different for each muscle on each person.[91,99] Also, there is a delay between the onset of the signal and the development of force by the muscle. This delay can be between 40 and 100 ms for a single fiber.[104] The EMG signal is quantified by measuring a maximum voluntary contraction and comparing the signal from gait to this maximum.[4,73] To obtain the best correlation of EMG with output, the maximum measurement is taken of the muscle at its length during gait and at the same shortening rate as occurs during gait.[73] This calibration of EMG signal to maximum voluntary contraction must be done for each subject; the results in one person may not work for another.[73] It is possible to predict the moment at joints from the EMG signal.[73] It was also observed that the variation between subjects is so high that a normal EMG pattern would be very difficult to establish.[4]

Combined measurements: force and motion and mechanical analysis

When utilizing the model approach to understanding injuries, it is necessary to calculate internal forces. This calculation requires knowledge of the external forces and the motion of the parts of the body. For example, both ground reactive force and the pull from the Achilles tendon contribute to the compressive force at the ankle joint and to the moment about the joint. The net moment about the joint determines the direction of motion of the joint. Ground reactive force can be measured and the tension in the Achilles tendon can be calculated from the motion that is seen.

Steps involved in the calculation of joint moment include determination of the direction and lever arm of ground reactive force, measurement of the motion, and calculation of the moment from the muscle. The lever arm of ground reactive force is dependent on joint position and the direction of the force[11] (Fig. 8-9). This moment is compared to the angular acceleration of the joint. The equation for angular acceleration is the following: net moment = moment of inertia × angular acceleration. If the moment from ground reactive force is not equal to the moment of inertia times the angular acceleration, then there must be a moment contributed by the muscles that can be found by subtracting the ground reactive force moment from the net moment. Returning to the example, the tension in the Achilles tendon could then be calculated using moment = force × lever arm, if the lever arm of the tendon is known. This assumes that the Achilles tendon is the only plantarflexor. For a more detailed discussion of link segment calculations, see Winter's text.[104]

There are several points that deserve further elaboration. The lever arm of the force from the tendon and from the ground has to be located relative to the joint axis. The position of the axis either has to be found or it has to be assumed.[84] The moment of inertia is a very important component of the equation and cannot be ignored.[74,97,100] Moments of inertia for specific body parts may be found in published tables.[27] It is also important to scale the moment of inertia, position of muscles, and position of joint axes to the subject's size.[97] The assumption that a muscle is the sole contributor to joint moment is not always an accurate one.[11,106] When there is more than one anatomical structure that can contribute to a moment, then this situation is called indeterminate. There exist an infinite combination of forces from the different muscles that could equal the net force. In addition to agonist contraction at the joint, there might also be contraction of an antagonist muscle at the same time. For example, at heel contact both knee extensors and flexors contract.[11,106] The indeterminate problem can be partially solved by EMG measurement of the muscles involved.[106]

Support moment and sagittal plane balance

Support moment is a concept that was introduced[100] and refined[103] by Winter and co-workers. It is

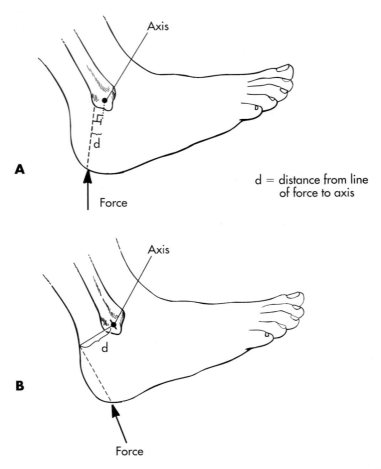

Fig. 8-9. The direction of force is important in determining the magnitude of the joint moment. The location and magnitude of the force in both diagrams is the same, but the lever arm of the force in **B** is greater, thus creating a larger moment.

defined as the sum of the moments from the hip, knee, and ankle. It represents the moment from these joints that is needed to keep the body upright. Winter examined the coefficient of variation of the moment of the joints that make up the support moment and found some interesting relationships.[100] The coefficient of variation is essentially a measurement of the percentage change that is seen with normal variation from stride to stride. Winter found that the coefficient of variation of ankle moments was 22%, that of knee moments was 67%, and that of hip moments was 72%. Surprisingly the coefficient of variation for the support moment was only 25%.[100]

The explanation for the low variation in the support moment was an inverse relationship between the hip and the knee moments.[103] The reason for the hip variation was attributed to the need to adjust for anteroposterior balance of the trunk.[100] If the trunk leans too far forward the hip extensors act to pull the trunk back. If the trunk leans too far back, the knee extensors move it forward. It was also found that there was a high correlation between hip

moment and trunk acceleration.[103] These changes in moment were present when there was very little change in the motion of the limbs.[100] In other words, the moment varied greatly even though the motion from that moment did not vary much. Another lesson from these data is that the moment at a single joint should not be measured by itself because the moment at one joint is interrelated with moments at other joints.[98,101,107]

Kinematics and kinetics

Kinematics is the measurement of motion without regard to the forces that cause the motion. Kinetics is measurement of motion and the forces that cause the motion. As was mentioned above the kinematic pattern may not change but there may be an infinite combination of moments at the joints that can produce the same motion. This can occur because an extension moment at the hip can produce extension of the knee, and an extension moment at the knee may produce extension of the hip. Kinematic analysis may be useful for monitoring progress, but is probably not as good as kinetics diagnostically.[101] In addition, it has been demonstrated that when weights are added to the legs, the motion of the swing leg while running remains the same, while both the moments at the joints and aerobic demand increase.[56] This study also found that the weights affected only the joints proximal to where the weights were placed. The body worked harder to keep the motion the same. This finding has dramatic implications for the use of motion measurements in diagnosis. There may be changes in how the body is working that may not be detected by motion measurements alone.

Joint power

Joint power is the moment at a joint multiplied by the angular velocity of the joint.[91] This is a measure of the contribution of the muscles of each joint to the total movement of the limb. The difference between joint moment and joint power can be illustrated by the fact that a joint moment may be high but there may be no angular velocity at that joint. In this situation the muscles at this joint are contributing to support but not to motion.[101] For this reason joint power does not correlate with aerobic demand because a large part of the effort of gait is used to support body weight and is not used for propulsion.[57] If a patient has difficulty with locomotion, joint power is a better diagnostic measurement.[101] Another reason why joint power is attractive in assessing gait is that it is something that cannot be seen with the unaided human eye, whereas many motion measurements can.

The following are examples of the use of joint power in analysis of gait. Comparison of the gait of people who had injured their anterior cruciate ligament of the knee with people without injury demonstrated that the previously injured patients walked more erectly. This was the result of the comparison from kinematic analysis only. After joint power analysis of the same subjects, it was seen that the knee absorbed less energy at contact and the hip was much more important in producing propulsion in the subjects with prior injury.[28] There was less knee extensor power and more hip flexor power. This correlates with the observation that EMG studies demonstrate that the hamstrings are more active in patients with a history of anterior cruciate injury.[33,86,87] In this example the kinematic analysis noted the change, but it was not effective in explaining the change.

Another example of the use of joint moment and joint power is the analysis of antagonistic muscles contracting at the same time. One of the most studied examples of this phenomenon is the contraction of the hamstrings and the quadriceps at the same time during the late part of the downstroke in bicycle pedaling.[91] The quadriceps are knee exten-

sors and the hamstrings are knee flexors. The explanation for the co-contraction was that the direction of the force that was needed is an important determinant in which muscles fire (Fig. 8-10). The reactive force from the pedal would tend to flex the knee so the extensors should be active. However, the direction of force applied to the pedal would require knee flexion. This study showed that hip power was directed to extend the hip and that knee power was zero. The hamstrings and the quadriceps cancel each other so that there is no motion at the knee. The cancellation of moments at the knee allow all the hip extensors to use the whole leg as a rigid lever to apply force to the pedal.[91] Using joint power allowed the researchers to see that the knee was locked by the co-contraction of the muscles. This information could not have been obtained visually or by EMG.

Power can also be used to assess the effects of loads carried by people while they walk.[74,75] It was found that the mass of the load of a backpack affects the power output of the joints. It was also suggested that the attachment of the load to the body is important in determining the magnitude of the effect of the power output. Different pack frames could be evaluated by this method.

A final example of the use of joint power is the comparison of the amount of propulsion from different prosthetic feet. Czerniecki et al.[24] found that there were large differences in the amount of "ankle power" among various prosthetic feet. An increase in ankle power correlated with a decrease in the hip flexion power needed to initiate the swing phase of gait.

The use of power to differentiate between ankle push-off and hip pull-off may be an important indicator of gait.[101] This measurement has great potential for evaluating the effectiveness of orthoses. Ankle power is a quantifiable measurement of propulsion. It has already been shown to be significantly different in the gait of elderly vs. younger subjects.[104,105,108] In these studies it was found that in order for elderly subjects to walk at the same speed as younger subjects, they had to decrease stride length and increase cadence. Ankle joint power is a factor in decreased stride length, because it helps push the leg forward for the next step. After the usefulness of ankle joint power is determined, it may not even be necessary to measure power for the monitoring of patients. Some of the components that determine power or that are the result of power may be good indicators of the success of treatment. When the ankle power is propelling the leg forward the anteroposterior component of ground reactive force will be high, as will the amount of plantarflexion of the ankle compared to when the leg is pulled forward by the hip muscles. Also, with more

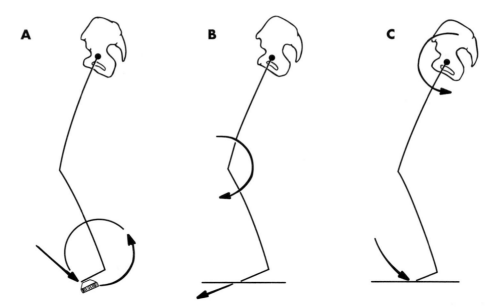

Fig. 8-10. Using power to explain muscle function. **A,** The direction of the force needed to move a bicycle pedal. **B,** The direction the foot would move with knee extension is opposite to the direction that is required. **C,** When the knee is held motionless by co-contraction of the flexors and extensors, the hip can provide the correct direction of force.

propulsion, stride length and cadence change and the results of propulsion could be indicators of a change in gait. However, joint power would be the important variable in explaining the change in the other indicators.

Summary

There have been two major limitations to the use of computerized gait analysis: the technical ability of machines to measure gait, and the documentation of the relationship between gait measurements and specific pathologic conditions. Many of the technical problems of measurement have been solved, but prospective studies are still needed on the relationship between the gait findings and pathologic changes.

The methods described in this chapter are adequate for measuring how a person walks. However, the devices cannot explain why a person walks the way he or she does. People choose how they walk, and they will alter their style when they have pain. Limping is an obvious example of this. There may be a question whether pain causes a particular style of gait or whether a particular style of gait causes pain. This question may be answered by the use of models to analyze stresses on anatomical structures.

In order to justify the time and cost of computerized gait analysis the results from the analysis must be used to alter the treatment plan. It is of no benefit to obtain a measurement when the clinical

process would be the same whether the measurement was taken or not. It is important that the practitioner understand the approach that is used in the analysis of the data obtained from the device. The modeling approach may lead to more accurate predictions of the type of treatment or the likelihood of success of treatment than the empirical approach. However, the difficulties of the modeling approach may make it impractical for use on every patient. If modeling is found to be successful, then perhaps a single measurement of the many that are used in the model may be utilized successfully empirically— that is, that through the use of models, empirical measures may be identified that may predict pathology or may be utilized to successfully evaluate treatment. In its use as a clinical instrument, computerized gait analysis is still in its early stages. A number of prospective studies need to be performed to prove its usefulness.

References

1. An KN, Chao EY: Kinematic analysis of human movement, *Ann Biomech Eng* 12:585–597, 1984.
2. Areblad M, Nigg BM, Ekstrand J, et al: Three-dimensional measurement of rearfoot motion during running, *J Biomech* 23:933–940, 1990.
3. Arsenault AB, Winter DA, Marteniuk RG: Treadmill versus walkway locomotion in humans: an EMG study, *Ergonomics* 29:665–676, 1986.
4. Arsenault AB, Winter DA, Marteniuk RG: Is there a "normal" profile of EMG activity in gait? *Med Biol Eng Comput* 24:337–343, 1986.

5. Bahlsen A: The etiology of running injuries: a longitudinal, prospective study, PhD thesis, University of Calgary, Calgary, 1988.

6. Bates BT: Comment on "The influence of running velocity and midsole hardness on external impact forces in heel-toe running," *J Biomech* 22:963–965, 1989.

7. Betts RP, Duckworth T, Austin IG: Critical light reflection at a plastic/glass interface and its application to foot pressure measurements, *J Med Eng Technol* 4:136–142, 1980.

8. Betts RP, Franks CI, Duckworth T: Analysis of pressure and loads under the foot. Part II. Quantitation of the dyanamic distribution, *Clin Phys Meas* 1:113–124, 1980.

9. Betts RP, Franks CI, Duckworth D: Foot pressure studies: normal and pathologic gait analysis. In Jahss MH (ed): *Disorders of the foot and ankle: medical and surgical management,* ed 2. Philadelphia, WB Saunders, 1991.

10. Bobbert MF, Schamhardt HC, Nigg BM: Calculation of vertical ground reaction force estimates during running from positional data, *J Biomech* 24:1095–1105, 1991.

11. Bobbert MF, Yeadon MR, Nigg BM: Mechanical analysis of the landing phase in heel-toe running, *J Biomech* 25:223–234, 1992.

12. Brodsky JW, Kourosh S, Mooney B: Objective evaluation and review of commercial gait analysis systems. Presented at 19th Annual Meeting of the American Orthopaedic Foot and Ankle Society, Las Vegas, 1989.

13. Carmines DV, Nunley JA, McElhaney JH: Effects of ankle taping on the motion and loading pattern of the foot for walking subjects, *J Orthop Res* 6:223–229, 1988.

14. Cavanagh PR: The biomechanics of lower extremity action in distance running, *Foot Ankle* 7:197–217, 1987.

15. Cavanagh PR: JB Wolffe memorial lecture. Biomechanics: a bridge builder among the sport sciences. *Med Sci Sports Exerc* 22:546–557, 1990.

16. Cavanagh PR, Henley JD: The computer era in gait analysis, *Clin Podiatr Med Surg* 10:471–484, 1993.

17. Cavanagh PR, Rodgers MM, Iiboshi A: Pressure distribution under symptom-free feet during barefoot standing, *Foot & Ankle* 7:262–276, 1987.

18. Cavanagh PR, Simoneau GG, Ulbrecht JS: Ulceration, unsteadiness, and uncertainty: the biomechanical consequences of diabetes mellitus, *J Biomech* 26(Suppl 1):23–40, 1993.

19. Cavanagh PR, Sims DS Jr, Sanders LJ: Body mass is a poor predictor of peak plantar pressure in diabetic men, *Diabetes Care* 14:750–755, 1991.

20. Cavanagh PR, Ulbrecht JS: Biomechanics of the diabetic foot: a quantitative approach to the assessment of neuropathy, deformity, and plantar pressure. In Jahss MH (ed): *Disorders of the Foot and Ankle: Medical and Surgical Management,* ed 2. Philadelphia, WB Saunders, 1991.

21. Cavanagh PR, Ulbrecht JS: Clinical plantar pressure in diabetes: rationale and methodology. Foot, in press.

22. Charteris J, Taves C: The process of habituation to treadmill walking: a kinematic analysis, *Percept Mot Skills* 47:659–666, 1978.

23. Close JR, Inman VT, Poor PM, et al: The function of the subtalar joint, *Clin Orthop* 1967.

24. Czerniecki JM, Gitter A, Munro C: Joint moment and muscle power output characteristics of below knee amputees during running: the influence of energy storing prosthetic feet, *J Biomech* 24:63–75, 1991 [erratum in *J Biomech* 24:63–75, 1991].

25. Dal Monte A, Fucci S, Manoni A: The treadmill used as a training and a simulator instrument in middle and long distance running. In Cirquiglini A, Benerando A, Wartenweiler J (eds): Biomechanics vol 3. Baltimore, University Park Press, 1973.

26. Dean E, Ross J, Bartz J, et al: Improving the validity of clinical exercise testing: the relationship between practice and performance, *Arch Phys Med Rehabil* 70:599–604, 1989.

27. Dempster WT: *The Space Requirements of the Seated Operator.* Ohio, Wright-Patterson Air Force Base, 1955, WADC TR 55-159.

28. Devita P, Hunter PB, Skelly WA: Effects of a functional knee brace on the biomechanics of running, *Med Sci Sports Exerc* 24:797–806, 1992.

29. Dhanendran M, Hutton WC, Klenerman L, et al: Foot function in juvenile chronic arthritis, *Rheum Rehabil* 19:20–24, 1980.

30. Dufek JS, Bates BT: Dynamic performance assessment of selected sport shoes on impact forces, *Med Sci Sports Exerc* 23:1062–1067, 1991.

31. Engsberg JR: A biomechanical analysis of the talocalcaneal joint in vitro, *J Biomech* 20:429–442, 1987.

32. Engsberg JR, Andrews JG: Kinematic analysis of the talocalcaneal/talocrural joint during running support, *Med Sci Sports Exerc* 19:275–284, 1987.

33. Grabiner MD, Weiker GG, Anderson TE, et al: Neuromotor synergies of the ligamentously injured knee. In Proceedings of the 13th Annual Meeting of the American Society of Biomechanics, Burlington, Vt, August 1989, pp 140–141.

34. Greig C, Butler F, Skelton D, et al: Treadmill walking in old age may not reproduce the real life situation, *J Am Geriatr Soc* 41:15–18, 1993.

35. Grieve DW, Rashdi T: Pressures under normal feet in standing and walking as measured by foil pedobarography, *Ann Rheum Dis* 43:816–818, 1984.

36. Gross TS, Bunch RP: Measurement of discrete vertical in-shoe stress with piezoelectric transducers, *J Biomed Eng* 10:261–265, 1988.

37. Gross TS, Bunch RP. Material moderation of plantar impact stress, *Med Sci Sports Exerc* 21:619–624, 1989.

38. Gross TS, Bunch RP: Discrete normal plantar stress variations with running speed, *J Biomech* 22:699–703, 1989.

39. Hamill J, Bates BT, Holt KG: Timing of lower extremity joint actions during treadmill running, *Med Sci Sports Exerc* 24:807–813, 1992.

40. Herzog W, Conway PJ, Willcox BJ: Effects of different treatment modalities on gait symmetry and clinical measures for sacroiliac joint patients, *J Manipulative Physiol Ther* 14:104–109, 1991.

41. Herzog W, Nigg BM, Read LJ, et al: Asymmetries in ground reaction force patterns in normal human gait, *Med Sci Sports Exerc* 21:110–114, 1989.

42. Hughes J, Clark P, Jagoe JR, et al: The pattern of pressure distribution under the weightbearing forefoot, *Foot* 1:117–124, 1991.

43. Hutton WC, Dhanendran M: The mechanics of normal and hallux valgus feet—a quantitative study, *Clin Orthop* 157:7–13, 1981.

44. Isacson J, Gransberg L, Knutsson E: Three-dimensional electrogoniometric gait recording, *J Biomech* 19:627–635, 1986.

45. Jefferson RJ, Whittle MW: Performance of three walking orthoses for the paralysed: a case study using gait analysis, *Prosthet Orthot Int* 14:103–110, 1990.

46. Kadaba MP, Ramakrishnan HK, Wootten ME, et al: Repeatability of kinematic, kinetic, and electromyographic data in normal adult gait, *J Orthop Res* 7:849–860, 1989.

47. Komi PV: Relevance of in vivo force measurements to human biomechanics, *J Biomech* 23(suppl 1):23–34, 1990.

48. Komi PV, Gollhofer A, Schmidtbleicher D, et al: Interaction between man and shoe in running: considerations for a more comprehensive measurement approach, *Int J Sports Med* 8:196–202, 1987.

49. Lafortune MA: The use of intra-cortical pins to measure the motion of the knee joint during walking, doctoral dissertation, Pennsylvania State University, University Park, 1984.

50. Lafortune MA, Hennig EM: Contribution of angular motion and gravity to tibial acceleration, *Med Sci Sports Exerc* 23:360–363, 1991.

51. Lanyon LE, Hamson WGJ, Goodship AE, et al: Bone deformation recorded in vivo from strain gauges attached to the human tibial shaft, *Acta Orthop Scand* 46:256–268, 1975.

52. Laughman RK, Askew LJ, Bleimeyer RJ, et al: Objective clinical evaluation of function: gait analysis, *Phys Ther* 64:1839–1845, 1984.

53. Lord M, Reynolds DP, Hughes JR: Foot pressure measurement: a review of clinical findings, *J Biomed Eng* 8:283–294, 1986.

54. Luethi SM, Frederick EC, Hawes MR, et al: Influence of shoe construction on lower extremity kinematics and load during lateral movements in tennis, *Int J Sport Biomech* 2:166–174, 1986.

55. MacKinnon CD, Winter DA: Control of whole body balance in the frontal plane during human walking, *J Biomech* 26:633–644, 1993.

56. Martin PE, Cavanagh PR: Segment interactions within the swing leg during unloaded and loaded running, *J Biomech* 23:529–536, 1990.

57. Martin PE, Heise GD, Morgan DW: Interrelationships between mechanical power, energy transfers, and walking and running economy, *Med Sci Sports Exerc* 25:508–515, 1993.

58. Matsusaka N: Control of the medial-lateral balance in walking, *Acta Orthop Scand* 57:555–559, 1986.

59. Michael RH, Holder LE: The soleus syndrome. A cause of medial tibial stress (shin splints), *Am J Sports Med* 13:87–94, 1985.

60. Mittlmeier TWF, Morlock MM: Pressure distribution measurements during normal gait: dependency on measurement frequency and sensor resolution (abstract). NACOB EMED Newsletter 3:20-21, 1992.

61. Morgan DW, Martin PE, Krahenbuhl GS, et al: Variability in running economy and mechanics among trained male runners, *Med Sci Sports Exerc* 23:378–383, 1991.

62. Morlock MM: *The Use of Pressure Distribution*. Minneapolis, Novel, 1992.

63. Motriuk HU, Nigg BM: A technique for normalizing centre of pressure paths, *J Biomech* 23:927–932, 1990.

64. Mueller MJ: Etiology, evaluation, and treatment of the neuropathic foot, *Crit Rev Phys Rehabil Med* 3:289–309, 1992.

65. Munro CF, Miller DI, Fuglevand AJ: Ground reaction forces in running: a reexamination, *J Biomech* 20:147–155, 1987.

66. Nachbauer W, Nigg BM: Effects of arch height of the foot on ground reaction forces in running, *Med Sci Sports Exerc* 24:1264–1269, 1992.

67. Nigg BM: The validity and relevance of tests used for the assessment of sports surfaces, *Med Sci Sports Exerc* 22:131–139, 1990.

68. Nigg BM, Bahlson AH, Denoth J, et al: Factors influencing kinematic and kinematic variables in running. In Nigg BM (ed): *Biomechanics of Running Shoes* Champaign, Ill, Human Kinetics, 1986.

69. Nigg BM, Bahlsen HA, Luethi SM, et al: The influence of running velocity and midsole hardness on external impact forces in heel-toe running, *J Biomech* 20:951–959, 1987.

70. Nigg BM, Bobbert M: On the potential of various approaches in load analysis to reduce the frequency of sports injuries, *J Biomech* 23(suppl 1):3–12, 1990.

71. Nigg BM, Fisher V, Allinger TL, et al: Range of motion of the foot as a function of age, *Foot Ankle* 13:336–343, 1992.

72. Nigg BM, Morlock M: The influence of lateral heel flare of running shoes on pronation and impact forces, *Med Sci Sports Exerc* 19:294–302, 1987.

73. Olney SJ, Winter DA: Predictions of knee and ankle moments of force in walking from EMG and kinematic data, *J Biomech* 18:9–20, 1985.

74. Pierrynowski MR, Norman RW, Winter DA: Mechanical energy analyses of the human during local carriage on a treadmill, *Ergonomics* 24:1–14, 1981.

75. Pierrynowski MR, Winter DA, Norman RW: Transfers of mechanical energy within the total body and mechanical efficiency during treadmill walking, *Ergonomics* 23:147–156, 1980.

76. Reinschmidt C, Stacoff A, Stussi E: Heel movement within a court shoe, *Med Sci Sports Exerc* 24:1390–1395, 1992 [erratum in *Med Sci Sports Exerc* 25:410, 1993].

77. Rodgers MM, Cavanagh PR: Pressure distribution in Morton's foot structure, *Med Sci Sports Exerc* 21:23–28, 1989.

78. Root ML, Orien WP, Weed JH: Normal and abnormal function of the foot. In *Clinical Biomechanics*, vol 3. Los Angeles, Clinical Biomechanics, p 137, 1977.

79. Rose NE, Feiwell LA, Cracchiolo A III: A method for measuring foot pressures using a high resolution, computerized insole sensor: the effect of heel wedges on plantar pressure distribution and center of force, *Foot Ankle* 13:263–270, 1992.

80. Sanders AP, Snijders CJ, van Linge B: Medial deviation of the first metatarsal head as a result of flexion forces in hallux valgus, *Foot Ankle* 13:515–522, 1992.

81. Sanfilippo PB II, Stess RM, Moss KM: Dynamic plantar pressure analysis. Comparing common insole materials, *J Am Podiatr Med Assoc* 82:507–513, 1992.

82. Schieb DA: Kinematic accommodation of novice treadmill runners, *Research Q Exerc Sport* 57:1–7, 1986.

83. Scott SH, Winter DA: Internal forces of chronic running injury sites, *Med Sci Sports Exerc* 22:357–369, 1990.

84. Scott SH, Winter DA: Talocrural and talocalcaneal joint kinematics and kinetics during the stance phase of walking, *J Biomech* 24:743–752, 1991.

85. Shereff MJ, Bregman AM, Kummer FJ: The effect of immobilization devices on the load distribution under the foot, *Clin Orthop* 192:260–267, 1985.

86. Shiavi R, Limbird T. The effect of anterior cruciate deficiency on EMG patterns during locomotion, In Proceedings of the Fifth Biennial Conference and Symposium of the Canadian Society of Biomechanics, Ottawa, Canada, August 1988, pp 142–143.

87. Sinkjaer TL, Arendt-Nielsen S, Kaalund P, et al: Muscle coordination in normal and anterior cruciate ligament (ACL) injured subjects. In Proceedings of the Eighth International Congress of the International Society of Electrophysiological Kinesiology, Baltimore, August 1990, p 45.

88. Stacoff A, Denoth J, Kaelin X, et al: Running injuries and shoe construction: some possible relationships, *Int J Sport Biomech* 4:342–357, 1988.

89. Stacoff A, Reinschmidt C, Stussi E: The movement of the heel within a running shoe, *Med Sci Sports Exerc* 24:695–701, 1992.

90. Stokes VP, Andersson C, Forssberg H: Rotational and translational movement features of the pelvis and thorax during adult human locomotion, *J Biomech* 22:43–50, 1989.

91. Van Ingen Schenau GJ: Some fundamental aspects of the biomechanics of overground versus treadmill locomotion, *Med Sci Sports Exerc* 12:257–261, 1980.

92. Van Ingen Schenau GJ, Boots PJ, de Groot G, et al: The constrained control of force and position in multi-joint movements, *Neuroscience* 46:197–207, 1992.

93. Van Langelaan EJ: A kinematical analysis of the tarsal joints. An x-ray photogrammatic study, *Acta Orthop Scand Suppl* 54:204, 1983.

94. Viitasalo JT, Kvist M: Some biomechanical aspects of the foot and ankle in athletes with and without shin splints, *Am J Sports Med* 11:125–130, 1983.

95. Wall JC, Charteris J: A kinematic study of long-term habituation to treadmill walking, *Ergonomics* 24:531–542, 1981.

96. Wang JW, Kuo KN, Andriacchi TP, et al. The influence of walking mechanics and time on the results of proximal tibial osteotomy, *J Bone Joint Surg [Am]* 72:905–909, 1990.

97. White SC, Yack HJ, Winter DA: A three-dimensional musculoskeletal model for gait analysis. Anatomical variability estimates, *J Biomech* 22:885–893, 1989.

98. Winter DA: Overall principle of lower limb support during stance phase of gait, *J Biomech* 13:923–927, 1980.

99. Winter DA: Pathologic gait diagnosis with computer-averaged electromyographic profiles, *Arch Phys Med Rehabil* 65:393–398, 1984.

100. Winter DA: Kinematic and kinetic patterns in human gait: variability and compensating effects, *Hum Movement Sci* 3:51–76, 1984.

101. Winter DA: Concerning the scientific basis for the diagnosis of pathological gait and for rehabilitation protocols, *Physiother Can* 37:245–252, 1985.

102. Winter DA: Biomechanics of normal and pathological gait: implications for understanding human locomotor control, *J Mot Behav* 21:337–355, 1989.

103. Winter DA: Sagittal plane balance and posture in human walking. *IEEE Eng Med Biol*, Sept. 1987.

104. Winter DA: *Biomechanics and Motor Control of Human Movement*, ed 2. New York, John Wiley & Sons, 1990.

105. Winter DA: Foot trajectory in human gait: a precise and multifactorial motor control task, *Phys Ther* 72:45–56, 1992.

106. Winter DA, Bishop PJ: Lower extremity injury. Biomechanical factors associated with chronic injury to the lower extremity, *Sports Med* 14:149–156, 1992.

107. Winter DA, Patla AE, Frank JS: Assessment of balance control in humans, *Med Prog Technol* 16:31–51, 1990.

108. Winter DA, Patla AE, Frank JS, et al: Biomechanical walking pattern changes in the fit and healthy elderly, *Phys Ther* 70:340–347, 1990.

109. Winter DA, Sidwall HG, Hobson DA: Measurement and reduction of noise in kinematics of locomotion, *J Biomech* 7:157–159, 1974.

110. Winter DA, White SC: Cause-effect correlations of variables of gait. In Jonsson B (ed): *International Series on Biomechanics*, vol 10-A. Champaign, Ill, Human Kinetics, 1987.

111. Wright DG, Desai SM, Henderson WH: Action of the subtalar and ankle-joint complex during the stance phase of walking, *J Bone Joint Surg [Am]* 46:361-383, 1964.

112. Young MJ, Cavanagh PR, Thomas G, et al: The effect of callus removal on dynamic plantar foot pressures in diabetic patients, *Diabetic Med* 9:55–57, 1992.

Suggested reading

Brand RA: Comment on criteria for patient evaluation tools, *J Biomech* 14:655, 1981.

Brunt D, Lafferty MJ, Mckeon A, et al: Invariant characteristics of gait initiation, *Am J Phys Med Rehabil* 70:206–212, 1991.

Davis BL, Cavanagh PR: Decomposition of superimposed ground reaction forces into left and right force profiles, *J Biomech* 26:593–597, 1993.

Hamill J, Bates BT, Knutzen KM, et al: Relationship between selected static and dynamic lower extremity measures, *Clin Biomech* 4:217–225, 1989.

Katoh Y, Chao EY, Laughman RK, et al: Biomechanical analysis of foot function during gait and clinical applications, *Clin Orthop* 177:23–33, 1983.

Morgan DW, Martin PE, Baldini FD, et al: Effects of a prolonged maximal run on running economy and running mechanics, *Med Sci Sports Exerc* 22:834–840, 1990.

Saltzman CL, Johnson KA, Goldstein RH, et al: The patellar tendon–bearing brace as treatment for neurotrophic arthropathy: a dynamic force monitoring study, *Foot Ankle* 13:14–21, 1992.

Simpson KJ, Shewokis PA, Alduwaisan S, et al: Factors influencing rearfoot kinematics during a rapid lateral braking movement, *Med Sci Sports Exerc* 24:586–594, 1992.

Stockley I, Betts RP, Getty CJ, et al: A prospective study of forefoot arthroplasty, *Clin Orthop* 248:213–218, 1989.

Strathy GM, Chao EY, Laughman RK: Changes in knee function associated with treadmill ambulation, *J Biomech* 16:517–522, 1983.

Veves A, Murray HJ, Young MJ, et al: The risk of foot ulceration in diabetic patients with high foot pressure: a prospective study, *Diabetologia* 35:660–663, 1992.

Warren BL, Jones CJ: Predicting plantar fasciitis in runners, *Med Sci Sports Exerc* 19:71–73, 1987.

neuromuscular examination

Michael O. Seibel, DO, DPM

Neurologic history
Neurologic examination
Conclusion

Many neuromuscular disorders completely or partially manifest themselves in the lower extremity. It may therefore be necessary to perform a comprehensive neurologic examination to assess these signs or symptoms. This chapter focuses on the components of the neurologic history and physical examination. The significance of normal and abnormal findings is discussed.

Neurologic history

The neurologic history (Table 9-1) can reveal information that is helpful in identifying the patient's disease process. By taking a comprehensive history, one may piece together important clues that ultimately reveal the diagnosis. For example, a chief complaint of numbness and paresthesias in the third and fourth toes sounds like a local Morton's foot until the examiner discovers that there are similar areas in both hands, which suggests a more systemic involvement. Additionally, important information regarding any compromise of the patient's functional abilities is obtained as well as progression or stability of the disorder.

Identification includes the patient's name, age, sex, handedness, race, and credibility as a historical reporter. Naturally, information on age, sex, and race is important in helping to identify certain groups at risk for various disorders. The patient's reliability in reporting symptoms and other history is an important indicator for weighting the credibility of the historical data.

The *chief complaint* should succinctly identify the reason why the patient is seeking your evaluation. The nature of the problem and its duration is documented.

Under *history of present illness*, all important information concerning the chief complaint should be uncovered. When was the onset of symptoms? Were they obviously related to any event? Did they come on insidiously or suddenly? What has happened since that time? What is the nature of the symptoms? Do they persist without variation or do they only appear intermittently? Are there factors that can be identified that exacerbate or relieve the problem? Do any other signs or symptoms accompany that of the chief complaint? Has treatment been given? With what results? Have any diagnostic tests been performed? With what results? What effect have medications had on the problem? Has the patient developed any secondary problems as a result of the chief complaint? Has he or she ever had any similar problems in the past?

In obtaining the *functional history,* one must note if the patient's activities of daily living (ADLs) have been impaired as a result of the neuromuscular complaint. If so, to what degree? Has the decline in ADLs been progressive or has it remained stable since the onset of the problem? Has the patient's ability to ambulate been impaired? Is the patient experiencing difficulty in performing occupational or avocational activities as a result of the complaint?

The *medications* that the patient is currently taking are listed, including dosage and duration. Additionally, all medicines taken from the time of onset of symptoms are likewise noted. Attention is given to whether any of the medicines identified alone or in combination could produce or contribute to the patient's symptoms.

Information obtained in the *past medical history* is evaluated for possible relationships to the current problem. Special attention is given to illnesses and conditions that can have neuromuscular manifestations (e.g., diabetes mellitus, spondylosis, acquired immunodeficiency syndrome [AIDS]). The *review of systems* later in the history serves a similar purpose. The *past trauma history* is important for the purpose of uncovering previously existing areas of neurologic deficit resulting from trauma. Some traumatic conditions may predispose to neuromuscular conditions (e.g., a fractured femur causing a limb length discrepancy which over time results in scoliosis and facet joint arthritis, producing a radiculopathy). The *past surgical history* is examined for possible relationships to the chief complaint (e.g., a coronary artery bypass graft using the saphenous vein in a patient who complains of numbness in the medial aspect of the foot and leg). The *immunization history* is relevant because some people will have neurologic sequelae from a reaction to the immunization.

A complete *family history* is necessary to understand which diseases with possible neurologic sequelae the patient may be prone to developing. The *social history* elicits habits (e.g., alcohol, tobacco,

Table 9-1
Neurologic history

1. Identification
2. Chief complaint
3. History of present illness
4. Functional history
5. Allergies
6. Medications
7. Past medical history
8. Past trauma history
9. Past surgical history
10. Immunization history
11. Family history
12. Social history
13. Review of systems

recreational drug use) that may be related to the chief complaint (e.g., alcoholic neuropathy). The most advanced grade level completed in school is ascertained. Avocational activities are evaluated for their potential impact on the chief complaint. The patient's occupation and occupational environment are likewise evaluated. Travel history and sexual orientation are noted.

Neurologic examination

The neurologic examination (Table 9-2) is a prototypal example of the fusion of art and science in medicine. Properly performed and understood, it will unveil the details of the picture suggested by the history. As with all physical examinations, a well-practiced routine will allow the examination to be performed with an economy of time and without omitting any important components.

Mental status

The patient's general level of arousal is noted (e.g., obtunded, alert) and orientation to person, place, and time is checked. Both short- and long-term memory are assessed. The former may be accomplished by reciting a list of four unrelated items and having the patient repeat them until he or she has done this twice without error. Then, after waiting 10 minutes, during which the patient is engaged in some unrelated activity, have the patient repeat the list and record how many items he or she has recalled. Normally, a person should be able to recall all four items. For long-term memory, a quick screening method is to ask the patient to name the U.S. Presidents starting from the most recent and working back. The patient should be tested for judgment with hypothetical situations (e.g., seeing smoke in a movie theater). Calculation ability should be tested in the context of the patient's educational background. Insight should be assessed by asking the patient to explain common proverbs. There are standardized brief mental status examinations that are available and useful for this component of the neurologic examination.[1,3]

Table 9-2
Neurologic examination

General mental status
Cranial nerves
Cerebellum
Motor
Reflexes
Sensation
Gait

Cranial nerve examination

The cranial nerve (CN) examination (Table 9-3) can be performed quickly and yield information that may be valuable. Diseases with systemic neurologic involvement may be revealed during this examination. Central disorders, such as strokes, may show cranial nerve involvement, with the limbs to later echo the same affliction. Table 9-4 gives a condensed screening evaluation of the cranial nerves that is useful for the general neurologic examination.

The olfactory nerve (CN I) can be evaluated using scents of common substances such as coffee, peppermint, soap, or chewing gum. Care should be taken not to use a substance (e.g., ammonia) that can produce irritation of the nasal mucosa and thus stimulate the receptors for the trigeminal nerve (CN V), which provide the sensory afferents for this region. Use of such irritating materials may yield erroneous results of olfactory function.

Table 9-3
The cranial nerves

I	Olfactory
II	Optic
III	Oculomotor
IV	Trochlear
V	Trigeminal
VI	Abducens
VII	Facial
VIII	Vestibulocochlear
IX	Glossopharyngeal
X	Vagus
XI	Accessory
XII	Hypoglossal

Table 9-4
Evaluation

Cranial nerve evaluation	Test
I	Smell
II	Visual fields, visual acuity, fundus examination
II—afferent III—efferent	Pupillary reflex
III, IV, VI	Extraocular movements
V_1, V_2, V_3	Facial sensation
V	Muscles of mastication
V—afferent VII—efferent	Corneal reflex
VIII	Hearing
IX, X	Pharyngeal gag reflex
XI	Sternocleidomastoid function
XII	Tongue active movement

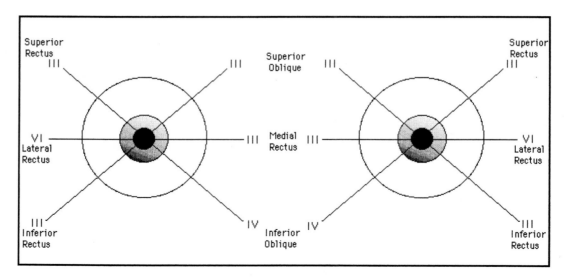

Fig. 9-1. Examination of extraocular movements. Eye rotations and relevant cranial nerves *(roman numerals)* are shown.

The optic nerve (CN II) is evaluated by visualizing the fundus, testing the visual fields, pupil size, and the pupillary reflexes. Visual field testing is most conveniently done by confrontation testing. This is performed with the examiner positioning his or her face at arm's length from the patient's face. The patient then covers one eye with his or her hand while the examiner covers his or her eye on the contralateral side (e.g., if the patient covers the right eye, the examiner covers his or her left eye). This should superimpose the patient's and examiner's visual fields. The patient is instructed to fixate on the examiner's open eye. A finger or other target is then slowly moved in from outside of the examiner's visual field, and the patient is instructed to indicate when the target is first seen. This should be about the same time that the examiner first perceives the target. This is repeated for all four quadrants. A deficit in the patient's ability to identify the stimulus at the same time as the examiner indicates a visual field deficit, which may then be related to either an optic nerve or brain lesion, depending on the type of field cut and related findings.

The pupillary reflex has CN II involved in its afferent loop, carrying the light stimulus back to the midbrain. The oculomotor nerve (CN III) then carries the motor efferent limb of the response back to the pupillary constrictors bilaterally. Normally, a light shined in one eye will elicit a pupillary constriction in both eyes. Accommodation will also cause pupillary constriction. This is tested by having the patient look at a distant object and then suddenly shift his or her focus to a near object (e.g., a finger held 12 in. away). Normally, both pupils will constrict as the near object is focused upon.

Pupil size should be documented. It is noteworthy, however, that up to 20% of the general population have pupils that are unequal in size (i.e., physiologic anisocoria). In physiologic anisocoria, however, there should be no more than 1 mm of difference between the two sides. More than this magnitude of difference indicates an underlying pathologic condition. The fundi should be examined for any abnormalities or asymmetry.

The examination of the extraocular movements assesses the oculomotor (CN III), trochlear (CN IV), and abducens (CN VI) nerves (Fig. 9-1). The patient is instructed to follow a target that is moved in the form of a broad H. This allows assessment of all extraocular muscles as the eyes are led through the cardinal fields of gaze. Simultaneously, the examiner notes whether there is any evidence of nystagmus, which, if present, can point to a variety of organic and metabolic disorders.

There are three sensory divisions of the trigeminal nerve. The ophthalmic division (V_1) is responsible for sensation of the forehead, upper eyelid, and anterior nose. The maxillary division (V_2) is responsible for sensation of the cheeks, upper lip, and lateral nose. The mandibular division (V_3) is responsible for sensation of the lower face and carries with it the motor division of the trigeminal nerve, which innervates the muscles of mastication (e.g., pterygoids, temporalis, masseter). Sensory assessment is carried out by testing sensation in each division on either side of the face by applying a wisp of cotton and comparing the perceived sensation. Additionally, the corneal reflex uses the trigeminal nerve as its sensory afferent limb and the facial nerve (CN VII) as its efferent limb. This reflex is elicited by

Table 9-5
Localizing significance of cerebellar signs

Signs	Cerebellar part affected
Truncal ataxia, disequilibrium	Basal and midline lesions
Stance and gait incoordination	Rostral midline lesion
Ipsilateral extremity incoordination	Hemispheric lesion

having the patient look up and to the contralateral side as the examiner slowly touches a wisp of cotton to the cornea from an inferolateral direction. Care should be taken not to allow the cotton to touch the skin or eyelashes and to make certain that it is on the sensitive cornea and not on the less sensitive sclera. Lastly, the muscles of mastication may be tested by palpating them as the patient clenches and unclenches the jaw.

The vestibulocochlear nerve (CN VIII) may be tested by Weber's test and the Rinne test. In the Rinne test, a 512-Hz tuning fork is struck and its base is applied to the mastoid process. The patient is asked to indicate when the sound can no longer be heard (through bone conduction). The head of the tuning fork is then placed next to the patient's ear with care taken not to touch the ear, and the patient is asked if he or she can hear the sound. Normally, since air conduction is better than bone conduction, the patient should still be able to hear the sound. In the case of nerve deafness (between the hair cells and the brainstem) the patient may likewise be able to hear the sound in the air longer than that conducted through the bone. If the patient's bone conduction is better than the air conduction, it indicates a problem with conduction loss (i.e., a deficiency in the conduction of sound and endolymph movement to the hair cells). Weber's test is performed by placing the vibrating tuning fork at the vertex and asking the patient if the sound is heard equally in both ears. Normally, the response is affirmative. If the sound is louder in one ear, it may indicate a conduction loss on that side or a nerve loss on the contralateral side.

The pharyngeal gag reflex uses the glossopharyngeal nerve (CN IX) as its afferent sensory limb and the vagus nerve (CN X) as its efferent motor limb. Since disorders of CN IX generally do not occur by themselves, but usually in combination with the vagus and the accessory (CN XI) nerves, this is a reasonable screening method for evaluating the glossopharyngeal as well as the vagus nerve. It is elicited by touching the posterior pharyngeal wall on each side with a tongue depressor.

The accessory nerve innervates both the sterno-cleidomastoid and upper trapezius muscles. Manual muscle testing of their strength bilaterally allows assessment of this cranial nerve. The hypoglossal nerve (CN XII) is easily evaluated by having the patient stick his or her tongue out and move it from side to side. If the tongue deviates to one side when the patient is asked to stick it straight out, a lesion of the nerve on the side the tongue points to is indicated. The strength can be assessed by having the patient push the tongue against the inside of the cheek and comparing this maneuver on both sides.

Cerebellar examination

The cerebellum is extremely important in equilibrium, in motor coordination of voluntary movement, and in its influence on muscle tone. A somatotopic organization exists in the cerebellum for different body parts, and thus the clinical examination has to include maneuvers and observations that take this into account (Table 9-5).

Cerebellar lesions will frequently cause *ataxia* (deterioration of the ability to perform smooth movements). This may be seen in the gait evaluation with the patient demonstrating an unsteady, broad-based gait, sometimes falling toward the side of the lesion. Ataxia may also be detected in the finger-to-nose and heel-to-shin tests. In the former, the patient touches the nose with the index finger. A positive test is demonstrated by deviation of the hand from the ideal course with attempted corrections interposed. Similar findings may be apparent with the heel-to-shin test in which the patient is asked to touch the knee with the heel of the opposite leg and then slowly run the heel down the anterior tibial surface. *Dysmetria* may be seen in which the patient has exaggerated movements in attempting purposeful activity, often missing the target. *Intention tremor* may also be seen in which the tremor worsens as the patient approaches the target.

Dysdiadochokinesia, an impairment of rapid alternating movements, may be seen with cerebellar disease. This is tested by having the patient rapidly pronate and supinate the hands on the thighs. *Hypotonia* is another frequently seen motor disorder that may be associated with cerebellar disease.

The observation of eye movement can be a telling indicator of cerebellar dysfunction. *Nystagmus,* a rhythmic biphasic oscillation of the eyes, can be due to lesions in the vestibular system, brainstem, or cerebellum, as well as to metabolic causes. It is named for its fast component. In cerebellar lesions, the fast component is toward the side of the lesion and increases when the subject looks to that side.

Table 9-6
Manual muscle grading systems

	System		
Percent[4]	Word[5]	Number[6]	Description
100	Normal	5	Active movement against maximum resistance (normal strength)
95	Normal −	5−	
90	Good +	4+	
80	Good	4	Active movement against some resistance
70	Good −	4−	
60	Fair +	3+	
50	Fair	3	Active movement against gravity only
40	Fair −	3−	
30	Poor +	2+	
20	Poor	2	Active movement with gravity eliminated
10	Poor −	2−	
5	Trace	1	Trace movement; can palpate muscle contraction
0	Zero	0	No movement

Motor examination

In undertaking the examination of the motor system, it is wise to review the anatomy of the motor unit, since any lesion along its anatomy can result in abnormalities. The motor unit is composed of the anterior horn cell (i.e., the motor neuron) and all of the muscle fibers supplied by its axons. Additionally, the motor unit can be affected by the neural pathways that interface with it directly or indirectly in the spinal cord. It should also be remembered that many systemic diseases (e.g., hypothyroidism, diabetes), as well as various medications (e.g., phenytoin, corticosteroids), can have pathologic effects on the motor system.

First, a general examination of the appearance of the muscles is performed. Asymmetry with atrophy or hypertrophy is noted, as is spasm or fasciculation. Any skeletal abnormality is recorded because it may cause compensatory motor abnormalities. Next, muscle tone is examined. *Tone* is defined as a muscle's resistance to passive joint movement. Systems at both the spinal and supraspinal levels govern muscle tone. In the most basic sense, disorders of tone can be divided into hypertonia and hypotonia. Hypertonia can manifest as spasticity or rigidity. In spasticity, there is a velocity-dependent increase in muscle tone due to an upper motor neuron lesion.[3] The tone is usually highest when the passive movement is initiated and decreases as the movement continues. This variation in tone is known as the clasp-knife phenomenon. Muscle stretch reflexes are also increased with spasticity. On the other hand, in rigidity, the hypertonic state remains the same regardless of the velocity or direction of movement. Muscle stretch reflexes are not increased as they are in spasticity. Types of rigidity that have been noted include cogwheel rigidity, in which there is a rachetlike yielding through the range of motion, and lead-pipe rigidity, in which there is an unchanging hypertonus. Cogwheel rigidity may be seen in Parkinson's disease. Paratonia (gegenhalten) refers to a condition seen with frontal lobe injury or diffuse cerebral involvement in which there is involuntary resistance to passive limb movement. Interestingly, there is normal tone when the limb is moved slowly. This is seen more commonly in patients who have sustained a stroke and in Alzheimer's dementia.

Many different systems have been described for grading muscle power through manual muscle testing.[2] Probably the most widely used are the word and number systems (Table 9-6). The key issue that governs these two similar systems is the ability of the muscle to produce active movement against the examiner's resistance or the force of gravity. When testing individual muscles (Table 9-7), it is important to check for symmetry in order to appreciate subtle differences in power. Additionally, it is necessary to note whether pain is a limiting factor in muscle strength. Generally, proximal weak-

Table 9-7
Mechanisms of manual muscle testing*

Muscle	Nerve	Position of foot or part	Patient applies this force	Examiner exerts this force
Flexor hallucis brevis	Tibial	STJ and MTJ in neutral positions; foot stabilized just proximal to MPJ	Plantarflexion of hallux at MPJ and IPJ	Dorsiflexion against plantar aspect of head of phalanx (see **Fig. 9-2**)
Flexor digitorum brevis	Tibial	STJ and MTJ in neutral positions; stabilized proximal phalanges	Plantarflexion of PIPJs	Dorsiflexion against plantar aspect of 2nd–5th middle phalanges (see **Fig. 9-3**)
Flexor hallucis longus	Tibial	MPJ and ankle joint in neutral positions	Plantarflexion of hallux at IPJ	Dorsiflexion against plantar aspect of hallux distal phalanx (see **Fig. 9-4**)
Flexor digitorum longus	Tibial	Foot and ankle joint in neutral positions; metatarsals stabilized	Plantarflexion of 2nd–5th DIPJs	Dorsiflexion against plantar aspect of 2nd–5th distal phalanges (see **Fig. 9-5**)
Interossei and lumbricales	Tibial	Foot and ankle joint in neutral positions; MTJ stabilized	Plantarflexion of 2nd–5th toes, avoiding IPJ plantarflexion	Dorsiflexion against plantar aspect of 2nd–5th proximal phalanges (see **Fig. 9-3**)
Extensor digitorum longus and brevis	Deep peroneal	Slight plantarflexion	Dorsiflexion of 2nd–5th toes (all joints)	Plantarflexion of toes (see **Fig. 9-6**)
Peroneus tertius	Deep peroneal	Distal leg supported	Dorsiflexion of ankle joint with foot eversion	Plantarflexion and inversion of dorsal-lateral aspect of foot (see **Fig. 9-7**)
Extensor hallucis longus and brevis	Deep peroneal	Foot and ankle stabilized in slight plantarflexion	Dorsiflexion of hallux IPJ and MPJ	Plantarflexion to dorsal aspect of hallux (see **Fig. 9-8**)
Anterior tibial	Deep peroneal	Distal leg supported with knee bent	Ankle joint dorsiflexion with foot inversion, avoiding hallux extension	Plantarflexion and eversion of ankle and foot applied to dorsum of foot (see **Fig. 9-9**)
Posterior tibial	Tibial	Distal leg supported	Ankle joint plantarflexion with foot inversion	Dorsiflexion and eversion of ankle and foot applied to plantar-medial foot (see **Fig. 9-10**)
Peroneus longus and brevis	Superficial peroneal	Distal leg supported	Ankle joint plantarflexion with foot eversion	Dorsiflexion and inversion of ankle and foot applied to plantar-lateral foot (see **Fig. 9-11**)
Soleus	Tibial	Distal leg supported; knee flexed ≥90 degrees	Ankle joint plantarflexion with foot neutral	Dorsiflexion of ankle joint applied to sole with foot maintained neutral (see **Fig. 9-12**)
Gastrocnemius	Tibial	Leg supported by examining table with patient prone	Foot plantarflexion	Dorsiflexion of foot with force applied to forefoot (see **Fig. 9-13**)
Medial-hamstring (semitendinosus and semimembranosus)	Sciatic, tibial branch	Thigh held down firmly on examining table	Flexion of knee to <90 degrees with hip and leg internally rotated	Knee extension, applied to distal leg

Continued.

Table 9-7
Mechanisms of manual muscle testing—cont'd

Muscle	Nerve	Position of foot or part	Patient applies this force	Examiner exerts this force
Lateral hamstring	Sciatic†	With patient sitting, thigh held down firmly on examining table	Flexion of knee to <90 degrees, with hip and leg slightly externally rotated	Knee extension, applied to distal leg
Quadriceps femoris	Femoral	With patient sitting, thigh held down firmly on examining table	Knee extension with care taken not to rotate thigh	Knee flexion, applied to distal leg
Iliopsoas	Femoral; lumbar plexus	With patient supine, contralateral iliac crest is fixated	Hip flexion with slight abduction and lateral rotation	Extension and slight abduction, applied to anteromedial leg
Tensor fasciae latae	Superior gluteal	Patient supine	Hip flexion, abduction, and internal rotation with knee extended	Extension and adduction, applied to anterolateral leg
Gluteus minimus	Superior gluteal	Patient in decubitus position, with pelvis stabilized	Hip abduction	Adduction with slight extension, applied to lateral-anterior leg
Gluteus medius	Superior gluteal	Patient in decubitus position, with pelvis stabilized	Hip abduction with slight extension and external rotation	Adduction and slight flexion, applied to leg
Gluteus maximus	Inferior gluteal	Patient prone	Hip extension, with knee flexed ≥90 degrees	Hip flexion applied to the posteroinferior thigh
Hip adductors	‡	Patient in decubitus position, with upper lower extremity held in abduction	Adduction of inferior lower extremity toward ceiling	Abduction, applied to distal-medial thigh (above knee)
Sartorius	Femoral	Patient supine	Flexion of knee with external rotation, abduction, and flexion of hip	Hip extension, adduction and internal rotation, applied at anterolateral aspect of inferior thigh; knee extension applied to distal leg

* STJ, subtalar joint; MTJ, midtarsal joint; MPJ, metatarsophalangeal joint; IPJ, interphalangeal joint; PIPJ, proximal interphalangeal joint; DIPJ, distal interphalangeal joint.
† Tibial branch to long head, and peroneal branch to short head.
‡ Obturator supplies adductor longus, brevis, magnus, pectineus, and gracilis. Pectineus also receives innervation from the femoral nerve, and the adductor magnus from the sciatic nerve.

ness is seen in myopathy and distal weakness in neuropathic disorders. When muscle power or distribution or both are variable over time, disorders of neuromuscular transmission and functional disorders should be entertained as possible diagnoses.

The gait examination is a substantive part of the motor examination and is covered elsewhere in this book. When evaluating gait, it is important to differentiate between biomechanical and neuromuscular disorders.[6]

Muscle stretch reflexes
The muscle stretch reflex (MSR; also the deep tendon reflex or myotatic reflex) is useful in distinguishing upper from lower motor neuron lesions as well as isolating the segmental level of involvement in a spinal root or plexus disorder (Table 9-8). Generally, a hyperreflexive state is reflective of an upper motor neuron lesion in which the normal descending corticospinal inhibitory impulses are diminished.[7] Clonus of over four beats (i.e., sustained clonus) may accompany a hyperreflexive state. A hyporeflexive state can result from a lesion anywhere along the monosynaptic reflex arc. Thus, hyporeflexia can result from peripheral neuropathy, spinal cord abnormalities at or close to the level of the reflex arc, and diseases of neuromuscular transmission. In addition, hyporeflexia may also be seen with cerebellar disorders, early stroke, and coma.

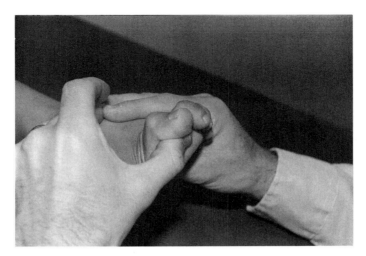

Fig. 9-2. Testing of the flexor hallucis brevis: dorsiflexory force is placed against the plantar aspect of the head of the proximal phalanx.

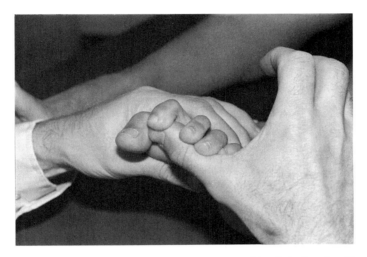

Fig. 9-3. Testing of the flexor digitorium brevis, interossei, and lumbricales: dorsiflexory force is placed against the plantar aspect of the middle phalanges of the lesser digits when testing the flexor digitorium brevis and against the plantar aspect of the proximal phalanges of the lesser digits when testing the interossei and lumbricales.

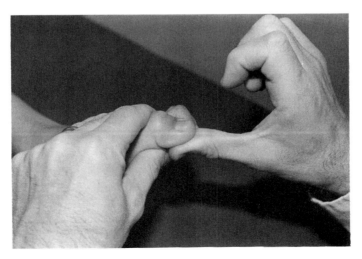

Fig. 9-4. Testing of the flexor hallucis longus: dorsiflexory force is placed against the plantar aspect of the hallux distal phalanx.

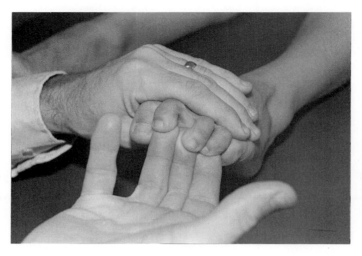

Fig. 9-5. Testing of the flexor digitorium longus: dorsiflexory force is placed against the plantar aspect of the proximal phalanges of the lesser digits.

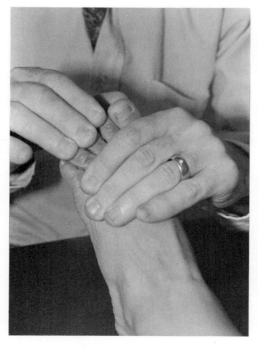

Fig. 9-6. Testing of the extensor digitorium longus and brevis: plantarflexory force is placed against the lesser digits.

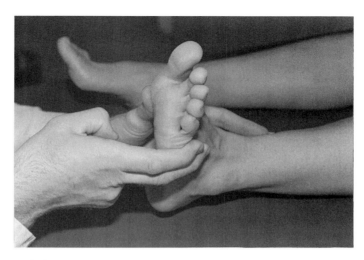

Fig. 9-7. Testing of the peroneus tertius: plantarflexory and inverting force is applied to the dorsal-lateral aspect of the foot.

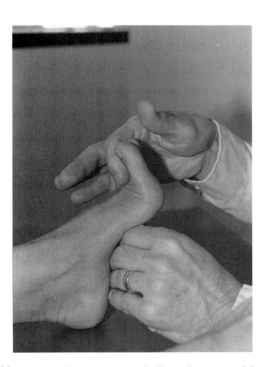

Fig. 9-8. Testing of the extensor hallucis longus and brevis: plantarflexory force is applied to the dorsal aspect of the hallux.

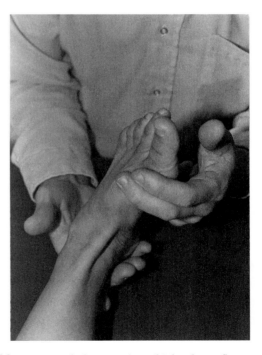

Fig. 9-9. Testing of the anterior tibial: plantarflexory and everting force is applied to the dorsum of the foot.

In evaluating reflexes, one should always compare for symmetry of a given reflex. The reflex should be assessed both by visual inspection of the reflex activity and palpation of the muscle that will contract with the reflex. Reflex activity should be graded (Table 9-9). Grades 0 and 4 are always pathologic. Reflexes should be symmetric. Asymmetry suggests an abnormality. If the asymmetry is limited to one reflex, a pathologic condition of the nerve root, plexus, or nerve is suggested. If there is asymmetry of one side of the body, a central upper motor neuron problem is suggested. When distal reflexes are diminished or lost, and the proximal ones remain relatively preserved, a polyneuropathy may be present. The latency of the response and duration of contraction should also be evaluated. In

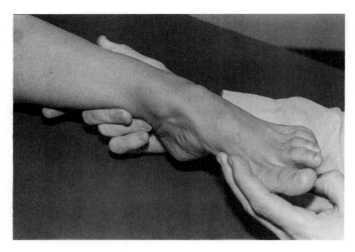

Fig. 9-10. Testing of the posterior tibial: dorsiflexory and everting force is applied to the plantar-medial aspect of the foot.

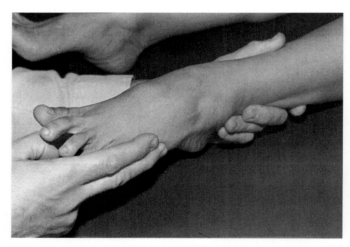

Fig. 9-11. Testing of the peroneus longus and brevis: dorsiflexory and inverting force is applied to the plantar-lateral aspect of the foot.

hypothyroidism, for example, there may be a lag time between the stimulus and the muscle contraction. In myoclonic dystrophy, there may be a prolonged contraction.

Superficial reflexes

Superficial (or cutaneous) reflexes are segmental responses that help to identify levels of dysfunction (Table 9-10). They are elicited by different methods. The corneal and gag reflexes have been described above under Cranial Nerves Examination. The superficial abdominal reflexes (i.e., epigastric, mid-abdominal, and hypogastric) are elicited by stroking the abdominal wall segment with a tongue depressor in an inferior and medial direction. Normally, the umbilicus will move toward the stimulus as the underlying muscle segment con-

tracts. Absence of umbilical movement indicates a segmental dysfunction of T9–T11, as shown in Table 9-11. The cremasteric response is elicited by stroking the inside of the thigh with a tongue depressor. Normally, the ipsilateral testicle retracts proximally. Absence of this action may indicate dysfunction at the L1–2 level. The bulbocavernosus reflex is elicited by lightly squeezing the glans penis in the male or the clitoris in the female and feeling a reflex contraction of the anal sphincter around the gloved examining finger. Absence of the contraction indicates a lesion at the S3–4 level. The plantar response is elicited by using a semisharp object (e.g., a key) to stroke the lateral aspect of the foot distally from the heel to the midmetatarsal area and then medially, curving toward the first metatarsal head. Normally, the toes contract in a plantarflexory direction. In the

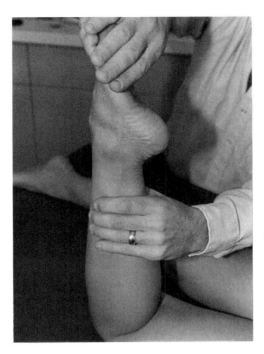

Fig. 9-12. Testing of the soleus: doriflexory force is applied to the sole of the foot with the knee flexed 90 degrees.

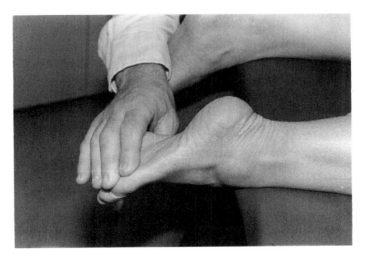

Fig. 9-13. Testing of the gastrocnemius: dorsiflexory force is applied to the forefoot with the knee extended.

abnormal Babinski's response, the lesser toes fan apart and the hallux dorsiflexes, indicating an upper motor neuron lesion. This response is conducted through the tibial nerve and the L5–S2 spinal segments.

Sensation

The sensory examination by necessity evaluates pathways and structures from the cerebral cortex distal to the cutaneous sensory receptors. Specific types of sensory input are carried in various spinal tracts (Table 9-11). The sensory examination is therefore divided into components which allow assessment of these different pathways. Radiations of these various pathways ultimately terminate in the primary sensory cortex.

All of the sensory tests described below are performed with the patient keeping the eyes closed

Table 9-8
Muscle stretch reflexes (MSR)

MSR	Spinal segment	Nerve
Biceps	C5-6	Musculocutaneous
Brachioradialis	C5-6	Radial
Pectoralis major	C6-7	Lateral pectoral
Triceps	C7-8	Radial
Patellar	L3-4	Femoral
Achilles	S1-2	Tibial

Table 9-9
Grading muscle stretch reflexes

Grade	Description
0	Absent (abnormal)
1	Decreased or present only with reinforcement manuever
2	Normal
3	Increased
4	Profoundly increased (abnormal)

Table 9-10
Location of various senses in spinal cord

Sense	Tract
Light touch	Anterior spinothalamic
Pain and temperature	Lateral spinothalamic
Deep touch and pressure, two-point discrimination, proprioception, vibration	Posterior column

Table 9-11
Superficial reflexes

Reflex	Segment
Corneal	Pons (CN, V, VII)
Gag	Medulla (CN IX, X)
Epigastric	T6–9
Midabdominal	T9–11
Hypogastric	T11–L1
Cremasteric	L1–2
Plantar	L5–S2
Bulbocavernosus	S3–4

to neutralize any inadvertent visual clues. Light touch (anterior spinothalamic tract) may be evaluated by a single stimulus to the skin with a wisp of cotton. This stimulus should be delivered irregularly. The patient indicates when he or she feels the stimulus. In this way, the peripheral nerve distributions and dermatomes may be evaluated. The same distributions should be evaluated with a safety pin (sharp vs. dull stimuli) or vials of hot and cold water (lateral spinothalamic tract). Vibration (posterior column) may be tested using a 128-Hz tuning fork applied to various bony prominences. Alternatively, two-point discrimination or joint position may be tested. The latter is most commonly tested using the thumb and hallux interphalangeal joints while grasping the distal phalanx on the sides, thus avoiding any pressure cues that might be perceived if the phalanx were held on its dorsal and palmar or plantar surfaces. The distal phalanx should be moved in short arcs (e.g., 5 degrees) and normally the patient will quickly report the movement in the correct direction. If this does not occur, the next major joint proximally can be assessed, and so on. Lastly, graphesthesia and stereognosis may be tested. To test graphesthesia, the patient's hand is opened and numbers are traced on the palm with a finger or closed pen. Normally, these are easily identifiable. Stereognosis refers to the ability to distin-

guish objects by feeling them with a hand while the eyes are closed. Problems with graphesthesia or stereognosis in the face of otherwise normal skin sensation suggest a parietal lobe lesion of the contralateral hemisphere.[3]

The Romberg test is used to evaluate position sense in the lower extremities. It is performed by having the patient stand erect with the feet together and the eyes first open and then closed. Normally, there should be almost no body sway with the eyes open and only a slight sway without falling when the eyes are closed. If there is excessive sway or falling with the eyes closed, this may indicate a problem with lower extremity joint position sense. If a lesion is in the cerebellum or vestibular system, there will usually be an increased sway when the patient has the eyes open that significantly increases when the eyes are closed.

When percussion over a nerve produces paresthesias in the distribution of that nerve, it is called *Tinel's sign*. This is indicative of nerve entrapment and may be seen anywhere along the course of a nerve, but is particularly prominent at areas where nerves pass through a relatively tight space. Examples of such areas are the carpal tunnel (median nerve), Guyon's canal (ulnar nerve), the cubital tunnel (ulnar nerve), and the tarsal tunnel (posterior tibial nerve).

Conclusion

The neuromuscular examination is a vital component of the clinical examination that should be undertaken in a patient with lower extremity complaints. A thorough neurologic examination, performed in a routine fashion so that no parts are omitted, will allow the discovery of neuromuscular deficits that may be integrally related to the patient's problem.

References

1. Folstein M, Folstein S, McHugh PR: "Mini-mental status." A practical method for grading the cognitive state of patients for the clinician, *J Psychiatr Res* 12:189, 1975.

2. Kendall FP, McCreary EK: *Muscles Testing and Function*, Baltimore, Williams & Wilkins, 1983.

3. Kokmen E, Naessens JM, Offord KP: A short test of mental status: description and preliminary results, *Mayo Clin Proc* 62:281–288, 1987.

4. Legg AT: Physical therapy in infantile paralysis. In Mock RM, editor: *Principles and Practice of Physical Therapy*, vol 2. Hagerstown, Md, WF Prior 1932.

5. Medical Research Council: *Aids to the Investigation of Peripheral Nerve Injuries*, War Memorandum No. 7, ed 2, revised. London, HMSO, 1943.

6. Seibel M: *Foot Function*, Baltimore, Williams & Wilkins, 1988.

7. Simon RP, Aminoff MJ, Greenberg DA: *Clinical Neurology*, Norwalk, Conn, Appleton & Lange, 1989.

limp and the pediatric patient

Leon Paul Smith, MD

Abnormal gait patterns
    Antalgic gait
    Neurologic gait
    Shortened extremity
    Loss of supporting structures and limp
    Contracture limp
    Mimicry

Specific disorders
    Dislocation of the hip
    Legg-Calvé-Perthes disease (coxa plana)
    Slipped capital femoral epiphysis
    Scoliosis
    Osteomyelitis
    Arthritis
    Knee problems

Summary

Normal childhood gait varies with age.[15] The child at onset of walking (Fig. 10-1) has a low center of gravity, a wide stance, more external rotation, and a nonpropulsive pattern compared to the normal older child or adult (Fig. 10-2). This pattern changes over approximately 2 years so that the typical 3-year-old has near-normal adult gait with a heel–toe-off pattern (Fig. 10-3). Children commonly have calcaneal eversion and a flexible flatfoot at the onset of ambulation, but the foot is comparable to that of an adult by 8 years of age. The subtle variations and the significant biomechanical variations from normal are discussed later in this chapter. This discussion reviews variations related to underlying pathologic conditions that go beyond biomechanical and functional problems. The patient may be symptomatic but may not complain and only be seen because of parental or teacher observations.

To define the problem, one needs to define normal gait and how variations differ from normal. The variations may technically be called a limp. *Limp* is not easy to define but has been said by Isadore Yablon[30] to be a deficiency, or an exaggeration, of normal gait. A number of gait patterns in normal people, particularly teenagers, may fit this definition. It is, therefore, loosely defined and deviations not ordinarily considered limp fulfill the definition. Nonetheless, in most circumstances it is clinically clear if a child has a gait abnormality. The next step is to determine why. This is obviously not

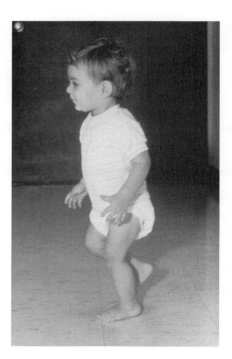

Fig. 10-2. Two-year-old with narrow base of gait. *(From Valmassy RL, Smith L, Koch T: Gait analysis in children: Diagnostic and therapeutic implications. Medcom Corp., New York, 1985.)*

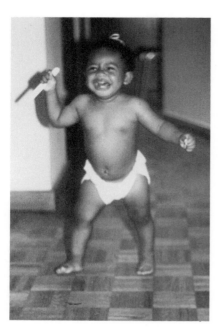

Fig. 10-1. Childhood gait at onset of walking (age 12–15-months). *(From Valmassy RL, Smith L, Koch T: Gait analysis in children: Diagnostic and therapeutic implications. Medcom Corp., New York, 1985.)*

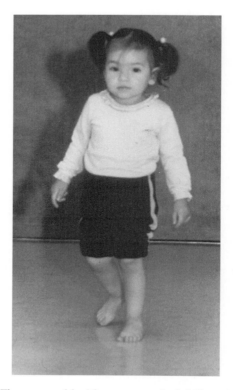

Fig. 10-3. Three-year-old with near-normal adultlike gait. *(From Valmassy RL, Smith L, Koch T: Gait analysis in children: Diagnostic and therapeutic implications. Medcom Corp., New York, 1985.)*

Table 10-1
Etiologic classification of the more common conditions causing limp

Congenital
    Spina bifida and meningomyelocele
    Scoliosis
    Neurologic disorders
        Cerebral palsy
        Spinal muscular atrophies
    Congenital dislocation of hip (CDH)
    Clubfoot
    Short extremity
    Absence or maldevelopment of part of an
        extremity (focal deficiency)
    Pseudarthrosis of tibia
    Hemiatrophy of hemihypertrophy

Vascular
    Hemangiomatosis
    Arteriovenous malformations
    Coagulopathies

Neoplastic
    Osteosarcoma
    Ewing's sarcoma
    Enchondromatosis

Traumatic
    Fractures
        Complete
        Incomplete (greenstick)
    Fracture complications
        Angulation
        Shortening
    Epiphyseal injuries

Neurologic
    Poliomyelitis
    Muscular dystrophy
    Cerebral palsy

Infections
    Osteomyelitis
    Septic arthritis

Metabolic
    Rickets
    Scurvy
    Morquio's disease
    Hurler's disease

Hyperimmune
    Rheumatoid arthritis

Ideopathic
    Legg-Calvé-Perthes disease
    Slipped capital femoral epiphysis
    Transient synovitis

Iatrogenic
    Avascular necrosis
    Premature epiphyseal closure
    Tight casts

Miscellaneous
    Skin infections of the foot
    Improperly fitting shoes
    Calluses and corns
    Ingrown toenails
    Psychogenic limp

Modified from Yablon IG: Problems in family practice: limp in childhood, *Fam Pract* 2:291–295, 1975. Used by permission.

easy if one reviews the literature. Children presenting with a limp to an emergency room most frequently leave with no specific diagnosis. Limp reflects serious disease until proved otherwise.*

History of onset and development of the limp is the most important aspect in arriving at a correct diagnosis. The age of the child and the pattern of limp are an added help diagnostically.[11] Radiographs and other imaging studies and laboratory tests may be confirmatory.[1]* The following is a discussion of a variety of pediatric disorders resulting in limp.

One can look at the pattern of limp and consider diagnoses that fit that pattern. Evaluation on an anatomic basis includes examining soft tissue, articular structures, bone, the central and peripheral nervous system, and the abdominal and pelvic structures. An alternative or additional approach is to consider whether the cause of limp is most likely genetic, congenital, developmental, vascular, neoplastic, traumatic, neurologic, infectious, metabolic, hyperimmune (collagen disorders), idiopathic, iatrogenic, degenerative, or miscellaneous[30] (Table 10-1) . An added guide is to consider the presence of pain (antalgic gait) or no pain in association with limp.

Jonathan Singer,[23] in an exquisite chapter in *Advances in Pediatrics* in 1979, outlined a long list of disorders causing gait disturbance in children under 5 years old (Table 10-2). To his list, one needs to add Lyme disease, and neuroradiculitis secondary to immunizations, particularly rubella vaccine. Beyond 5 years of age a number of conditions occurring in the school-age child and adolescent may cause limp.

In childhood and adolescence, the patient may lurch laterally over the affected hip because the hip abductors cannot contract adequately to elevate the pelvis on the opposite or nonweightbearing side (Trendelenburg lurch) (Fig. 10-4**A**). In stance, the

_____
* References 1, 6-10, 13, 14, 19, 20, 24-28.

Table 10-2
Causes of gait disturbance in children less than 5 years of age

Osseous

　　Trauma
　　Osgood-Schlatter's disease
　　Legg-Calvé-Perthes disease
　　Meyer's dysplasia
　　Köhler's disease
　　Osteomyelitis*
　　Sacroiliac infection
　　Intervertebral disk infection,
　　　　discitis
　　Pott's disease
　　Paraspinal abscess*
　　Intervertebral disk herniation
　　Tumors*
　　Sickle cell disease
　　Bone marrow necrosis
　　Vitamin A poisoning
　　Rickets
　　Caffey's disease
　　Blount's disease

Soft tissue

　　Sprain, strain, hematoma
　　Embedded foreign body
　　Calluses, corns, ingrown toenails
　　Myositis, viral and trichinous
　　Cellulitis
　　Postimmunization disease
　　Injections
　　Erythema nodosum
　　Sexual abuse
　　Erythromelalgia
　　Baker's cyst
　　Scurvy

Peripheral nervous system

　　Guillain-Barré syndrome*
　　Poliomyelitis
　　Acute transverse myelopathy
　　Juvenile diabetes mellitus
　　Heavy metal intoxication
　　Drug intoxication
　　Tick paralysis*
　　Periodic paralysis, electrolyte
　　　　imbalance
　　Causalgia

Articular

　　Pyarthrosis*
　　Transient synovitis
　　Systemic lupus erythematosus
　　Dermatomyositis
　　Scleroderma
　　Childhood polyarteritis
　　Juvenile rheumatic fever
　　Acute rheumatic fever
　　Henoch-Schönlein purpura
　　Inflammatory bowel disease
　　Hepatitis
　　Serum sickness
　　Hemophilia
　　Dislocated hip
　　Brucellosis
　　Rat-bite fever
　　Congenital syphilis
　　Kawasaki's disease

Central nervous system

　　Cerebral vascular accident
　　Cerebral abscess*
　　Meningitis, encephalitis*
　　Acute infantile hemiplegia
　　Complicated migraine–alternating
　　　　hemiplegia, basilar artery migraine
　　Acute cerebellar ataxia
　　Drug intoxication
　　Malingering

Intraabdominal

　　Appendicitis*
　　Appendiceal abscess*
　　Retroperitoneal abscess
　　Iliac adenitis
　　Retroperitoneal fibrosis

Modified from Singer J: Evaluation of acute and incidious gait disturbance in children less than five years of age. In Barness L, editor: *Advances in Pediatrics*, vol 26. St Louis, Mosby–Year Book, 1979. Used by permission.
*Conditions that demand immediate recognition.

pelvis drops to the opposite side (Trendelenburg sign) (Fig. 10-4**B**). The young child in gait may drop the pelvis to the nonweightbearing side rather than lurch (Trendelenburg gait). If bilateral, it has been referred to as a "Marilyn Monroe" gait. It can be subtle and easily missed if the child is not observed in shorts or a bathing suit. The age of the child makes certain causes more likely. In the child beginning to walk, hip dysplasia, congenital or developmental dislocation, and neurologic disorders are common causes of limp. In the child 3 years old through early school years, trauma or infection of bone or joints becomes a serious consideration, but an undiagnosed congenital dislocated hip, a developmental dislocated hip, and cerebral palsy are still possibilities. In the early school-age years, Legg-Calvé-Perthes disease (coxa plana) is an important consideration in addition to the previously mentioned possibilities. In adolescence, slipped capital femoral epiphysis becomes a significant possibility. It is more likely in heavy-set, active males but can be seen in short, thin girls.

In mid- to late adolescence, knee problems become a more common cause of limp, particu-

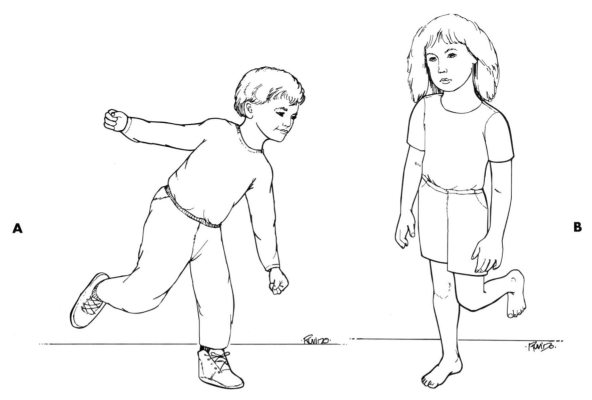

Fig. 10-4. Gluteus medius weakness or paralysis. **A,** Congenital dislocated hip results in the Trendelenburg lurch (the child lurches to the affected side to bear weight and avoid pelvic drop). **B,** Trendelenburg's sign (pelvis drops on side opposite disease).

larly in girls, presumably because of their wider pelvis. At this age, malignancy, though rare, always has to be considered, especially when the knee area is involved. A cardinal rule is always to consider knee pain to be referred from above the knee (i.e., the hip, pelvis, or spine) until proven otherwise.

Let us now consider in more detail the evaluation of the patient, how gait can be altered, and specific conditions and their diagnosis and management. History is essential in evaluating the child who limps. Past history, birth history, development, trauma, prior surgery, duration of limp, constancy, family history of limp, pain, presence of fever, weight loss, systemic symptoms, other joint involvement, and recent immunizations may all help in determining the diagnosis.

Physical examination begins with a routine evaluation with careful neurologic and spine examination prior to extremity and gait evaluation. Evaluating gait involves separate and combined evaluation of the lower extremities, pelvis, and trunk during locomotion. Gait and extremity evaluation should be made with the child undressed except for underclothing. Leg length should be measured and the circumference of the thigh and calf recorded. Palpate for tenderness any areas of increased warmth. Place the feet, ankles, knees, hips, and back through a full range of motion, actively and passively. Restriction or pain suggests the area of involvement. Then note stance, walk, run, and response to squat and to standing on one leg at a time. Observe the patient from the side, front, and back. A positive Trendelenburg test indicates weakness of the abductors or a deficiency of supporting structures around the hip. When reclining, abduction must be tested with the hip in extension as the flexors can simulate abduction if the hip is in flexion. To test for hip flexion contracture, lock the hip you are testing in a neutral position by flexing one thigh on the abdomen while attempting to extend the hip in question. The knee is examined in extension as well as in 15 and 90 degrees of flexion to differentiate collateral ligament and cruciate ligament laxity. In extension, laxity with valgus-varus strain indicates injury to collateral or cruciate ligaments or both. The same maneuver with 15 degrees of flexion isolates the collateral ligaments. With the knee flexed to 90 degrees and with the foot flat on the examining table, a push-pull maneuver against the tibia in the sagittal plane, resulting in increased motions, indicates cruciate ligament involvement. Evaluate sensation and proprioception in the usual manner.

Table 10-3
Probable cause of limp according to age groups

Age at which limp presents (yr)	Short leg gait	Contracture gait	Instability of supporting structures	Antalgic gait	Paralytic gait
Birth–4	Congenital absence or shortening Coxa vara CDH* Hemiatrophy Infection	Spina bifida Cerebral palsy CDH* Infection	Focal femoral deficiency Coxa vara Spina bifida CDH* Trauma	Infection Trauma	Spina bifida Spinal muscular atrophies Cerebral palsy
5–10	Spina bifida CDH* Rheumatoid arthritis Trauma Infection	Trauma Legg-Calvé-Perthes disease CDH* Rheumatoid arthritis Infection	Trauma Infection Muscular dystrophy Poliomyelitis	Trauma Infection Rheumatoid arthritis Hemophilia Legg-Calvé-Perthes disease	Muscular dystrophy Spina bifida Poliomyelitis Cerebral palsy
11–14	Trauma Slipped capital femoral epiphysis Infection Neoplastic	Trauma Legg-Calvé-Perthes disease Infection Slipped capital femoral epiphysis	Trauma Slipped capital femoral epiphysis Inadequate treatment of CDH* (subluxating hip)	Trauma Transient synovitis Slipped capital femoral epiphysis Legg-Calvé-Perthes disease	Muscular dystrophy Neoplasm of central nervous system Peripheral nerve trauma Poliomyelitis Ischemic contracture

Modified from Yablon IG: Problems in family practice: limp in childhood, *Fam Pract* 2:291–295, 1975. Used by permission.
*CDH, congenital dislocated hip.

Normal gait can be altered in several basic ways[30] (Table 10-3):

1. Pain
2. Neuromuscular abnormaility (paralysis, spasticity, ataxia)
3. Shortened extremity
4. Loss of supporting structures
5. Contracture
6. Mimicry

Abnormal gait patterns

The basic variations in gait pattern are the following:

I. *Antalgic (Painful) Gait*

The patient attempts to avoid weightbearing on the painful side, or if walking, bears weight on the affected extremity for the shortest time possible during stance phase. If the hip is involved, the patient tends to plantarflex the foot to act as a shock absorber and to slightly flex, abduct, and externally rotate the hip to increase the volume of the joint and to pivot on the ball of the foot as the normal leg swings forward (to avoid a forceful push-off and internal rotation.) With knee pain, the ankle is plantarflexed, with the knee held in mild flexion without extension during push-off. Stance phase is short, but there is no Trendelenburg lurch or trunk oscillation. With ankle pain, the foot will most likely be planted flat in the sagittal plane and slightly everted and externally rotated (particularly with the typical talofibular sprain). Stance phase is short with no push-off. With subtalar or forefoot pain, the patient will heel-walk or walk flat, with virtually no push-off, and may invert and supinate slightly. With rearfoot pain the patient will toe-walk on the affected side.

II. *Neurologic Gait*

A. *Paralytic Gait*

1. *Gluteus medius paralysis:* This muscle is the chief abductor of the hip. Paralysis causes a Trendelenburg gait (see Fig. 10-5), as in loss of hip-supporting

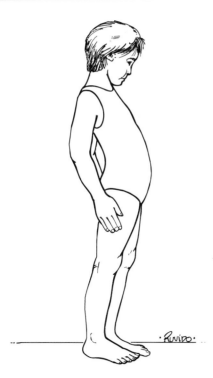

Fig. 10-5. Gluteus maximus weakness or paralysis (rare) (pelvis thrusts forward arms back to place center of gravity farther posterior to keep from falling forward).

structures, but in this case, one cannot feel the contracting muscle during abduction.

2. *Gluteus maximus paralysis* (Fig. 10-5): The loss of stability of the trunk forces the patient to keep the center of gravity behind the hip to keep from falling forward.

3. *Quadriceps paralysis:* This muscle extends the knee. Weakness of the quadriceps, especially with no other muscles involved, may produce a noticeable limp, which may be one of three types:
   a. Locking of the knee by placing the center of gravity in front of the knee by tilting the trunk and pelvis forward (Fig. 10-6**A**).
   b. Placing the hand on the distal thigh at heel strike and pushing backward to lock the knee in extension (Fig. 10-6**B**).
   c. Externally rotating the extremity so the medial knee faces forward preventing flexion (Fig. 10-6**C**).

4. *Hamstrings weakness* (Fig. 10-7) usually causes a genu recurvatum without significant limp, but may result in greater hip flexion and knee hyperextension.

5. *Calcaneus gait* (Fig. 10-8): A weakened Achilles tendon results in some external rotation and pronation, with the

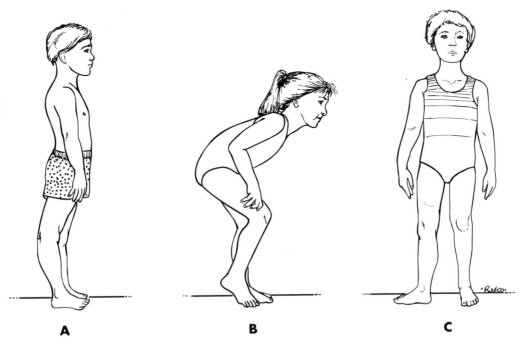

A   **B**   **C**

Fig. 10-6. Quadriceps paralysis compensated by (**A**) genu recurvatum or (**B**) by pushing on the distal thigh to prevent collapse and maintain equilibrium or (**C**) by externally rotating the leg.

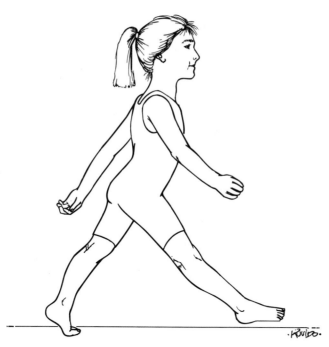

Fig. 10-7. Hamstring paralysis. The hamstring muscles act at the termination of the swing phase to slow hip flexion and prevent hyperextension of the knee, and at stance phase to aid in hip extension. This results in greater hip flexion and hyperextension at the knee.

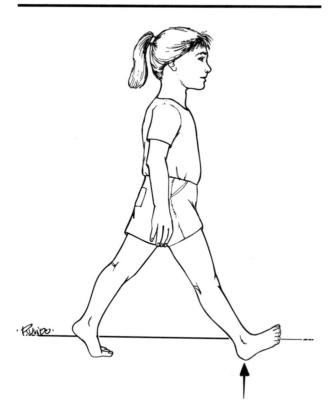

Fig. 10-8. Calcaneus gait caused by contraction of the anterior motor group, by severe weakness of the posterior muscles, or by persistent talipes calcaneovalgus. The foot is held in dorsiflexion throughout gait.

foot pushing off as a unit with an exaggerated rise of the pelvis on that side, so the foot can clear the ground.

6. *Footdrop gait* (Fig. 10-9) results in loss of dorsiflexion of the foot and ankle. In the swing phase, the affected leg must be raised higher for the foot to clear the ground as the trunk moves forward. The toes strike and then the foot and heel, causing the so-called steppage gait.

B. *Spastic gait* (Fig. 10-10) is secondary to an upper motor neuron lesion that results in hypertonicity and an overplay of the stronger muscle groups. This usually causes adduction, internal rotation, and flexion of the hip, with the knee slightly flexed and the ankle and foot in equinus.

C. *Ataxic gait* results in loss of balance.

D. *Primary muscle disease* is manifested by weakness that depends on the muscle groups involved.[1,6]

III. *Shortened Extremity*

Leg length inequality is a common orthopedic condition and has many basic causes.

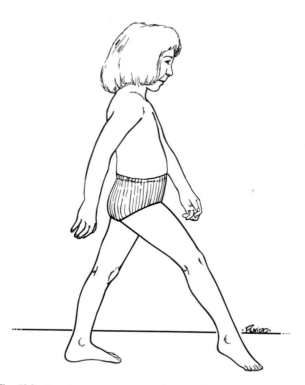

Fig. 10-9. Footdrop gait caused by weak foot dorsiflexors (anterior tibial and peroneals). The foot remains in plantarflexion in the swing phase with anterior weakness or in plantarflexion throughout weightbearing with posterior contracture.

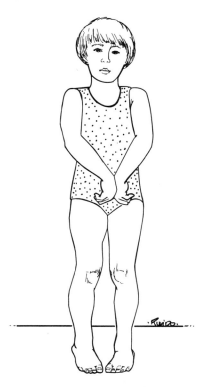

Fig. 10-10. Spastic gait. An overplay of the stronger muscle groups results in adduction, internal rotation, hip and knee flexion, and ankle foot equinus.

Understanding this condition necessitates a knowledge of normal longitudinal bone growth.

A. *Anatomy of Bone Growth:* A long bone is made up of the shaft consisting of the diaphysis and metaphysis, the physis (growth plate), and the epiphysis at the end. Pressure epiphyses enter into joint formation and contribute to bone growth. Traction epiphyses serve as sites for muscle or tendon attachment and do not contribute to length growth. The major long bones have an epiphysis and physis at both ends. The short tubular bones have them at only one end. It is proximal in the first metatarsal and distal in the other metatarsals. In the physis, the zone of resting cartilage grows by apposition increasing the transverse diameter, while the zone of proliferation cartilage grows by interstitial division increasing the length of the bone. The metaphysis is funnel-shaped, narrowing as it approaches the diaphysis, where cortical remodeling is a lifelong process.

B. *Rate of Bone Growth:* This is rapid in infancy, decreasing in rate until adolescence, when a second spurt occurs lasting about 2 years. Bone growth then decreases to zero over another 4 years. Limb growth is usually complete at about 14 years in girls and 16 years in boys. Prior to the adolescent growth spurt, the lower limbs grow faster than the spine, but following that, the spine grows faster. Sixty-five percent of the lower limb growth occurs at the knee (35% femur, 30% tibia), another 15% occurs at the proximal femur, and 20% occurs at the distal tibia.

C. *Clinical and Radiographic Evaluation:* Measurements include (1) absolute length as measured by radiograph; (2) clinical length measured from the anterior superior iliac spine to the lateral malleolus, weightbearing or supine; (3) apparent length measured from the umbilicus to the medial malleolus while supine and standing; (4) pelvic tilt measured in stance; and (5) gait evaluation. Subtalar joint pronation may be a cause of, or compensation for, leg length discrepancy. In minor discrepancies, a patient may supinate on the short side and pronate on the long side. Shoe wear may readily demonstrate this compensation. Conversely, a unilateral pronated foot will lead to a functional short limb while a unilateral supinated foot will lead to a functional long limb. Skeletal age, as evidenced by radiographs of the hands and wrists and compared to standards, is an indicator of maturity and an aid in predicting subsequent growth. Prediction charts allow for projection of correction obtainable by epiphysiodesis (stapling). Clinical measurement of the lower limbs is only approximate, and radiographic evaluation is necessary for accuracy.

D. *Etiology* of leg length discrepancy includes a long list:
  1. *Structural* inequality is the result of shortening (or lengthening) of one or more bones due to growth retardation or growth stimulation.
  2. *Functional* inequality is due to soft tissue contracture, with bony structures being equal bilaterally. Shortening may be congenital or secondary to the following: infection, neuromuscular disorders, tumors, trauma, or miscellaneous disease (Legg-Calvé-Perthes disease, arteriovenous fistula, neurofibromatosis, etc.). Lengthening due to growth stimulation may be congenital or associated

with vascular abnormalities, trauma, infection, or tumors. Clinically, the patient presents with abnormal gait or limp. Evaluation should include: (a) leg length measurement reclining, sitting, and standing; (b) pelvic tilt; (c) ranges of motion of the joints of the lower extremity; (d) neuromuscular evaluation of muscle mass, tone, strength, sensation, and tenderness; and (e) laboratory evaluations including x-ray films, electromyography (EMG), telemetry, computed tomography (CT) scans, and magnetic resonance imaging (MRI).

E. *Compensation in Response to Leg Length Discrepancy:* The child with a shortened lower extremity in stance will tilt the pelvis down to the side of the affected extremity. If the shortening is less than 3.5 cm (about 1.3 in.) the child tends to supinate or to plantarflex the foot on the short side and walk with the foot in equinus. With shortening in excess of 3.5 cm, the child will, in addition, tend to flex the normal hip and knee. Evaluation of the shoe wear pattern may be helpful in diagnosis. Treatment of leg length discrepancy may involve:

1. Arrest of growth of the longer limb (permanent) by epiphysiodesis.
2. Retardation of growth of the longer limb (epiphyseal stapling).
3. Shortening of the longer limb surgically.
4. Lengthening of the shorter limb by osteotomy and distraction or by stimulating growth of the epiphysis.
5. A lift on the short side in minor cases.

F. *Hemihypertrophy:* This represents a rare and special factor in leg length discrepancy; treatment, however, is the same as for other forms of leg length inequality. Congenital hemihypertrophy is probably a defect in the process of twinning that bilateral structures normally undergo. Classically, all tissues on the hypertrophied side are enlarged (crossed and segmental hypertrophy may occur). Mental retardation is associated in about 20% of cases and anomalies in 50%, particularly syndactyly, polydactylism, and nail deformities. About 75% of these cases require surgery to correct the length discrepancy.

IV. *Loss of Supporting Structures and Limp:* This is caused by an abnormal relationship of the acetabulum to the femoral head and neck. This prevents abductor stability and results in a Trendelenburg gait. Causes include (1) congenital or developmental hip dislocation; (2) Legg-Calvé-Perthes disease; (3) slipped capital femoral epiphysis; (4) arthritis; (5) osteomyelitis; (6) tuberculosis; and (7) tumor (e.g., Ewing's sarcoma). The type of limp gives a significant clue to the cause, as does the patient's age (see Table 10-3). After arriving at a reasonable differential diagnosis, appropriate laboratory tests and radiographs should be obtained. Laboratory work should include a complete blood cell count (CBC), urinalysis, and erythrocyte sedimentation rate (ESR). The ESR is normal in trauma, Osgood-Schlatter's disease, Legg-Calvé-Perthes disease, Köhler's disease, and slipped capital femoral epiphysis. If the ESR is elevated, one should consider malignancy; osteomyelitis; and septic arthritis or collagen disease, especially rheumatoid arthritis; and perform the appropriate tests. Radiographs should include anteroposterior (AP) and lateral views of the area in question and comparison views of the uninvolved side. If referred pain from the back is suspected, obtain appropriate films of the spine and pelvis. Early in osteomyelitis, radiographs may be negative. Technetium scanning is useful early and is more helpful than radiographs in following the patient later. (Fine fractures may not be demonstrated until periosteal reaction has occurred, approximately 10 days after the injury.) Additionally, the type of pain may provide a clue to the cause. It is usually mild with slipped capital femoral epiphysis, Legg-Calvé-Perthes disease, Osgood-Schlatter's disease, juvenile rheumatoid arthritis (JRA), and transient synovitis. Pain is more likely to be severe with fractures, dislocations, septic joints, and acute osteomyelitis. Fever may also be suggestive of the cause. High fever is more apt to occur in osteomyelitis or joint sepsis. Low fever is associated with tuberculosis, smoldering osteomyelitis, Gaucher's disease and Ewing's sarcoma.

V. *Contracture Limp:* Contractures result in flexion at the hip or knee, in effect shortening the extremity, and may resemble short-legged gait. The hip, however, cannot extend, and this results in an abnormal pelvic tilt anteriorly in swing phase, which reverses in the stance phase. With flexion contracture at the knee, the affected knee does not fully extend at push-off.

VI. *Mimicry:* Occasionally, psychogenic limp may occur in children, in which case the child mimics the limp of someone he or she knows. If this is the case, the physical examination is normal and a person the patient has contact with should demonstrate a similar limp. From the pediatrician's viewpoint, limp takes on a different perspective from that seen by the podiatrist or orthopedist. Legg-Calvé-Perthes disease, Sever's disease, and Köhler's disease are somewhat rare. Osteomyelitis, foot fractures, and dislocation of the hip are seen occasionally, while ankle sprains, lower extremity trauma, synovitis, Osgood Schlatter's disease, jumper's knee, and soft tissue infections (secondary to puncture wounds and ingrown toenails) are frequent. Plantar warts as a cause of pain and slight limp, and foreign bodies in the foot are common.

Specific disorders
Dislocation of the hip

Hip dislocation may be: (1) congenital, (2) developmental, or (3) traumatic.

Terminology

1. *Dislocation:* the femoral head is completely displaced from the acetabulum.
2. *Dislocatable hip:* the femoral head is normally in the acetabulum, but can be forcibly displaced.
3. *Subluxation:* the femoral head can be partially displaced from its normal position in the acetabulum.
4. *Dysplasia:* abnormal development of the acetabulum or femoral head.

In the United States the incidence of the above is: dislocation, 1/1,000 livebirths; dislocatable-subluxable hips, greater than 10/1,000 livebirths. The incidence is higher in Italy, Israel, and Japan. The reason for this is uncertain.

Etiology

1. Heredity. The first child of normal parents has a risk of about 1/1,000. If there is one affected child a male offspring has a risk of 1 in 100, and a female offspring a risk of 1 in 10. If one parent has a history of congenital dislocation of the hip (CDH), a male offspring has a risk of about 6 in 100 and a female offspring, about 17 in 100. If one parent and one child are affected, the risk to the next child is approximately 40%.
2. Environmental influences include (a) breech position (associated in up to 40% of cases), (b) first pregnancy, and (c) swaddling with the legs in extension.
3. Hormonal. Relaxin from the mother during labor is questionably related to increased frequency in girls. Dislocation is nearly eight times more common in females. Children with metatarsus adductus and torticollis have an increased incidence of CDH. (These abnormalities are also associated with breech position and constraint in the uterus).

Diagnosis

Early diagnosis of dislocated hip generally means satisfactory treatment; late diagnosis may mean lifetime disability.[26]

History

A dislocated hip is more commonly associated with first pregnancy; breech position; female sex; Italian, Israeli, or Japanese descent; family history; prematurity; Ehlers-Danlos syndrome; and Marfan's syndrome. The primary defect in the last two is related to soft tissue laxity.

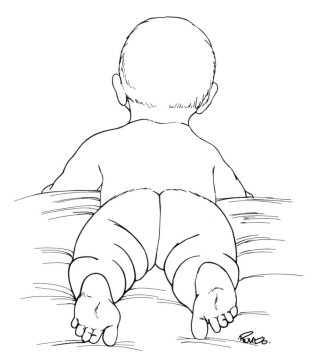

Fig. 10-11. Congenital dislocated hip demonstrating accentuation of skinfolds on the affected side. The folds are asymmetric. In this illustration, the hip is dislocated on the left side.

Clinical signs

1. Asymmetric inguinal and buttock skinfolds (Fig. 10-11) are suggestive. (Appear in approximately 20% of normal infants).

2. Restriction of abduction and external rotation (Fig. 10-12) is *the most significant sign*. Normal hips abduct greater than 60 degrees. Anything less should arouse suspicion.

3. Galeazzi's sign (Fig. 10-13): With dislocation, when the child is placed supine on the examining table and the hips and knees are flexed with the feet placed flat on the table,the knee on the displaced side is at a

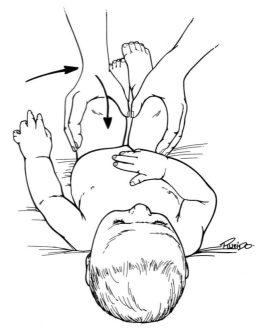

Fig. 10-14. Congenital dislocated hip. Barlow's maneuver to dislocate a dislocatable hip. The baby's thigh is adducted and internally rotated with gentle, superoposterior pressure. Dislocation is felt as the femoral head moves out of the acetabulum.

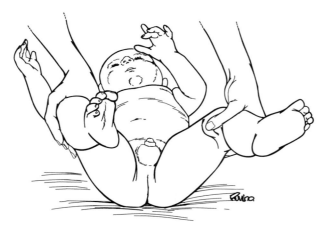

Fig. 10-12. Congenital dislocated hip. Limitation of abduction is caused by contraction of hip adductor muscles. After a few months of age, restriction of abduction becomes the most suggestive sign.

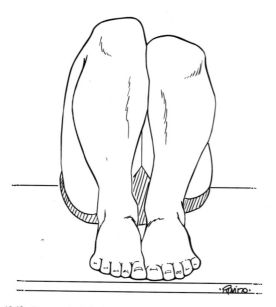

Fig. 10-13. Congenital dislocated hip. Galeazzi's (or Allis') sign: the knee is lower on the affected side when the knees and hips are flexed.

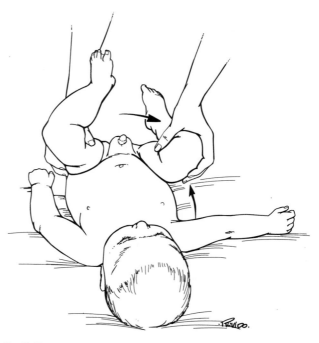

Fig. 10-15. Congenital dislocated hip. *Ortolani's test* to reduce a dislocated hip. The hips and knees are flexed to 90 degrees and then examined one at a time by grasping the thigh with the middle finger over the greater trochanter (lifting the thigh while simultaneously abducting it by reducing the femoral head into the acetabulum). The examiner will feel a "bumping" sensation or "clunk."

lower level. Galeazzi's sign is absent in bilateral dislocation.

4. Barlow's maneuver (Fig. 10-14): From a supine position, with the hips and knees flexed, the leg is adducted and internally rotated with laterally directed pressure on the medial thigh and gentle downward pressure on the knee. With this maneuver, a dislocatable hip can be displaced from the acetabulum. The advisability of this test is now in question. Sidney Gellis of Tufts University has questioned the wisdom of intentionally dislocating any joint.

5. Ortolani's sign (Fig. 10-15): With the infant supine, the hips and knees flexed, the middle finger over the greater trochanter, and the thumb on the medial aspect of the thigh, the thigh is lifted anteriorly and then abducted and externally rotated. As the head of a displaced femur moves into the acetabulum a "clunking" sensation is felt. This sign has been described as a click, but as Ortolani described it, it is not an audible sign, but rather a palpable sensation. Audible clicks can be heard in normal hips.

After a few months, these signs, except for Galeazzi's sign and the restriction of abduction and external rotation, which is the best sign, are not useful. An ambulatory child should present with a positive Trendelenburg sign and Trendelenburg gait or abductor lurch with a tendency to hold the affected extremity in external rotation, resisting internal rotation.

Laboratory diagnosis
Radiographs. Films of newborns may be false-negative because of (1) infant positioning or (2) lack of ossification of the femoral head and only fuzzy ossification of the innominate. This makes interpretation difficult.

Infants. In infants lateral and superior displacement of the femur may be obvious. Without obvious displacement, the following measurements are helpful (Fig. 10-16):

1. A horizontal line (Hilgenreiner's line) or the Y line through the center of both triradiate cartilages.
2. A vertical line from the lateral margin of the acetabulum (Ombredanne's or Perkin's or X line).
   The intersection of these two lines delineates four quadrants. The head of a normal femur lies in the medial inferior quadrant.
3. Acetabular index: A line drawn along the acetabular roof and crossing the Y line forms an angle, which, in the infant less than 1 year of age, should not exceed 30 degrees. A higher angle suggests acetabular dysplasia and increases the possibility of a dislocated hip.
4. Shenton's line: On the AP projection, a line drawn along the medial border of the femur and femoral neck and continued along the superior margin of the obturator foramen. The line is disrupted with femoral displacement.[18,26]

Ultrasound. This is now the preferred diagnostic laboratory test if experienced interpreters are available.[19,22,23,26,27] The technique involves short-focus transducers using high-frequency, high-resolution, real-time equipment, taking linear images in a coronal plane. In a normal hip, more than 50% of the femoral head is covered by the acetabulum. In dislocation, the femoral head is displaced laterally and invariably uncovered. By rotating the transducer 90 degrees, the hip can be seen in the transverse plane. In dislocation, it is displaced posteriorly toward the ischium. The test has a sensitivity of about 95%. If a follow-up clinical examination is suggestive in the face of a negative sonogram, a repeat sonogram should be done, stressing the hip by performing Barlow's maneuver.

Radiographs are still valuable in monitoring treatment. A recent article[29] recommends that all patients with risk factors have ultrasound or radiographic studies of the hips, even though the clinical examination is normal.

Treatment
The principle is to maintain the leg in flexion, external rotation, and abduction. Early treatment includes

1. Pavlik harness (at present the most popular) (Fig. 10-17)
2. Ilfeld splint (Fig. 10-18)
3. Von Rosen splint
4. Frejka splint

Care should be exercised with all these splints as forced abduction can impair femoral blood flow, leading to necrosis of the femoral head.

In general, treatment time is twice the child's age in months from the time treatment is started. If diagnosis is delayed beyond 6 to 12 months, traction and surgery may be necessary. Diagnosis delayed beyond the age of walking will almost always result in major deformity and some degree of lifetime disability. Deformities resulting from delayed diag-

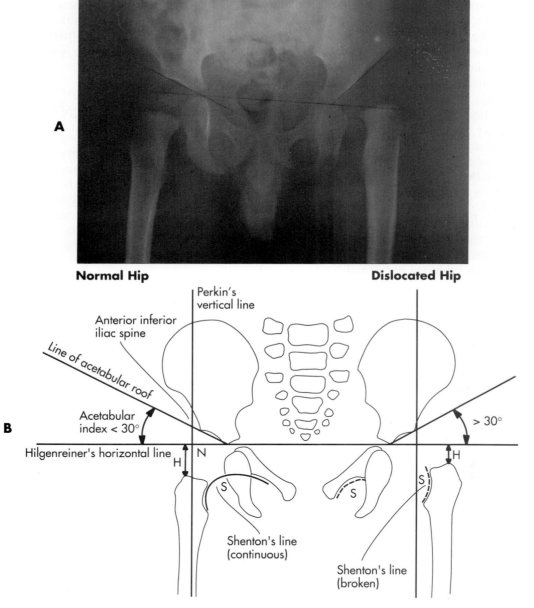

Fig. 10-16. A, Radiograph of dislocated hip. **B,** Diagrammatic representation. *H,* Distance from highest point of femoral neck to Hilgenreiner's line; *N,* ossific nucleus of femoral head, if present; *S,* Shenton's curved line (broken in hip dislocation).

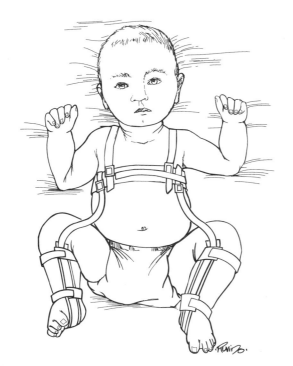

Fig. 10-17. The Pavlik harness allows safe abduction.

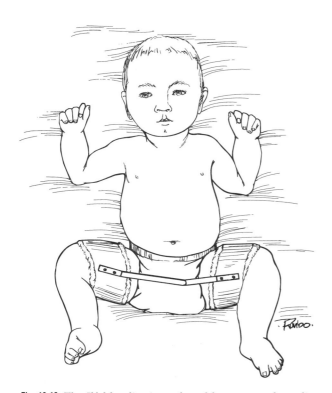

Fig. 10-18. The Ilfeld splint is preferred by some orthopedists.

nosis until after the age of walking include deformed acetabulum, false acetabulum, misshapen femoral head, and a thickened capsule blocking relocation.

Legg-Calvé-Perthes disease (coxa plana)

This is a self-limited disease. Radiographic signs of avascular necrosis of the capital femoral epiphysis are evident. The incidence is approximately 1/750 children. About 15% of cases are bilateral. The cause is unknown, but a factor that interferes with blood supply is a probable cause. It occurs in boys four to five times more frequently than in girls with many of the children being premature at birth. The age of occurrence is most commonly 4 to 5 years, which correlates with the stage of isolated blood supply of the capital femoral epiphysis. Skeletal age and height are less than normal, and the feet tend to be small. It is rare in blacks and when it does occur, is most often associated with hemoglobinopathies. Limp and pain are vague in the early stages. Pain is usually in the groin, medial thigh, or occasionally referred to the knee via the obturator nerve. An antalgic limp is typical. The weightbearing phase is short, with a lurch toward the affected side. Range of motion is decreased in abduction and external rotation, and there may be local tenderness over the hip joint. Atrophy of the thigh muscles is common as the disease progresses. Radiographs vary with the stage of involvement (Fig. 10-19). Early in the process there is intracapusular fluid, followed by demineralization of the femoral head and neck, and later, increased density, fragmentation, flattening of the head of the femur and broadening of the femoral neck. Later, the vascular supply returns and the radiographic pattern returns to normal except for the flattening of the femoral head (coxa plana). Initially, treatment includes bed rest, analgesics, and slings. Traction may be hazardous. Typically, the disease heals within 2 years. Prognosis is better the earlier the age of onset and the earlier the diagnosis. Once the acute phase is over, the child can ambulate using a brace that maintains the femoral head in the acetabulum by abduction and internal rotation. The greater the degree of epiphyseal involvement, the poorer the results, generally. *Catterall's classification* is as follows[5]:

Group I: Anterior head involvement with no other changes; the disease heals without sequelae.

Group II: Greater head involvement—intact lateral pillar and epiphyseal metaphyseal area; results are good.

Group III: Three fourths of the epiphysis is affected with early collapse. This often ends

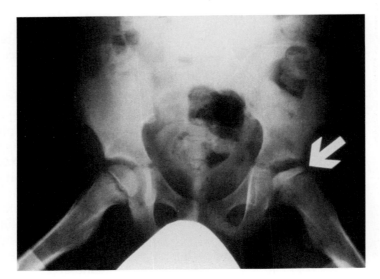

Fig. 10-19. Radiograph of Legg-Calvé-Perthes disease of the left hip *(arrow)*. *(From Valmassy RL, Smith L, Koch T.:* Gait analysis in children: Diagnostic and therapeutic implications. *Medcom Corp., New York, 1985)*

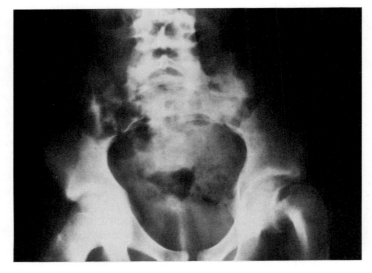

Fig. 10-20. Radiograph showing slipped capital femoral epiphysis of the left hip.

poorly; the metaphyseal area and plate are involved.

Group IV: The entire epiphysis is involved with severe collapse, and the plate is involved early; results are almost universally poor.

Treatment should probably be continued until reconstitution of the subchondral bone plate is complete.

Slipped capital femoral epiphysis

An acute or chronic disruption of the structural integrity of the epiphyseal cartilage plate of the proximal femur, this is the most common hip disorder in adolescence, albeit rare. The result is displacement of the head relative to the neck of the femur. It occurs most commonly in the growth spurt in adolescence, and it is much more frequent in boys. Growth hormone increases the thickness of the plate and decreases the shear strength. Also, the plate in adolescence is more vertical, allowing greater shearing force. Obesity is an aggravating factor, with more than half the patients above the 95th percentile in weight, increasing the shear load. The majority have delayed bone ages. In some cases, underlying connective tissue disorders, such as Ehlers-Danlos or Marfan's syndrome, or endocrine abnormalities, such as hypothyroidism, may be associated. Symptoms include pain, much as in Legg-Calvé-Perthes disease. There is an antalgic limp with lurch to the affected side and a short weightbearing period. The leg is held in external rotation. The pain is increased on all forced motion. The hip cannot be internally rotated because the neck strikes against the anterior rim of the acetabulum. (There is an upward and anterior movement of the femoral neck in relation to the head.) There may be tenderness over the anterior hip joint. Radiographs (Fig. 10-20) are confirmatory and should be taken in the AP and frog-leg lateral views.

Comparison films are important. If the disease is suspected, the patient should be kept off weightbearing until the diagnosis is excluded (an acute slip may exaggerate a chronic slip). Bilateral involvement is reported in approximately 25% of cases. Slips are classified as grade I, II, or III. A slip less than one third of the diameter of the growth plate is a grade 1 slip; from one third to one half is grade II; and greater than one half of the diameter is grade III. With grade I and II slips, in situ pinning with threaded pins is preferred. Epiphyseal closure occurs in about 6 months. With a grade III deformity, trochanteric osteotomy may be indicated. Femoral neck osteotomy and manipulation under anesthesia carry a high risk of avascular necrosis. Chondrolysis is more common in the black child and in grade III slip with a high risk of chronic disability.

Scoliosis

Scoliosis is any lateral tilt of the spine from the normal. A functional type (i.e., short leg) disappears on reclining. The structural type relates to a spine defect (wedging of the vertebrae or intervertebral disks). The most frequent type is idiopathic, most common in adolescent girls. It is hereditary, transmitted as an autosomal dominant trait with incomplete penetrance. In adolescent idiopathic scoliosis, 90% of cases are familial, with 90% having only convex thoracic curves which are usually to the right, and 70% progressing to some degree (one third demonstrate no progression; one third, insignificant progression; and one third, significant progression). The progression of the curve defect will generally stop when growth is complete. Curves under 50 degrees can usually be managed in the Boston or a comparable brace. This needs to be worn for an average of 3 years. The brace should be fitted by an experienced orthotist in conjunction with an orthopedist who is experienced in scoliosis. Surgery may be indicated for scoliosis with a curve greater than 50 degrees (Fig. 10-21), with neurofibromatosis, or in those children who cannot tolerate the brace. If the onset is early in the child's

Degrees of scoliosis as measured by x-ray

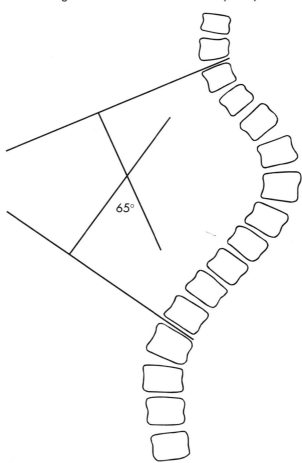

Fig. 10-21. Cobb's angle (degree of scoliosis as measured by radiograph). Approximately 90% of adolescent idiopathic scoliolsis curves are thoracic only and most commonly convex to the right.

development, or if the curve is progressing rapidly, bracing or surgery may be indicated at a younger age and at lesser degrees of curvature. Rapidly progressing curves should be considered for fusion.

Electric stimulation of muscle on the convex side at night has been a popular method of preventing progression, although it has poor patient acceptance. Most authorities believe exercise is of no help, although most patients say they feel more comfortable if they exercise regularly. Nonsurgical treatment methods will not permanently reduce the curve. The curve will return to the degree it was when first diagnosed and treated, which is why early diagnosis is so important.

The patient is examined undressed except for an examination gown. The level of the pelvis, the height of the scapula, and the spine with the patient bent over (Fig. 10-22), straight, and in the half-bent position are evaluated. There is an associated rota-

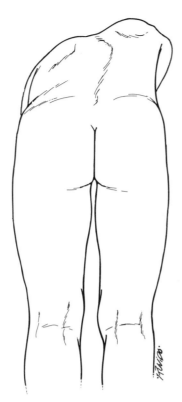

Fig. 10-22. Forward bending magnifies the curve and the rib humping.

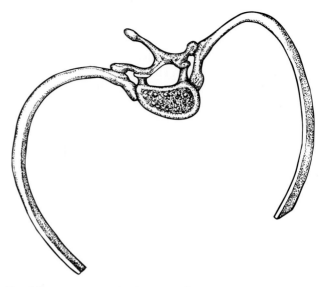

Fig. 10-23. The spine not only curves but rotates.

tional deformity that accounts for the humping (Fig. 10-23). Back sensation is evaluated with a pin. The skin is examined for hairy nevi or dimples, which could suggest diastematomyelia or other defects. Café au lait spots are associated with neurofibromatosis. The absence of a Trendelenburg sign will rule out hip abnormalities. Neuromuscular disease is ruled out by having the patient walk on the heels and toes, perform head raises, and sit up from a reclining position. Radiographs of the entire spine, recumbent and standing, are taken if there is any suggestion of a curve. If the iliac crest apophysis has appeared, the patient is probably nearing completion of growth and the curve may be near its maximum. Curves can progress rapidly to a very deforming degree and should be followed at frequent intervals from the onset. If the curve exceeds 20 degrees, the child should be referred to an orthopedist.

Osteomyelitis

This occurs most commonly in 5- to 14-year-old boys. While any organism is possible, *Staphylococcus aureus* is most common, and a primary lesion often exists (impetigo, boil, etc.). It is usually manifested by localized pain, tenderness, and swelling. Fever occurs in only about 50% of cases. Leukocytosis is common, and the ESR and C-reactive protein values are elevated. Radiographic changes may not be apparent for 10 or more days. Early diagnosis may be determined with a three-phase scan. A technetium scan may be helpful early and is a better aid in follow-up than radiographs. Treatment includes surgical drainage and appropriate antibiotics. The most common sites involved are the distal femur (25%), proximal tibia (25%), and distal humerus, distal ulna, or wrist and foot bones (14%). Approximately 75% are due to hemolytic *S. aureus*, coagulase-positive. In the sickle cell patient, salmonella is an occasional cause but staphyloccus is still more common.

Arthritis

Arthritis is characterized by nonbony swelling of a joint. If there is no clinical swelling, three other conditions must be met: (1) pain and tenderness, (2) heat, and (3) decreased range of motion. Cellulitis, tenosynovitis, and bone pain can mimic the condition. Analysis of joint fluid is indicated in monoarticular arthritis except in hemophilia. The fluid is withdrawn in a heparinized syringe. Associated fever suggests infection or malignancy and possibly collagen disease. Migrating polyarthritis with a *rash* and tenosynovitis in a sexually active teenager should be considered gonococcemia until excluded. Arthritis of over 3 months' duration is probably JRA if other conditions have been excluded. A girl with polyarthritis and sacroiliac disease probably has ulcerative colitis, whereas a boy with the same symptoms most likely has ankylosing spondylitis. Other chronic bowel diseases may be associated (e.g., Crohn's disease), and the joint symptoms may precede any evidence of bowel disease.

Septic arthritis occurs 40% of the time in children

less than 2 years of age, with a distribution most common at the knee, hip, elbow, ankles, and wrist. Joint aspiration typically demonstrates more than 50,000 white blood cells per cubic millimeter and less than 50 mg/dL glucose. About one third of patients are culture negative; the most common organisms are gonococcus, hemolytic staphylococcus, *Haemophilus influenzae*, group B streptococcus, and pneumococcus. Pseudomonas, other gram-negative organisms, and tuberculosis, are also seen. *Haemophilus influenzae* as a cause is rapidly disappearing since the advent of vaccine.

Knee problems

Knee problems are common in the pediatric age group, typically involving acute and chronic injury. A complete history is often as important as the clinical examination in determining the diagnosis. A detailed history of activity at the time of injury is crucial. Straightforward movement seldom results in injury. However, any lateral, uphill, downhill, or deceleration movements may relate to injury, especially to the menisci or anterior cruciate ligament. If the patient was not weightbearing, injury is usually limited to the extensor mechanism. Direct blows usually result in posterior cruciate injury or patellar contusion or fracture. A noise at the time of injury suggests serious injury (i.e., anterior cruciate ligament) until proved otherwise. A locking of the knee may be due to structural obstruction (i.e., loose body or meniscal tear) or a stiffness after being flexed for a period of time, as in "theatre knee." If the patient is unable, or feels that he or she is unable, to bear weight, it suggests serious injury. Rapid swelling also indicates serious injury.

The practitioner should attempt to establish the exact location of the pain. Initially, it is usually at the site of injury (i.e., meniscal tears at the joint line; anterior cruciate on either side of the patellar tendon, etc.). Injury to internal structures, for example, menisci, are not associated with ecchymoses. Bruising not related to direct trauma also suggests serious injury.

Overuse syndromes typically cause a more diffuse pain. Patellofemoral syndromes, frequently referred to simply as anterior knee pain syndrome, are more common in teenage girls. They have a variety of causes associated with patellofemoral joint structures. Pain may be reproduced by pushing the patella distally while compressing it against the femoral groove. The patient is usually asymtomatic on arising in the morning, in contrast to the arthritis patient who is stiff in the morning. There is often a quadriceps weakness and atrophy of the vastus medialis. Overpronation is often noted as the primary cause. Treatment primarily involves quadriceps strengthening exercises plus nonsteroidal anti-inflammatory drugs and functional foot orthoses. Distal superficial patellar pain is typical of Larsen's syndrome (so-called jumper's knee), most common in basketball players. Osgood-Schlatter's disease is characterized by mild pain, swelling, and tenderness at the tibial tubercle. It is typically present more often in boys than in girls, and it is most common in adolescence, particularly in physically active teenagers.

Femoral anteversion, external tibial torsion (which is not common), patella alta, genu valgum, and severe pronation of the feet may contribute to patellofemoral syndromes.

The sine qua non of patellofemoral syndromes is quadriceps weakness, and therefore the mainstay of treatment is quadriceps strengthening exercises and stretching before and after exercise.

Summary

This has been a brief and somewhat superficial look at childhood limp. It is a challenging diagnostic problem. Many of the conditions causing it represent critical but curable problems if proper diagnosis is made and appropriate therapy instituted in a timely fashion.

References

1. Abbott G, Carty H: Pyogenic sacroiliitis, the missed diagnosis? Br J Radiol 166:120–122, 1993.
2. Alexander JE, Siebert JJ, Glasier CM, et al: High-resolution hip ultrasound in the limping child. J Clin Ultrasound 12:19–24, 1989.
3. Aronson J, Garvin K, Seibert J, et al: Efficiency of the bone scan for occult limping toddlers, J Pediatr Orthop 12:38–44, 1992.
4. Blatt SD, Rosenthal BM, Barnhart DC: Diagnostic utility of lower extremity radiographs of young children with gait disturbance, Pediatrics 87:138–140, 1991.
5. Catterall A.: The natural history of Calvé-Perthes disease, J Bone Joint Surg [Br]. 53:37, 1971.
6. Chobin S, Killian JT: Evaluation of acute gait abnormalities in preschool children, J Pediatr Orthop 10:74–78, 1990.
7. Ducroquet R, Ducroquet J, Ducroquet P: Walking and Limping, J B Lippincott, 1968.
8. Fields L: The limping child, a review of the literature, J Am Podiatr Assoc, 71:2, 1981.
9. Gavalas M: Bone infection and the limping child in the accident and emergency department: a diagnosis to be considered, Arch Emerg Med 9:323–325, 1993.
10. Grattan-Smith JD, Wagner ML, Barnes DA: Osteomyelitis of the talus: an unusual cause of limping in childhood, AJR 156:785–789, 1991.
11. Greenstein N: Acute limp in childhood—"jumping jack syndrome" (letter), Clin Pediatr, 14:7, 1975.
12. Howard C, Eihoran M, Dagan R, et al: The use of ultrasound in children with pain around the hip and thigh, Isr J Med Sci 29:77–81, 1993.
13. Hunsinger R: Limp, Pediatr Clin North Am 723–730, 1977.

14. Illingworth CN: 128 limping children with no fracture, sprain, or obvious cause, *Clin Pediatr* 17:2, 1978.

15. Inman V, Henry R, Frank T: *Human Walking,* Baltimore, Williams & Wilkins, 1981.

16. MacEwen GD, Dehne R: The limping child, *Pediatr Rev* 12:268–274, 1992.

17. Martinez A: *Sonography of the painful hip in children: 500 consecutive cases, AJR* 152:579–582, 1989.

18. McCrea JD: *Pediatric Orthopedics of the Lower Extremity,* Mt Kisca, NY, Futura, 1985.

19. Miralles M, Gonzales G, Pulpeiro JR, et al: Pelvic muscle abcess. An unusual cause of gait disturbance in young children, *Clin Pediatr* 32:298–299.

20. Murtagh J: Hip pain in children. *Aus Fam Physician* 21:1018–1021, 1992.

21. Oestreich AE: Imaging of the skeleton and soft tissues in children *Curr Opin Radiol* 4:55–61, 1992.

22. Rose SA, Ounpuu S, DeLuca PA: Strategies for the assessment of pediatric gait in the clinical setting, *Phys Ther* 71:961–980, 1991.

23. Singer J: Evaluation of acute and insidious gait disturbance in children less than five years of age. In Barkness L, editor: *Advances in Pediatrics,* vol 26. St Louis, Mosby–Year Book, 1979.

24. Singer J, Towbin R: Occult fractures in the production of gait disturbance in childhood, *Pediatrics* 64:2, 1979

25. Staheli LT: Pain of musculoskeletal origin in children, *Curr Opin Rheumatol* 4:748–752, 1993.

26. Sutherland D: *Gait Disorders in Childhood and Adolesence,* Baltimore, William & Wilkins, 1984.

27. Swischuk LE: Limp in young child, *Pediatr Emerg Care* 6:65–66, 1990.

28. Swischuk LE: Painless limp, *Pediatr Emerg Care* 8:105–106, 1992

29. Treadwell SJ: Neonatal screening for hip joint instability: Its clinical and economic relevance, *Clin Orthop* 281:63–68, 1992.

30. Yablon IG: Problems in family practice: limp in childhood, *J Fam Pract* 2:4, 1975.

biomechanical evaluation of the child

Ronald L. Valmassy, DPM

Initial visit
Perinatal history
Neuromuscular developmental landmarks
Family history
Sleeping and sitting positions
Growing pains
Shoe wear
Level of activity
Participation in sports

Clinical examination
Head tilt
Shoulder and pelvis level
Patellae position
Angle of gait
Calcaneal position
Examination of the hip
Examination of the knee and tibia
Examination of the foot and ankle joint

The practitioner involved in treating lower extremity pediatric problems should have a sound knowledge of the normal and abnormal development of the child's lower extremities. As structural and positional developmental changes take place in a dynamic and continuous fashion, the practitioner must have a thorough knowledge of when and how the changes occur during normal maturation. Once a practitioner becomes comfortable with this knowlege, successful diagnosis and treatment of pediatric lower extremity gait abnormalities may be accomplished. As many have stated, the early years of development represent the golden years of treatment when the practitioner may favorably influence lower extremity development and gait. Therefore, the practitioner's ultimate goal should be to identify the conditions that may spontaneously improve and resolve over time vs. those problems that will require treatment. Although the practitioner will be called upon to treat a variety of traumatic or dermatologic problems in the pediatric patient, the vast majority of parental concerns regarding the developing child focus on angle of gait, flatfooted gait, and unstable and unsteady gait problems. When evaluating the pediatric patient, one should not consider undertaking any form of treatment until a complete and developmentally pertinent history has been obtained and an appropriate physical examination completed. The intent of this chapter is to provide a systematic and logical approach to examining the pediatric patient from a musculoskeletal and biomechanical standpoint.

Initial visit

Prior to the actual "laying on of hands," the practitioner should acquire certain historical information pertaining to the child's development. A patient information sheet may be mailed to the parents before the child's initial visit to facilitate the introduction of the patient into the practice. Any measures that will shorten the overall office time, along with creating a welcoming environment for the child, are helpful. The most reliable clinical information is generally obtained when the child is cooperative and alert. A tired, restless child who has spent a prolonged period of time in a crowded waiting room is not likely to be cooperative. Although valuable information may be obtained by having the parent fill out an information sheet in the office, more specific questioning should be conducted at the time of the office visit. This line of questioning is directed toward specific areas involving the likelihood of an abnormal musculoskeletal condition. The parents should be thoroughly questioned in the following areas prior to the actual physical examination:

- Perinatal history
- Neuromuscular development landmarks
- Family history
- Sleeping and sitting positions
- Growing pains
- Shoe Wear
- Level of activity
- Participation in sports

Perinatal history

The practitioner should ask whether the child was delivered following full-term pregnancy or if the child was born prematurely. In cases where the child was born prematurely, it is essential to determine to what extent the child was premature and if immediate medical problems were apparent. Often, children who are born markedly premature sustain increased risk of neurologic deficit which may ultimately affect their lower extremity function. Additionally, it is appropriate to determine whether the child was delivered in a standard procedure or by a cesarean section. If the infant was delivered by cesarean section, the reason for this delivery should be explored. If the child could not pass through the birth canal owing to its size or limitation of available space, then most likely there is no probable association with lower extremity abnormality. However, two other factors may have an adverse effect on lower extremity development. First, if the cesarean section was performed because there was some distress to the child during labor, there is a possibility of some neurologic process that might interfere with the development of normal gait. Second, if the infant was delivered via cesarean section due to a breech presentation, careful evaluation for the presence of a dislocated or dislocatable hip should be carried out, as an increased incidence of this condition occurs with breech presentation. Careful questioning often elicits a history of a cesarean section being performed primarily because the previous child or children may have been delivered in the same fashion. This generally does not include any increased likelihood for the presence of lower extremity abnormalities.[81,83,85]

Neuromuscular developmental landmarks

In order to assess whether a child is undergoing normal neuromuscular development, a line of questioning regarding specific developmental landmarks should be employed. Any significant deviation from the following should be considered suspicious for the possibility of a lower extremity musculoskeletal or neuromuscular disorder. Most prewalkers initiate crawling at approximately 5 to 6 months of age. At the same time, the child is capable of rolling from a supine to a prone position. Additionally, the parents should note if the child can support his or her body weight while standing with assistance. At 9 to 10 months children can pull themselves into an upright position, and by 12 months are generally capable of standing in an unassisted fashion. The child can walk with assistance at that age. By 15 months, the child should be walking easily with a classic broad-based, knee-flexed, and full-footed contact type of gait pattern. By 18 months, most toddlers are capable of running. By the time the child has reached 24 months, he or she can run without difficulty or unsteadiness, and is generally capable of walking up and downstairs without parental assistance.[24] By age 3 years, a child can balance briefly on one foot and can run and jump easily. At 4, the child generally can climb up or downstairs, one stair after the other, rather than placing both feet simultaneously on each step. This typically corresponds with the onset of a heel-to-toe type of propulsive gait pattern. At age 5, most children are capable of skipping and balancing on one foot. During subsequent examination of the child in the office, the child may be asked to perform tandem walking. An inability to perform this normally is suggestive of subtle cerebral pathologic changes. Additionally, the child may be asked to hop. If this is successfully accomplished, the practitioner may assume that the sensory, cerebellar and lower limb motor functions are essentially within normal limits.[24]

Although the normal range for the onset of ambulation ranges from 10 to 16 months, most children ambulate at approximately 1 year of age. A delayed onset of abulation to 14 to 18 months absent any previously diagnosed neuromuscular disease process should alert the practitioner to a musculoskeletal problem affecting the lower extremity. Most typically, a talipes calcaneovalgus deformity or an external femoral or tibial torsion or position problem will result in such a delayed onset of ambulation.[81]

Family history

A careful and complete history of any lower extremity abnormalities in the family should be obtained. The history should include the parents, aunts, uncles, and siblings. If a positive history is elicited, then the extent of the problem, the treatment employed, and the outcome of that treatment should be ascertained.[81] Additionally, it is appropriate to observe the parents' gait as well as their lower extremities to determine if any adult deformity exists. If an extensive family history for

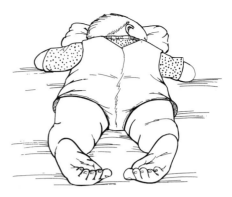

Fig. 11-1. Children who sleep on their stomach with their feet adducted will reinforce an internally deviated leg or foot. night splints are often effective in altering sleeping positions.*

specific lower extremity deformity exists—for example, a transverse plane deformity—then the child falls into the small percentage (approximately 10%) of children whose deformity will most likely persist regardless of the treatment employed.[81,85]

Sleeping and sitting positions

Parents should be questioned regarding their child's typical sleeping and sitting positions. Transverse plane deformities generally cause the child to assume positions of comfort, which generally reinforce the deformity. Children with internally deviated limbs will generally sleep on their stomachs with their legs internally rotated, and their feet adducted (Fig. 11-1). Conversely, children with a marked external limb deviation sleep on their stomachs with their legs externally rotated, and their feet abducted.

The older child typically assumes sitting positions that tend to reinforce his or her pathologic conditions. These generally result in positions where either the femoral, tibial, or pedal components are maintained in an internally rotated position (Figs. 11-2 and 11-3). The practitioner can make specific recommendations regarding night splint therapy to alter the sleeping position, as well as specific recommendations pertaining to more appropriate sitting positions (Fig. 11-4). Generally, the latter requires the child to sit cross-legged or straight-legged.

---

* The following figures are reproduced with permission from Valmassy RL, Smith L, Koch T: *Gait Analysis in children: Diagnostic and therapeutic implications.* Medcom Corp.: Figs. 11-6, 11-7, 11-8**A** and **B**, 11-11**A** and **B**, 11-13**B**, 11-14, 11-17, 11-19, 11-20, 11-21**A** and **B**, 11-24, 11-25, 11-26, 11-27**A** and **B**, 11-28, 11-31, and 11-32.

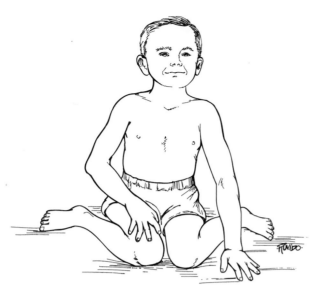

Fig. 11-2. Abnormal sitting positions such as this reinforce an internal femoral torsion or position.

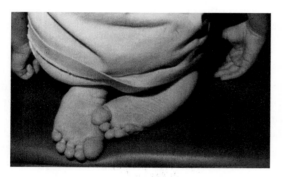

Fig. 11-3. A child with an internal tibial torsion or position or metatarsus adductus is most comfortable sitting or playing in this position.

Growing pains

Often practitioners tend to dismiss "growing pains" as a normal and transient finding that all children experience. Although this is certainly the case in most instances, the practitioner must be concerned when these complaints persist for a protracted period of time. Although growing pains lasting 3 to 4 months may be considered normal, discomfort persisting for a longer period is generally considered abnormal. A child who undergoes a rapid spurt in skeletal development may grow several inches over a relatively short period and typically experience posterior leg muscle cramping or knotting. This continues until soft tissue development and lengthening have compensated for the osseous growth increase.[78,85,87] On the other hand, the practitioner must be alert to a history of prolonged or excessive cramping. A child who chronically complains of muscle cramping and tightness, to the point where

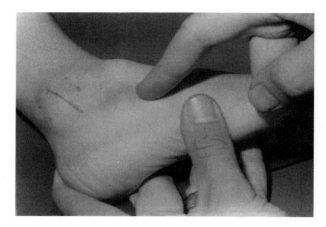

Fig. 11-4. A hyperkeratotic or hyperpigmented area overlying the lateral aspect of the talar head appears when children chronically sit on their feet. Careful monitoring of this dermatologic sign will indicate whether the parents have been successful in altering their child's sitting patterns.

minimal activity causes discomfort or night cramps, should not be dismissed as "normal."[28] Commonly, a congenital muscle tightness primarily involving the gastrocnemius or the gastrocnemius and soleus muscles is the precipitating factor.

Shoe wear

The practitioner should question the parents regarding shoe replacement. Are the child's shoes outgrown or are they excessively worn during the course of normal activities? One should note that up to the age of 7 or 8 years, the wear pattern on a child's shoes should be located on the central portion of the heel. This is due to the normal amount of calcaneal eversion that is present in the developing child's foot. After the age of 7 or 8 years, the presence of tibial varum along with a more normal calcaneal stance position will generally place the heel in an inverted position at heel contact, a condition which normally persists throughout adulthood.[81] If the child breaks down the counters of the shoes quickly or develops predominantly medial wear on the soles, this may indicate marked abnormal pronation (Fig. 11-5). Therefore, the extent and location of wear should be evaluated before conducting the lower extremity biomechanical evaluation.

Level of activity

After the child has been able to initiate ambulation on a regular basis, he or she should be able to run, play, and be normally active without hesitation. The practitioner should be alert to a history that the child is easily fatigued, or wants to be carried, or be transported in a stroller for extended periods of time. Although a normally developing child will periodically fall into this category, especially when participating in such activities as shopping, a chronic

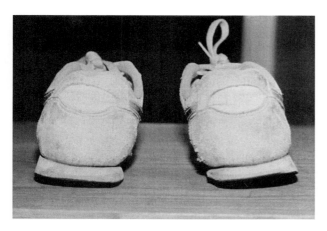

Fig. 11-5. Medial heel and sole wear associated with broken-down heel counters indicate marked abnormal foot pronation, typically observed in compensated transverse plane deformity or compensated gastrocnemius equinus.

history of this should be considered abnormal. Parents may note that this type of behavior exists even in cases where the child is particpating in enjoyable activities such as going to an amusement park, circus, etc. Although it is uncommon for a child under 5 or 6 to complain of chronic pain or discomfort such as that perceived by adults, they are able to perceive and complain of fatigue. This type of situation usually occurs in cases of abnormal flexible pes planus deformities occurring secondary to any of the more common causes. Furthermore, the parents may note a tendency for prolonged instability in gait coupled with tripping and falling. Although this occurs normally as the child develops a normal gait pattern, a continuation of this presentation is most often noted consistently with compensation for transverse plane deformities. Prolonged unsteadiness in gait accompanied by easy fatigability often indicates the presence of some degree of abnormal lower extremity musculoskeletal deformity.

Participation in sports

Most normally developing youngsters are active and participate in some type of game or sports activity without difficulty. However, children with lower extremity musculoskeletal problems may have difficulty in being as active as their peers. At times this leads to reluctance or inability to successfully participate in games or sports. Certainly, this history in the older child, coupled with positive findings from the previous history, indicates the presence of a longstanding functional or developmental problem.[84]

Clinical examination

Before performing the lower extremity musculoskeletal examination, observation of the child's gait

and posture are helpful in forming the initial diagnostic impression. The child is evaluated in diapers or shorts and allowed to walk independently without parental support. It may be helpful to have the child carry a small toy back and forth between parent and examiner in order to function in a more comfortable and normal fashion. At this time, the examiner should carefully note five specific areas of observation: These are (1) head tilt, (2) shoulder and pelvis level, (3) patellar position, (4) angle of gait, and (5) calcaneal position.[81,83]

Head tilt

Although an obvious head tilt is an unusual finding in the early walker, it is appropriate to observe the head position during gait. An obvious tilting of the head away from the midline of the body is consistent with scoliosis, limb length inequality, or dislocated hip.

Shoulder and pelvis level

If the child walks with an obvious shoulder drop, the examiner should concurrently note the level of the pelvis. Any deviation from the transverse plane at either level is consistent with scoliosis, limb length inequality, or dislocated hip. The presence of a lowered shoulder in a young child may be consistent with a shortened limb on that side. Generally, in a child under 12 to 13 years of age, the shoulder drop is to the short leg side, as there is typically no developmental scoliosis present until after that age.[77-79] Conversely, in older children and adolescents where longstanding compensation for a limb length discrepancy results in a functional scoliosis, the shoulder drop is to the long leg side.

Patellar position

During the examination of a child with an in-toed gait pattern, the examiner must determine the structural level responsible for the deformity. The examiner should note the position of the patella relative to the frontal plane. Normally, the patella functions in a slight external position up to the age of 5 or 6, and then essentially on the frontal plane thereafter (Fig. 11-6). Because of this, the patella becomes an important landmark to observe when evaluating the child with a transverse plane deformity. If the child ambulates with one or both patellae facing internally, leading to the classic "squinting patella" appearance, the examiner may correctly conclude that the adducted gait stems at least in part from the femoral component.[14,64,83] This indicates an internal femoral torsion or an internal femoral position (Fig. 11-7). However, if the patellar position is on the frontal plane or slightly externally rotated and the foot is adducted, then the probable cause lies outside of the femoral component. In this case, the examiner should suspect an in-toed gait second-

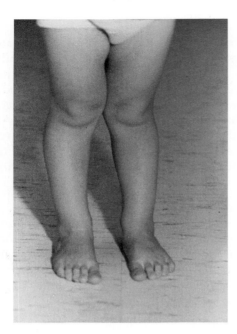

Fig. 11-6. Normal patellar position in a 3-year-old child.

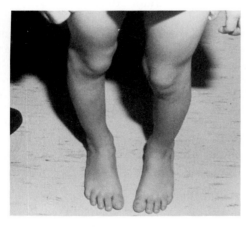

Fig. 11-7. "Squinting patella" sign with each patella internally rotated secondary to bilateral internal femoral torsion. Note the prominent talar head present bilaterally, indicative of marked subtalar joint compensation for an internally deviated limb.

ary to an internal tibial torsion, internal tibial position, metatarsus adductus, talar head adductus, rigid forefoot valgus, or a rigid plantarflexed first-ray deformity. Although it is difficult to determine the full extent of involvement at each level, the examiner will minimally develop suspicion for the level of deformity based on this assessment.

Angle of gait

The angle of each foot relative to the line of progression is termed the child's *angle of gait*. Typically, a marked internal or external torsional abnormality is reflected in an abnormal angle of

gait. During normal development, the child's angle of gait is in a more external position, especially during the first few years of ambulation. This generally corresponds with the presence of a high degree of external hip rotation, a condition which gradually decreases with normal development.

If a child's gait is adducted on the transverse plane owing to a torsional deformity, that angle is generally consistent. However, in some cases, the examiner will note that the angle of gait varies consistently from step to step. Since this type of gait pattern is typically associated with an internal tibial position, careful attention should be directed to the amount and direction of transverse plane knee rotation during the off-weightbearing examination. In other instances, the examiner will note that rather than exhibiting an "adducted gait," some children demonstrate an "adducting gait," which occurs at heel contact. This type of dynamic in-toeing is often associated with tight or contracted medial musculature. Therefore, special attention should be directed to the adductor muscle group and medial hamstring muscles during the off-weightbearing portion of the examination. It should be noted that this movement is quite distinct from the marked adduction noted in children with spastic adductors or hamstrings that are associated with various forms of neurologic deficits.[17,72,74]

Calcaneal position

The examiner should note that the developing child's foot is "fat, flat, and floppy" — an appropriate description of the normally appearing pes planus that most children develop upon weightbearing.[83] When a child initiates ambulation, no medial arch is apparent, a fact emphasized by the amount of fat present in the area. Additionally, the child's calcaneus may be normally everted from 5 to 10 degrees at the onset of ambulation.[56] During normal development, calcaneal eversion generally reduces by approximately 1 degree per year. Therefore, a heel everted 5 to 10 degrees (average, 7–8 degrees) may be acceptable at 1 year of age; this should reduce to a perpendicular attitude by 7 to 8 years of age (Fig. 11-8). A practical formula for evaluating the calcaneal stance position is to subtract the child's age from the number 7. This provides an approximation of the normal amount of pronation and calcaneal eversion that should be present at any specific age. For example, the formula for a 4-year-old child is:

$$7 - 4 = 3 \text{ degrees of calcaneal eversion}$$

Marked deviation from this value should lead to careful clinical evaluation of the possible causes of this condition. Additionally, a normal degree of cal-

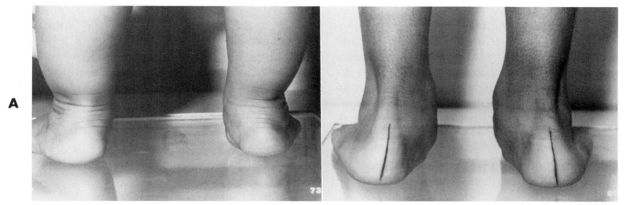

Fig. 11-8. A, Normal calcaneal stance position with an acceptable degree of heel eversion in a 24-month-old child. Note the significant medial fat pad in the arch increasing the overall flattened attitude of the foot. **B,** Abnormal calcaneal stance position in a 10-year-old child. At this age the calcaneus should appear vertical. Any significant calcaneal eversion that is noted beyond the age of 7 or 8 should be considered abnormal.

caneal eversion associated with a significant pronatory force (e.g., gastrocnemius equinus, transverse plane deformity) generally warrants treatment, as the deforming force will prevent the calcaneal eversion from improving over time.

Examination of the hip

Once the gait evaluation is completed, the examiner evaluates the lower extremity with the child initially supine. The prewalker may be examined in the parent's lap. The examination begins with the hip joints and progresses distally. The importance of repeated examinations of the hip in the infant, prewalker, and early walker cannot be overemphasized. As the status of the hip joint stability may change spontaneously, it is essential to evaluate that segment's position even when recent examination by other practitioners may have been normal. Clinical signs indicative of a possible dislocated hip include redundant skinfolds of the thigh associated with an apparently shortened limb and asymmetric gluteal folds (positive anchor sign). A Trendelenburg-type gait associated with mild shoulder and hip drop along with a unilateral externally positioned limb is often suggestive of a dislocated hip in the early walker.[23,70,71] A complete discussion pertaining to the evaluation, diagnosis, and treatment regimen for a dislocated or dislocatable hip is found in Chapter 10.

Femoral component

Transverse plane evaluation. Rotational abnormalities of the developing child's femoral segment are responsible for a great number of gait-related problems. A complete understanding of the development of this segment coupled with sound clinical evaluation techniques will allow the practitioner to implement an appropriate treatment regimen when indicated.

During normal development of the child in utero, internal rotation and flexion of the hip occurs during the closing months of pregnancy. This position has been attributed to a combination of factors including hereditary and intrinsic factors of muscle force and bone growth as well as uterine pressure. Of note is the fact that unilateral internal complaints involving the femoral segment occur in a ratio greater than 2:1 in favor of the left limb. This left-sided propensity is attributable to the fact that most babies are carried with their backs to the left side of the mother, thereby causing the child's left leg to abduct and overlie the right leg.[85]

Upon reviewing the literature dealing with rotational problems affecting the femoral component, one notes that the terms *antetorsion* and *anteversion*, as well as *retrotorsion* and *retroversion*, are often used interchangeably. In 1979 the Subcommittee on Torsional Deformity of the Pediatric Orthopedic Society attempted to standardize these definitions. As a result of this, the following definitions were adopted[73]:

Version. The angular difference between the transverse axis of each end of a long bone. This represents the normal angular difference.

Torsion. This is present when version is increased and occurs when the value for a given measurement falls outside the norm by 2 SD.

Femoral anteversion is the angle of femoral version made when the femoral head and neck axis is directed forward or anteriorly from the femoral shaft. Femoral retroversion is the angle of femoral version made when the femoral head and neck axis is directed in a slightly backward direction from the femoral shaft. Therefore, femoral torsion and antetorsion represent abnormal increases in the femoral version angle. Lateral femoral torsion and retrotorsion represent an abnormal decrease in anteversion or an abnormal increase in retroversion. Although most clinicians understand the concept on which this terminology is based, the interchangeable use of these terms in the literature has led to confusion. In an attempt to clarify and simplify the process of examination, the various causative factors involving rotation of the femoral component are divided into two groups: (1) torsional, or bony, changes and (2) positional, or soft tissue, changes. With this grouping, the examiner is able to more clearly understand and define the structures involved in the development of the abnormal gait pattern.

Although femoral torsion is considered the most common cause of the development of an in-toed gait in the early walker up to the age of 10 years, a host of conditions influence the overall function of the femoral component.[18,41,69,71] In 1968 Kleiger,[40] reporting that a variety of factors were most likely responsible for an adducted gait, developed the term *anteversion syndrome.* The factors in this syndrome that led to an adducted gait pattern included an anteriorly located acetabulum, a tight hip capsule, a tight iliotibial band, or short or tightened anterior hip muscles.

The following is an overview of the various components most likely to affect femoral torsion and positional changes in the developing child. Torsional development of the femur is most easily understood if one visualizes an isolated femur lying on a flat surface. Close inspection of the bone indicates that there is a 30-degree internal angulation of the femoral condyles relative to the head and neck of the femur. As normal development of this segment occurs, there is a gradual "unwinding" of this relationship so that by the age of 5 or 6 a 20-degree external twist has occurred, leading to the normally accepted 8- to 12-degree angle of femoral antetorsion. In other children, this torsional growth may occur very slowly and the angle may not completely reduce until the age of 13 or 14. In this instance, the change may occur at an almost imperceptible rate of 1 to 3 degrees per year. This slow change explains why some children who appear pigeon-toed for a long period of time ultimately appear "normal" when they become teenagers.[85] Additionally, it has been observed that children being treated for torsional problems of the femur often demonstrate angle-of-gait changes which seem to correspond to overall growth spurts and increases in height. This is a readily observable phenomenom which may be noted by the parents as well as the practitioner. It is

postulated that growth spurts not only affect the length of the long bones of the body but also are responsible for contributing in part to transverse plane alterations of those structures. In cases where the normal transverse plane change within the long axis of the femur does not occur, or occurs very slowly, an in-toed type of gait is noted.[7,14,41] The factors that influence this condition include heredity, abnormal sleeping and sitting positions, and ligamentous laxity. Sommerville[70,71] described how the normally taut ligaments of the hip capsule assist in molding away antetorsion. He reported that when the hip is maintained in its extended position, the anterior capsule tightens, leading to an external torsional strain on the femoral neck, an area which grows rapidly and is therefore considered extremely malleable. If these ligaments are generally lax, the forces necessary to assist in reduction of the femoral torsion will not be present. Clinically, it is important to note that there is typically a generalized joint laxity in most cases of persistent internal femoral torsion.[41,70,71] Statistically, it is important to note that approximately 90% of children having an internal femoral torsion will outgrow it by adolescence unless there is a significant familial tendency for transverse plane deformities of this type. In these instances, there is little likelihood of the torsional component improving spontaneously over time, either with or without treatment.[72,76,87]

In other instances, there may be excessive external torsional growth (retrotorsion) of the femoral segment which may ultimately result in an external femoral torsion. Since this represents an overgrowth or overdevelopment in the transverse plane of the femoral component, there is generally no treatment that can easily be provided to reverse the situation. The practitioner must be cautious in informing parents which problems are most likely to resolve with time, as an external femoral torsion may appear potentially worse at age 13 or 14, depending on subsequent rotational tendencies of the lower extremities.

The other component involving transverse plane development of the femoral segment is associated with the soft tissue or positional changes that occur over the first few years of life. This soft tissue change involves an internal positioning of the femoral component relative to its position within the acetabulum. As this gradual internal rotation of the entire femur occurs, the long axis of the shaft is externally rotating or unwinding. This positional adaptation is generally attributed to the child's abducted and externally rotated position in utero. At birth, the ratio of external to internal rotation is approximately 3:1, with the total range of motion approaching 100 degrees. As normal development occurs, the overall range of motion, as well as this external position, gradually decreases. Although a tendency toward an externally rotated position persists throughout the first few years of life, this should decrease by age 5 or 6, at which time each patella is typically functioning on the frontal plane throughout gait.[83,85,86,87]

A gradual reduction of the external femoral position is accompanied by a variety of changes affecting the soft tissue structures about the hip. These include the capsule, ligaments, and muscles. Contracture of the iliofemoral and pubofemoral ligaments causes an internal femoral position, while contracture of the ischiofemoral ligament produces an external femoral position. Contracture of the following muscles may be responsible for persistent internal femoral position: iliopsoas, tensor fascia lata, gluteus medius, and gluteus mini-

mis. A persistent external femoral position may result from contracture of the gluteus maximus, obturator externus, obturator internus, gemelli, quadratus femoris, piriformis, sartorius, adductor magnus, adductor longus, and adductor brevis.[85]

Acetabular position may also influence rotational leg position. Skeletal variations in acetabular position have been reported. The most common variation, and certainly a normal variant, is one in which the acetabulum is more externally rotated, which complements the overall externally rotated femoral position that is present in the infant. If, however, the acetabulum is significantly internally placed or located, it will contribute to an internally positioned limb, a factor that many authors consider to be significant, though commonly overlooked, in the overall development of the child's angle of gait.[34,72,87]

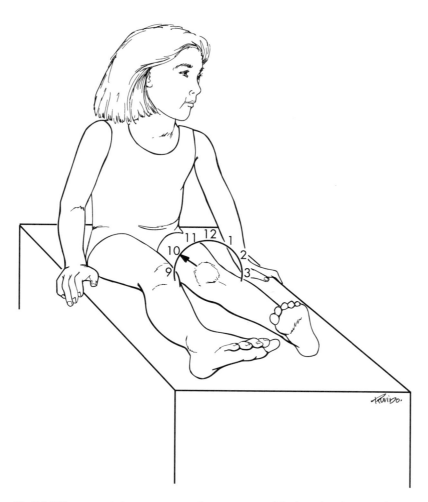

Fig. 11-9. When examining transverse plane rotation of the hip, the clinician should envision the face of a clock behind the child's knee. Patellar position relative to the hour on the clock will provide an approximation of internal or external leg rotation. In this illustration, the left limb internally rotates to 10 o'clock, which represents approximately 60 degrees of internal rotation.

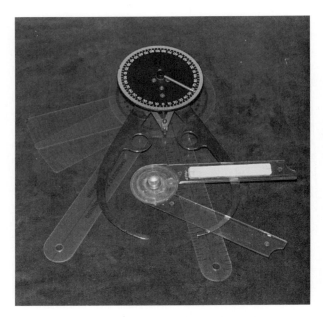

Fig. 11-10. Instruments that may be effectively used to measure lower extremity ranges of motion.

Clinical evaluation of the hip

There are numerous methods for determining the ranges of motion of the hip within the transverse plane. The child is examined prone or supine, sitting up, or lying down, with the knee either extended or flexed. One effective method for determining the transverse plane range of motion of the hip involves measuring the internal and external rotation available at the hip with the child in both a hip-flexed and hip-extended position. Although it may be necessary to perform the examination with the child on the parent's lap, it is generally more accurate to perform this with the child sitting and then lying supine on the examining table. Initially, the range and ratio of available motion is assessed by placing the hips through their range of motion. This may be performed without instruments to allow orientation to the overall limb rotation. A general impression of the available ranges of motion may be achieved by envisioning the face of a clock proximal to the child's patella with the hour hand perpendicular to the center of the patella. When the patella is parallel to the supporting surface, the hour hand is at the 12-o'clock position or zero degrees. Therefore, with internal or external leg rotation, each hour designates a 30-degree angular change. For example, if internal rotation of a child's left limb placed the patellar position at 10 o'clock, then 60 degrees of internal rotation is present (Fig. 11-9). Again, this is a cursory examination, and is carried out to obtain an initial impression before performing a more complete examination.

When obtaining more accurate measurements, the examiner may use whatever he or she is most comfortable with. A gravity goniometer, devil's level, or tractograph are all capable of providing an accurate measurement of femoral rotation (Fig. 11-10). Initially, the child is be placed in a hip-flexed position with internal and external hip rotation recorded for both limbs. (Fig. 11-11). When measuring internal hip rotation, care is taken not to elevate the buttock on measurement of the ipsilateral side, as this would erroneously increase the apparent amount of internal rotation (Fig. 11-12). Conversely, when measuring external rotation of the limb, care is taken that the contralateral buttock does not rise from the examining table, as this would increase the apparent amount of external rotation. Visualization of either buttock rising during the examination indicates that excessive force is being used. Next, internal and external rotation are assessed with the child in a hip-extended position. Following recording of the degrees of external and internal rotation, it must also be noted whether the ends of the ranges of motion were soft and spongy or abrupt and bony.[81,83,85,87] As a rule, if the ends of the range of motion are abrupt or bony, a torsional abnormality is suspected. In cases where the end of the range of motion is soft and spongy, a positional deformity is most likely present. It should be noted that children generally demonstrate greater external than internal rotation of the femoral segment up until the age of 6 or 7, with anywhere from two to three times as much external rotation normally being present.[64,77–79] The total range of motion available on the transverse plane may range from 100 to 120 degrees at birth. Over the following years, the general tendency is for internal and external rotations to become more symmetric, with the total range of motion generally decreasing to approximately 80 degrees. Any significant variation in these values may be accompanied by lower extremity gait disturbances.

Upon performing the range-of-motion examination of the hips, specific clinical oberservations are noted by the practitioner. These are extremely useful in establishing a diagnosis for marked internal or external femoral rotational problems. As previously mentioned, the quality of the end of the range of motion is recorded. For example, if one measures 80 degrees of internal hip rotation and 30 degrees of external hip rotation in both the hip-extended and hip-flexed positions and the end of the range of motion is abrupt or bony, then

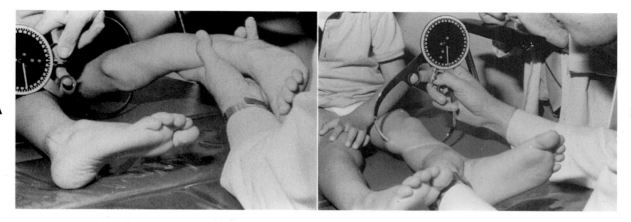

Fig. 11-11. Examination of internal **(A)** and external **(B)** hip range of motion with a goniometer. Note that there is 80 degrees of internal rotation and 25 degrees of external rotation present. These findings are consistent with either an internal femoral torsion or position.

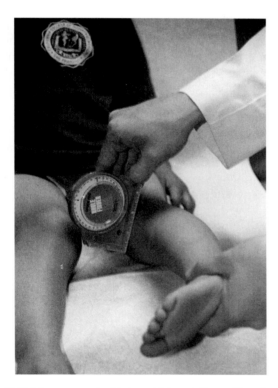

Fig. 11-12. Measurement of internal hip rotation with a devil's level. Care is taken not to elevate the buttock on the ipsilateral side during the examination, as this would increase the observable internal measurement.

that patient's clinical presentation is consistent with an internal femoral torsion. Conversely, 90 degrees of external rotation with 10 degrees of internal rotation in both the hip-extended and hip-flexed position with that same bony feel to the end of the range of motion is consistent with an external femoral torsion.[41,83]

In cases where there is a marked difference in the measured rotations and the examiner feels that the ends of the range of motion are generally "spongy" or "yielding," muscle or ligamentous involvement is suspected. A clincial example of this is the following. If clinical examination reveals 60 degrees of internal rotation and 30 degrees of external rotation with the hip extended, and a similar amount of internal rotation with 60 degrees of external rotation with the hips flexed, soft tissue involvement is likely. Specifically, the pubofemoral ligament, the iliofemoral ligament, or the ligamentum teres is suspected of limiting the external rotation. This is due to the fact that these structures, if contracted, limit external rotation with the hip extended. However, once the hip is flexed and the structures relax, increased available external rotation is noted.[83,85]

Conversely, if the same apparent change existed in external vs. internal rotation produced by examining the child first in the hip-flexed and then in the hip-extended position, the hamstrings should be suspected of being involved in restricting external rotation. In this instance, specific evaluation of the hamstrings is necessary to complete the examination. In order to appropriately assess the flexibility of the hamstrings, the child should lie supine on the examining table. Initially, the hip and knee are flexed with the child's knee then gradually moved into an extended position. Full extension of the legs should be noted in the developing child through adolescence. Any significant reduction in the degree of flexibility indicates primary or secondary contracture of the medial or lateral hamstrings or both. In this instance, the flexibility of the medial hamstrings is assessed by flexing the hip and internally

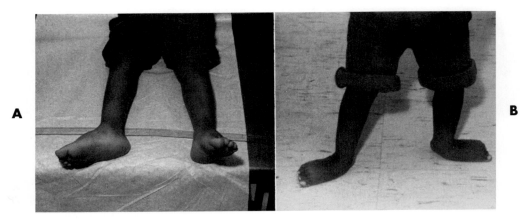

Fig. 11-13. A and **B,** Marked bilateral external femoral position with associated talipes calcaneovalgus led to a marked delay in the onset of ambulation in this 17-month-old boy.

rotating the leg. The knee is then extended to its end of range of motion. Conversely, the flexibility of the lateral hamstrings is assessed by flexing the hip, externally rotating the leg, and then extending the knee.

With respect to external femoral position problems (Fig. 11-13), one should note the following clinical possibilities. An external hip position is present if the internal rotation available increases with the hip moving from an extended to a flexed position, or vice versa. Specifically, if a limited amount of internal rotation is noted only with the hip flexed and knee extended, a tight or shortened lateral hamstring is present (see above). If limitation of internal rotation is only present with the hip extended, one must suspect a contracture of the iliopsoas.[79,87]

As a rule, a measured range of motion that remains essentially unchanged regardless of hip position, accompanied by a bony or abrupt feeling at the end of its range of motion, is typically a femoral torsion problem (internal or external). Conversely, a range of motion that is obviously altered in its external or internal measurement, depending on whether the hip is flexed or extended, accompanied by a spongy feel at the end of its range of motion, typically reflects a femoral position problem (internal or external).

Needless to say, the preceding may be compounded by the fact that there may be a combination of the above-stated deformities. Although a soft tissue problem typically presents and continues to function primarily as a soft tissue problem throughout development and treatment, the same might not hold true for a problem that was originally torsional. This is due to an internal or external femoral torsion leading to some degree of secondary internal or external femoral position as well. Similarly, primary

contracted ligaments lead to secondary tightness of the surrounding musculature. Because the soft tissue structures crossing the hip joint will most likely contract and adapt to an externally or internally deviated femoral segment, they often add to the overall deformity.

Additionally, ranges of motion may vary significantly from individual to individual, and even within the same individual over a period of years. Regardless of what the off-weightbearing measurements indicate, the most important factor is evaluation of the overall gait presentation along with any subsequent compensatory changes generated by the alternation of that gait. With regard to frontal plane changes associated with the femur, the development of coxa vara or coxa valga is the most clinically significant. Although most changes associated with frontal plane alterations of the head and neck of the femoral segment are rare, it is still appropriate to discuss them. The angle of femoral inclination is the angle formed in the frontal plane between the long axis of the head and neck of the femur and the long axis of the femoral shaft. In neonates the angle is 140 to 150 degrees, decreasing to 120 to 132 degrees (average, 128 degrees) by age 6 years.

Coxa vara

Coxa vara exists when the angle of femoral inclination has decreased to beyond 128 degrees. Typically this represents an overgrowth that may sometimes be seen in association with a slipped capital femoral epiphysis. Additionally, it may be caused by trauma or it may be developmental. Coxa vara is difficult to evaluate in radiographs of very young infants, and is usually first noticed when the child begins to walk. When this occurs, the leg appears shorter on the affected side, and adduction as well as internal rotation of the leg is restricted. Coxa vara may result in genu valgum.[64,87]

Coxa valga

When the angle of femoral inclination has not decreased to 128 degrees, then coxa valga exists. The etiology may be associated with a lack of development of the head and neck of the femur relative to the shaft of the femur resulting from dysplasia (generally bilateral) or trauma (generally unilateral). Typically, there is an awkward gait, and frequently a degree of hip dislocation is present in this rare, usually congenital condition. There may be a concomitant genu varum. In either case, a marked frontal plane deviation of the femoral segment should be further evaluated via standard anteroposterior (AP) hip radiographs in the older child.

Examination of the knee and tibia

Tibial torsion

Evaluation of the transverse plane rotation of the tibia relative to the fibula allows the examiner to evaluate the influence of this segment on the patient's angle of gait. The overall placement of the foot relative to the supporting surface may be affected by a series of rotational components involving the lower leg. In 1955 Rosen and Sandick[60] defined *tibial torsion* as the change that occurs in the axial rotation of the foot relative to the leg. They noted a series of levels of deformity:

1. Rotation of the knee (see Tibial Position below)

2. Twisting within the longitudinal axis of the leg itself. This includes rotation of the fibula relative to the tibia at its proximal aspect, its distal aspect, or both. Additionally, either bone is capable of twisting on its own.

3. Rotation at the ankle joint. Most researchers agree that there is little or no external rotation of the tibia relative to the fibula at birth. A study by Khermosh et al.[34] demonstrated an outward deflection of approximately 1.3 degrees per year, with the most rapid development occurring from 16 to 21 months. Staheli and Engel[74] noted that by adulthood tibial torsion was approximately 14 degrees, and believed the most rapid increase occurred during the first year of life. A study conducted by Valmassy and Stanton[88] in 1989 of 281 children between 1 1/2 and 6 years of age confirmed what a variety of other authors reported: that a gradual external positioning of the tibia relative to the fibula occurs. Their study indicated an external malleolar position of 5.5

degrees at 18 months of age, with an average of 11.2 degrees at 6 years of age.[88]

Postnatal development of the tibia relative to the fibula is external and generally results in an average angle of 18 to 23 degrees for true tibial torsion. True tibial torsion may be measured radiographically or through computed tomography (CT). As it is not possible to clinically measure true tibial torsion, the examiner must evaluate malleolar position, which is represented by a line bisecting both malleoli relative to the frontal plane position of the patella. Malleolar position or tibial-fibular rotation is a clinical representation of tibial torsion and changes gradually through the first several years of development, with approximately 13 to 18 degrees of measurable external malleolar position being noted by the age of 7 or 8. Although various authors have reported that tibial torsion may be completed by the age of 2 or 3, by age 7, or in adolescence, most studies indicate that, in fact, the vast majority of normal development occurs by age 7 or 8.[69] The practitioner should note that there is a difference between a low tibial or malleolar torsion and an internal tibial or malleolar torsion. An internal or negative tibial torsion (e.g., −10 degrees) in a 3-year-old child is considered significant, as it is unlikely that it will be outgrown. In this instance, the tibia has not even attained the position that should have been present at birth (0 degrees). However, a lesser deformity would be present in the 3-year-old with 2 to 3 degrees of external tibial torsion. Although this is less than the anticipated 7 to 8 degrees of external tibial torsion, it is not as significant as the child with a minus value and is more likely to be outgrown.

Clinical measurement of tibial torsion or malleolar position is accomplished with the child supine or seated with the knee extended. If the measurement is obtained with the knee flexed to 90 degrees, the tibia will internally rotate and the measurement of the degree of tibial torsion or malleolar position will be lower than that actually present. Additionally, if an element of internal tibial position (see Tibial Position below) is present, the measurement will be lower. Next, the femoral condyles are placed parallel to the supporting surface. Once in this position, the child's tibial torsion is assessed by placing the thumb and index finger anterior and posterior to each malleolus (Fig 11-14). This allows the examiner to note whether an internal or external tibial torsion is present. Next, each malleolus is bisected. Care is taken to mark the actual bisection of each malleolus rather than to use the more prominent crest. Finally, the foot is held at a 90-degree angle to the leg with the subtalar joint maintained in its neutral position. The transmal-

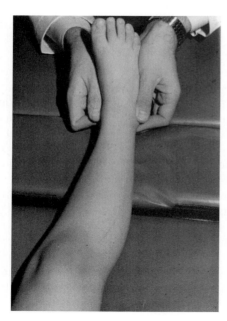

Fig. 11-14. The thumb and index finger are used to note the approximate level of the malleoli. This will demonstrate the presence of either an internal or external position of the medial malleolus relative to the lateral malleolus.

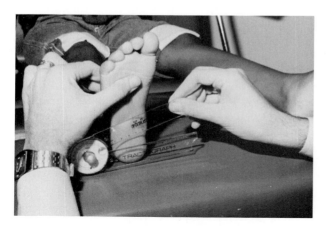

Fig. 11-15. Measurement of tibial torsion utilizing a tractograph. Note that the knee is placed on the frontal plane, and the subtalar joint is maintained in its neutral position.

leolar axis is then measured relative to the frontal plane with either a tractograph or goniometer[58] (Fig. 11-15).

It is important to remember that, in obtaining the measurement, a closed kinetic situation is brought about by the examining technique. Therefore, it is essential to maintain the foot in its neutral position while obtaining this measurement. Inadvertent pronation of the subtalar joint leads to internal rotation of the tibial segment, which results in the recording of a lower value for tibial torsion. Conversely, inadvertent supination of the subtalar joint leads to external rotation of the tibia, which may mask the presence of a low tibial torsion.

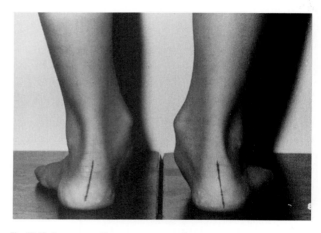

Fig. 11-16. Longstanding pronatory changes associated with an internal tibial torsion. Note the significant degree of subtalar joint and midtarsal joint compensation. Oblique axis midtarsal joint compensation has led to marked abduction of the forefoot relative to the rearfoot.

An abnormal tibial torsion is generally attributed to retention of an abnormal intrauterine position exacerbated by soft tissue accommodation as well as improper sleeping and sitting positions. Marked involvement of this segment leads to an adducted gait pattern with possible abnormal compensatory pronation (Fig. 11-16). The compensation is secondary to an internally positioned tibia, causing the talus to adduct and plantarflex, thereby leading to closed kinetic chain pronation of the foot. If marked compensation occurs, treatment aimed at improving foot function and increasing tibial torsion should be initiated (see Chapter 20). Operative correction may be indicated when the deformity is greater than 4 SD, there is persistence of the torsion into middle and late childhood, and a significant cosmetic disability is present.[7] It should be noted, however, that in a study by Weiner and Weiner in 1979,[90] no cases of abnormal tibial torsion requiring surgical derotation had been reported to that time.

Tibial position
Careful evaluation of the transverse plane rotation of the early walker's knee is necessary, particularly when diagnosing the cause of an adducted gait pattern. The examiner must be aware that the overall range of motion of this joint is capable of changing significantly over the first 3 to 4 years of life. As in other joints of both the upper and lower extremities, the available range of motion in the knee is increased at birth and throughout infancy, with a marked decrease in motion noted over the first few years. The total transverse plane range of motion may range from 0 to 20 degrees with the knee extended, with up to 35 to 45 degrees available with the knee flexed.[64,78]

When the knee joint and its surrounding ligamentous and muscular attachments develop normally, so does the gait pattern. However, when there is a tightening or contracture of the medial structures due to retention of an abnormal intrauterine position, accompanied by a resultant weakness of the lateral musculature, the normal transverse plane development of the knee will be affected. In this instance, a developmental and functional asymmetry of internal vs. external knee rotation occurs. The position of the tibia relative to the femur will develop and function in an internally rotated attitude. Just as one can differentiate between an internal femoral torsion and an internal femoral position, it is possible to diagnose internal tibial position vs. internal tibial torsion.[85,87]

Originally referred to by Sgarlato[64] as a pseudo-lack of malleolar torsion or pseudo-malleolar torsion, and classically described as an increase in the overall range of knee rotation, the deformity should be evaluated and considered from a different clinical perspective. All clinicians agree that if an early walker were to ambulate in an adducted fashion with the patella lying on the frontal plane, the deformity would always lie distal to the femoral segment. If a child demonstrates a normal tibial torsion and is absent any pathologic changes in the foot (e.g., metatarsus adductus, talar head adductus, rigid forefoot valgus, or rigid plantarflexed first ray),[5] the problem is most likely within the knee joint itself. This internal tibial position was originally described as the aforementioned pseudo-lack of malleolar torsion. The original term, although often confusing to practitioners, actually was an accurate representation of what was occurring, that is, an adducted foot in a child whose knee functioned within the frontal plane, giving the *pseudo* appearance of a low or internal tibial torsion.

On clinical examination of a child with this presenting problem, the examiner would note that besides the presence of an adducted gait pattern, the affected foot appears to strike the ground in different positions with each step. This is due to the presence of contracted soft tissue structures affecting the medial aspect of the knee. Additionally, there is a greater tendency toward tripping and instability in gait due to this gait disturbance.

When performing the nonweightbearing examination of this specific segment, it is not necessary for the examiner to use any specific measuring instrument. Clinical interpretation of the amount or extent of the available rotation is adequate, particularly when considered in light of the presenting complaint and initial gait evaluation.

In a normally developing infant or child below the age of 3 or 4 years, one would expect that little transverse plane rotation of the knee is present in the extended or locked position. However, with knee

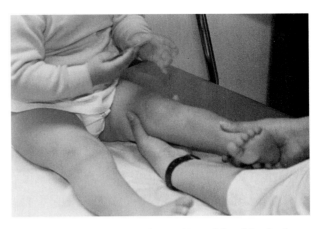

Fig. 11-17. When determining the position of the tibia, the femur is stabilized with one hand while the tibia is placed through its range of internal and external motion with the other. Assessment of available motions are noted relative to the tibia's original resting position.

flexion, a marked increase in the overall range of motion is appreciated. Examination of the knee in this position normally yields approximately equal amounts of internal and external rotation of the tibia relative to the distal aspect of the femur. However, if greater external than internal rotation is available from the initial "resting position" of the tibia, an internal tibial position is present (Fig. 11-17). This is the result of tight medial structures placing the resting or functional position of the tibia in an internal attitude. Subsequent attempts at eliciting internal rotation of the tibia relative to the femur does not yield appreciable movement, as the tibia is already held in its maximally internally rotated attitude. The overall range of motion of the knee is generally unaffected, with the actual deformity representing an excessive degree of internal rotation of the tibia. Therefore, the abnormality, as it should be understood, indicates excessive internal rotation of the tibia relative to the femur, leading to an adducted gait pattern.

Following initial assessment of the amount of available transverse plane motion of the knee, the child's knee is evaluated in both the hip-flexed and hip-extended position. If the available rotation of the tibia relative to the femur changes with hip extension and flexion, the musculature crossing the knee is most likely the primary deforming force. Although this generally indicates a contracture of the medial hamstrings, contracture of the gastrocnemius, popliteus and plantaris may also exist.[64,87] However, if the tibial rotation were to remain essentially unchanged with both hip extension and flexion, the primary etiologic factor would most likely be ligamentous. Some associated secondary muscle contracture would also be expected in those instances, much in the same manner as when there is some muscle contracture at the hip in the case of an internally rotated femoral segment. It should be noted that an internal tibial position is often associated with other internal transverse plane deformities, such as an internal femoral torsion, internal femoral position, low tibial torsion, or metatarsus adductus.

Although an external tibial position is uncommon, its presence must be considered when evaluating children that function in an abnormally abducted position. In these cases, the available tibial rotation occurs primarily in the internal direction, with little or no external rotation available. This deformity may be found in association with other transverse plane deformities such as an external femoral torsion, external femoral position, external tibial torsion, or talipes calcaneolvalgus.

A greater appreciation of this pathologic condition may be obtained if one understands the biomechanical changes associated with the development of the knee. This will further clarify why this deformity is only present in the early walker and is often a self-limiting process. The beginning walker's gait pattern is one of knee flexion with whole-foot contact at "heel strike." Knee extension occurs much later than at heel contact and only for a brief period of time.[64,85,87] Thus, when the knee remains flexed for a prolonged period of time in the early walker, especially at heel contact, one can appreciate the effect of tight medial structures. Specifically, the foot adducts with each subsequent step. As the child matures and develops, a more normal type of gait pattern develops by the age of 3 or 4 years. This includes development of a distinct heel contact with full knee extension as the foot approaches the supporting surface. This, combined with the overall reduction of normal transverse plane knee rotation to 0 to 5 degrees, causes this deformity to ultimately become self-limiting. Treatment is based on the child's age and his or her ability to ambulate efficiently. In milder cases, an improved gait pattern is achieved with the use of in-shoe, triplane, or varus wedging. This stabilizes the child's gait and places a mild external force on the tibia.[54,87] In more severe instances, where the child's gait is markedly adducted and unstable, more aggressive treatment may be appropriate. In these cases, serial plaster immobilization or night splints and braces may allow the child to ambulate and develop more normally (see Chapters 19 and 20).

Genu recurvatum

With the child standing, examination for an excessive degree of genu recurvatum is carried out. The normal degree of posterior deflection of the femur relative to the tibia is 5 to 10 degrees until the age of 5 years. Any deflection greater than that in children less than 5, or the presence of that amount of deflection in a child above 5, may indicate a lower extremity abnormality. It should be noted that the most common cause of this condition is a congenital gastrocnemius equinus. In instances where inadequate subtalar joint and midtarsal joint pronation do not allow normal compensation for the equinus deformity, a genu recurvatum may develop. The recurvatum position allows the foot to assume a plantarflexed attitude relative to the lower limb, thereby decreasing the effect of the contracted posterior musculature. If this type of compensation continues for some time, the abnormal deflection of the posterior surface of the knee becomes progressively worse and most likely symptomatic.[64]

Additionally, careful and repetitive monitoring of this angular deflection is essential when prescribing functional foot orthoses for the treatment of a marked pes planus associated with a clinically contracted posterior muscle group. If the orthosis can reduce subtalar and midtarsal joint pronation, the tightened posterior musculature will be placed under an even greater dynamic tension. If the tightness is due to an accommodative contracture, the Achilles tendon will stretch, and a measurable increase in ankle joint motion may be achieved. No alternation in the original angle of genu recurvatum should be noted during this change. However, if the angle of genu recurvatum increases with the use of functional foot orthoses, congenital equinus should be suspected (see Examination of the Foot and Ankle Joint, below).

Genu varum and genu valgum

Parents often express concern over their child's bowlegged or knock-kneed appearance. The practitioner should understand when and to what degree normal frontal plan changes of the knee may occur so that decisions regarding further diagnostic tests may be made. The physiologically normal genu varum that is present in infants and children is the result of a combination of the inherent lateral bowing of the femur and tibia combined with a normally occurring coxa valga. This relationship may be noted at birth and is present through the first 4 years of development. The degree of normal bowing that is present at this age is often exacerbated by an internal femoral or tibial torsion or position which leads to an extremely deviated position of the posterior musculature of the calf. This increases the overall varus attitude of the child's lower limb. Other disease processes such as rickets, Blount's disease, and asymmetric epiphyseal development may exacerbate the normal frontal plane bowing of the knee and must be considered when a greater-than-normal amount of bowing is present or persists beyond the age of 4.

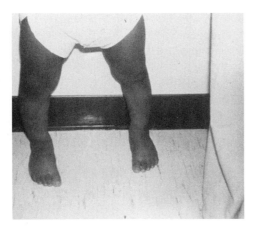

Fig. 11-18. Marked genu varum may be associated with rickets or Blount's disease. Radiographic evaluation of the child's knees is necessary to rule out an abnormality.

Although rickets is not a common finding, it must be considered when establishing a differential diagnosis for a marked degree of genu varum (Fig. 11-18). The cause may be vitamin D deficiency. This is typically due to chronic renal insufficiency, malabsorption problems, hypophosphatasia, or malnutrition.[87] The child with rickets is typically weak, lethargic, and may demonstrate other musculoskeletal abnormalities. If rickets is suspected, radiographic diagnosis will confirm its presence as the resultant changes in phosphorus and calcium metabolism diminishes calcification of the soft tissue matrix. As this is radiographically most evident at the ends of long bones, a thickened and hazy physis, along with a widened epiphysis with irregular femoral and tibial metaphyseal borders, is noted. This results in the characteristic trumpet-shaped flaring of the knee joint, a radiographic site consistent with this disease process.[76,77,79]

Blount's disease, which is due to a growth disturbance of the medial aspect of the proximal tibial epiphysis, results in progressive medial angulation of the tibia at the proximal medial epiphysis and metaphysis of the tibia. This is typically associated with failure of epiphyseal growth combined with changes in the stress forces affecting the area. Two forms of Blount's disease may occur, one in infancy, and the other in adolescence. The infant form may be present in the 1- to 3-year-old and is typically associated with the chubby child who also initiated ambulation at an early age, for example, at 9 months. It is suggested that the combination of excessive weight along with early ambulation leads to increased pressure at the proximal medial physis. The adolescent type generally occurs following trauma and is associated with an arrest of the physes. Radiographs confirm the presence of Blount's disease, demonstrating acute medial angu-

lation of the proximal tibia with associated beaking, as well as widening of the medial physis and metaphysis in the infant type.[47,79,87]

Physiologic genu valgum occurs normally to some extent in most children between the ages of 3 and 5, and is generally outgrown by the age of 8 years. This condition is generally associated with a normally occuring coxa vara and is noted following the previously discussed genu varum. As the child develops, the normal-appearing genu valgum is due to an obliquity of the femur when the medial femoral condyle is lower than the lateral condyle. Additionally, normal development and weightbearing lead to overgrowth of the medial femoral condyle, contributing to this position. According to Tax,[79] this, combined with varying rates of development of the medial and lateral aspects of the tibial epiphyses, leads to a valgus position and may be associated with curvature of the femoral or tibial shaft as well. Additionally, other factors such as the child's weight, trauma, or infection may precipitate varying degrees of genu valgum.

As the child develops, the lateral femoral condyle bears more weight than the medial femoral condyle, which increases the pressure on the lateral physes of the knee joint. As a result, gradual reduction of normal genu valgum occurs. Some authors note that a second physiologically normal episode of genu valgum may occur in the 12- to 14-year-old, depending on the presence of concomitant rotational deformities influencing the femoral segment. In cases where severe musculoskeletal deformities exist, for example, abnormal coxa vara or marked internal femoral torsion or position, epiphyseodesis or osteotomy may be considered.[83,87]

The degree of genu varum or genu valgum present may be measured either clinically or radiographically with the child either supine or standing. During normal development, angular measurements of between 15 and 30 degrees are obtained. Any measurement above 30 degrees or persistence of the angular deviation beyond the years of normal occurrence warrants additional evaluation. Additionally, indirect measurements may be obtained by measuring the separation of the knees in genu varum or the separation of the malleoli in genu valgum. In the classic study of genu valgum in 1000 children by Morley in 1957,[49] the following grading system was established:

Grade I: Intermalleolar distance less than 2.5 cm
Grade II: Intermalleolar distance, 2.5 to 5.0 cm
Grade III: Intermalleolar distance, 5.0 to 7.5 cm
Grade IV: Intermalleolar distance greater than 7.5 cm

It should be noted that increased angles of genu valgum shift overall body weight to the medial aspect of the developing foot, thereby increasing the tendency for abnormal foot pronation. Persistent abnormal genu valgum leads to some contracture of the lateral hamstrings, increased rotation of the tibia, and continued pronation. It should be noted that if marked abnormal pronation exists as the primary abnormality, an associated abnormal genu valgum may also be present.[64,87]

Tibial varum

Tibial varum is often associated with genu varum and contributes to the overall normal physiologic bowing that is clinically evidenced in the 2- to 4-year-old. Normal ranges for frontal plane bowing of the tibia are 5 to 10 degrees at birth, with a gradual reduction to 2 to 3 degrees by the age of 2 to 4 years. The latter is the normal adult value for tibial varum. Tibial bowing greater than 5 degrees requires some degree of subtalar joint compensation in order to allow the calcaneus to maintain a normal vertical position relative to the supporting surface. If the degree of tibial varum exceeds available subtalar joint eversion with pronation, the calcaneus will function in a varus attitude throughout the gait cycle. For example, a patient may exhibit 20 degrees of inversion with supination, 5 degrees of eversion with pronation, and 10 degrees of tibial varum. In this instance, the patient's foot functions in a 5 degree inverted position, which represents its maximally pronated attitude. This foot type is classified as a partially compensated rearfoot varus and is likely to lead to chronic ankle instability or to the development of a retrocalcaneal exostosis or "pump bump."[85,87]

Tibial valgum

A marked tibial valgum is rare. The clincial presentation is usually seen following physeal injury or malunion of a tibial fracture. It is not the result of overreduction of the normally occurring tibial varum. In evaluating the various causes of flexible flatfoot, the practitioner must obtain an AP radiograph of the ankle to rule out an abnormal force generated by a valgus ankle joint with or without tibial valgum.[47,85]

Examination of the foot and ankle joint

Ankle range of motion

Careful assessment of ankle joint motion is essential in order to detect any significant deforming force on the developing child's lower extremities. At birth, one should note unrestricted ankle joint dorsiflexion so that the dorsum of the foot may be dorsiflexed against the anterior aspect of the tibia at an angle of approximatley 75 degrees. As the child develops, this amount of dorsiflexion rapidly decreases to approximately 20 to 25 degrees by the age

of 3, to 15 degrees by the age of 10, and to 10 degrees by the age of 15. Although this last value was considered the adult norm for a number of years, clinical experience indicates that dorsiflexion in the range of 5 to 10 degrees with the knee extended may be considered normal.[64,81,87] If a congenital tightness is present, there is a consistent lack of dorsiflexion present from birth, with virtually no or minimal measurable dorsiflexion. Additionally, throughout normal development, one should always note ankle joint dorsiflexion greater than 15 degrees with the knee in its flexed position.

An *equinus* condition may be defined as a limitation of normal ankle joint dorsiflexion with the subtalar joint maintained in its neutral position. An equinus can be present while the knee joint is extended, flexed, or in some cases in both positions, depending on the etiologic factors involved. One should note that the gastrocnemius muscle originates above the knee joint, while the origin of the soleus is below the knee. In order to clinically differentiate between the tightness of the two muscles, the ankle joint range of motion is measured with the knee in both its extended and flexed position. There are four types of congenital equinus conditions that may be present in the developing child's lower extremities[46,58,78,79]:

1. **Congenital gastrocnemius equinus.** The most common type of congenital equinus involves primary involvement of the gastrocnemius muscle and tendon. In this case, a limitation of ankle joint dorsiflexion is noted with the subtalar joint in its neutral position and the knee fully extended. Flexion of the knee demonstrates normal range of motion.

2. **Congenital soleus equinus.** In this instance, a limitation of dorsiflexion is present with the knee in its flexed position. Generally, similar limitation is noted with the knee extended, even in cases of a normal gastrocnemius muscle and tendon. This type of deformity is rare.

3. **Congenital gastrocnemius-soleus equinus.** When both muscle tendon units are congenitally tight, one notes a limitation of ankle joint dorsiflexion with the knee in both its extended and flexed positions. Although there is generally some increase in the available dorsiflexion noted with the knee flexed, it is generally less than 10 degrees. In the older child or adolescent, this may be attributable to an osseous or bony block of the talotibial articulation. In this instance, the range of motion is also decreased with the knee in both its extended and flexed positions. However,

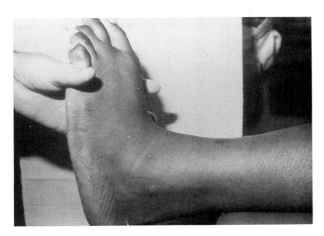

Fig. 11-19. Marked limitation of ankle joint range of motion with the knee extended and the subtalar joint maintained in its neutral position.

while the soft tissue equinus feels "spongy" at the end of its range of motion, the bony equinus is more abrupt. Radiographic changes consistent with the osseous deformity are demonstrated when comparing weightbearing lateral films with weightbearing stress lateral films. The two films are superimposed, and a bisection of each tibia is drawn on the films. If the deflection of the tibia on the stress film relative to the standard lateral film is greater than 15 degrees, a soft tissue contracture is suspected. If it is less than 15 degrees, a bony equinus is present. Additonally, inspection of the films often demonstrates the appearance of an obvious osseous block.

4. **Spastic equinus.** This type of ankle joint limitation is commonly associated with spastic diplegia (cerebral palsy), diastematomyelia, or hyperkinesia. A marked limitation of ankle joint motion is noted in both the knee-extended and knee-flexed attitudes. This may be accompanied by increased Achilles reflexes and an unsustained, reproducible ankle clonus. In addition, posterior muscle group contraction may also occur with a variety of other conditions such as Duchenne's muscular dystrophy. In this instance, the posterior musculature appears enlarged (pseudohypertrophy) and eventually develops myostatic contractures. Deep tendon relfexes are diminished.[24,32,87]

When obtaining this measurement, certain guidelines should be followed to ensure accurate and reproducible results. It is generally best to perform the maneuver with the patient supine. The hip may be either flexed or extended. The foot is then maximally dorsiflexed to the leg with the subtalar joint maintained in its neutral position (Fig. 11-19). This is essential because the pronated subtalar joint allows the midtarsal joint to unlock, thereby introducing excessive dorsiflexion of the forefoot relative to the rearfoot. Because of this, it is best to maintain the rearfoot slightly supinated, as this will decrease the likelihood of any pronation occurring. Although one should be concerned that pronation of the rearfoot will create an apparent normal degree of dorsiflexion via midtarsal joint dorsiflexion, mild supination of the rearfoot does not decrease the actual amount of available dorsiflexion. Occasionally, some children plantarflex their foot as the practitioner attempts to passively dorsiflex it. In these cases, one may stroke the plantar aspect of the foot and then maximally dorsiflex the child's foot as it is being withdrawn. If this is unsuccessful, the practitioner may initially flex the knee, dorsiflex the foot with the gastrocnemius now in its relaxed position, and then slowly extend the knee. When obtaining the actual measurement, care must be taken in placement of the tractograph so that one arm extends along the lateral aspect of the foot and the other accurately bisects the lower one third of the leg. If this measurement is within normal limits for the child's age, it is not necessary to retake the measurement with the knee flexed. As previously noted, however, if there is a marked lack of dorsiflexion, one should determine to what extent, if any, the soleus is implicated. When ankle joint dorsiflexion is limited with the knee extended but greater than 15 degrees with the knee flexed, the child most likely has a gastrocnemius equinus. If the limitation is present in both the knee-flexed and the knee-extended positions, a gastrocnemius soleus equinus is most likely responsible.

Alteration in gait associated with true congenital gastrocnemius equinus is classified as either compensated, partially compensated, or uncompensated. The classic compensated form is characterized by a maximally pronated gait with marked calcaneal eversion. This may occur from the onset of ambulation and persist through adulthood if untreated. In order for the condition to occur, a full, unrestricted range of subtalar joint pronation without significant rearfoot varus must be present. If compensation is to occur, then eversion of the calcaneus beyond a vertical position is necessary to allow the oblique axis of the midtarsal joint to unlock. When this occurs, independent dorsiflexion of the forefoot relative to the rearfoot takes place, thereby allowing dorsiflexion of the foot relative to the leg. This dorsiflexory motion may result in a rocker-bottom type of flatfoot deformity. This can lead to a host of musculoskeletal and postural

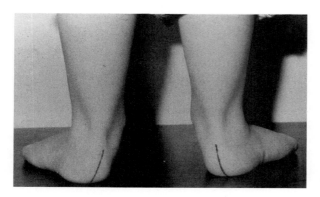

Fig. 11-20. Compensated congenital gastrocnemius equinus. Note the marked calcaneal eversion and forefoot abduction secondary to subtalar and midtarsal joint pronation.

disorders affecting the lower extremities, (Fig. 11-20), including hallux abducto valgus, tailor's bunion, hammer toes, heel spurs, and plantar fasciitis. Postural complaints such as muscle cramping and fatigue, as well as knee, hip, and lower back pain, may be noted.[15,21,57,64]

In cases where there is a low degree of available subtalar joint pronation associated with a high degree of rearfoot varus, the foot is unable to fully compensate as previously described. If, for example, the developing child or adolescent has a subtalar joint with 35 degrees of inversion with supination and 7 degrees of eversion with pronation along with 9 degrees of tibial varum, the maximally pronated position of this foot will be 2 degrees inverted. This represents a stable rearfoot with a relatively stable midtarsal joint. Since the midtarsal joint is unable to unlock fully and allow midfoot compensation, alternative forms of compensation must be adopted. The resultant gait patterns are considered as representative of a partially compensated type of congenital gastrocnemius equinus. These include an abducted gait, an early heel-off, a flexed-knee position during gait, and the development of genu recurvatum. All will allow the lower extremity to function without the requisite 5 to 10 degrees of ankle joint dorsiflexion. An uncompensated gastrocnemius equinus may occur with extreme muscle shortage or tightness and is characterized by no heel contact whatsoever. This is relatively rare and must be distinguished from idiopathic toe-walking, which is typically benign.[87]

If the child is being examined because he or she is a toe-walker, extreme care must be exercised in measuring dorsiflexion. Although most children with a tendency towards toe-walking have no specific lower extremity abnormality, the practitioner must rule out musculoskeletal as well as possible neurologic conditions. A tiptoe type of gait

is often demonstrated at the onset of ambulation in normal children and may be present intermittently up to the age of 6 or 7 years.[87] Idiopathic toe-walking is generally demonstrated two to three times more frequently in boys than in girls and is generally associated with lack of ankle joint dorsiflexion.[24,87] These children are more comfortable walking on their toes and continue to do so unless instructed to do otherwise. In these instances, they are capable of placing weight on the heels and walking with a heel-to-toe type of gait (which is not the case in spastic disorders or in uncompensated gastrocnemius equinus). The differential diagnosis of idiopathic toe-walking includes cerebral palsy, Duchenne's muscular dystrophy, spinal cord tumor, peroneal muscle atrophy, limb length discrepancy, and congenital dislocation of the hip.[87] Interestingly, a positive family history of toe-walking and learning disabilities has been reported.[32,87,93] Although the cause of toe-walking is unknown, it may be associated with a subclinical central nervous system abnormality, with a mild contracture due to abnormal intrauterine position, or habit, complicated by secondary adaptation and contracture.[87]

Treatment. Early identification of a suspected congenital equinus allows the practitioner to initiate therapy via night splinting or serial plaster immobilization. Initially, a below-knee splint may be worn at night with the foot maintained at an angle of 90 degrees to the leg. This could be a posterior splint or a Wheaton brace* (see Chapter 20). If no progress is noted after 8 to 12 weeks, an above-knee cast may be worn, with the cast changed every week in the child under 1 year of age. The cast may be changed every 10 to 14 days in the older child. In the older child, a below-knee cast may be worn because the child will extend the knee during gait. Gradual dorsiflexion of the foot may be carried out as tolerated, with the entire casting series typically lasting 6 to 8 weeks. Extreme caution must be exercised in maintaining the subtalar joint in its neutral or supinated position to ensure that midtarsal joint compensation does not occur during dorsiflexion of the foot. This may result in the development of a rocker-bottom flatfoot after the casts have been applied. Although this technique is not always effective in resolving cases of congenital gastrocnemius equinus, it is generally successful in treating the contracture state associated with idiopathic toe-walking. In cases where an equinus condition persists or is first diagnosed in the older child, initial treatment consists of aggressive stretching and the use of functional foot orthoses. Stretching is carried out vigorously with

---

* Wheaton Brace Co., Carol Stream, IL.

parental supervision. It is advisable to have at least one session with a physical therapist to ensure that this is being carried out appropriately. In some instances, long-term, regularly scheduled visits with a physical therapist are beneficial. Generally, the exercises are carried out as follows: The feet are maintained straightforward or slightly adducted to lessen the likelihood of subtalar joint pronation. The knees are extended, the back is straight, and child is instructed to lean forward into the wall until a comfortable tension is felt in the gastrocnemius muscle belly. This position is maintained for approximately 30 seconds and repeated ten times. Morning and evening sessions are recommended. In addition, functional foot orthoses are worn in cases where abnormal subtalar joint pronation is present.[87]

When using functional foot orthoses in children who demonstrate both a flexible flatfoot deformity and an apparent lack of dorsiflexion, two separate conditions may exist:

1. The child may have had a developmental flexible flatfoot that resulted in excessive subtalar joint and midtarsal joint pronation. In children with marked dorsiflexion and abduction of the forefoot, a gradual reduction in ankle joint motion and a concomitant posterior muscle group contracture may occur. This is due to shortening of the muscle as the foot assumes a more everted position. Additional shortening occurs because the requisite amount of foot-to-leg dorsiflexion is now at the expense of midtarsal joint mobility and flexibility. In these cases, the implementation of aggressive stretching exercises and functional foot orthoses improve foot position and function. Specifically, the functional foot orthosis locks the midtarsal joint, thereby eliminating the ability of the forefoot to independently dorsiflex on the rearfoot. Thus, the functional foot orthosis dynamically stretches the posterior musculature with each foot strike. In this instance, the device is a dynamic method of stretching the involved musculature. Generally speaking, contracted muscles may be stretched from 5 to 10 degrees over a 6-month period with the combined treatment.[46,57,64]

2. In other instances, the child being evaluated may have had a primary posterior muscle group tightness which resulted in compensation by means of a flexible flatfoot deformity, as previously described. In this case, the child's ability to compensate for the equinus is restricted by the effect of the functional foot orthosis. Typically, this results in the following: (a) an inability to tolerate the device, (b) repeated breakage of the device due to the marked pronatory force, (c) the development of a marked early heel-off, or (d) the development of genu recurvatum. The development of genu recurvatum is the most significant sequela. If a child with a congenital gastrocnemius equinus is able to tolerate the device, the lower extremity must develop some level of compensation for the unyielding posterior muscle group contracture. A posterior deflection of the femur relative to the tibia may occur in order to maintain the heel in contact with the ground. As this process often develops over several months, it may go unnoticed until significant compensation has occurred in the posterior compartment of the knee. Therefore, it is essential that when utilizing a functional foot orthosis to treat a flexible pes planus associated with a possible gastrocnemius equinus, that the angle of genu recurvatum be evaluated and documented at the time of the initial lower extremity biomechanical examination. The angle must then be remeasured and carefully monitored throughout the treatment by means of functional foot orthoses. If at any time the practitioner notes an increase in this angle, then the clinical assumption may be made that a true congenital equinus exists and surgical intervention should be carried out.

When surgical correction is carried out, the child will be immobilized in a below-knee cast for approximately 3 to 4 weeks. Appropriate physical therapy to restrengthen the posterior musculature is carried out vigorously to ensure maximum muscle strength as early as possible. In the older child and adolescent, a marked hip drop or Trendelenburg-type gait follows the surgical procedure. In cases of a bilateral lengthening, a bilateral hip drop is noted, while unilateral lengthening results in a hip drop on the opposite side. This hip drop is due to instability of the lower extremity to properly load the lateral column of the foot to assist in propulsion. This is due to the surgically weakened posterior musculature. Because of this situation, weight is immediately shifted to the opposite limb throughout gait, thereby causing an observable hip drop.[57,64] Resolution of the hip drop indicates that normal muscle strength and tone have been achieved. Functional foot orthoses are used following this procedure to assist in stabilizing the subtalar joint and improving whatever midtarsal joint subluxation may have occurred during the early years of compensation. Although the device may be used for only a short period of time in some cases, a significant degree of midtarsal joint subluxation dictates that it be used indefinitely. One should be aware of the admonition that although it is not in the patient's interest to delay or avoid performing a posterior lengthening procedure when a congenital tightness is present, the opposite situation represents a potentially worse situation. This is the case when a flexible flatfoot deformity causes the posterior contracture. If the practitioner assumes that there is a primary congenital tightness and chooses to lengthen the tendon before implementing conservative care, a normal muscle would be significantly lengthened. This is a clinically unacceptable situation, in that it would be most difficult to develop normal muscle strength following such a procedure. In such cases, flexor digitorum longus substitution and peroneus longus contracture occur, leading over time to a dynamic pes cavus deformity.[57,59,85,87]

Assessment of the ankle mortise

When evaluating a pediatric patient for possible flatfoot surgical correction, the ankle joint must be evaluated not only for a congenital vs. acquired posterior contracture, but also for frontal plane deviations. The practitioner should note that some children demonstrate an abnormally positioned valgus attitude of their ankle. Although this may be caused by a more proximal deformity such as a marked genu valgum, the deformity exists as a primary problem in some children. In these cases, a congenitally short fibula, an improperly reduced fibular fracture, or an aberration involving the tibial epiphysis may be implicated. If any of these are noted, surgical intervention to reestablish normal frontal plane positioning of the ankle mortise must be carried out separately or in combination with a surgical procedure directed to the foot. Failure to adequately assess the frontal plane position of the ankle mortise before surgical intervention for a flexible flatfoot deformity may lead to failure of the surgery.[81,85,87]

Subtalar joint range of motion

In most instances, functional foot orthoses are only used in pediatric patients after they have initiated a heel-to-toe type of gait, a situation that generally occurs between 3 and 4 years of age. Prior to that time, there is typically a full-foot contact with an apropulsive type of gait pattern. Although it is essential to assess the total range of motion of the child's subtalar joint, an accurate assessment of subtalar joint motion is not generally beneficial until

functional foot orthoses are prescribed. In order to properly assess subtalar joint motion, the child is placed in a prone position with the posterior surface of the calcaneus lying on the frontal plane. This may necessitate internally or externally rotating the child's limb. The examiner then palpates the medial and lateral borders prior to bisecting the calcaneus. If the posterior surface is irregularly shaped, making it difficult to establish an appropriate bisection, the bisection is placed parallel to the medial border of the calcaneus. Next, the foot is placed through its full range of motion and a measurement for inversion with supination and eversion with pronation is noted. This measurement is taken relative to the distal one third of the leg. Care is taken to maintain the foot at an angle of 90 degrees with the leg, as a plantarflexed foot position will reflect extraneous frontal plane ankle motion. The examiner notes the presence of approximately 40 to 50 degrees of total range of motion of the subtalar joint in the child as opposed to the normal adult range, which is generally between 20 and 30 degrees. As in the other major joints of the lower extremity, the range of motion of the child's subtalar joint is much greater than the normally accepted adult values.[56,59] Further evaluation of the functional position of the subtalar joint is assessed via weightbearing, in the resting calcaneal stance position (Fig. 11-21). The extent of abnormal calcaneal eversion may be determined by applying the previously described formula (7 minus the child's age equals a normally acceptable degree of heel eversion).

Complete examination of the subtalar joint includes not only an appreciation for the complete range of motion available, but also some appreciation for the location of the subtalar joint axis of motion. In a normally developing lower extremity, the motion that occurs at the level of the subtalar joint involves a gliding movement of the talus relative to the calcaneus. The average subtalar joint axis generally passes at a 16-degree angle from the sagittal plane and a 42-degree angle from the transverse plane of the foot.[59,64] The axis normally passes through the head of the talus in a posterolateral-inferior to anteromedial-superior direction, as described by Manter[45] and Root et al.[59]

Since the axis of motion may vary considerably from individual to individual, the examiner should be aware of variations likely to be associated with an abnormally functioning foot. As a rule, the subtalar joint axis passes through the talar head, and extends distally in line with either the second digit or first interspace. A pronated foot generally demonstrates a more medially displaced subtalar joint axis, while a supinated foot develops a more laterally displaced subtalar joint axis.[36,37] Kirby[35,36] devised a method

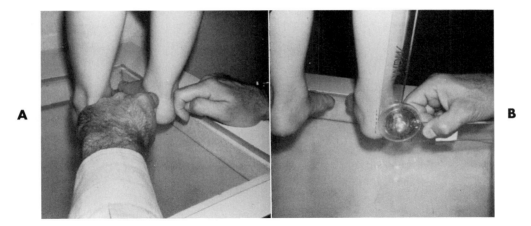

Fig. 11-21. A, The medial and lateral borders of the calcaneus are palpated prior to drawing the calcaneal bisector. **B,** The calcaneal bisector in place. The calcaneal stance position is measured with the tractograph.

of assessing the appropriate angle of the subtalar joint axis of motion that enables the examiner to ascertain the extent of deviation. As a rule, the more medially deviated the subtalar joint axis of motion, the greater the degree of supination that is required to allow the foot to function more normally. From a clinical perspective, the following is noted: when the talus has rotated into a more medial position relative to the calcaneus, there will be a greater degree of pronation present with a greater supinating force required to improve the foot's position.

Kirby's method[36] of clinically determining the location of the subtalar joint axis is performed as follows: First, the patient is placed in the supine position. The plane of the forefoot is maintained in the patient's transverse plane, and the feet are positioned to reproduce their functional base of gait. If necessary, the patient's limbs are rotated internally or externally until the second digit appears vertical relative to the rearfoot (the foot neither abducted nor abducted). The position of the subtalar joint axis is determined by noting those points on the plantar surface of the foot that do not produce inversion or eversion upon plantar pressure.[36] In examining the right foot, the right hand is used to place plantar pressure on the calcaneus while the left hand is used to duplicate the allowable subtalar joint motion. Subtalar joint supination occurs when thumb pressure is placed medial to the subtalar joint axis. Subtalar joint pronation occurs when thumb pressure is placed lateral to the subtalar joint axis, while no subtalar joint motion occurs when thumb pressure is placed directly on the subtalar joint axis. The location of the subtalar joint axis may then be visualized by placing an X at each point where no discernible rotation occurs (Fig. 11-22). This information, coupled with an assessment of concomitant ligamentous and structural abnormalities, allows the examiner to determine those cases of flexible flatfoot deformity which might ultimately require a more aggressive treatment regimen.

Talipes calcaneovalgus

This condition is a positional deformity in which the child demonstrates a dorsiflexed, abducted, and everted position of the forefoot and heel relative to the leg. The dorsum of the foot often lies against the anterior aspect of the tibia with varying degrees of soft tissue contracture and adaptation. Although this deformity occurs in approximately 1% to 2% of livebirths, this figure may be low because the positioning of the foot may occur as a normal variation. A talipes calcaneovalgus may be either flexible or rigid, and is generally attributed to an abnormal intrauterine position and compression. The deformity is classically present in the first-born child of a young mother who is most likely to demonstrate tight uterine musculature, thereby decreasing available space for the developing fetus. Other causative factors include congenital dislocation of the peroneal tendons, which often results in a more rigid deformity requiring more aggressive treatment.[22,67] Although this apparent valgus attitude of the foot relative to the leg is a common positional variation noted at birth, it generally reduces spontaneously.[77] However, if there is a marked contracture of the peroneal musculature along with prolonged positioning of the forefoot in an abducted and dorsiflexed position, some treatment is required. If the deformity does not spontaneously resolve in the first few weeks of life, certain characteristic clinical findings quickly become evident.

The osseous structures are generally not impli-

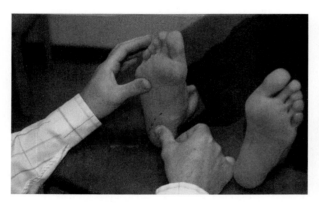

Fig. 11-22. Kirby's method for determining the axis of the subtalar joint. Subtalar joint supination will occur when thumb pressure is placed medial to the subtalar joint axis. Subtalar joint pronation will occur when thumb pressure is placed lateral to the subtalar joint axis. The location of the subtalar joint axis may be visualized by placing an X at each point where no discernible rotation occurs.

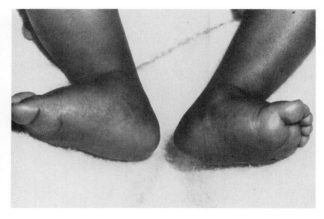

Fig. 11-23. Clinical presentation of a talipes calcaneovalgus in the infant.

cated and demonstrate normal relationships with the exception of the navicular, which assumes a slightly laterally displaced position relative to the talus. The talus typically is plantarflexed and adducted, with the distal aspect of the calcaneus appearing laterally displaced. The forefoot is dorsiflexed and everted (Fig. 11-23) and the talar head is prominent medially and plantar. The Achilles tendon is normal, without any contracture, while the anterior and lateral muscles demonstrate a mild to severe contracture. Besides the abnormal foot position, the practitioner will also note marked redundancy of the lateral skinfolds of both the foot and ankle, as well as a decreased ability to actively move the foot into a corrected, adducted, inverted, and plantarflexed position.[81,83,85] A hallmark of a more severe deformity may be noted if the examiner directs the foot into a corrected position and then, allowing the foot to fall freely, it immediately returns to its abnormal position. If the foot remains in the corrected position for several seconds and then slowly moves back into the abnormal valgus attitude, the problem is less severe. Additionally, if the child is noted to intermittently actively adduct or plantarflex the foot, or do both, this generally indicates a more flexible deformity which may reduce spontaneously or following completion of short-term treatment with manipulation and splints.

If radiographs are obtained, they should be obtained with the foot closely resembling the foot in a weightbearing position. This may be accomplished in the infant or prewalker by artificially placing the foot into the desired position relative to the x-ray cassette. This positioning is maintained either by the parent or clinician during exposure. A talipes calcaneovalgus deformity demonstrates a severely plan-

tarflexed (not vertical) talus with a low calcaneal inclination angle. The talar axis passes through the sole of the foot, and the first metatarsal axis passes dorsal to the talar head. The forefoot appears dorsiflexed relative to the rearfoot. On the AP view, the talocalcaneal angle appears abnormally increased with visible forefoot abduction noted. In order to determine that the deformity is indeed flexible, the foot may be maintained in a corrected position, and a lateral radiograph retaken in the stress lateral view. This should indicate a readily observable reduction of the forefoot position with a more normal metatarsal alignment, this being when the talar and first metatarsal axes are parallel.[46]

If the deformity is left untreated, the child is typically a late walker. When accompanied by an external torsion or position of the femoral or tibial component, this combination makes initial attempts at ambulation an extremely difficult undertaking. When the child finally is able to stand and walk, often as late as 16 to 20 months, the deformity does not spontaneously resolve owing to the abducted, everted, and apropulsive positioning and function of the foot.[81,87] The child's foot then proceeds to develop in a markedly pronated and abducted fashion which persists into adulthood. It is for this reason that early treatment, ranging from parental manipulative exercises and shoe therapy in the more flexible cases to serial plaster immobilization in the more significant cases, is recommended (see Chapter 19). One must note that even if a more severe presentation is successfully treated with serial plaster immobilization, night splints, and prescription shoes, prolonged treatment with functional foot orthoses, (Fig. 11-24), often for life, may be an appropriate long-term adjunctive treatment (see Chapter 20). Owing to its clinical presentation, the talipes calcaneovalgus foot type requires differ-

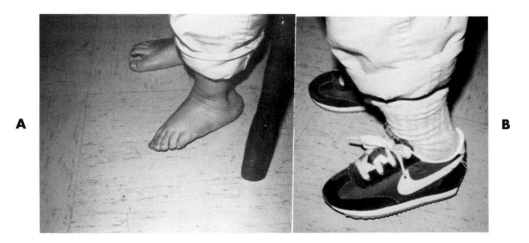

Fig. 11-24. A, A 3-year-old child with undiagnosed and untreated talipes calcaneovalgus. **B,** Note the improved position of the foot in both the frontal and transverse planes with the use of the Blake inverted orthosis (45-degree inverted orthosis with a 4-mm Kirby skive).

entiation from the more severe congenital convex pes valgus foot deformity.[67,81]

Congenital convex pes valgus

Although this is a relatively rare form of flatfoot deformity, the practitioner should be capable of making the diagnosis, because delayed treatment generally results in marked abnormal sequelae. The incidence of congenital convex pes valgus (vertical talus) is less than 1% of livebirths, with no sex distinction.[37,77,78,79] The majority of reported cases are bilateral. The deformity is classically described as a rigid dislocation of the talocalcaneal navicular joint with the navicular typically being locked in a position dorsal to the talar neck. Various authors have reported on this deformity, including Henken in 1914, Rocher and Pouyanne in 1934, and Lamy and Weissman in 1939.[67] Of note is the fact that fewer than 500 cases have been reported in the English literature. In 18 years of clinical practice, I have treated only two cases.

The etiologic factors involved include intra-uterine and developmental muscular imbalance, a developmental delay in limb embryogenesis, inheritance, and associated genetic defects. Most researchers believe that developmental muscular imbalances are the most typical findings associated with this deformity. In this case, there is a contracture of the gastrocnemius-soleus muscle group leading to marked plantarflexion of the calcaneus, with subsequent plantarflexion of the talus. After this initial abnormal positioning of the rearfoot, the secondarily contracted dorsiflexors and peroneals force the forefoot into dorsiflexion. Ultimately, the navicular is positioned against the dorsal aspect of the talar deformity, rigidly locking the deformity in

place. At birth the deformity is generally rigid. The sole of the child's foot appears convex with the classic rocker-bottom appearance (Fig. 11-25). Both the talar head and anterior plantar surface of the calceneus are easily palpable beneath the skin's surface. Radiographs should be obtained with the foot in a simulated weightbearing attitude as previously described. A radiograph typically demonstrates that the calcaneus is in a marked plantarflexed position with the talus lying parallel to the tibia, and the forefoot dorsiflexed. The talar axis passes through the sole of the foot, and the first metatarsal axis passes dorsal to the talar head (Fig. 11-26). In the stress lateral view, the axes remain abnormally aligned owing to dislocation of the navicular. An AP view demonstrates an increased talocalcaneal angle along with a forefoot valgus. With magnetic resonance imaging (MRI), the dorsal dislocation of the navicular may be demonstrated in the infant and young child prior to the normal age of ossification (3–4 years).[67]

Treatment consists of initial gentle manipulation followed by serial plaster immobilization with the forefoot held in a plantarflexed, inverted, and adducted position. The casts are changed twice-weekly for approximately 6 to 8 weeks, with closed reduction of the rearfoot dislocation carried out at that time. If closed reduction is performed, the foot is pinned in the corrected position and maintained for approximately 8 weeks.[78] Unfortunately, as this more conservative therapy is generally not successful, open reduction is generally required.[85] The most successful long-term results are achieved when a pantalar release is performed in a child less than 1 year old. If treatment is delayed or a rigid deformity persists following the reduction, navicular excision

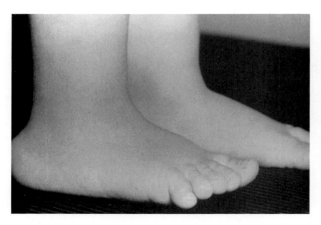

Fig. 11-25. Undiagnosed bilateral congenital convex pes valgus in a 2-year-old boy.

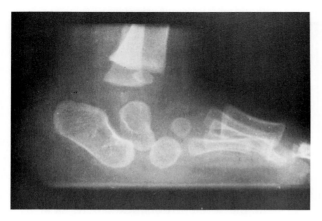

Fig. 11-26. Congenital convex pes valgus (vertical talus) weight-bearing lateral radiograph demonstrating marked plantar-flexion of the talus. Although not visible at this age radiographically, the deformity involves dislocation of the navicular onto the talar neck.

is recommended. If the child is diagnosed at a later stage or previous procedures are unsuccessful, a triple arthrodesis may be performed at the age of 10 to 13.[67,78]

Tarsal coalitions

This restriction of motion may be the child's chief complaint, or may be noted within the course of the lower extremity muscuskeletal examination. In some instances the practitioner will note a restricted or asymmetric range of subtalar joint motion. Restriction of rearfoot motion associated with a valgus foot in apparent spasm secondary to a tightness of the peroneus brevis muscle is consistent with a tarsal coalition. Tarsal coalitions may be congenital or acquired and are generally associated with numerous other pathologic conditions affecting the lower extremity. A congenital coalition may be associated with either incorporation of accessory ossicles into adjacent tarsal bones or the more commonly accepted failure of mesenchymal differentiation. Heredity has also been implicated as a cause owing to reporting of various combinations of family members demonstrating this condition. Acquired forms are generally associated with juvenile rheumatoid arthritis, rheumatoid arthritis, juvenile ankylosing spondylitis, subtalar joint fractures, or significant rearfoot infections.[75]

Although tarsal coalitions have been reported in the medical and anatomic literature for over 225 years, the extent of their involvement within the complex arrangement of rearfoot articulations has only recently been fully realized. The recent use of tomography and computed cross-sectional imaging has increased the practitioner's ability to identify and delineate the extent of this abnormality.[50]

The incidence of tarsal coalitions occurs in less than 1% of the population, with studies demonstrating various male-to-female ratios.[75] Overall, most studies indicate a slight predilection for males. Talocalcaneal coalitions are most commonly involved, the next most common involvement being calcaneonavicular coalitions. Interestingly, appoximately 50% of talocalcaneal coalitions and approximately 60% of calcaneonavicular, calcaneocuboid, and talonavicular coalitions are present bilaterally. Talocalcaneal coalitions most often involve the middle facet. The posterior facet is next most commonly involved, with the anterior facet being the least affected.[50,75]

Clinically, a tarsal coalition may be either a true coalition with intraarticular fusion of the bones or a bar or bridge which occurs when the bones are joined in an extraarticular fashion. Although the clinical picture typically involves an apparent spasm of the peroneus brevis muscle, a coalition may exist without such spasm. Conversely, a peroneal spastic flatfoot is not always associated with a tarsal coalition, as rheumatoid arthritis, infection, talar head fractures, and neoplasms may all cause this clinical picture.

Although some children present with a chief complaint of pain or discomfort associated with their rearfoot, or a complaint of limitation of foot motion, a tarsal coalition may be identified during the course of a routine lower extremity biomechanical examination. A marked limitation of the subtalar and midtarsal joint ranges of motion are noted. In some instances, no rearfoot motion may be elicited. Careful clinical evaluation of this entity involves maintaining the foot at a 90-degree angle to the leg to fully assess the available subtalar joint range of motion. If in fact the foot is evaluated with the ankle plantarflexed, the frontal plane ankle joint motion will mask any decreased subtalar joint limitation.

Generally speaking, rearfoot motion appears greater in cases of a calcaneonavicular coalition as opposed to a talocalcaneal coalition. Clinical evidence of peroneal spasm may also be identified.[11-13] This generally occurs when a coalition has fractured during activity or after intense physical activity without actual fracture. In other instances, the peroneals may be contracted secondary to a prolonged rearfoot valgus which may be due to a chronic limitation of subtalar joint motion.[6] Bilateral standard radiographs including AP, lateral, and medial oblique views are obtained. Comparison views are considered appropriate to delineate the extent of the abnormality. In most instances, the presence of a calcaneocuboid, talonavicular, and navicular-cunieform coalition is readily confirmed with these views. Talocalcaneal coalitions are best viewed with Harris and Beath posteroanterior (PA) axial projections obtained at the standard 35-, 40-, and 45-degree projections. Typically, one notes the classic secondary signs of tarsal coalitions when evaluating the standard films. These include talar beaking, a ball-and-socket ankle joint, a visible "halo effect" caused by sclerotic alterations surrounding the subtalar joint, narrowing of the posterior talocalcaneal facet, and apparent obliteration of the middle facet. CT has expanded the clinician's ability to not only determine the presence of a coalition but also its relative size and effect on surrounding structures.[11-13]

Since most diagnoses are made following the onset of pain, the treatment is conservative. The first goal is to reduce pain and associated peroneal spasm, if present. Injection into the sinus tarsi of a local anesthetic or a common peroneal nerve block followed by a series of casts may reduce discomfort. Once this has been accomplished, a pronated off-weightbearing suspension cast is obtained. A pronated, rigid, functional foot orthosis with a high medial and lateral heel cup is then prescribed. A flat rearfoot post with 0 degrees of motion is added. This type of device is generally effective in reducing symptoms and allowing resumption of normal activities. If conservative care is ineffective, surgical intervention becomes the alternative. This generally includes excision of the coalition or fusion of the rearfoot, depending on the patient's age and the extent of the deformity.[77,78]

Midtarsal joint

A significant varus or valgus deformity that is often related only to the adult foot may be readily demonstrated in the developing child's foot. Therefore, it is essential that the practitioner fully assess the position of the child's forefoot-to-rearfoot relationship. This examination is carried out as in the adult foot.

The child is placed in the prone position with the calcaneus properly bisected as a reference point. The leg is positioned so that the posterior portion of the calcaneus lies within the frontal plane. The subtalar joint is placed in the neutral position, and the midtarsal joint is then locked. This is accomplished by placing a dorsiflexory force on the plantar surface of the fifth metatarsal just proximal to the metatarsal head. In this fashion, the two axes of the metatarsal joint (oblique and longitudinal) cross each other and limit extraneous midtarsal joint mobility.[56,57] In the rearfoot-to-forefoot view, a measurable varus or valgus deformity becomes apparent. In no instance should the forefoot be "loaded" with pressure directed plantar to the first metatarsal head. This unlocks the midtarsal joint and supinates its longitude axis, thereby initiating a false degree of forefoot varus deformity. A structural forefoot varus or valgus is generally not outgrown and should be addressed. In most cases, supporting an everted forefoot deformity improves the child's gait and overall lateral stability. If the child demonstrates a rigid forefoot valgus deformity, he or she will invert the rearfoot and adduct the forefoot in an attempt to achieve weightbearing on the lateral column of the foot. In these cases, a functional foot orthosis designed to support the lateral column will not only support the deformity but will also place the heel in a vertical position and decrease the adducted position of the forefoot.[56,57,83,85] This results in improved function as well as an improved cosmetic appearance of the foot during gait. It has been noted by Ganley and others that any attempt to support the inverted or varus attitude of the forefoot in a pediatric patient will result in maintaining the foot in an abnormal position throughout the child's development.[72] In these instances, appropriate positioning of the child's foot in applying casts for functional foot orthoses will reduce the deformity and improve overall development of the segment (see Chapter 20).

Metatarsus adductus

One of the most common pediatric abnormalities that responds well to early conservative treatment is metatarsus adductus, a transverse plane deformity at Lisfranc's joint (Fig. 11-27). This deformity is characterized by adduction of the metatarsals toward the midline, with the severity of the adduction being present medially. Metatarsus adductus occurs in approximately 1 in 1000 births, with no apparent sex predilection, although some authors report a female-to-male ratio of 0.76 to 1.94. According to Wynn-Davies,[94] there is a 4% to 5% transmission rate to the second child regardless of the cause of the initial problem. This deformity was initially de-

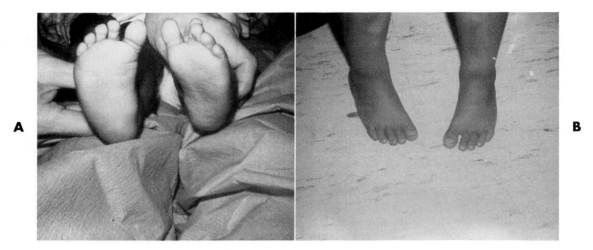

A and **B**

Fig. 11-27. A and **B,** Bilateral metatarsus adductus.

scribed by Henke in 1863[21] and first reported in the English literature by Bankart in 1921.[1] The most significant causative factor is an abnormal intrauterine position with increased uterine wall compression. Other factors associated with metatarsus adductus are a congenitally tight or malinserted abductor hallucis tendon or a tight or malpositioned anterior tibial tendon. Thomson[80] was the first to report involvement of the abductor hallucis; Ponsetti and Becker[52] first described the abnormal insertion of the anterior tibial into the base of the first ray. Bankhart[1] postulated that an absent medial cuneiform is the most likely cause. Implication of other soft tissue structures such as contracted capsules and ligaments were later reported by Reimann and Werner.[21] Anterior tibial contracture secondary to weak peroneals was suggested by Kite.[39] Browne and Patton[8] believed that an abnormal insertion of the posterior tibial was the more likely cause and Diaz and Diaz[16] believed that arrested development of the foot in utero at 8 to 9 weeks of gestation was the pathogenesis.

Since some elements of all of the preceeding are noted in most feet displaying a metatarsus adductus, there are most likely a number of etiologic factors involved. The clinical picture of a metatarsus adductus is best visualized by placing the child's foot into a V formed by the second and third fingers of the examiner's hand. In metatarsus adductus, the following signs may be evident: a concave medial border, a convex lateral border, a prominent styloid process, and an increased metatarsus primus adductus[82] (Fig. 11-28) There is no abnormal subtalar or midtarsal joint range of motion in the nonweight-bearing position. Clinically, the deformity may be classified as mild (flexible), moderate, or severe (rigid). In order to more easily record the various

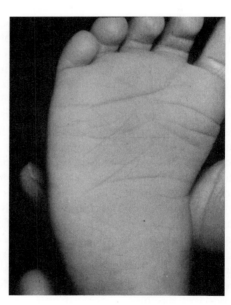

Fig. 11-28. Clinical appearance of a metatarsus adductus. Note concave medial border, convex lateral border, prominent styloid process, and metatarsus primus adductus.

forms of metatarsus adductus, Bleck[4] described an efficient, clinically reproducible classification. The child's heel is bisected with the line of bisection extending through the forefoot. In a normally developing child's foot, this line typically exits between the second and third digits. If the bisection falls through the third toe, a mild deformity is present. If the bisection falls between the third and fourth toes, a moderate deformity is present. In cases of a severe deformity, the line extends between the fourth and fifth toes (Fig. 11-29). To monitor clinical progress, the child's foot may be outlined on a piece of paper, the appropriate lines drawn, and the paper maintained as part of the treatment record.

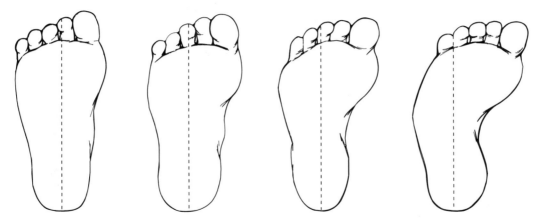

Fig. 11-29. Bleck's classification of metatarsus adductus deformities relative to the position of a heel bisector. *From left,* a normal foot, and a mild, moderate, and severe deformity. (Redrawn with permission De Valentine S. (Ed) Foot and Ankle Disorders in Children. Churchill Livingstone Inc., 1992.)

To determine the flexibility of the forefoot position relative to the rearfoot, the foot is stroked medially and laterally. If there is no visible change in position, the forefoot is actively mobilized. The examiner places the subtalar joint in a slightly inverted and plantarflexed attitude to maintain a neutral position. The forefoot is then abducted to resistance. Pressure is applied at the level of the first metatarsal head, not at the hallux. The other hand locks the lateral column of the foot by applying pressure at the level of the cuboid. At this point, one may observe the reducibility of the deformity and additionally assess the extent of force required to produce changes.[21,79,81,82] If a vertical cleft is noted along the medial border of the foot, one may anticipate that the deformity will be more rigid. By far, the mild to moderate forms are most prevalent, and therefore responsive to conservative therapy. In addition to the more common types of metatarsus adductus deformities already noted, the practitioner must also consider the functional type, which is generally associated with a tight or malinserted abductor hallucis tendon, or with a tight flexor hallucis longus. As this form often goes unnoticed until the child initiates weightbearing, it is essential that the infant be placed into a weightbearing attitude in order to determine the presence of such pathologic changes. The resultant loading of the forefoot causes the tight abductor hallucis brevis to pull the hallux into an adducted postion.[82,87]

Although radiographs may not be necessary when treating the milder forms of metatarsus adductus, they are appropriate when a more rigid deformity is present. Radiographs are useful for two reasons: (1), the radiograph allows the determination of the measurable extent of the metatarsus adductus, and (2) it provides a baseline of the

relative stability of the foot prior to treatment. It is essential to document this measurement, as it allows the practitioner to determine if any subluxatory changes are being initiated through overaggressive or improper treatment with serial plaster immobilzation. These baseline films are especially useful in the more rigid type of deformity, as the practitioner might anticipate exerting a more aggressive force during treatment.

The standard weightbearing dorsal plantar film is obtained. It is generally necessary to have the parent or clinician press the child's foot against the x-ray cassette. In other instances, a better image may be obtained by taping the child's foot directly to the cassette. The radiographic angle of metatarsus adductus is measured by bisecting the second metatarsal shaft relative to a perpendicular bisection of the lesser tarsus. D'Amico[15] in 1976 and then Lepow et al.[43] in 1987 described a useful and practical method of determining the angle of metatarsus adductus in the pediatric foot. Since the osseous anatomical landmarks used to determine the angle of metatarsus adductus in the mature foot are not visible in the prewalker or early walker, this method has proved successful in providing an appropriate measurement of the degree of the deformity. Rather than attempting to actually bisect the lesser tarsus via the normal anatomical landmarks, this method uses the bases of the first and fifth metatarsals as reference points to establish a perpendicular bisection of the lesser tarsus (Fig. 11-30A). In addition to this measurement, the practitioner also measures the angle of the forefoot adductus on the same dorsal plantar film. This measurement is obtained by bisecting the second metatarsal shaft and intersecting it with a line representing the longitudinal bisection of the rear-

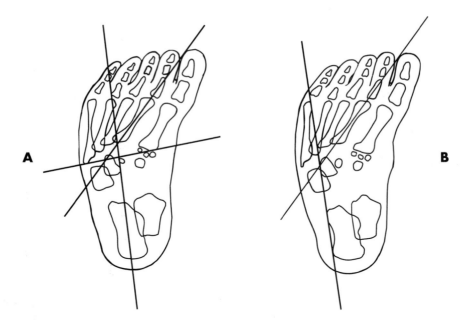

Fig. 11-30. Prior to treatment of a metatarsus adductus by means of serial plaster immobilization, the practitioner measures and documents the angles of metatarsus adductus **(A)**, and forefoot adductus **(B)**. Monitoring of these angles on subsequent radiographs will demonstrate if correction is being accomplished at the appropriate joint level. (**A** is redrawn with permission De Valentine, S. (Ed) Foot and Ankle Disorders in Children, Churchill Livingstone Inc., 1992.)

foot.[64] This measurement is most easily reproduced by drawing a line parallel to the lateral border of the calcaneus (Fig. 11-30**B**). Once these two angles have been recorded, they are monitored on subsequent exposures.

Generally, the next radiograph is obtained after the foot has gone through a series of four casts. If, for example, the intitial angle of metatarsus adductus was 40 degrees and the forefoot adductus angle was 38 degrees, and the subsequent film demonstrates that the angles are 35 and 20 degrees, respectively, this indicates inappropriate correction. Although the clinical picture of the child's foot shows an improved position, the measurable radiographic changes indicate that the correction occurred at the level of the midtarsal joint. As this could lead to a subluxed midtarsal joint and possibly a rocker-bottom type of flatfoot deformity, the practitioner must decide whether or not to continue with the treatment regimen at that time. If the decision is made to continue treatment via serial plaster immobilization, increased caution must be exercised to properly maintain the subtalar and midtarsal joints in a more stable position during the series of casts. The following values for metatarsus adductus are acceptable during normal development:

- Birth: 15 to 35 degrees
- Beginning walker (9–16 months): 20 degrees

- Four years: 15 degrees
- Adult: 15 degrees

Positive radiographic findings associated with a metatarsus adductus deformity are the following[64,82,87] (Fig. 11-31):

- Increase in the metatarsus adductus angle
- Apparent decrease of the adductus laterally
- Increased metatarsal base superimposition laterally
- Hypoplasia of the medial cunieform
- Associated metatarsus primus adductus

A metatarsus adductus is a signficant lower extremity congenital abnormality. Failure to arrive at an early diagnosis and to initiate appropriate treatment may result in any of the following in the older child [56,64,77,78]:

1. Painful styloid process
2. Difficulty with shoe fitting in the more rigid deformity
3. Retrograde pronatory influence in the rearfoot as the flexible type accommodates itself to footwear; typically, this results in the Z-foot or skewfoot-type deformity often seen in the compensated forms of metatarsus adductus
4. Early bunion formation

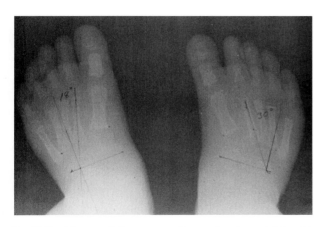

Fig. 11-31. AP weightbearing radiograph of a child with metatarsus adductus.

The first line of defense in the mild-to-moderate form of metatarsus adductus that is diagnosed within the first few months of life is passive stretching done by the parents. This approach serves two purposes. It may correct the mild form of metatarsus adductus or, minimally, it promotes flexibility before the initiation of further treatment. The parents are instructed on how to maintain the subtalar joint in its neutral or supinated position and on abducting the forefoot on the rearfoot for a count of 10 to 20 seconds. This maneuver is repeated 10 times per session and is performed at a minimum at each diaper change.

In the moderate-to-severe deformity, serial plaster immobilization is the most effective method for treating metatarsus adductus. Although a host of other splinting and bracing techniques are available, serial plaster immobilization remains the most common treatment for the more severe deformity. Whenever serial plaster immobilization is used, it is best to initiate it prior to ambulation, as the deformity will generally be less rigid, and the casts will not hamper the child's initial attempts at walking. If the decision is made to use plaster casts, it is best to manipulate the foot into the corrected position before applying the cast. This loosens the foot and lessens the likelihood of the practitioner exerting excessive and possibly subluxatory pressure against the foot. Generally, a below-knee cast is used in the nonabulatory child. If, however, the child is ambulating, an above-knee cast is used for at least the last two or three applications. This is recommended because the abulatory child will otherwise tend to circumduct the below-knee cast. This tends to cause excessive transverse plane motion at the knee that will eventually lead to an internally deviated limb position in gait. Clinically this most closely resembles the internal tibial position deformity noted

previously in this chapter. If this occurs, there may be no apparent improvement in the child's overall angle of gait. As a rule, serial plaster immobilzation becomes less successful as the child becomes older, with only minimal positive results attained in the child over 24 months of age. Although serial plaster immobilization may be carried out in the 2- or 3-year-old child, one should not anticipate complete resolution of the deformity. This is due to the degree of soft tissue and osseous adaptation that occurs over the first or second year of life.

At the point at which correction becomes clinically apparent and is confirmed by radiographics, serial plaster immobilization is carried out for at least half again as many times in order to decrease the likelihood of recurrence.[79,82] If at any time during the sequence of casts, a marked and rapid reduction of the deformity is noted, a radiograph should be taken to rule out midtarsal joint subluxation. As previously discussed, this is a common problem created by overzealous abduction of the forefoot relative to the rearfoot during the series of casts and is to be avoided. This type of subluxation generally persists into later life, with the pathologic changes being potentially greater than the original presenting complaint.

Following successful treatment with plaster immobilization, measures are taken to maintain the correction. This is essential in that the correction was achieved following manipulation and retention of soft-tissue structures which can revert to their original abnormal position without adequate follow-up care. The Ganley splint* is the most appropriate technique for this, because it maintains the forefoot in a corrected position relative to the rearfoot.[46,81,82] The splint is worn for approximately twice as long as the serial plaster immobilization period to provide the best possible results. In addition, since metatarsus adductus deformities may be associated with other transverse plane deformities of the lower extremities, this type of splint may be used successfully to treat those problems as well. Additionally, a Wheaton brace may be used as a retentive splint following serial plaster immobilization. In other cases, the Ganley splint or Wheaton brace may be used as the primary mode of therapy if the deformity appears to be flexible. In conjunction with this splinting process, the child should also be placed in a straight-last type of shoe for 1 to 2 years following correction.

Reverse-last shoes or tarsal-pronator shoes should be avoided, if possible, as these may place a constant subluxatory force on the developing child's forefoot. Although these shoes provide apparent

_____
* Ganley Splint, Chicago Medical, Chicago.

cosmetic changes, they are generally not functionally stable owing to their pronatory effect. However, in cases where residual deformity is noted or in cases of a mild deformity, these shoes may be appropriate for a short period.

The goal of treatment for metatarsus adductus deformities is to improve the position, function, and appearance of the foot while maintaining normal functional and anatomical integrity. However, there are instances where it may appropriate to slightly sublux or pronate the foot while reducing the deformity. It has been argued that a child will eventually function better with a slightly pronated foot with no metatarsus adductus than he or she would if any significant adductus deformity persisted.[64] The reasoning here is that a residual adductus creates longer-lasting problems with fitting shoes. In cases where there is a residual amount of metatarsus adductus present post-treatment, and the child's foot exhibits abnormal compensatory pronation, rigid functional foot orthoses should be used to decrease the likelihood of more significant secondary forms of compensation.[56,82] If the child's problem is refractory to conservative therapy or is initially diagnosed at a later age, surgical correction is called for. Surgical alternatives range from soft-tissue release to a variety of osteotomies depending on the child's age and the severity of the condition.

Juvenile hallux valgus

Following examination of the midtarsal joint, the practitioner should direct his or her attention to the forefoot. Evaluation of the foot should include investigation for the presence of a juvenile hallux abducto valgus deformity. Although this may often present as the chief complaint in the older child or adolescent, the earlier stages of this deformity often go unnoticed by parents and typically do not present any problem for the developing pediatric patient. The earlier, more formative stages of this deformity may appear shortly after the onset of ambulation. Since hallux valgus is a dynamic condition that generally worsens over time, early treatment is mandatory.

The literature is full of attempts to determine the incidence of juvenile hallux valgus. Piggott[2] reported that 57% of adult patients with the deformity noted that they had the problem in their teenage years, with many relating a history even earlier into their first recollections of childhood; Hardy and Clapham,[19,29,95] reported that 46% of their adult patients noted that they had at least some degree of deformity before age 20.[2,19,29,95] Cole reported an incidence of 36% in children aged 6 through 18, with girls making up approximately 75% of the sample studied.[95] Helal noted that 92% of his patients with

juvenile hallux abducto valgus, aged 9 to 19, were girls.[78] A host of factors appear to contribute to the development of this condition, the most notable factors including malposition of the metatarsophalangeal joint and abnormalities of the first metatarsal, medial cuneiform, or metatarsal cunieform joint itself.[25,47] Associated mechanical problems such as metatarsus adductus, compensated congenital gastrocnemius equinus, and pes planus conditions arising from flexible forefoot valgus deformities, forefoot varus deformities, or compensated transverse plane deformities have all been implicated. In a study by Meier and Kenzora,[77,78] analysis demonstrated a family history for bunion problems in greater than 80% of the patients which they surveyed, while Glynn found a family history in 68% of his sample.[95] Although various authors subscribe to the theory of heredity being involved in this process, it is generally the inherited foot function that predisposes a child to the development of a bunion deformity. An adult patient with flatfeet and bunions generally has children with flatfeet and an abnormal gait pattern. Ultimately, this leads to the onset or exacerbation of a hallux valgus deformity.

Although shoes have proved to be an aggravating factor in the development of a hallux valgus or associated bunion pain, juvenile hallux valgus has been reported in non-shoe-wearing populations.[19,29] The intermetatarsal angle has been reported on by several investigators. Some studies indicate marked hallux valgus deformities with intermetatarsal angles as low as 7 degrees. In 1988, Kalen et al.[32] noted that metatarsus primus varus was infrequently found in adolescents, with only 27% demonstrating an increased intermetatarsal angle.[32] Hardy and Clapham[95] reported that hallux valgus occurred primarily in children under the age of 14, while the intermetatarsal angle did not increase until age 15.[95] These studies are supplemented by Root et al.,[57] who reported on the four stages of the development of hallux abducto valgus. They noted that the first stage—abduction of the base of the proximal phalanx away from the dorsiflexed inverted and adducted first-ray segment noted on standard dorsoplantar radiographs of a developing child's foot. Stage 2 involves abduction of the hallux, and only in stage 3 after the hallux valgus deformity had been present for a number of years does an increased intermetatarsal angle actually develop.[59] Obviously, there are cases when abnormal structural findings might affect the intermetatarsal angle. For example, an abnormal development of the first metatarsal-cuneiform articulation causing the first metatarsal to deviate medially from birth would cause an increased intermetatarsal angle and most

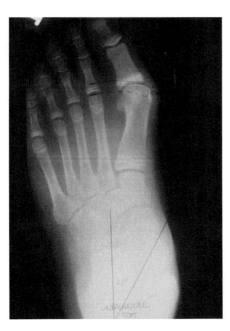

Fig. 11-32. Dorsoplantar weightbearing radiograph demonstrating a juvenile hallux abducto valgus deformity.

likely lead to a hallux valgus deformity.[47] A long or short first metatarsal may also contribute to the deformity.

This deformity may be classified as static or dynamic. The static type of hallux valgus deformity demonstrates a marked early appearance of an increased intermetatarsal angle. The abnormally increased intermetatarsal angle is considered to be the primary cause of the deformity and leads to a dynamic, ever-increasing deformity as the child develops. Abnormal development of the first metatarsal-cuneiform joint is the suspected cause. In the dynamic type, the deformity occurs at the conclusion of development of the first metatarsal and is associated with hypermobility of the first ray.[47] This is commonly considered to be the more functional cause of a juvenile hallux valgus.

Evaluation of the juvenile bunion should entail a complete clinical and radiographic examination. If specific questioning in regard to the presence of the hallux valgus was not conducted at the time of the initial history taking, then at this point the practitioner should obtain the answers to a series of relevant questions. The line of questioning should elicit a history regarding the extent of the symptoms if present; the extent or severity of the deformity; the rate of progression as noted by the parents; the family history for the same condition or other familial foot, ankle, or leg problems; and the overall effect of the deformity on the child's ability to stand, walk, and exercise comfortably.

Radiographs are obtained using the standard weightbearing angle and base of gait—dorsal plantar, lateral, and plantar axial views (Fig. 11-32). Evaluation of the films includes the following: hallux valgus angle, intermetatarsal angle, metatarsus adductus, metatarsus primus adductus, tibial sesamoid position, proximal articular set angle, distal articular set angle, hallux abductus interphalangeus angle, and an overall impression regarding osseous development and the status of growth plates, primarily of the first metatarsal. Additionally, other radiographic observations such as measuring the calcaneal inclination angle, the talar declination angle, the talo-calcaneal angle, and the presence of talar beaking should be noted.[26] This helps in assessing the extent of any concomitant foot abnormality such as a flexible pes planus, compensated transverse plane deformity, or compensated congenital gastrocnemius equinus.

Treatment for juvenile hallux valgus is an often-debated topic with a wide range of opinions. Treatment recommendations include the use of hallux splints, toe wedges, and bunion shields.[68] Additionally, it has been recommended that functional foot orthoses be used in some cases, while corrective foot surgery should be recommended in others.[77,79] Since there is no appropriate long-term study on the response of juvenile hallux valgus to treatment, the practitioner must rely on his or her own knowledge, skills, and experience to determine which treatment is most appropriate for each individual case. There is no one treatment for juvenile bunions. There should be a balanced use of all treatment plans, conservative or surgical. As a rule, functional foot orthoses are effective in milder, more flexible deformities, especially in the earlier stages. In cases where a specific biomechanical entity such as a flexible forefoot valgus, forefoot varus, or other form of flexible flatfoot is noted, functional foot orthoses are the most effective form of treatment. Surgical management of juvenile hallux valgus is appropriate in the more severe, symptomatic cases, or when there is marked progression over a short period of time. This is evidenced radiographically and by clinical signs consistent with limitation of first metatarsophalangeal joint motion, or by pain elicited on joint movement in the corrected position. Skeletal bone growth and epiphyseal development must also be evaluated; the most common procedures involve placement of an osteotomy at the base of the first metatarsal. If associated structural and mechanical influences are also noted, such as severe metatarsal adductus, pes planus, or congenital equinus, they should be addressed surgically as well.[94] Failure to recognize and eliminate significant pronatory forces on the developing foot may result in eventual failure of hallux valgus surgery. Many experts believe that

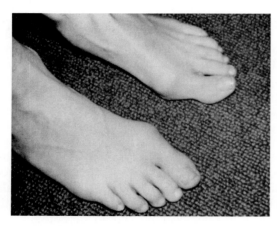

Fig. 11-33. Bilateral juvenile hallux abducto valgus in a 13-year-old girl. This deformity was present in association with a congenital gastrocnemius equinus.

surgical intervention in the child aged 10 to 15 years is most appropriate when the deformity is progressing rapidly, when marked adaptive changes are noted, and when associated functional and structural abnormalities exacerbate the condition (Fig. 11-33). In these instances, surgical intervention is appropriate even in the absence of marked symptoms.[68] In all cases, the newly repositioned joint, sesamoids, and intermetatarsal angle should be maintained through long-term use of functional foot orthoses. This will provide the most efficacious and long-standing results.

The evaluation and treatment of pediatric lower extremity problems is both a rewarding and challenging experience for the practitioner. Hopefully, the information presented in this chapter will allow the clinician to deliver care effectively and efficiently.

References

1. Bankhart B: Metatarsus varus, *Br Med J* 2:685, 1921.
2. Barnicot NA, Hardy RH: The position of the hallux in West Africans, *J Anat* 89:355, 1955.
3. Beckley DE, Anderson PW, Pedjana LR, et al: Radiology of the subtalar joint with special reference for talocalcaneal coalition, *Clin Radiol* 26:333, 1975.
4. Bleck E: Metatarsus adductus — classification and relationship to outcome of treatment, *J Pediatr Orthop* 3:2, 1983.
5. Bleck E, Minaire D: Persistent medial deviation of the neck of the talus — a common cause of in-toeing in children, *J Pediatr Orthop* 3:149, 1983.
6. Braddock GTF: A prolonged follow-up of peroneal spastic flatfoot, *J Bone Joint Surg [Br]* 43:566, 1961.
7. Briggs RG, Carlson WO: The Management of Intoeing—a Review, SD, 1990, pp 13–16.
8. Browne R, Patton D: Abnormal insertion of the posterior tibial tendon in congenital metatarsus varus, *J Bone Joint Surg [Br]* 61:74, 1979.
9. Cholmeley JA: Hallux valgus in adolescents, *Proc R Soc Med* 51:903, 1958.
10. Close JR, Inman VT, Poor DM, et al: The function of the subtalar joint, *Clin Orthop* 50:149, 1967.
11. Conway JJ, Cowell HR: Tarsal coalition — clinical significance and roentgenographic demonstration, *Radiology* 92:799, 1969.
12. Cowell HR: Talocalcaneal coalition and new causes of peroneal spastic flatfoot, *Clin Orthop* 85:16, 1972.
13. Cowell HR: Diagnosis and management of peroneal spastic flatfoot, *Instr Course Lect* 24:94, 1975.
14. Crane L: Femoral torsion and its relation to toeing-in and toeing-out, *J Bone Joint Surg [Am]* 41:255, 1959.
15. D'Amico JC: Developmental flatfoot, *Clin Podiatr Med Surg* 1:535–546, 1984.
16. Diaz A, Diaz J: Pathogenesis of idiopathic clubfoot, *Clin Orthop* 185:14, 1984.
17. Elftman H: Torsion of the lower extremity, *Am J Phys Anthropol* 3:255, 1945.
18. Engel GM, Staheli LT: The natural history of torsion and other factors influencing gait in childhood, *Clin Orthop* 99:12, 1974.
19. Engle ET, Morton DJ: Notes on foot disorders among natives of the Belgian Congo, *J Bone Joint Surg [Am]* 13:311, 1931.
20. Ertel AN, O'Connell FD: Talonavicular coalition following avascular necrosis of the tarsal navicular, *J Pediatr Orthop* 4:482, 1984.
21. Fagan J: Metatarsus adductus. In DeValentine S (ed): *Foot and Ankle Disorders in Children*, New York, Churchill Livingstone, 1992, pp 175–192.
22. Ganley J: Calcaneovalgus deformity in children, *J Am Podiatr Med Assoc* 65:407, 1975.
23. Ganley JV: Lower extremity examination of the infant, *J Am Podiatr Assoc* 71:92–98, 1981.
24. Grant R, Harris E: Neurology. In Thomson, editor: *Introduction to Podopaediatrics*, London, WB Saunders, 1993, pp 175–200.
25. Green DR, Carol A; Planal dominance, *J Am Podiatr Med Assoc* 74:98, 1984.
26. Haas M: Radiographic and biomechanical consideration of bunion surgery. In Gerbert J, editor: *Textbook of Bunion Surgery*, Mt Kisco, NY, 1981, Futura.
27. Haber J: Surgical treatment of metatarsus adductus, *Arch Podiatr Med Foot Surg* 20: 189–193, 1981
28. Hawksley JC: The nature of growing pains and their relation to rheumatism in children and adolescents, *Br Med J* 2:155, 1939.
29. Hoffman P: Conclusions drawn from a comparative study of the feet of barefooted and shoe wearing people, *Am J Orthop Surg* 3:105, 1905.
30. Hutter CG Jr, Scott W: Tibial torsion, *J Bone Joint Surg [Am]* 31:511, 1949.
31. Jayakuman S, Cowell HR: Rigid flatfoot, *Clin Orthop* 122:77, 1977.
32. Kalen V, Adler N, Bleck EE: Electromyography of idiopathic toe walking, *J Pediatr Orthop* 6:31, 1986.
33. Kelikian H: *Hallux Valgus. Allied Deformities of the Forefoot and Metatarsalgia*, Philadelphia, WB Saunders, 1965.
34. Khermosh O, Lior G, Weissman SL: Tibial torsion in children, *Clin Orthop* 25:679, 1971.
35. Kirby KA: Methods for determination of positional changes in the subtalar joint axis, *J Am Podiatr Med* 77:228, 1987.
36. Kirby KA: Rotational equilibrium across the subtalar axis, *J Am Podiatr Med Assoc* 79:1, 1989.
37. Kirby K, Green D. Evaluation and non-operative management of pes valgus. In De Valentine S, editor: *Foot and Ankle Disorders in Children*, New York, Churchill Livingstone, 1992, pp 295–327.
38. Kite J: Torsion of the legs in young children, *Clin Orthop* 16:152-163, 1960.
39. Kite J: Errors and complications in treating foot conditions in children, *Clin Orthop* 53:31, 1967.

40. Kleiger B: The anteversion syndrome, *Bull Hosp Joint Dis* 29:22, 1968.

41. La Porta G: Torsional abnormalities, *Arch Podiatr Med Foot Surg* 1:47–61, 1973.

42. Le Damany P: Congenital luxation of the hip, *Am J Orthop Surg* 11:541, 1914.

43. Lepow G, Lepow R, Lyson R, et al: Pediatric metatarsus adductus angle, *J Am Podiatr Med Assoc* 77:529, 1987.

44. Mahan KT, Yu GV: Juvenile and adolescent hallux valgus. In McGlamany R, editor: Podiatry Institute Surgical Seminar. Atlanta, Doctors Hospital Podiatric Education and Research Institute, 1985.

45. Manter JT: Movements of the subtalar and transverse tarsal joints, *Anat Rec* 80:397, 1941.

46. McCrea J: *Pediatric Orthopedics of the Lower Extremity.* Mt Kisco, NY, 1985, Futura.

47. McCrea JD, Lichty TK: The first metatarsocuneiform articulation and its relationship to metatarsus primus adductus, *J Am Podiatr Med Assoc* 69:700, 1979.

48. McDonough M: Angular and axial deformities of the legs of children, *Clin Podiatr* 1:601–620, 1984.

49. Morley AJM: Knock knee in children, *Br Med J* 2:976, 1957.

50. Oloff L, Heard J: Tarsal coalitions. In DeValentine S (ed): *Foot and Ankle Disorders in Children.* New York, Churchill Livingstone, 1992, pp 193–217.

51. Outland T, Murphy ID: The pathomechanics of peroneal spastic flatfoot, *Clin Orthop* 16:64, 1960.

52. Ponsetti I, Becker J: Congenital metatarsus adductus — the results of treatment, *J Bone Joint Surg [Am]* 48:702, 1966.

53. Purnell M, Drummond D, Engber A: Congenital dislocation of the peroneal tendons in the calcaneovalgus foot, *J Bone Joint Surg [Br]* 65:316, 1983.

54. Rendall G, Stuart PR, Hughes PF: Orthopaedics In Thomson P, editor: *Introduction to Podopaediatrics* London, WB Saunders, 1993, pp 201–230.

55. Ritter MA, De Rosa GD, Babcock JL: Tibial torsion? *Clin Orthop* 120:159, 1976.

56. Root ML: A discussion of biomechanical considerations for treatment of the infant foot, *Arch Podiatr Med Foot Surg* 1:41–46, 1973.

57. Root ML, Orien WD, Weed JH: Normal and Abnormal Function of the Foot. Los Angeles, Clinical Biomechanics Corp, 1977.

58. Root ML, Orien WD, Weed JH, et al: Biomechanical Examination of the Foot. Los Angeles, Clinical Biomechanics Corp, 1971.

59. Root ML, Weed JH, Sgarlato TE, et al: Axis of motion of the subtalar joint, *J Am Podiatr Med Assoc* 56:149, 1966.

60. Rosen H, Sandrick H: The measurement of tibiofibular torsion, *J Bone Joint Surg [Am]* 51:847, 1955.

61. Schoenhaus HD, Poss KD: The clinical and practical aspects in treating torsional problems in children, *J Am Podiatr Assoc* 67:620-627, 1977.

62. Schuster RD: A history of orthopedics in podiatry; *J Am Podiatr Medical Assoc* 64:332, 1974.

63. Schuster RD: In-toe and out-toe and its implications, *Arch Podiatr Med Foot Surg* 3:25-31, 1976.

64. Sgarlato T: A Compendium of Podiatric Biomechanics. San Francisco, California College of Podiatric Medicine, 1971.

65. Shands AR, Steele MK: Torsion of the femur, *J Bone Joint Surg [Am]* 40:47–61, 1958.

66. Shield LK: Toe walking and neuromuscular disease (letter). *Arch Dis Child* 59:1003, 1984.

67. Silvani S: Congenital pes valgus. In DeValentine S, editor: *Foot and Ankle Disorders in Children.* New York, Churchill Livingstone, 1992, pp 157–174.

68. Simmonds FA, Menelaus MB: Hallux valgus in adolescents, *J Bone Joint Surg [Br]* 42:761, 1960.

69. Sobel EC, Levitz SJ: Torsional development of the lower extremity — implications for in-toe and out-toe treatment, *J Am Podiatr Med Assoc* 81:344–357, 1993.

70. Somerville EW: Development of congenital dislocation of the hip, *J Bone Joint Surg [Br]* 35:568, 1953.

71. Somerville EW: Persistent frontal alignment of the hip, *J Bone Joint Surg [Br]* 39:106–113, 1957.

72. Staheli, L: Rotational problems of the lower extremities, *Orthop Clin North Am,* 11:127-132, 1967.

73. Staheli LT: Report of the Pediatric Orthopedic Society (POS), Subcommittee on Torsional Deformity, *Orthop Trans* 4:64, 1980.

74. Staheli LT, Engel GM: Tibial torsion, a method of assessment and a survey of normal children, *Clin Orthop* 86:183-186, 1972.

75. Stormont DM, Reterson HA: Relative incidence of tarsal coalition, *Clin Orthop* 181:28, 1983.

76. Swanson AB, Greene DW, Allis HD: Rotational deformities of the lower extremity in children and their significance, *Clin Orthop* 27: 1963.

77. Tachdjian M: *The Child's Foot.* Philadelphia, WB Saunders, 1985.

78. Tachdjian MO: *Pediatric Orthopedics.* Philadelphia, WB Saunders, 1972.

79. Tax H: *Podopediatrics.* Baltimore, Williams & Wilkins, 1980.

80. Thomson S: Hallux varus and metatarsus varus, *Clin Orthop* 16:109, 1960.

81. Valmassy RL: Lower extremity pediatric examination. Perspectives in Podiatry, Podiatry Arts Laboratory Newsletter, winter 1981.

82. Valmassy RL: Conservative treatment of metatarsus adductus. Perspectives in Podiatry, Podiatry Arts Laboratory Newsletter, summer 1981.

83. Valmassy RL: Biomechanical evaluation of the child, *Clin Podiatr* 1:563-579, 1984.

84. Valmassy RL: Children's sports injuries. *Child and Adolesc Social Work J* 10:403–410, 1993.

85. Valmassy RL: Torsional and frontal plane conditions of the lower extremity. In Thomson P, editor: *Introduction to Podopaediatrics,* London, WB Saunders, 1993, pp 27–46.

86. Valmassy RL, Day S: Congenital dislocation of the hip, *J Am Podiatr Med Assoc* 75:466–471, 1985.

87. Valmassy RL, DeValentine SJ: Torsional and frontal plane conditions of the leg and idiopathic toe walking. In DeValentine S, editor: *Foot and Ankle Disorders in Children.* New York, Churchill Livingstone, 1992, pp 277–294.

88. Valmassy RL, Stanton B: Tibial torsion — normal values in children, *J Am Podiatr Med Assoc* 79:432–435, 1989.

89. Weiner DS, Weiner SD: The management of developmental femoral anteversion — sham or science, *Orthopedics* 2:492, 1979.

90. Weiner DS, Weiner SD: The natural evolution of internal tibial torsion, *Orthopedics* 2:583, 1979.

91. Wenger DR, Mauldin D, Speck G, et al: Corrective shoes and inserts as treatment for flexible flatfoot in infants and children, *J Bone Joint Surg [Am]* 71:800, 1989.

92. Weseley MS, Berenfeld PA, Einstein AL: Thoughts on in-toeing and out-toeing — twenty years experience with over 5000 cases and a review of the literature, *Foot Ankle* 1:2:41–46, 1981.

93. Whitman R: Observations of forty-five cases of flat-foot with particular reference to etiology and treatment, *Boston Med Surg J* 118:598, 1988.

94. Wynn-Davies R: Family studies and the causes of congenital clubfoot, talipes equinovarus, talipes calcaneovalgus and metatarsus varus, *J Bone Joint Surg [Br]* 46:445, 1964

95. Yu G, Landers P, Lu K, et al: Juvenile and adolescent hallux abducto valgus deformity. In DeValentine S, editor: *Foot and Ankle Disorders in Children.* New York, Churchill Livingstone, 1992, pp 369–405.

impression casting techniques

James M. Losito, DPM

Negative casting techniques
Materials and preparation
Subtalar joint neutral position
Casting techniques

Impression casting with plaster is currently the most widely used and accepted means by which a negative model of the foot can be captured for subsequent fabrication of a functional or accommodative orthosis. Within the last 10 years there has been research and development into alternative methods designed to capture the topographic characteristics of the foot maintained in any desired position. One such technology employs a "scanner" which digitizes and records the characteristics of the foot while it is held in the neutral position and produces a computer-generated image.[2,23] The digitized image can be evaluated and corrected on the computer and the information transferred to the orthotic laboratory via telephone. The computer transmits the data to an apparatus which mills out a corrected positive wax cast. The orthosis is then produced directly from this cast. Although several orthotic laboratories currently employ this computer-automated design and manufacturing, the optical scanner has not become standard office equipment, and consequently plaster casting remains necessary. Although the automated technology is potentially more accurate and less time consuming than traditional plaster casting, due to the cost it remains distant.

Negative casting techniques
Selection of technique

There exist several methods by which a satisfactory negative impression may be rendered. All of these methods fall into two categories: (1) weightbearing or (2) nonweightbearing. Which technique is most appropriate depends on several factors: (1) the type of orthosis desired, functional or accommodative; (2) the style of shoe to be worn; and (3) the ease of achieving the desired subtalar and midtarsal joint position.

The most basic question that must be answered is that of the functional vs. the accommodative type of orthosis. A true functional orthosis attempts to do one or all of the following: limit abnormal midtarsal and subtalar joint motion; immobilize the subtalar or midtarsal joint complex; increase subtalar joint motion; cant the foot in a more functional or stable position; compensate for any lower extremity malalignment; and support ("balance") any existing forefoot deformity. Ultimately, the functional orthosis prevents any compensation from the midtarsal or subtalar joint and possibly the lower leg.[1,3,16,17,19,25] In order for these goals to be met, the foot must be cast with the subtalar joint in its neutral position, with the midtarsal joint maximally pronated or "locked."[1,14,17,19,26] Any existing forefoot deformity, such as a forefoot varus or valgus, must be captured by the negative cast in its uncompensated position.

It is widely accepted that these goals can best be achieved through one of the nonweightbearing casting techniques.[1,17,25,26]

The principle behind accommodation is redistribution of vertical and shearing forces away from painful areas. The goal of the accommodative orthosis consists in supporting the arch, increasing stability, and reducing pressure under painful areas and prominences. There is no attempt to support any forefoot deformity, reduce or increase subtalar joint motion, or resist abnormal joint motion. For these reasons, a weightbearing or semiweightbearing casting technique, which is technically easier than the nonweightbearing methods, is the casting technique of choice.[1,17,25,26]

Based on this discussion of functional vs. accommodative orthoses, one can appreciate why a functional orthosis is generally composed of rigid or semirigid materials, utilizes a rearfoot post, and involves intrinsic or extrinsic forefoot posting. In contrast, an accommodative orthosis is generally composed of softer, more flexible materials and usually involves no posting or balancing of any kind. However, there exist orthoses that utilize both accommodative and functional qualities to some degree.[7,10,11]

The shoe type also influences the choice of casting technique. If the patient plans on wearing high-heeled or tight-fitting shoes, or specialized footwear such as roller or ice skates, the in-shoe vacuum technique is preferred.[1,4,5,25,26]

Morphologic differences from patient to patient may require an alternative method of casting. For example, in some patients, the subtalar neutral position is more easily visualized in the prone instead of the supine position. Additionally, in the case of a patient with a large, heavy foot and leg, the practitioner might find it easier and less cumbersome to use the prone technique instead of the supine method.

Materials and preparation

Extra-fast-setting plaster of Paris in 5-in. splints or rolls allows for adequate coverage of the foot and solidifies quickly, thus preventing practitioner fatigue and loss of the desired positioning. Using warm water will further decrease the time required for the cast to harden. However, one must allow enough time for plaster application and proper positioning of the ankle, subtalar, and midtarsal joints prior to plaster solidification or the impression will not be accurate. If a nonweightbearing method is used, a pillow or sandbag may be necessary to maintain the knee in the frontal plane. Failure to do this may result in a supinated or pronated cast. If a

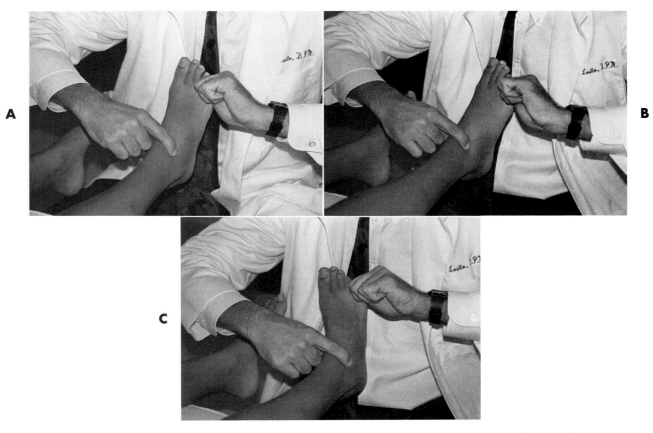

Fig. 12-1. Palpation of the subtalar joint. **A,** Neutral position. **B,** Pronated position. **C,** Supinated position.

weightbearing method is used, a 4- to 6-in. foam block is necessary. In all cases, it is recommended that the subtalar neutral position be located prior to the actual plaster application. Once the plaster is wet, the practitioner must work quickly to apply it and correctly position the foot before it begins to set. Furthermore, it is important that the practitioner and patient remain quiet during casting. This minimizes the occurrence of random movements or alteration of proper foot positioning.

Subtalar joint neutral position

When a true functional orthosis is desired, accurate palpation of the subtalar joint neutral position must be performed during casting. There are three established methods[1,7,18,25]: With the patient prone or supine, the practitioner's thumb and index finger are placed just anterior and distal to the medial and lateral malleoli respectively. The medial landmark corresponds to the talonavicular joint, and the lateral, the sinus tarsi. With the other hand, the forefoot is gripped just proximal to the fifth metatarsophalangeal joint. The subtalar joint can then be

moved through its range of motion (Fig. 12-1A–C). With pronation of the subtalar joint, the practitioner should be able to palpate the head of the talus medially as it protrudes from the posterior margin of the navicular. As the subtalar joint is supinated, the protruding talar head "disappears" as it becomes totally congruent with the navicular. The point of complete talonavicular congruence constitutes the subtalar joint neutral position. Additionally, the curvatures above and below the lateral malleolus should be relatively equal in appearance. This is generally best seen with the patient prone. A pronated subtalar joint will result in a greater curvature below than above the lateral malleolus (Fig. 12-2A–C). When the patient is supine, the skin lines overlying the sinus tarsi should be neither taut nor folded if the subtalar joint is neutral (Fig. 12-3A–C). If the skin is taut, it could represent a supinated subtalar joint position. Finally, when the subtalar joint is taken through its range of pronation and supination, an "arc" of motion can often be perceived which may be helpful in visualizing the neutral position. Typically, a series of repetitive movements through

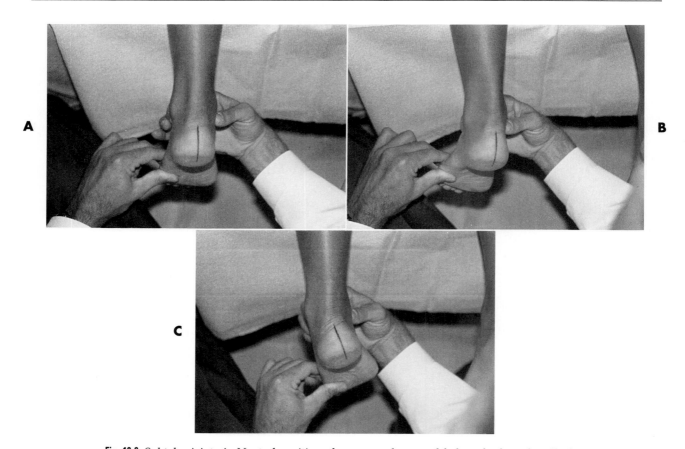

Fig. 12-2. Subtalar joint. **A,** Neutral position; the curves above and below the lateral malleolus appear equal. **B,** A pronated subtalar joint. Note the increased concavity below the lateral malleolus. **C,** A supinated subtalar joint. Note the decreased concavity below the lateral malleolus.

this arc will allow the practitioner to "feel" the neutral position. Use of all three of these techniques each time one attempts to locate the subtalar joint neutral position will provide the most accurate clinical picture.

Casting techniques
Neutral suspension casting technique
Indications and patient positioning

This technique was originally described by Merton Root and is considered the classic method for the fabrication of a functional orthosis.[1,3,16,17] The technique is performed with the patient supine and lying flat or sitting upright in an examination chair. The knee must be maintained in the frontal plane during casting. Slight flexion of the knee aids in patient comfort and allows the foot to be properly positioned with less force. If the knee is externally or internally rotated during casting, the subtalar joint will be supinated or pronated, respectively. As previously mentioned, a pillow may be used under the hip or a sandbag wedged against the knee to

help maintain the knee in the frontal plane. Additionally, the patient should be completely relaxed and not contracting any lower extremity muscles. Muscle firing during casting may alter the critical subtalar and midtarsal joint positioning and distort the cast. For example, firing of the extensors results in subtalar joint pronation. Activity of the anterior tibial muscle during casting may alter the position of the first metatarsal, thereby introducing or increasing an inverted forefoot-to-rearfoot angulation.[8] It is often helpful to ask the patient to let the extremity drop free from the hip down. This allows the patient to easily relax the entire leg and foot. The practitioner should avoid asking the patient specifically to relax the foot, as this often increases muscle activity and further interferes with proper positioning.

Technique

The practitioner grips the forefoot with the thumb placed firmly in the sulcus of the fourth and fifth digits and the index finger gripping the base of the digits dorsally[1,17,25,26] (Fig. 12-4A). The subtalar joint can be taken through its range of motion easily

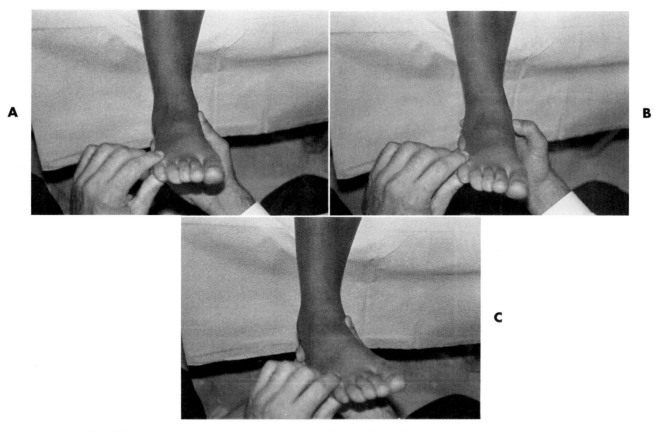

Fig. 12-3. A, Subtalar joint neutral position. The skin overlying the sinus tarsi appears relaxed. **B,** A pronated subtalar joint. The skin overlying the sinus tarsi appears folded. **C,** A supinated subtalar joint: The skin overlying the sinus tarsi appears taut.

from this position. The practitioner may sit or stand, but should maintain the foot at approximately chest level. With the other hand, the subtalar joint neutral position is then palpated and maintained, the wrist pronated, and the leg lifted slightly, thereby "suspending" the foot (Fig. 12-4**B**). Lifting the foot results in dorsiflexion of the foot and ankle, which effectively "locks" the midtarsal joint in a fully pronated position. Only a gentle dorsiflexory force should be applied and the ankle joint need not be at 90 degrees during positioning. If the foot is forcibly dorsiflexed, pronation of the subtalar joint may result. An alternative method exists in which the foot is loaded via pressure applied directly beneath the fifth metatarsal head in lieu of grasping the fourth and fifth digits (Fig. 12-4**C**). While this alternative method is technically easier, it is not recommended because it distorts the fifth metatarsal head impression, which is a critical landmark in orthosis fabrication. Care must be taken not to grasp the digits too aggressively. If the patient is made uncomfortable by excessive digital pressure, he or she may inadvertently contract the anterior tibial muscle, thereby supinating the cast.

Plaster application

Two pieces of extra-fast-setting plaster of Paris are used and may be applied in either a one- or two-step method. If the one-step method is chosen, the plaster is applied all at once. With the two-step method, the plaster is cut so that one piece encompasses the rear and midfoot, while a second piece is applied to the forefoot and overlaps the first piece. Although both techniques may yield a neutral negative cast, the one-step method may result in separation of the plaster from the arch when the foot is loaded. However, this can be avoided by applying a small piece of dry plaster to reinforce the arch just prior to positioning the subtalar joint.

Following measurement and cutting of the plaster (two-piece method), the plaster is immersed in lukewarm water, the excess water removed by squeezing it, and the plaster then smoothed between the fingers. One edge is then folded over lengthwise by approximately 0.25 in., creating a rim which will aid in removal of the cast when it has set. The rim edge of the plaster is then applied along the medial-dorsal aspect of the foot, around the heel, and onto the lateral-dorsal aspect of the foot (Fig.

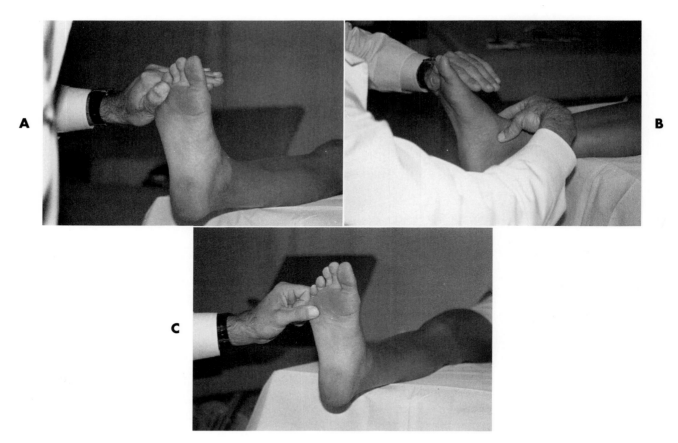

Fig. 12-4. The neutral suspension casting technique. **A,** Correct thumb position. **B,** The leg is lifted slightly while maintaining the subtalar joint in its neutral position and the midtarsal joint in a "locked" or maximally pronated position. **C,** The direct pressure method.

12-5**A**). The plaster should be high enough to incorporate the tip of each malleolus and is smoothed onto the skin so that it adheres well. The remaining plaster is then folded, one side at a time, onto the plantar aspect and smoothed in (Fig. 12-5**B–D**). If the two-piece method is used, the process is repeated with care taken to ensure that the two pieces connect well (Fig. 12-5**C**). If the one-step method is chosen, a small piece of dry plaster is incorporated into the arch region of the negative cast prior to positioning the foot (Fig. 12-6**A–C**). The foot is then grasped in the appropriate manner, the subtalar joint neutral position located, the midtarsal joint locked, and the foot held in place until the plaster has set (Fig. 12-6**D–F**). A small piece of paper towel or gauze can be helpful in gripping the fourth and fifth digits with the thumb.

Removal of the cast should not be undertaken until the plaster is fully set. Premature removal may result in loss of the neutral positioning or distortion of the cast. The rim edge of the plaster should first be freed from the dorsal-lateral and dorsal-medial skin (Fig. 12-7**A**). The skin overlying the ankle, midfoot, and forefoot is then squeezed together to separate the skin from the cast (Fig. 12-7**B** and **C**). Once this has been accomplished, the fingertips are placed along the rim of the cast and the cast is gently pulled downward until the heel is exposed (Fig. 12-7**D** and **E**). The cast is then gently pulled forward and off the foot. The cast should separate easily and not require any significant force. Forceful removal of the cast or pulling the cast away from the heel will typically plantarflex the forefoot on the rearfoot, resulting in supination of the cast.

Advantages and disadvantages

The neutral suspension technique allows for excellent visualization of the subtalar joint neutral position and adequate locking of the midtarsal joint during casting. Additionally, the technique maintains the existing forefoot-to-rearfoot relationship and produces elongation of the pedal soft tissue,

Text continues on page 288

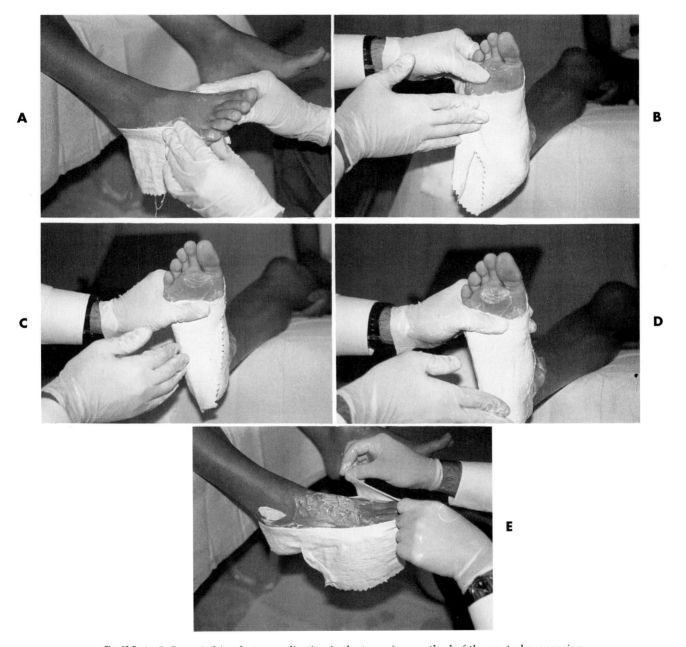

Fig. 12-5. **A–C,** Steps 1–3 in plaster application in the two-piece method of the neutral suspension technique. **D,** Step 4: Note that the plaster is smoothed onto the posterior aspect of the heel. **E,** Application of the second plaster bandage.

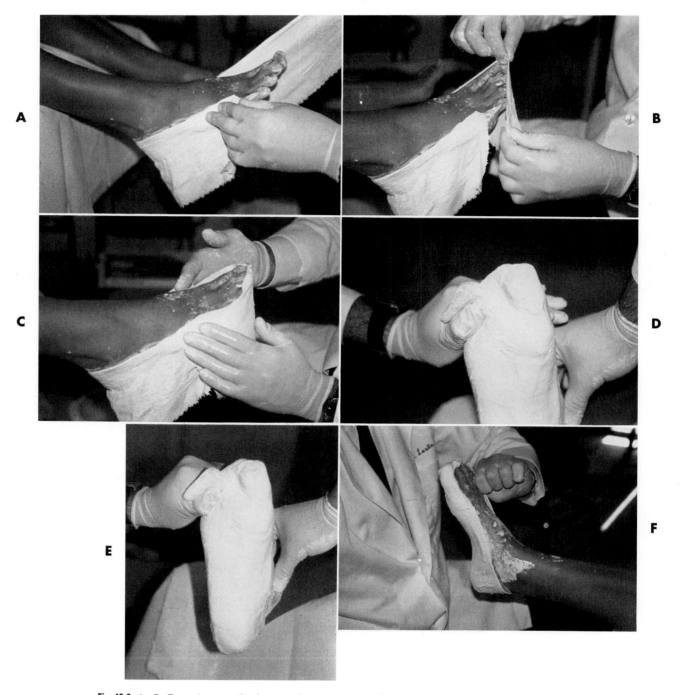

Fig. 12-6. A–C, One-piece method, neutral suspension technique. **D–F,** Correct thumb and hand position.

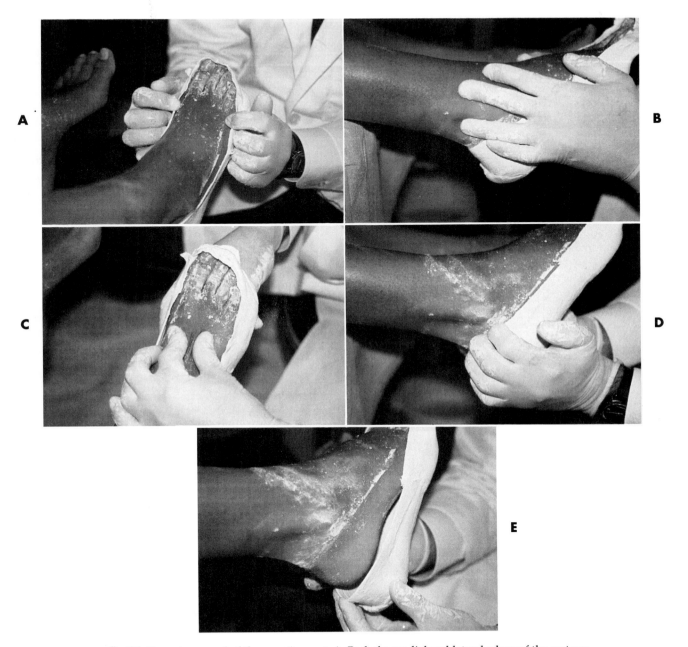

Fig. 12-7. Correct removal of the negative cast. **A,** Both the medial and lateral edges of the cast are freed from the skin. **B** and **C,** The skin is separated from the cast. **D** and **E,** Gentle downward pressure is applied until the heel is visible. The cast is then pulled forward and off the foot.

which is very similar to that which occurs during weightbearing.[1,25,26] The neutral suspension technique has no distinct disadvantage, other than its difficulty.

Evaluation

There exist several criteria by which the accuracy of the casting technique may be judged.[1,17,26] If the negative cast does not meet all of the criteria, the orthosis may not function properly. Careful inspection of the internal and external surfaces of the negative cast will identify casting errors.

1. The cast should accurately reflect the patient's specific plantar dermatoglyphics (skin lines, "wrinkles") and be a quality plaster impression that is a mirror image of the patient's foot. Of special importance are the first and fifth metatarsal heads and the heel region, as these areas represent the proximal and distal boundaries of the orthosis. If a proper first metatarsal head impression is not captured, the longitudinal axis of the midtarsal joint may not have been adequately loaded. If excessive wrinkles are present in the arch and are in a radiant or "sunburst" configuration, this may represent a supinated subtalar joint. When several short transverse lines are noted along the course of the first ray just proximal to the first metatarsal head, the anterior tibial may have been firing during casting. Small crevices and imperfections caused by trapped air can be corrected later but should be kept to a minimum.

2. Within the cast, the arch should be divided lengthwise into thirds and evaluated in the frontal plane (Fig. 12-8**A**). The lateral one third should be flat, the middle one third sloped upward slightly, and the medial one third sloped upward steeply. If the middle one third is not sloped upward enough or is flat, this may indicate that the subtalar joint was pronated during casting. If the middle one third has a steep slope, this may indicate a supinated subtalar joint.

3. Externally, the plaster should have been applied high enough dorsally to incorporate the tip of each malleolus. If the two-step method was used, the pieces should be tightly adherent to each other.

4. The plantar surface of the cast should be examined, and the lateral border of the cast should be straight (Fig. 12-8**B**). If the lateral border is curved or C-shaped, the subtalar joint may have been supinated during casting, thereby unlocking the midtarsal joint oblique axis. However, if the patient has residual metatarsus adductus or a prominent styloid process, do not confuse this with a supinated subtalar or midtarsal joint. Careful evaluation of the plantar aspect of the patient's foot at this time will confirm any structurally significant adduction. If the lateral border is abducted slightly, this may reflect a pronated subtalar or oblique midtarsal joint.

5. The fifth digit should be straight and in-line with the fifth metatarsal shaft when viewed from lateral (Fig. 12-8**C**). This ensures accurate representation of the fifth metatarsal head. If the fifth digit is dorsiflexed relative to the fifth metatarsal shaft during casting, plantarflexion of the metatarsophalangeal joint results and therefore distorts the actual forefoot-to-rearfoot position. Conversely, excessive plantarflexion of the digits may abnormally dorsiflex the metatarsal.

6. The external impression of the thumb should be restricted to the sulcus of the fourth and fifth phalanges (Fig. 12-8**D**). There should be no evidence of pressure medially or laterally. If the thumb was placed too far medially, such as in the sulcus of the third or second phalanges, the longitudinal axis of the midtarsal joint may have been supinated during casting. If the thumb or thenar eminence was resting on the lateral border of the foot, a pronated oblique midtarsal joint may result.

7. When placed on a flat and even surface, the cast should represent the forefoot-to-rearfoot position observed during the examination. If a forefoot valgus or plantarflexed first-ray deformity is present, the heel of the cast should be inverted relative to the ground (Fig. 12-8**E**). When the heel is everted upon inspection, a forefoot supinatus or varus must be present. The measured position of the cast must correspond within 2 degrees of the clinically observed deformity. If there is a discrepancy between "what you observed on the examining table and what the cast is telling you," and the cast meets all the other criteria, then the cast is most likely accurate and you should reexamine the patient. However, if any of the other negative cast criteria are not met, then the cast is probably faulty and you should recast the patient. This criterion does not apply when the semiweightbearing method is used.

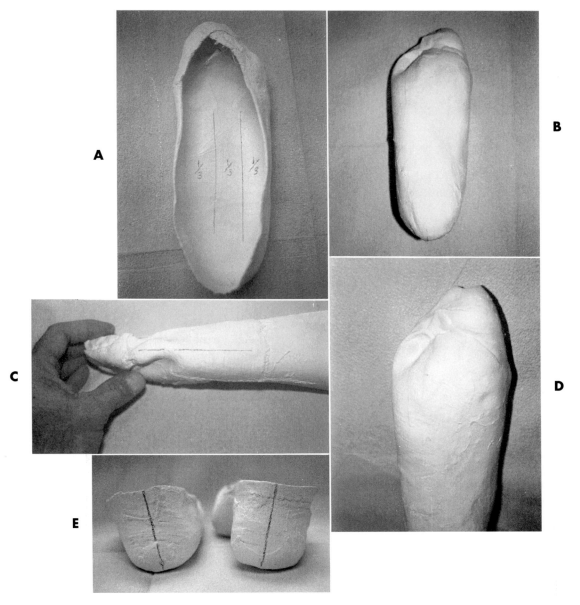

Fig. 12-8. Evaluation of the negative cast. **A,** The arch region is divided into thirds. **B,** A straight lateral border consistent with correct positioning of the subtalar and midtarsal joints. **C,** The fifth digit is in line with the fifth metatarsal. **D,** The external thumb impression is restricted to the sulcus of the fourth and fifth digits. **E,** Evaluation of the forefoot-to-rearfoot position. *Left,* a forefoot supinatus deformity; *right,* a forefoot valgus deformity.

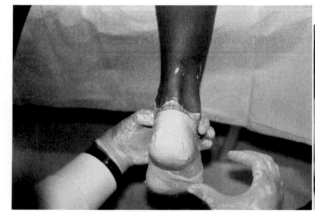 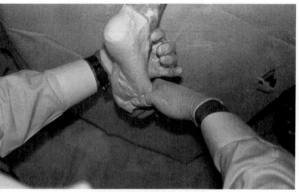

Fig. 12-9. Prone casting technique. **A,** The direct pressure method. **B,** The preferred method.

Although the negative cast provides information regarding any forefoot deformity that may exist, the negative cast cannot be used to establish or confirm the true rearfoot position (relaxed calcaneal stance position). Therefore, it is imperative that information regarding the relaxed and neutral calcaneal stance position be provided on the orthotic prescription form so that the cast is poured appropriately.

Prone casting technique

Indications and patient positioning

The prone casting or modified suspension technique is executed in much the same manner as the supine method, but with the patient prone.[1,17,25,26] The examiner then sights down the rearfoot to the forefoot while positioned above the foot (Fig. 12-9A). This allows for good visualization of the subtalar joint range of motion and neutral position. Once the subtalar joint neutral position is located, the foot may be loaded (locking the midtarsal joint) in one of two ways: a slight dorsiflexory force is placed below the fifth metatarsal head until resistance is felt, or the fourth and fifth digits may be grasped in much the same manner as with the supine technique and the foot dorsiflexed slightly with concomitant supination of the wrist (Fig. 12-9B). More effort must be made to dorsiflex the foot slightly, which is what happens automatically as the foot is lifted using the suspension technique. The direct pressure method locks the midtarsal joint well but results in deforming the fifth metatarsal head impression. Grasping the digits does not generally distort the cast but is often awkward and insufficient to lock the midtarsal joint in position.

The plaster is applied in the identical manner as previously described for the supine technique. As before, the plaster may be applied in one or two steps. If plaster application is difficult with the patient prone, apply the plaster with the patient

supine. Removal of the cast is performed in the previously described stepwise manner.

Advantages and disadvantages

The prone technique offers good visualization and accurate positioning of the foot during casting. It may be more comfortable for some patients because the foot need not be suspended. The midtarsal joint can be effectively locked and the forefoot-to-rearfoot relationship maintained. If the practitioner elects to load the foot via direct pressure below the fifth metatarsal head, this can be considered a disadvantage of the technique. Otherwise, the prone technique has no distinct disadvantage.

Vacuum casting technique

Indications

The vacuum casting technique is a relatively new nonweightbearing neutral casting method which allows increased specificity of the orthosis for a particular type of shoe.[1,4,5,25,26] If the patient requires a functional orthosis to be worn in a high-heeled (>1 in.) shoe, ice or roller skates, cleats, or any extremely tight-fitting or "atypical" shoe, the vacuum technique is useful and recommended. The vacuum technique allows for good visualization of the subtalar joint neutral position and therefore is appropriate for any functional orthosis, regardless of shoe type.

Materials and positioning

The vacuum technique requires some special equipment, including a vacuum pump, Velcro straps, and contoured plastic bags. Apply plaster only to the plantar aspect and less around the outside of the foot in order to allow for shoe fit during casting. The patient is positioned supine, sitting upright with the knee flexed slightly and the lower leg extended downward and off the ground by 1 to 2 feet. The leg to be cast is positioned in the

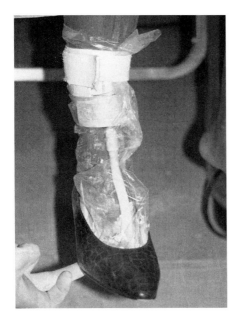

Fig. 12-10. The vacuum casting technique. Note that the subtalar joint is maintained in its neutral position and the midtarsal joint is "locked" via pressure directly plantar to the fifth metatarsal head.

center of the chair with the knee maintained in the frontal plane.

Technique

Liquid hand soap is first applied to the foot to aid in removal of the cast. This is an optional step but one that is encouraged. The ankle portion of the vacuum hose is then put in place and the subtalar joint neutral position is palpated. As before, extra-fast-setting plaster is then applied to predominantly the plantar aspect of the foot. A contoured plastic bag is then carefully slipped on the foot and ankle, and the excess bag is gathered and made airtight with a Velcro strap placed around the leg. The foot is then held in maximum subtalar pronation as the pump is activated. If a "specialized" shoe is to be worn, it is now gently slipped over the plastic and onto the foot. The subtalar joint neutral position is then palpated and maintained. The midtarsal joint is locked and the foot supported via pressure applied plantar to the fifth metatarsal head until the plaster has set (Fig. 12-10). Removal of the cast involves gentle separation of the "foot from the cast," as previously described.

Advantages and disadvantages

The vacuum technique has several clear advantages including excellent visualization of the subtalar joint neutral position and locking of the midtarsal joint. The method is nonweightbearing and is satisfactory for fabrication of a functional orthosis. When extra tight-fitting, specialized, or high-heeled

shoes are to be worn, the vacuum technique has unmatched advantages and is the casting technique of choice.[1,4,5,25,26] The only conceivable disadvantage is perhaps the additional time and steps required to perform the technique and the expense of owning a vacuum pump.

Semiweightbearing technique

Indications

The semiweightbearing technique is a fundamental weightbearing method of negative casting.[1,25,26] Emphasis is not placed on finding and maintaining subtalar joint neutral position or capturing any existing forefoot-to-rearfoot malalignment. The goal is basically to capture an accurate impression of the size and shape of the foot. With this kept in mind, the cast produced via the semiweightbearing technique is most appropriate for accommodative orthoses and not for a true functional orthosis. An exception exists in patients with a high degree (>5 degrees) of flexible or rigid forefoot valgus, who often respond well to a functional orthosis fabricated from a semiweightbearing cast.[1,25,26] The flexible forefoot valgus compensates via the midtarsal longitudinal axis while the rigid forefoot valgus compensates primarily via the oblique axis of the midtarsal and subtalar joints.[19,25] In rigid forefoot valgus, there is virtually no motion available at the midtarsal longitudinal axis. Because the longitudinal midtarsal joint is rigid, it does not supinate upon weightbearing (as it normally should), and therefore the forefoot valgus deformity is not distorted when the semiweightbearing technique is used. Secondarily, owing to the increased first metatarsal declination encountered in a foot with a severe rigid or flexible forefoot valgus, an orthosis fabricated from a nonweightbearing cast may not be tolerated by the patient. Additionally, patients who have severe equinus or require a pronated type of orthosis generally benefit from the semiweightbearing technique.[1,17,25]

Materials and positioning

The semiweightbearing technique requires a foam block of the desired thickness, usually between 2 and 6 in., covered by plastic. Semisolid plaster ("puddle" casting) and compressible foam (BioFoam, Smithers Biomedical Systems, Kent, Ohio) are some reported variations. The patient is supine and seated in an upright position with the hip, knee, and ankle joints maintained at approximately 90 degrees. The plaster is applied in the same manner as in the neutral suspension technique, and the chair is lowered until the foot contacts the foam block (Fig. 12-11). Prior to contact with the foam block, the subtalar joint neutral position may easily

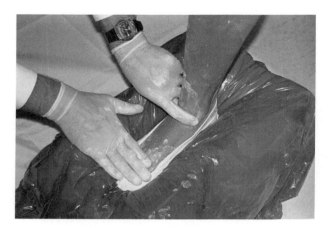

Fig. 12-11. The semiweightbearing technique.

be palpated but is difficult to maintain once the foot bears weight. The practitioner should palpate the medial and lateral landmarks of the subtalar joint and attempt to maintain the subtalar joint neutral position as the foot bears weight. The amount of weight to be placed on the foot may vary from one fourth to one half of the body weight. Gentle downward pressure is applied manually, to the dorsum of the forefoot while the plaster is setting. When set, the cast is removed using the appropriate stepwise method.

Advantages and disadvantages

Although the semiweightbearing technique allows for good visualization of the subtalar joint neutral position, any positioning is usually lost upon even partial weightbearing. As the foot loads onto the foam block, ground reactive force supinates the midtarsal joint around its longitudinal axis. This results in distortion of the forefoot-to-rearfoot relationship: the supinated position of the first metatarsal may increase or decrease the amount of varus or valgus angulation perceived. The supinated first metatarsal is unstable and may function in a hypermobile state with resulting deformities, including hallux valgus, hallux limitus, and digital deformities.[12,26]

The semiweightbearing technique usually produces an excellent impression suitable for fabricating a custom accommodative insole or orthosis. Although the subtalar joint neutral position is easily located, it is very difficult to maintain on weightbearing because of forefoot compensation and the influence of the lower leg. The ground reactive force of weightbearing effectively locks the midtarsal oblique axis but supinates the longitudinal axis. For these reasons, a semiweightbearing or any weightbearing technique is not appropriate for the fabrication of a true functional orthosis.

However, there exist modifications of the semiweightbearing method which attempt to offset some of the inherent problems of compensation. One such modification is simply reducing the amount of body weight placed on the foam block. If the foot is placed on the foam block with only the force of gravity, compensation generally does not occur.[22] However, if the semiweightbearing technique is used for a functional orthosis, the practitioner must understand the shortcomings of the technique and have satisfactory clinical solutions.

Modified casting techniques

Pronated casting technique

Pronated casting refers to positioning the subtalar joint in a semi- or maximally pronated position during casting instead of the customary neutral position.[1,25,26] The basic clinical indications include painful subtalar joint arthritis, inoperable tarsal coalition, severe ankle equinus, and unstable gait.[21,24] The pronated position immobilizes the subtalar joint and effectively stabilizes the foot. However, the patient will have a diminished capacity to absorb shock due to the absence of subtalar joint motion.[11,16,19]

The pronated method is best performed using the neutral suspension technique, although all of the aforementioned methods could conceivably be used. The examiner palpates the subtalar joint range of motion, applies the plaster, positions the subtalar joint in maximum pronation, and locks the midtarsal joint (Fig. 12-12). Depending on the abnormality and available subtalar range of motion, an intermediate pronated position may be chosen.

The supinatus foot

Forefoot supinatus is an acquired positional adaptation to increased ground reactive forces secondary to some other pronatory force.[1,20] Specifically, it occurs secondary to forces that create continuous supination of the longitudinal axis of the midtarsal joint. Clinically, supinatus appears as an inverted forefoot. However, this inverted position is easily reducible with gentle plantarflexory pressure applied at the base of the first metatarsal. This contrasts with a true forefoot varus, which is a fixed primary deformity and results in pronatory subtalar joint compensation during gait.[1,19,20] Forefoot varus is a clinically unmistakable flatfoot with a nonreducible inverted forefoot.

When treating the supinatus foot, the practitioner may elect to "cast out" (reduce) the existing forefoot supinatus by applying a plantarflexory force on the first metatarsal while holding the subtalar joint in neutral position during casting (Fig. 12-13). The first metatarsal is plantarflexed until the forefoot appears

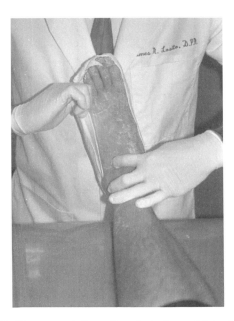

Fig. 12-12. The pronated casting technique. Note that the subtalar and midtarsal joints are positioned in their maximally pronated position.

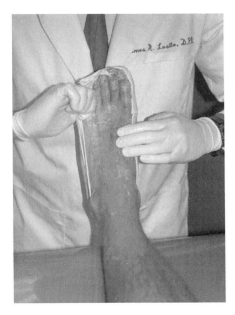

Fig. 12-13. Reduction of a forefoot supinatus deformity during neutral suspension casting.

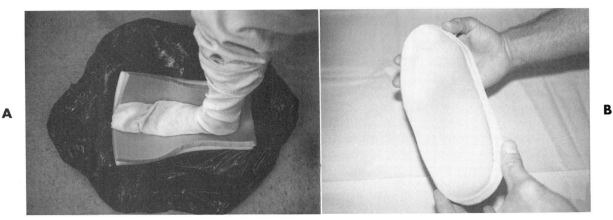

A   B

Fig. 12-14. A and B, Fabrication of an accommodative insole composed of Plastazote 1 and 2 directly from a patient's foot.

neutral (perpendicular to the rearfoot).[20] The heel of the resulting negative cast should then rest perpendicular to the ground. The resulting orthosis, when placed against the patient's foot held in the neutral position, should flare away from the first metatarsal head. The concept of reducing the supinatus during casting is based on the idea that once the pronatory forces acting on the forefoot are eliminated by the orthosis, the supinated position of the first metataral (and forefoot) will begin to reduce (plantarflex). If the supinatus was reduced during casting, the first metatarsal can plantarflex onto the orthosis, which

contours to a neutral forefoot. However, if the supinatus was not "cast out," the first metatarsal is supported in the supinated position by the orthosis and therefore cannot plantarflex. This may result in pain along the first ray within 6 months of orthotic therapy.

There is little concrete documentation delineating the superiority of one method over the other. The concept follows logically and merits further clinical trial. If the practitioner elects to not "cast out" the supinatus, the patient should be told of the potential need for a new orthosis within 6 to 8 months.

Positive casting (impression) methods

Positive casting refers to the production of an orthosis directly from the patient's foot. Utilizing semiweightbearing casting principles, the orthotic material is heated, placed on a 4- to 6-in. foam block and stepped on by the patient with the desired amount of body weight. An accommodative insole of Plastazote, Pelite, Nickoplast, Ortho-cork, or crepe can be easily fabricated in this manner (Fig. 12-14**A** and **B**). These materials are thermoplastic and generally heat mold easily. Plastazote 1 and 2 (closed cell polyethylene foam) and Pelite (polyethylene foam) are appropriate for use directly against the patient's skin.[6,15] Spenco (microcellular rubber) and Poron (ppt) may serve as excellent topcover material but are not as shock-absorbent as Plastazote 1 and 2. Plastazote may be laminated together prior to heating for increased strength and longevity. Plastazote 3, Evazote (ethyl vinyl acetate), Ortho-cork, Nikoplast (an ethylene vinyl acetate copolymer) and crepe are used as midsole or base layers only and never applied directly against the foot.

Leather (cowhide) has been used to capture an impression of the foot by weightbearing, semiweightbearing and nonweightbearing means.[9] The leather (1/16–1/8-in. thickness) is immersed in water, manipulated until pliable, and formed to the foot. Once completely dry, the leather shell is an excellent template for further laminations and additions.

Additionally, there exists an orthotic system which uses a prepackaged "sandwich" composed of two or three semirigid thermoplastic materials (Subortholene, polypropylene) which, when heated and molded to the foot, yields an "instant orthosis." Low-temperature thermoforming plastics such as Aquaplast and Manorthos (both WFR/Aquaplast Corp., Ramsey, N.J.) become flexible in hot water and mold to the foot on weightbearing, producing a semirigid device.[9] Yet another system utilizes a polyvinylchloride shell and liquid polyurethane foam which solidifies on weightbearing, yielding a similar semirigid device. These represent an attempt to produce a more functional type of orthosis, via weightbearing, which may prove satisfactory for a patient with only mild biomechanical flaws, or for use as an interim orthosis.

The obvious advantage of any positive casting method is that it is generally less expensive and the patient obtains the device immediately. This is crucial when managing the neuropathic foot.[13] The disadvantages of the positive method are those of any weightbearing method: difficulty maintaining subtalar joint neutral position and distortion of the forefoot. Consequently, most positive impression methods are recommended for accommodative orthoses and insoles only.

References

1. Anthony RJ: *The Manufacture and Use of Functional Foot Orthosis*, Basel, Karger, 1991, pp 17–34.
2. Bergmann J: The Bergmann foot scanner for automated orthotic fabrication, *Clin Podiatr Med Surg* 10:363–375, 1993.
3. Blake RL, Ferguson H: Limb length discrepancies, *J Am Podiatr Med Assoc* 82:33–38, 1992.
4. Brown D, Smith C: Vacuum casting for foot orthoses, *J Am Podiatry Assoc* 66:583–585, 1976.
5. Brown D, Smith C: Bio Vac In-Shoe Casting Technique Manual. Northwest Podiatric Laboratory, Blaine, WA, 1992.
6. Frykberg RC: Podiatric problems in diabetes. In Kozak, editor: *Management of Diabetic Foot Problems*. Philadelphia, WB Saunders, 1984, pp 45–67.
7. Gross MJ, Napoli RC: Treatment of lower extremity injuries with orthotic shoe inserts, *Sports Med* 15:66–70, 1993.
8. Kendall F, McCreary E: *Muscles, Testing and Function*, Baltimore, Williams & Wilkins, 1983, pp 129–140.
9. Levitz SJ, Whiteside LS, Fitzgerald TA: Biomechanical foot therapy, *Clin Podiatr Med Surg* 5:728–729, 1988.
10. Lockard MA: Foot orthosis, *Phys Ther* 68:1866–1873, 1988.
11. McPoil TG, Cornwall MW: Rigid vs soft foot orthosis: A single subject design, *J Am Podiatr Med Assoc* 81:638–642, 1991.
12. Merrill TJ, Weeber K: Biomechanical basis of forefoot derangement. In McGlamry ED, editor: *Comprehensive Textbook of Foot Surgery*, Baltimore, Williams & Wilkins, 1987, p. 544.
13. Meuller M, Minor S, et al: Relationship of foot deformity to ulcer location in patients with diabetes mellitus, *Phys Ther* 70:356–352, 1990.
14. Philps JW: *The Functional Foot Orthosis*. New York, Churchill Livingstone, 1990, pp 25–26.
15. Reed JR, Koziatek E: Materials. In Coleman WC (ed): The Insensitive Foot Seminar, Course Syllabus. Carville, La, 1990, pp 58–70.
16. Root ML: Indications for the use of functional orthosis. Podiatry Arts Lab Winter 1982.
17. Root ML, Weed J, Orien W: Neutral Position Casting Techniques, vol 3, Los Angeles, Clinical Biomechanics Corp, 1971.
18. Root MI, Weed J, Orien W: Biomechanical Examination of the Foot, vol 1. Los Angeles, Clinical Biomechanics Corp, 1971.
19. Root ML, Weed J, Orein W: Normal and Abnormal Function of the Foot. Los Angeles, Clinical Biomechanics Corp, 1977, p. 77.
20. Roy KJ, Scherer P: Forefoot supinatus, *J Am Podiatr Med Assoc* 76:390–394, 1986.
21. Schelfman BS: Tarsal coalition. In McGlamry ED (ed): *Comprehensive Textbook of Surgery, vol 1*. Baltimore, Williams & Wilkins, 1987, p 500.
22. Skliar DJ: Personal communication, November 1993.
23. Stats TB, Kriechbaum MP: Computer aided design and computer aided manufacturing of foot orthoses, *J Prosthet Orthot* 1:182–186, 1989.
24. Thompson J, Jennings M, Hodge W: Orthotic therapy in the management of osteoarthritis. *J Am Podiatr Med Assoc* 82:136–139, 1992.
25. Valmassy RL: Orthoses. In Subotnick SI (ed): *Sports Medicine in the Lower Extremity*, New York, Churchill Livingstone, 1989, pp 425–436.
26. Valmassy RL: Advantages and disadvantages of various casting techniques, *J Am Podiatr Assoc* 69:707–712, 1969.

prescription writing for functional and accommodative foot orthoses

Lester J. Jones, DPM, MS

Introduction
Lower extremity range of motion study
Casting for foot orthoses
Orthotic fabrication process
Extrinsic corrections to the orthosis

Introduction

Over the past 30 years, the art of fabrication of functional and accommodative foot orthoses has experienced numerous technical advances. Newer and more durable plastics, reinforced fiberglass, and various resin-reinforced materials have been developed by podiatric biomechanical laboratories with the goal of producing better and longer-lasting products for patient care and compliance. For all practical purposes, functional and accommodative orthoses are prescriptive medical devices that are utilized to lend assistance in realigning lower extremity joint malfunctions. Orthoses have additionally proved to aid effectively in maintenance of structural realignment following invasive reconstruction of the foot.

Orthoses in general tend to decrease the amount of abnormal stress and strain on the lower extremity. Abnormalities secondary to joint malfunction and muscle tendinous malposition are successfully addressed via functional orthoses. A functional foot orthosis best achieves its goal by maintaining normal function at the level of the subtalar and midtarsal joints, thereby allowing more improved functioning for the more distal and proximal articulations of the lower extremity. Properly fabricated orthoses help not only to improve abnormal foot function but also produce:[6]

1. Normal ankle joint dorsiflexion and plantar flexion
2. Normal knee flexion at the moment of heel contact for more efficient shock absorption
3. Proper hip flexion and extension
4. Efficient internal and external lower extremity motion
5. Proper subtalar and midtarsal joint pronation and supination

Once properly fabricated, functional and accommodative orthoses have the ability to effectively reduce and eliminate painful excrescences and dermatologic hypertrophied lesions beneath weightbearing pressure points. Typically, these are some of the most common presenting complaints that necessitate the patient's seeking professional foot care. Orthoses likewise provide significant relief of painful symptoms associated with arch fatigue. Typically this results from stress and strain of the plantar structures associated with the fascial, tendinous, and muscular tissue of the foot.

Although the title of this chapter is "Prescription Writing for Functional and Accommodative Foot Orthoses," one cannot ignore the topic of shoe gear. A properly prescribed and manufactured orthosis used in conjunction with an ill-fitted shoe renders the orthosis relatively ineffective. Shoes are manufactured from a variety of materials such as animal skins, and man-made materials, which include vinyls, urethane (which are softer than vinyls), and poromerics, which are leatherlike with good breathability.[7] Other materials used in shoe construction consist of various polymers, polyesters, and synthetic rubber–type materials. These man-made products are advantageous in terms of production owing to their versatility in colors, ease of mass production, water-resistance, and their relatively low manufacturing costs. However, the major disadvantage is their lack of breathability. The inability of these types of materials to dissipate heat and moisture may tend to promote and prolong skin rashes, maceration, and bacterial and fungal conditions. Careful consideration and sound judgment should be exercised in using this type of shoe gear to alter the function and mechanics of the patient's lower extremity, especially in the insensate foot. Even though one should carefully consider the above-mentioned drawbacks to man-made material, many of these circumstances can be at least partially overcome. Proper or improved venting can certainly improve the breathability of man-made shoe gear to some degree.[7] In any event, in considering the type of prescriptive orthoses for a particular condition, malfunction or malalignment of the foot and proper shoe size in terms of length, width, and style should be reviewed and evaluated before prescribing.

Lower extremity range of motion study

An appropriately prescribed orthosis emanates from a well-planned and thorough biomechanical evaluation, following a detailed description of the presenting complaint, along with the history of the presenting illness. Past medical history, systems review and physical examination, a list of positive and pertinent findings, diagnosis, and a treatment plan must all be completed prior to determining whether or not orthoses are appropriate for the patient's pathologic condition.

The biomechanical evaluation should document the range of motion of each major joint affected by ground reactive forces during normal standing and walking. The range of motion of the hip joint should document the range of internal and external rotation. The total range of motion should be noted. The effective neutral position should likewise be documented as it may be a significant influential factor that needs to be controlled for effective foot function. The malleolar position should be evaluated by placing the posterior aspect of the knee joint on the frontal plane and the subtalar joint neutral, with the midtarsal joint pronated. The angle formed by a line passing through the transverse plane of the medial and lateral malleoli and to the frontal plane of the knee is noted and measured to reflect the malleolar position. Ankle joint dorsiflexion is measured with the knee joint fully extended and the subtalar joint in its neutral position.[23] The subtalar and midtarsal joints are fully assessed. The first-ray range of motion is evaluated in reference to movement above and below the level of the adjacent second ray. Although this measurement is difficult to quantify, the practitioner can effectively evaluate and identify the existence or absence of either a dorsiflexed or plantarflexed first ray.[4,5]

Following the biomechanical evaluation, a gait analysis is performed which chronicles the visible moments of motion each foot and extremity produce during the swing and stance phases of gait.

Based on an interpretation of the gait analysis, along with the positive and pertinent findings in the biomechanical examination, a determination is made as to what type of device should be prescribed.

Casting for foot orthoses

The particular casting procedure is certainly deserving of ample time and discussion for it is this procedure that has the tendency to radically influence the success or failure of the treatment plan. Careful positioning and procuring of the negative impression slipper cast stands as the single most important procedure in this process. Most essential is development of the ability to produce an accurate negative cast with the subtalar joint neutral and the midtarsal joint fully pronated about both axes of motion. This is achieved by first positioning the patient on the examining chair or table with the knee slightly flexed. The lower leg may be slightly internally rotated. This position helps to prevent the extremity from externally rotating as the foot is held in the casting position. If the leg externally rotates, a supinatory force would produce a supinated negative impression cast. This would necessitate the need to repeat the casting process. The examiner should take care to be positioned comfortably so as to prevent fatigue or postural stress during the procedure. As the prepositioning process continues, the examiner simulates grasping the fourth and fifth digits properly in order to efficiently suspend the foot during the casting process. Care is taken to ensure that the examiner's thumb does not protrude beneath the patient's third metatarsophalangeal joint. This can inadvertently produce a supinatory force at the level of the longitudinal axis of the midtarsal joint,

thereby lessening the opportunity to produce an accurate impression of the patient's foot.

Following the prepositioning process, plaster bandage splints (5 × 30 in.) are applied to the patient's foot. This can be achieved by using two splints coupled with a 1/4-in. fold to offer rigidity to the posterior aspect of the cast. The plaster then is layered circumferentially around the medial, lateral, and plantar aspect of the foot. An alternative approach is to use two plaster splints each doubled in half. The first splint has a 1/4-in. fold for rigidity around the heel of the slipper cast. This splint is then applied around the posterior aspect of the heel, ending medially at the base of the first metatarsal and laterally at the base of the fifth metatarsal. The casting plaster is smoothed and attached to the plantar-medial and plantar-lateral aspect of the foot by gently but vigorously smoothing the plaster with the palm. The second splint is applied in a similar fashion to the distal, medial, lateral, and plantar surfaces of the foot with careful smoothing to produce a jointless slipper cast. Without hesitation, the examiner assumes the position of suspending the patient's foot by grasping the fourth and fifth digits as described during the repositioning process to help identify the subtalar joint neutral position. All that is necessary at this point is to lift the foot in a vertical direction by grasping the toes. This aids in locking the midtarsal joint about both axes of motion.

After the plaster impression is set, it is safe to remove the plaster cast from the foot, taking care to avoid any alterations to the captured contours contained within the body of the cast. The impression cast is then compared with the foot while the foot is again placed in the casting position. All contours visualized in the plaster impression cast are compared with the involved foot. The contours captured in this impression cast most accurately duplicate the contours of the soft tissue alignment around the posterior, medial, lateral, and plantar aspects of the foot (i.e., subtalar joint neutral position, midtarsal joint longitudinal and oblique axes).

Although alternative casting techniques similar to the above were described by Root et al.,[4,5] some are quite possibly much easier to master. The important goal to remember is that you must obtain a negative cast that places the foot in the best functional position. That position is most often with the subtalar joint in its neutral position and the midtarsal joint fully pronated about both axes of motion. (For a complete discussion regarding various casting techniques, see Chapter 12.)

Once an acceptable cast is obtained, the impressions are allowed to dry overnight before shipping to the orthotics laboratory. The prescription should

Jones Functional Orthotic Laboratory

Log No:_____   Date: _____

Doctor's Name:_____

Doctor's Address: _____

          City: _____ State:_____ Zip:_____

Account No: _____

Patient's Name:

          Age: _____ Sex: _____ Height: _____ Weight: _____

          Shoe Size: ___ Width: _____ Style: ____ Heel Height: _____

Diagnosis: _____

Description of Plantar Lesions: _____

Morphological Data	**Left**	**Right**
1. Rearfoot		
a. Varus	_____	_____
b. Valgus	_____	_____
2. Forefoot		
a. Varus	_____	_____
b. Valgus	_____	_____

Positive Cast Correction
- ☐ 1. Medial Arch Filler   ☐ Normal   ☐ See special instructions
- ☐ 2. Lateral Expansion   ☐ Normal   ☐ See special instructions
- ☐ 3. Intrinsic Forefoot Balancing   ☐ Heel Vertical
  - a. Balance heel inverted   ☐ Left ___°   ☐ Right ___°
  - b. Balance heel everted   ☐ Left ___°   ☐ Right ___°

Orthotic Construction
1) Heel Cup Height   ☐ Normal   Left__mm   Right__mm
2) Orthotic Width   ☐ Normal   ☐ Wide   ☐ Narrow
3) Plantar Fascia Accommodation   Left__mm   Right__mm
4) Top Cover___ Specify: _____
5) Bottom (over-specify): _____
6) Forefoot Accommodation (specify): _____
7) Material Required (specify): _____
8) Posting: Forefoot   Left___°   Right___°
                        Varus__   Valgus__ (Check one)
              Rearfoot   Left___°   Right___°

Fig. 13-1. Prescription form for a functional and an accommodative foot orthosis.

be clear and detailed. All intrinsic as well as extrinsic modifications to the positive cast should be detailed to minimize and limit any unnecessary laboratory judgments which may increase the opportunity for laboratory error and lead to malfunctioning of the final product (Fig. 13-1).

Once the negative cast is received by the laboratory, it is inspected for assurance that the cast has not been distorted during packaging and shipping.

Orthotic fabrication process

The following discussion relates to the fabrication of a functional foot orthosis. A reference line is inscribed bisecting the posterior surface of the cast (Fig. 13-2**A**). Separating media are used to prevent the negative cast from adhering to the positive cast during the curing process. A wedge is used to tilt the forefoot of the cast, which positions the heel bisector vertical to the supporting surface (Fig. 13-2**B**). Liq-

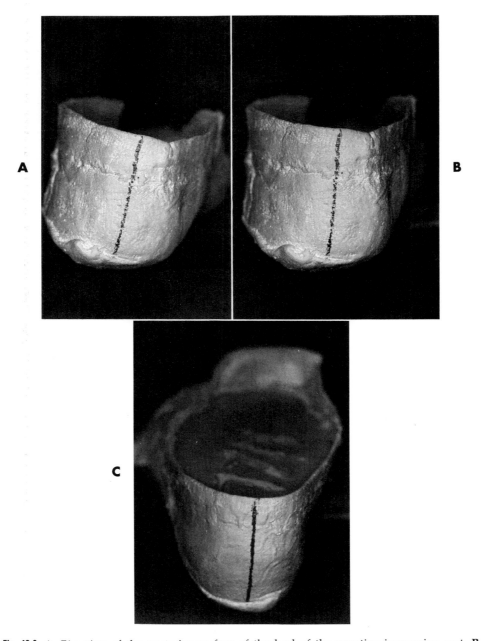

Fig. 13-2. A, Bisection of the posterior surface of the heel of the negative impression cast. **B,** Positioning the heel bisection vertical to the supporting surface by wedging the forefoot of the cast. **C,** Positive cast before removal of the negative cast.

uefied plaster material is then poured to fill the entire interior of the cast. The cast is then tapped or jogged gently, releasing any trapped air pockets, thereby allowing for a stronger, smoother, setting. After the cast has set, a reference marking is transferred to the positive cast (Fig. 13-2C). This reference marking is used to correct or balance the positive cast in preparation for fabrication of the orthosis. This reference marking can be the transfer of the heel bisector from the negative cast to the positive cast. An alternative method suggested by Root et

al.[4,5] places a devil's level transversely on the superior surface of the positive cast as the forefoot of the cast is wedged to bring the superior surface of the cast into a level position. This position is the reference mark.

The negative cast is then stripped from the positive cast. The meniscus found on the superior surface of the positive cast is removed with a file or cutting instrument which helps to ensure that the cast sits firmly on the pressing apparatus during fabrication of the orthosis.

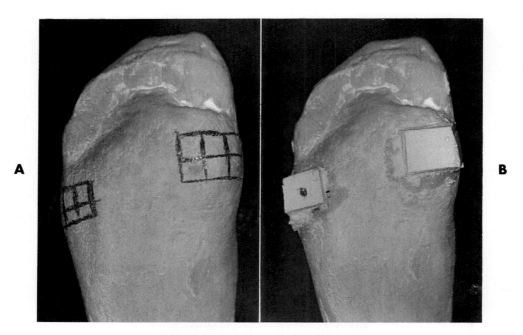

Fig. 13-3. A, Reference marking for intrinsic forefoot balancing during the positive cast correction technique. **B,** Reference and corrective platforms for intrinsic balancing of the positive cast.

The forefoot correction is achieved by two methods. These methods use either an intrinsic or extrinsic balancing technique. The intrinsic technique requires application of a reference or noncorrective platform and a balancing, or corrective, platform. For example, when balancing a cast that contains a forefoot varus deformity, the reference platform is located beneath the fifth metatarsal head of the cast and the balance platform is located beneath the first metatarsal head. The reverse is the case for a forefoot valgus deformity (Fig. 13-3**A**). There are variations that should be noted. A structurally plantarflexed or excessively long third metatarsal requires that the third metatarsal head be the reference platform, and that the first and fifth metatarsal heads be wedged to properly balance the negative cast. A cast that contains a perpendicular forefoot-to-rearfoot relationship does not require a corrective platform but rather two reference platforms, one each beneath the first and fifth metatarsal heads. In cases of severe midtarsal joint subluxation as seen in the rocker-bottom type of foot, the reference platform may be located at a more proximal location at the styloid process of the fifth metatarsal.[5]

The corrective and reference platforms are applied to the properly identified region of the positive cast (Fig. 13-3**B**). Following application of the platforms, a filler consisting of the same plaster mixture is applied between the medial aspect of the lateral platform and the lateral aspect of the medial platform. A gentle curvature should be apparent with its apex located at the center of the platform. This helps to support the transverse metatarsal arch on the finished orthosis. Following application of the filler, additional plaster is applied to the lateral and medial aspects of the positive cast. This addition is applied to allow for soft tissue expansion on the orthosis during weightbearing. The expansion material helps to bend the edge of the orthosis away from the lateral and medial border of the foot during weightbearing without distorting the normal contour of the orthosis as it aligns with the foot. All irregular surfaces are filled with plaster in the form of a light wash in the final smoothing process[2] (Fig. 13-4**A–E**).

The orthosis is fabricated by first outlining the dimensions of the cast on the orthotic blank. The excess material around this perimeter can be sharply removed to facilitate the pressing process (Fig. 13-5**A**, p. 302). When using acrylics, plastics, or a polyethylene foam–like material, a convection oven can be used to evenly heat the material to the desired flexibility. Once heated sufficiently, the blank is aligned with the positive cast and formed under mechanical or vacuum pressure until sufficiently cooled (Figs. 13-5**B** and **C**, p. 302). Once formed, the orthosis is fashioned by using a grinding instrument (Fig. 13-6**A**) to remove all redundant material until the orthosis meets the predetermined dimensions of the positive cast (Fig. 13-6**B–G**, p. 303). The orthosis is finished by polishing and buffing.

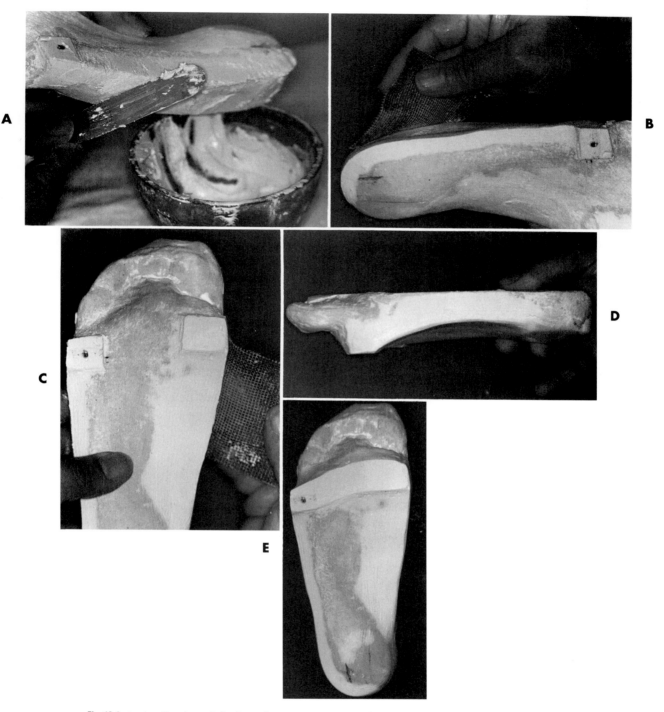

Fig. 13-4. A, Application of the lateral expansion. **B,** Fine finishing by wet-sanding excess plaster material in completing the lateral expansion. **C,** Application of the medial arch filler. **D,** Observation of the maintenance of the longitudinal curvature of the medial arch following application of the medial arch filler. **E,** Completion of the preparation process of the positive cast.

Rearfoot posting is used to stabilize the foot against ground reactive forces during the initial contact phase of gait. The rounded or curved surface of the plantar aspect of the plastic or nonflexible acrylic-type orthosis, termed the *heel contact point,* does little to effectively stabilize the foot up to forefoot contact. Therefore, a rearfoot post is used to limit the amount of motion during the initial contact

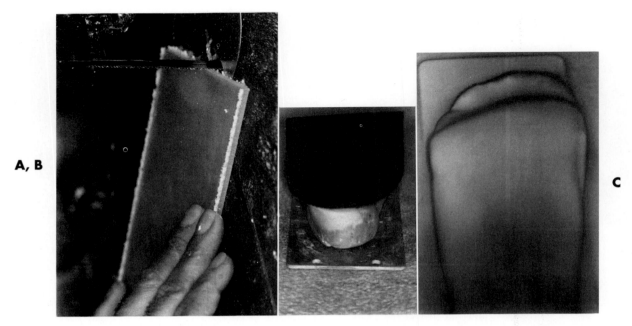

A, B

C

Fig. 13-5. A, Shaping the plastic blank before fabrication of the orthosis. **B,** Placement of the plastic blank on the positive cast for formation of the orthosis. **C,** Pressing of the orthosis by vacuum pressure.

phase of gait. The degree of control can be determined by the rigidity of the material used. An acrylic-type post limits motion significantly during the contact phases of gait. Owing to its rigidity, however, shock absorption is poor. One way to improve shock absorption is to grind into the post a specific degree of motion. This is accomplished by angling the medial side of the post to the lateral side.

Crepe, composition cork-nylon, and moldable polyethylene foam of firmer dimension can be used effectively as a rearfoot post. This type of post tends to compress with time, and is quicker to lose effectiveness in controlling heel contact motion. Often these materials are reinforced with a thin layer of plastic such as polypropylene to improve the life expectancy of the post. The overall purpose of the rearfoot post is to allow at least 4 to 6 degrees of calcaneal eversion during heel contact subtalar joint pronation to achieve the mobile adaptability function of the foot during this phase of gait.

The same material can be used extrinsically on the anterior edge of the orthosis when considering extrinsic forefoot posting. The use of extrinsic forefoot posting is limited owing to the difficulty in fitting the orthosis in shoe gear when dealing with large forefoot deformities. The plaster cast correction uses two reference platforms, one each beneath the first and fifth metatarsal heads. The unfinished and formed orthosis is wedged and marked beneath the positive cast until the reference surface is level. The balancing material is applied and allowed to

cure with the cast in the corrected position. Once cured, the fabrication is completed to produce the finished product.

Extrinsic corrections to the orthosis

There are occasions when it is necessary to use rearfoot corrective posting on an orthosis to significantly or totally restrict heel contact motion. This is achieved by instructing the laboratory to eliminate the normally prescribed medial grind which allows for normal subtalar joint motion during the initial contact phase of gait. This special instruction—"no motion"—is used in situations where a functional orthosis is prescribed for treatment of conditions such as peroneal spastic flatfoot, post calcaneal fracture, post talar and transchondral fractures of the talus, and post fibular fracture. It is often necessary to use this posting technique to limit axial loading stress through these areas. When using this technique, it is advisable to incorporate it with a deep heel cup both medially and laterally with these borders as high as the shoe will accommodate.[5]

Since it is often necessary to use a rearfoot post on a functional orthosis to control pronation at heel contact, it is important to ensure that the orthosis and post interface properly with the interior of the shoe. To achieve this goal, a posting elevator or adjustor is used to raise the heel seat of the orthosis relative to the anterior or distal edge of the orthosis when the rearfoot post is applied and allowed to

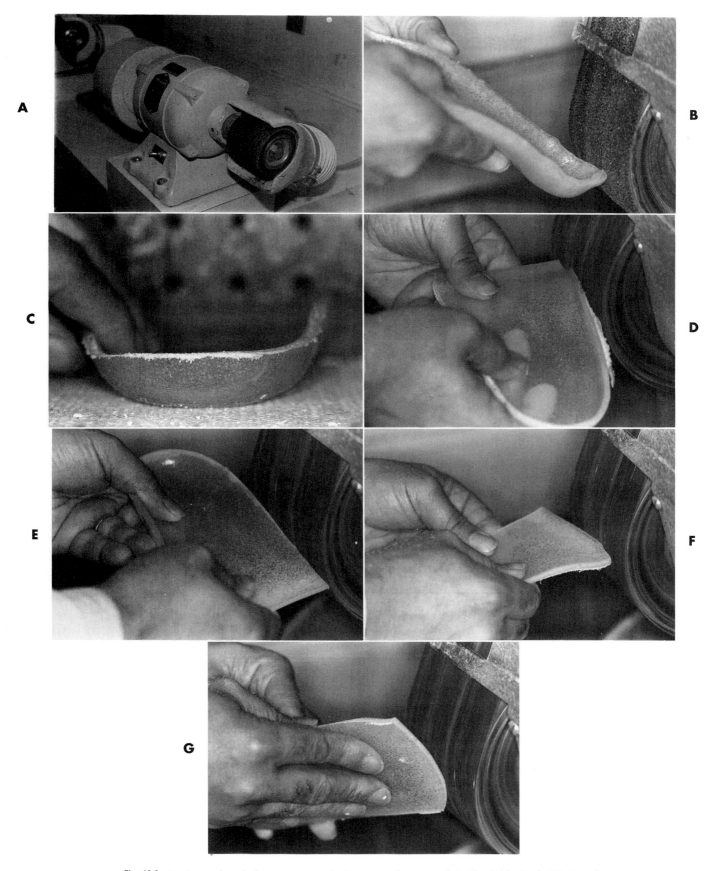

Fig. 13-6. **A,** A one-fourth horsepower grinder properly secured to the table to facilitate safe grinding of the orthosis. **B,** Removing the excess plastic material to develop the superior margin of the heel seat of the orthosis. **C,** Completion of the perimeter of the heel seat. **D,** Establishing the lateral margin. **E,** Establishing the medial margin. **F,** Establishing the distal limit. **G,** Application of a 45-degree bevel around the perimeter.

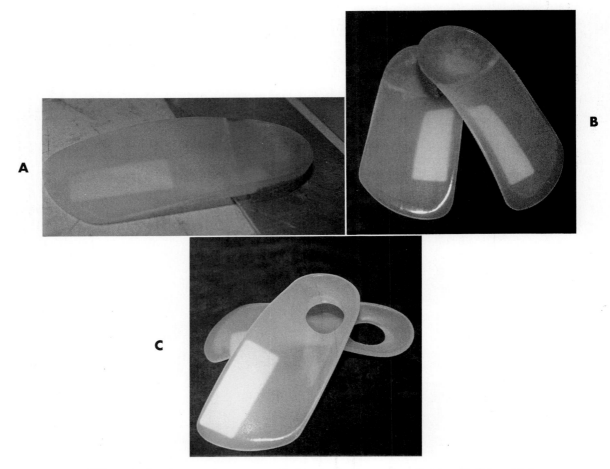

Fig. 13-7. **A,** Cork-nylon rearfoot post applied on a 4-mm posting elevator. **B,** Polypropylene functional foot orthoses with cork-nylon rearfoot posts. **C,** Polypropylene orthoses with the contact point ground out to facilitate use in women's flats and pumps.

properly cure. The elevator or height adjustor minimizes the possibility of the post being unstable. When using an acrylic posting material, which is often more rigid than the thermoplastic type of material such as Rohadur or Polydur, the elevator selection becomes relatively important in helping to prevent breakage of the orthosis. This may be caused by stress, which usually forces the orthosis to bend just distal to the anterior edge of the rearfoot post. The height of the elevator usually ranges from 4 to 12 mm. Jogging shoes, wedge-heeled shoes, and most Oxford-style shoes generally require no more than a 4-mm elevator for efficient function. (Fig. 13-7**A**). Higher-heeled shoes generally require higher elevators. It should be noted that the more flexible materials such as composition cork-nylon, crepe, and vacuum-formed polypropylene–type rearfoot posts have eliminated this problem (Fig. 13-7**B**). It should be noted, however, that often there is less heel contact pronation control with these less

rigid posting materials. In instances where shoe fit is a problem, the rearfoot post may be eliminated and the heel contact point ground out to allow the device to ride lower in the shoe (see Fig. 13-7**C**).

Other conditions, such as limb length inequality, can be accommodated either partially or completely by adding additional posting material to the rearfoot position. It is often necessary to modify either the exterior sole or inner lining of the shoe to fully accommodate limb length inequalities and improve overall lower extremity function in gait. When using an elevated rearfoot post to accommodate for a limb length discrepancy, shoes with a fairly deep heel counter are used to prevent the heel from rising above the rim of the heel counter, thereby creating further instability in gait.[5]

This chapter has centered around the construction of orthoses for the neutral suspension casting technique originally described by Root et al.[5] The heel of this cast is bisected for reference balancing

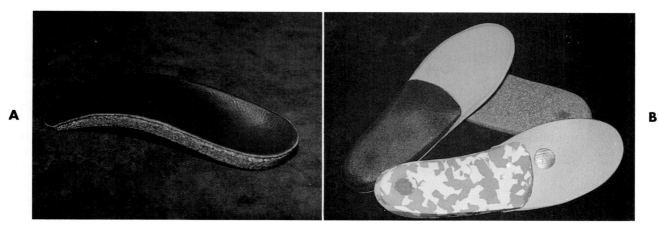

Fig. 13-8. A, Leather and Korex accommodative foot orthosis. **B,** Three accommodative devices. *From Top Clockwise,* Leather and Korex, ethylene vinyl acetate and Poron with additional accommodation for prominent second metatarsal head, and firm Plastazote and Poron.

during the pouring process for conversion of the negative cast to a positive cast. The superior surface of the positive cast is used as the level reference surface by which all intrinsic balance corrections are achieved during the preparatory process. The expansion modification for the medial-lateral surfaces of the cast have been described with reference to the necessity that the orthotic material mold correctly to the shape of the positive cast. All these are basic steps in the development of a functional orthosis.[5]

There are a few modifications that one should consider prescribing under special instances. A medial arch filler is used to bend the medial edge of the orthosis away from the medial longitudinal arch in cases where a large metatarsus adductus or forefoot adductus is present. Casts that demonstrate less of an adductus type will ultimately need less of a medial arch filler. A plantar fascial accommodation may be useful in accommodating this condition. When prescribing functional foot orthoses for rigid or semirigid cavus feet, care must be taken not to irritate the plantar fascia. Since the apex of the deformity in this foot type is most often at the region where the orthosis has its greatest rigidity, a plantar fascial groove in the orthosis helps to lessen the pressure. Other common uses of this modification include conditions of acute chronic plantar fasciitis and an abnormally bowstrung plantar fascia. The prescription should indicate the depth of the accommodation in millimeters as well as having the accommodation appropriately delineated on the negative cast. An average amount of plantar fascial accommodation is 2 to 4 mm.

The elimination of the filler between the platforms is usually prescribed when treating congenital plantarflexed first-ray and uncompensated forefoot varus deformities. Elimination of the filler increases the amount of weightbearing borne by the lesser metatarsals. A cuboid filler is used to accommodate for a foot with a plantarflexed cuboid. This is demonstrated in the negative cast by the accentuated contour of the lateral arch, which should be gentle. With this filler, the orthosis is prevented from exerting undue pressure during weightbearing. In cases where there is a prominent styloid process resulting from severe subluxatory changes in the foot, a plaster filler is added to this region of the cast. This alters the contour of the cast and reduces the possibility of irritation when walking.[5]

There are alternative casting techniques that may be used for fabricating accommodative orthoses. The neutral suspension cast, as first described by Root et. al., can likewise be used with specific instructions for accommodations.[4,5] The alternative casting techniques are (1) semiweightbearing casting, and (2) in-shoe vacuum casting described by Brown and Smith.[9] Although there are many other modifications, the remainder of this discussion centers around these two techniques.

The semiweightbearing casting technique is relatively simple to perform. No specialized equipment is needed. The patient is seated on a regular chair, with the thigh perpendicular to the lower leg and the foot placed on the floor perpendicular to the lower leg. The lower leg is slightly rotated in the transverse plane so that the foot is aligned with the subtalar joint neutral and in the patient's normal angle of gait. Beneath the foot is a foam block which supports the foot during the casting procedure. The heel region of the foam block has a 1/4-in. heel elevator to reproduce the pitch of the interior of a standard shoe. The plaster splints are applied to the foot in the same manner as described for the suspension casting technique. The foot is then placed on the cast foam block at the desired angle of gait. Care is taken to ensure that the foot is perpendicular to the lower leg. The plaster is allowed to harden with care taken to ensure that the plaster has not withdrawn from the foot since the foot is dependent. Prior to application of this casting technique, any areas needing accommodation should be well circumscribed with a marker to ensure proper duplication onto the plaster material. Since the foot is dependent during this casting process, the cast, in contrast to the suspension cast, will demonstrate broader and less well-defined contoured surfaces. This occurs because it places the plantar soft tissue structures under pressure, allowing the medial and lateral perimeters to expand. This produces less of a need for corrective positive plaster cast expansion or filler modifications.

Once the laboratory has prepared the positive cast, the accommodative dimensions are designed in preparation for production of the accommodative orthoses. This casting technique is particularly useful in the insensate foot where functional control is not the paramount focus. This type of device provides some degree of balance and relief of pressure beneath a bony prominence or lessens the stress on an area of excrescence or depression. This technique also facilitates development of an orthosis from a variety of materials such as leather and Korex, with Silastic reinforcement. This is a fairly standard orthosis which has withstood the test of time. The leather is durable and breathable. Korex provides good shock absorption during ambulation and provides for appropriate accommodations. The Silastic reinforces the strength and durability of the device. This type of device falls within the category of a semirigid orthosis. (Fig. 13-8**A** and **B**). A similar device is the Levymold. This device is composed of wood flour, granulated cork, and liquid latex. It too is very durable and has withstood the test of time. The laboratory may increase the rigidity of this device by increasing the ratio of wood flour to granulated cork in the mixture or make the device more flexible by reversing the process. Once the material has solidified on the cast and the excess has been removed by grinding, the interior is covered with 5-oz. strap leather and trimmed to fit the dimensions of the patient's shoe. This orthosis is usually a full-foot orthosis. Remnants of this material may be used and applied to the plantar surface of the orthosis to further accommodate or post the device at a later date.

The final casting procedure to be discussed is the vacuum casting or Biovac® system.[1] This procedure was initially described by Smith and Brown during the mid-1970's as an alternative negative casting system. The system is reproducible with less chance for error in proper subtalar joint and midtarsal joint positioning. Another advantage is that this is an in-shoe casting technique which allows the laboratory to actually see how the foot must adapt to the particular shoe style with an orthosis. The technique is particularly appropriate when prescribing functional orthoses for women who for professional or other reasons must wear high-heeled shoes. It should be noted that this is an acceptable alternative to the negative casting techniques used for functional or accommodative orthoses.

One of the most popular types of orthoses used for "fashionable" shoes are those made from materials similar to fiberglass combined with epoxy resins. This process consists of various layers of these similarly laminated materials which can produce a varied range of orthoses in terms of flexibility or rigidity. Added accommodations, forefoot extensions, or heel accommodations can be incorporated.

In conclusion, this chapter has covered a broad range of information involving the biomechanical evaluation, various casting procedures, and the process of fabrication of orthoses. Production of an effective orthosis stems from a thorough evaluation of the presenting condition of the patient. The thoroughness of the evaluation coupled with the accuracy of the practitioner's negative cast are the major determinants as to whether or not laboratories are able to fabricate an appropriate functional orthosis.

The same may be remarked concerning the fabrication of a prescriptive accommodative orthosis. It is the practitioner's evaluation and casting that separate these professionally fabricated devices from over-the-counter nonprescription arch supports.

References

1. Brown D, Smith CE: Vacuum casting for foot orthoses. J Am Podiatry Assoc 66:585–1587, 1976.
2. Hicks JH: The mechanics of the foot. J Anat 87:345, 1953.
3. Inman V: The Joints of the Ankle. 1976.
4. Root ML, Orien WP, Weed JH: Normal and Abnormal Function of the Foot, vol 2. Los Angeles, Clinical Biomechanics Corp, 1977.
5. Root ML, Orien WP, Weed JH, et al. Biomechanical Examination of the Foot, vol I. Los Angeles, Clinical Biomechanics Corp, 1971.
6. Sgarlatto T: A Compendium of Podiatric Biomechanics. California College of Podiatric Medicine, San Francisco: Board of Trustees of the California College of Podiatric Medicine Corporation. 1971.
7. Wu KK: Foot Orthoses: Principles and Clinical Applications. Baltimore, Williams & Wilkins, 1990, pp 49–142.

orthotic materials

William R. Olson, DPM

History
Efficacy of functional orthoses
Materials
Comparison of materials for functional foot orthoses
Summary

The functional orthosis is an orthopedic device that is designed to promote structural integrity of the joints of the foot and lower limb by resisting ground reaction forces that cause abnormal skeletal motion to occur during the stance phase of gait.[1] This working definition of a functional orthosis accurately describes not only what a functional orthosis is, but establishes the basic design objectives which have effectively been in place since the time of the earliest attempts at foot orthosis fabrication. Achieving these stated objectives in a clinical setting has proven to be an elusive goal for practitioners, as indicated by the many modifications in the design and construction of the functional foot orthosis down through the decades. These modifications and advancements have, however, largely been the result of a rapidly expanding body of clinical and laboratory research which has effectively refined the level of understanding of how ground reaction forces generated during closed kinetic chain activities affect the musculoskeletal units of the lower extremity. A significant part of this evolution in the understanding and management of lower extremity biomechanical function is in the area of materials research.

History

Originally, foot orthoses were designed primarily to redistribute the pressures on the plantar aspect of the foot.[104] While effective in this capacity, they had limited benefit in controlling the abnormal biomechanical forces causing lower extremity pathology. This inadequacy in the design of the early arch supports led to the eventual development of devices that were designed to control motion at specific joints as opposed to merely redistributing plantar pressures.[59] One of the first such devices was described by Whitman,[126] who used a metal foot brace incorporating a high medial and lateral flange. Subsequently, Roberts developed a metal device similar to the one described by Whitman, but in an effort to reduce bulk, eliminated the flanges and attempted to control the rearfoot through the use of medial and lateral heel clips along with a deeply inverted heel cup.[105] Schuster later combined the features of the Whitman and Roberts devices to make the Roberts-Whitman brace. This device made use of the deep, inverted heel cup of the Roberts-Whitman orthosis, as well as the flanges, which were a key feature of the Whitman brace. Again, steel was the material of choice.

As experimentation with early orthotic design continued, fundamental biomechanical relationships were beginning to appear in the literature. Jones[60] and later Hicks[56] described the association

between tibial rotation and subtalar motion. Rose[100] developed a model of the foot incorporating the axes of the ankle, subtalar, and first- and fifth-ray joints.

By the late 1950s and early 1960s, many of the key fundamental principles of lower extremity biomechanical function had been discovered and described. It was also during this time that the functional foot orthosis was developed by Root.[1] The result of extensive laboratory and clinical research, the design for the prototype Root functional orthosis is still firmly established as the standard for the vast majority of foot orthoses made today. While the materials used for the original Root functional device were a mixture of oak wood flour and latex, plexiglass soon became the material of choice for this device.[1]

Research in the area of lower extremity bone and joint motion continued to move forward, advanced by gait studies performed using two (2-D)- and three-dimensional (3-D) cinematographic techniques as well as x-ray stereophotogrammetric analysis.* These studies brought significant advancements in the understanding of specific joint motion as related to ground reaction forces incurred during gait,† in the determination of subtalar neutral position,[37,99] and in joint axis position in static stance[62] and as related to joint motion.[23]

The significant contributions made by these researchers in the understanding of human locomotion and specific lower extremity joint function during gait brought forth modifications of the original Root functional orthosis. The inverted functional orthosis introduced by Blake[11] resulted from attempts to control excessive pronation not responsive to the standard Root device. Based on dynamic measurements of pronation rather than on the static alignment of the foot obtained from a nonweightbearing examination, kinematic analysis has shown the Blake technique to control excessive pronation when traditional orthoses have failed.[2] Polysectional triaxial posting, described by Lundeen,[68] and the medial skive technique, described by Kirby,[63] also represented significant modifications in the design of the basic functional orthosis, which enhances the ability of the functional orthosis to control abnormal foot motion in certain instances.

Efficacy of functional orthoses

The clinical relevance of advancements in lower extremity biomechanical research and functional

---

* References 2–9, 23, 26, 27, 32–34, 37, 45, 62, 96, 99, 108, 111, 112, 119, 122.

† References 3–5, 23, 33, 45, 112, 119, 122.

foot orthosis design is found in numerous studies documenting both the objective efficacy of functional orthoses in controlling excessive pronation, as well as in subjective reports documenting the frequency of symptomatic relief achieved through the use of these devices. A review of the literature reveals numerous reports of successful outcomes when functional foot orthoses are used to treat overuse injuries and malalignment syndromes of the lower extremities.

Subjective reports documenting the success of functional foot orthoses in providing symptomatic relief can be found in the podiatric, orthopedic, family practice, and physical therapy literature.* Campbell and Inman,[22] in a study of patients presenting with a chief complaint of plantar fasciitis, reported that 31 of the 33 (94%) patients receiving functional orthoses reported symptomatic improvement. Donatelli et al.[41] studied 53 patients and used a questionnaire to collect information regarding the success of "semirigid" orthoses in relieving various lower extremity conditions. In this study, semirigid orthoses were described as being made from "plastic and fiberglass." In the population described, orthotic intervention was effective in relieving pain in 51 (96%) patients. James et al.[57] showed that 78% of runners were able to return to their running program after being fitted with orthoses to treat various injuries. D'Ambrosia and Douglas[40] reported a similar success rate using foot orthoses. Blake and Denton[12] performed a retrospective study of patients receiving functional foot orthoses, 98% of which were described as "rigid." The success rate of the orthoses in these patients was 70% as determined by a response of "definitely helped" on a questionnaire. Ferguson et al.[46] performed another prospective study comparing TL-61 (Medical Materials Corp., Camarillo, Calif.) and Rohadur orthoses in the specific treatment of heel spur syndrome. In this study, 85% of the patients reported improvement of symptoms and no difference was noted in the patient response between TL-61 and Rohadur. Richie and Olson,[95] in a prospective study of 40 athletes, reported a 72% rating (29/40) of good-excellent in terms of a symptomatic relief in a study comparing TL-2100 Semi-Flexible and 3/16-in. polypropylene. The effectiveness of orthoses in the treatment of patients with patellofemoral pain syndrome was investigated by Eng and Pierrynowski.[44] In this study, a subject population of 20 adolescent female patients were treated, with 10 patients receiving orthoses in addition to an exercise rehabilitation program and a control group of 10

* References 12, 13, 17, 22, 36, 40, 42, 43, 44, 46, 52, 57, 67, 78, 80, 81, 90, 93, 95, 103, 116, 118, 120.

patients receiving the rehabilitation program alone. Their findings revealed that overall improvement of symptoms was noted in both groups, but the improvement in the group receiving orthoses was significantly greater than that in the group not receiving orthoses. In this study, "soft" orthoses were used. Santoro et al.,[103] in a survey of seven alpine skiers wearing functional orthoses made from unspecified materials, reported improved performance and relief of fatigue in four (57%) and improved comfort in five (71%) of subjects questioned.

Subjective benefit is also documented in the clinical management of acute and chronic symptomatic manifestations of osteoarthritis in studies by Thompson et al.[120] and Moskowitz et al.[80]; however, mention of materials from which the orthoses were made was limited and nonspecific. The largest study documenting the effectiveness of functional foot orthoses was that by Moraros and Hodge.[78] A total of 453 patients were followed for a 14-week period after receiving functional foot orthoses to treat a wide variety of lower extremity abnormalities. General satisfaction with the orthotic therapy was reported by 83% of the subjects. At the end of the 14-week period, 62% of the subjects reported that the initial chief complaint had been fully resolved, while 32% reported partial resolution of symptoms. Although a wide variety of orthosis types with various material compositions were used in this study, the authors made no mention of any correlation of clinical improvement with any particular type of orthotic material.

Also of note in a review of the literature is the near absence of reported complications resulting from the use of foot orthoses. While the incidence of "no improvement" ranged from 4.0% to 12.5%[12,46,52] in the aforementioned studies, no direct injury was documented as the specific result of wearing orthoses. Further, in the few studies where strictly rigid orthoses were used, 85% to 89% of the patients surveyed reported that their symptoms improved "definitely or somewhat," while no complications were reported.[12,46] These studies indicate that the opinion expressed by Baxter,[7,8] that the wearing of rigid orthoses may result in complications, addresses only the rare and exceptional case and pales in the face of the overwhelming evidence that supports the efficacy of functional foot orthoses in the alleviation of lower extremity musculoskeletal symptoms. It seems, however, that where poor outcomes are reported through the use of functional orthoses, shortcomings on the part of the practitioner, such as lack of knowledge or understanding of prescription details and materials selection, errors in impression casting, and failure to recognize foot deformities that require specific orthosis modification, and errors or imprecision on the part of the laboratory in positive cast correction and orthosis fabrication, are sufficient to explain these occasional occurrences.[109,117] These errors must be considered when interpreting the results of any study documenting either the subjective or objective results of orthotic therapy.

In addition to the subjective reports of positive patient response to the use of functional foot orthoses, the literature also is replete with objective evidence documenting the efficacy of functional orthoses in controlling foot and leg motion.* Frontal plane movement of the calcaneus has been the primary indicator for measurement of foot pronation in studies on foot orthoses, while control of excessive foot pronation has been the primary objective in the prescription of functional foot orthoses.[41,90] The assumption that heel counter movement represents actual calcaneal movement has been validated by Clarke et al.,[33] Stacoff et al.,[113] and Nigg et al.,[82] but questioned by Cavanagh and Edgington.[28] Reinschmidt et al.[94] also questioned the accuracy of shoe markers in the evaluation of foot motion in a shoe, but their study was limited to lateral motion sports.

Motion control has been documented through the use of orthoses made from materials described as soft,[34,111] semirigid,[34,52,96,111,119] and rigid.[2,52,108] Clarke et al.[34] reported a 2.5-degree decrease in maximum pronation, while Smith et al.[111] showed a decrease in pronation velocity, both using what they termed "soft" orthoses. This finding was similar to that of Cavanagh et al.,[27] where four subjects showed a decrease of 2 degrees in the amount of maximum pronation with each layer of 6-mm-thick adhesive felt applied to the medial border of the subject's shoes. Cavanagh et al. also showed a progressive decrease in the peak angular velocity of pronation as increasing thickness of the felt was applied. Functional orthoses described as "semiflexible" by their researchers have also been proven effective in controlling the total amount of pronation in various studies. The maximal pronation during support has been reported to be decreased by 1 to 2 degrees with the use of semirigid orthoses in studies employing 10 or more subjects.[96,111,119] In a study by Cornwall and McPoil,[38] a reduction in force-time integral was reported through the use of "semirigid" orthoses. In this case, the material from which the orthoses were made was described, consisting of laminated Aliplast (Alimed Inc., Dedham, Mass.) of different densities. Through the use of "rigid"

orthoses, Sims[108] demonstrated a mean decrease of 2.5 degrees in midstance pronation. Baitch et al.,[2] also documented, through kinematic evaluation, a significant reduction in tibiocalcaneal eversion with standard Root functional and 25-degree Inverted orthoses. In this study, the material used was 4-mm Rohadur.

While the subjective benefits of functional foot orthoses are well documented, as is their ability to control excessive pronation, the optimal type of orthosis to be used to achieve the desired effects reported in these studies remains somewhat obscure. It is, however, through the efforts of researchers seeking to determine whether or not the use of functional foot orthoses results in measurable physiologic benefit, that a significant variable in the material from which orthoses may be made is revealed.

While some studies have shown a physiologic benefit in terms of oxygen consumption (Vo_2) from the use of functional orthoses,[55,87] most studies indicate that, at least in runners, Vo_2 is actually increased with functional orthosis use.[19,115] In a study[19] comparing absolute Vo_2 in 21 male runners wearing a shoe only versus wearing a shoe with a 160-g orthosis, an increase of 1.4% in absolute Vo_2 was noted. The orthoses used in this study were reported to be made using polypropylene and were classified as "semirigid" by the authors.[19] It is hypothesized that where diminished running economy is noted with orthosis use, that the sheer weight of the device is the reason for this finding.[25,39,54,109] Catlin and Dressendorfer[25] found that the addition of 100 g of mass per shoe resulted in a 1.9% increase in absolute Vo_2, while 175 g per shoe of added weight resulted in a 3.3% increase. Support for this theory comes from the work of several investigators who have shown that the metabolic cost of a load carried on the foot is approximately six times the cost of the same load carried on the waist.[47,77] Further insight into the effects of foot orthoses on running economy comes from Frederick et al.,[48] who reported a 2.8% energy savings for treadmill running using well-cushioned shoes vs. poorly cushioned shoes of similar weight. Frederick et al. further hypothesized that a possible explanation for this is that greater muscular effort is exerted to provide cushioning when the shoe itself does not provide adequate shock absorption. It may be inferred from the studies performed on the effects on running economy with orthosis use that the optimal material for use in functional orthosis fabrication would be a material of minimal weight, yet sufficiently rigid and strong so as to resist abnormal forces. It would also provide the ability to

---

* References 2–6, 13, 27, 33, 34, 38, 72, 75, 96, 108, 111, 119.

Table 14-1
Classification of orthotic materials by various authors

| Authors | Classification | | |
	Soft	Semirigid	Rigid
Anthony[1]			MMA
			TL-2100
Baitch et al.[2]			MMA
Baxter[7]	Felt Cork Leather	Plastazote	MMA
Blake and Denten[12]; Blake and Ferguson[13]			MMA TL-2100 Polypropylene
Burkett et al.[19]			Polypropylene
Clarke et al.[34]	Polyethylene foam		
Cornwall and McPoil[38]		Aliplast	
Donatelli et al.[41]	Aliplast	Plastic with fiberglass	
Ferguson et al.[46]			MMA
Mann[71]	Felt Cork Leather	Plastazote Orthoplast	MMA
McPoil and Cornwall[76]	Plastazote		Polyethylene
Novick et al.[83]			Polyethylene
Olson[85]		Polypropylene Polyethylene	TL-61 MMA
Richie and Olson[95]		Polypropylene TI-2100 Semi-Flexible	
Schwartz[106]			Steel Polypropylene Polyethylene MMA Laminated plastics

absorb shock ideally via resilience in the material itself whereby it could store elastic or strain energy and return it to the body.[95] Such a material, it is hypothesized, could more than offset the negative effects of its weight and cause a net decrease in oxygen uptake,[8,49] while providing the designed beneficial effect of controlling pathogenic motion.

The efficacy of functional foot orthoses is well documented throughout the literature of virtually all of the medical specialties that deal, in some form With lower extremity musculoskeletal pathology. However, specific descriptions of the materials used in the fabrication of the orthoses is generally vague, if described at all, leaving some controversy about the optimal material from which functional foot orthoses should be made. In the remainder of this chapter we examine the various materials from which foot orthoses are made, their mechanical properties, and their properties as they relate to foot function.

Materials

Orthotic materials are typically classified as soft, semirigid, and rigid.* There is, however, no established standard by which one may classify orthotic materials by these terms. Furthermore, since the basis for rendering an orthotic material to one of these categories is, by definition, highly subjective and arbitrary, confusion and disagreement must be the ultimate outcome of such a grouping. This point is well illustrated by the classifications to which various materials are assigned by their respective authors (Table 14-1). Clearly a more in-depth understanding of the properties inherent to the materials used in the fabrication of foot orthoses, as well as the prescription variables that affect their performance in controlling imposed forces, is necessary if the clinician is to attain more consistent, predictable, and reproducible results in their prescriptions of

* References 7, 8, 44, 53, 67, 73, 84, 93, 101, 106.

functional foot orthoses. Possibly of greater significance, however, is that a working knowledge and understanding of these variables will help the clinician avoid the potential complications that may result from errors in the prescription process, particularly as it pertains to material selection and performance.

While there is considerable disagreement as to what constitutes a "soft," "semiflexible," or "rigid" orthosis, there does seem to be a modicum of agreement as to those material properties and performance features that are desirable in an orthotic material. Features such as durability, shape retention, and sufficient rigidity so as to control motion are consistently reported to be important characteristics.* In addition, minimal weight[85,95,106] and ease of fabrication[22,85] are considered important features. Of the vast number of materials that have been used in the fabrication of functional foot orthoses, the composite thermoplastics and a few of the homogeneous thermoplastics manage to achieve all of these criteria. Specifically, TL-2100 (Medical Materials Corp.), the only thermoplastic composite currently available for use in orthosis fabrication, and the polyolefins, polypropylene and polyethylene, represent the only materials which satisfy the rather stringent criteria for foot orthosis fabrication. Rohadur, a long-time standard for functional foot orthosis fabrication, ceased to be produced in 1990, and despite the introduction of several polymethyl methacrylate acrylic polymers since, none, to date, have proven to satisfy the demands of foot orthosis application.

The behavior of orthotic materials, as with all materials subjected to defined forces, depends not only on the fundamental laws of Newtonian mechanics that govern the equilibrium of the forces, but also on the physical characteristics of the materials themselves.[88] In order to understand the relevant physical properties of the materials from which functional foot orthoses are made, it is first necessary to define certain items and principles of basic material analysis with respect to load-bearing behavior.

1. **Force.** *Force* (F) is defined as a unit mass (M) subjected to a unit of acceleration (A) and is determined by the equation $F = M \times A$, with force designated in newtons. An understanding of this relationship is most important in clinical application when assessing the response of orthotic materials to applied stresses, since a material that effectively decelerates the velocity of a mass effectively diminishes the actual force imposed by that

mass. It can therefore be said that an orthosis that provides effective deceleration of motion diminishes the pronatory forces imposed, even if the change in degree of actual measured calcaneal eversion is minimal, and can most definitely result in subjective efficacy through symptomatic improvement or relief. Such is the case with materials that are compliant yet sufficiently resilient to rebound quickly to their original shape. The relatively recent emergence of 2-D and 3-D kinematic studies have been most helpful in assessing the ability of functional foot orthoses of various degrees of stiffness to decelerate pronatory motion, as the steepness of the motion-vs.-time curve indicates the speed and deceleration of pronation over a defined segment of the gait cycle.

2. **Stress.** *Stress* is the force that is applied over an area of a given object and is quantified in newtons per square centimeter (N/cm^2).

3. **Strain.** *Strain* is the elongation or deformation of a part per unit of length when stress is applied. Strain is dimensionless, that is, it has no units. It is simply expressed as a ratio or percentage of the original shape or position of the unit. The relationship between increasing degrees of stress and the strain that results in the material to which the stress is applied is denoted by the *stress-strain* curve for that particular part (Fig. 14-1).

Almost all materials have a deformation that is proportional to the imposed stress over a finite range of applied stress. It is therefore a fact that, for a certain distance from the point of origin, the experimental values of stress vs. strain lie essentially on a straight line. This fact generally holds true for virtually all materials. *Hooke's law* is the statement of that proportionality, and is quantified for a given material by the equation stress/strain = E, where E represents a constant for that particular plastic. That constant is referred to as the *elastic modulus, modulus of elasticity,* or *Young's modulus,* and is unique for not only every plastic, but also for every thickness of a given plastic (see Fig. 14-1). The elastic modulus is, therefore, the slope of the initial straight portion of the stress-strain curve, and defines the *elastic region* for a given material. When stress is applied to a material that is functioning within its elastic region and therefore functioning according to Hooke's law, it will return to its original shape once that load is removed. With these basic principles established, the technical definition of the *elasticity* of material

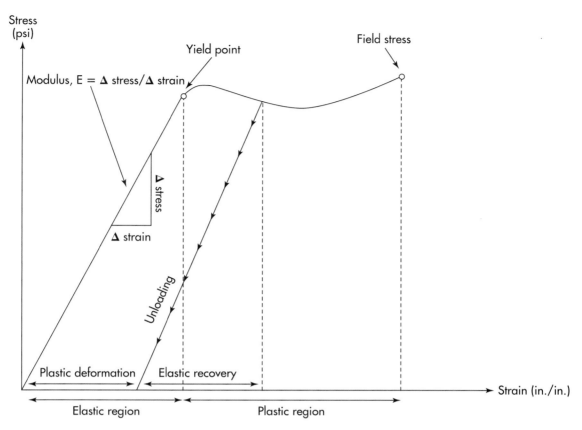

Fig. 14-1. Stress-strain curve for typical plastic materials.

may be made. In such usage, it means that a material is able to regain completely its original dimensions upon removal of the applied forces.

The transition point for a material that defines the end of its elastic region is termed the *yield point*. If stress continues to be applied beyond the yield point for that material, the degree of strain relative to stress will significantly increase and will cease to be proportionate to the applied stress. At this point, that material will perform inelastically and will no longer be performing according to Hooke's law. At this degree of imposed stress, that material will be said to have entered what is referred to as the *plastic region* for that material. When a plastic is loaded to the point that it enters its plastic region, it will not return to its original shape or length. This phenomenon is referred to as *plastic deformation* (see Fig. 14-1).

In orthotic application, materials fail in two ways when stressed. The perfectly elastic material has no plasticity and, therefore, will fracture when stressed to failure rather than permanently deform. That point of failure is represented by the terminal point of the stress-strain curve for that particular material. When the material that is not perfectly elastic is stressed past its yield point, it will fail through plastic elongation. In this case, stresses that exceed the yield point for that material will cause the material to behave inelastically, causing permanent deformation to occur in the shape of that part. Through an analysis of the stress-strain curves for a particular material, the degree of stress required to produce failure can be somewhat quantified, as can the method of failure for that particular material. The relative stress-strain curves for the polyolefins and TL-2100 may be found in Figure 14-2. It should be noted that the steepness of the curve indicates the rigidity of that particular material, while the area under the curve defines the capacity of that material to store energy.

4. **Creep.** *Creep* is defined as the deformation in the shape of a part or structure that occurs as the result of the application of a constant load over time. It can also be defined as increasing strain over time in the presence of constant stress. The rate of creep for a material depends on the amount of applied stress, temperature, and time. In application, this manifests as shape deformation as well as diminished ability of the part to resist load (Fig. 14-3).

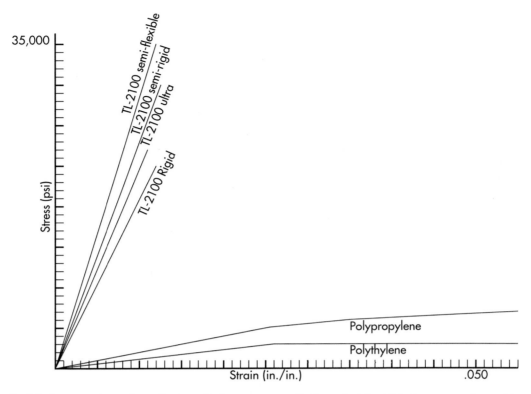

Fig. 14-2. A comparison of tensile strength for common orthotic materials. All tests were performed in accordance with the American Society for Testing and Materials D638-87b test.

5. **Glass transition temperature.** *Glass transition temperature (Tg)* is usually defined as the temperature below which the molecular chain of a particular polymer is frozen and above which there is sufficient energy to permit motion and undulations in the chain.[85] Materials existing above their Tg exhibit short-range orientation changes of portions of their molecules, resulting in a slow return to the predeformed shape when stress is removed. This is referred to as *viscoelasticity,* and is similar in general terms to the behavior of rubbery materials.[61] In polymers existing above their Tg, the relatively high degree of chain motion results in a material which tends to be soft, flexible, nonbrittle, and nonresilient, and which generally functions in a plastic manner. Materials existing below their Tg are rigid, hard, and generally brittle, yet resilient. These materials exhibit Hookean elasticity, which means that the material exhibits completely reversible, low deformations as a reaction to applied forces (Table 14-2).

6. **Poisson's ratio.** *Poisson's ratio* is the measure of the ability of a material to change its

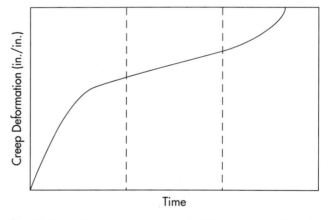

Fig. 14-3. Typical creep curve for nonbrittle material subjected to a constant stress over time.

shape when a stress is applied to it. In orthotic application, it is Poisson's ratio that provides the material information which defines, in part, the compatibility of an extrinsic rearfoot post of a particular material with the orthosis shell to which it is applied. When materials used to fabricate a rearfoot post and orthosis shell possess significantly dissimilar Poisson's ratios, as in the case

Table 14-2
Glass transition temperature (Tg) of some common orthotic materials

Material	Tg (°C)
TL-2100 Semi-Flexible	93
TL-2100 Semi-Rigid	93
TL-2100 Rigid	93
TL-2100 Ultra	93
Methyl methacrylate	105
Polypropylene	−20
Polyethylene	−25

Table 14-3
Material properties comparison for standard orthotic materials*

Material	Thickness (%)	Stiffness (%)	Flexible load (%)
TL-2100			
Ultra	100	113	127
Rigid	100	100	100
Semi-Rigid	82	62	78
Semi-Flexible	64	23	56
Polypropylene			
1/8 in.	114	11	7
3/16 in.	170	38	17
1/4 in.	227	91	30

* Tests were performed in accordance with the American Society for Testing and Materials D-790 test. Values are compared to TL-2100 Rigid.

of an acrylic rearfoot post applied to a relatively flexible polyolefin or TL-2100 shell, forces are concentrated at the interface between the two materials and failure can be expected at an accelerated rate. As previously noted, failure occurs either through fracture or permanent shape deformation, depending on the stress-strain relationship for that material.

7. **Stiffness.** *Stiffness* is the ability of a fabricated part to resist deformation under load and is a factor of material composition, temperature, thickness, shape, and length of the part. Stiffness is defined by the flexural rigidity for a given material, and is the product of the elastic modulus (E) and the moment of inertia (L), which is a function of the thickness. In terms of a functional orthosis, effective stiffness is significantly affected not only by the thickness of the material, but also by the use of a rigid rearfoot post, since the relatively flexible portion of that orthosis is only that portion distal to the rearfoot post. As stiffness relates to length, stiffness is proportional to the inverse of the length of the span cubed (stiffness = 1/span length cubed). In practical application, therefore, lengthening any portion of the rearfoot post will significantly increase the stiffness of the orthosis shell distal to that portion of the rearfoot post. If, for instance, the medial aspect of the rearfoot post was designed to be 1 cm longer than the lateral aspect, the orthosis shell would be significantly stiffer longitudinally along the medial aspect of the device. In this same manner, lengthening of the entire post would result in making the entire orthotic device distal to the post stiffer. This principle, of course, applies to the use of

extrinsic forefoot posts as well. Complex contours in the shape of the fabricated part also significantly enhance stiffness of that part. In orthotic application, the use of flanges, fascial accommodations, or extended or extra-deep heel cups can be expected to significantly stiffen the final orthosis, far beyond what would be expected simply by evaluation of the relative stiffness of each material as it relates to a given thickness (Table 14-3).

8. **Hardness.** *Hardness* may be defined as the resistance of a given material to compression. Different methods of evaluating hardness have been developed which give different ratings because they measure somewhat different characteristics of the material.[98] There is no absolute scale for hardness, and hardness, in fact, represents an agglomeration of various properties that are somewhat related to one another.[97]

Based on these definitions of the basic terminology necessary for an accurate analysis of the properties inherent in the materials most commonly used in the fabrication of functional orthoses, those materials, polypropylene, polyethylene, and the thermoplastic composite TL-2100, may be described.

Polypropylene

Polypropylene is an olefin polymer derived from the polymerization of the monomer butadiene. It is synthesized by using a Ziegler-type stereospecific

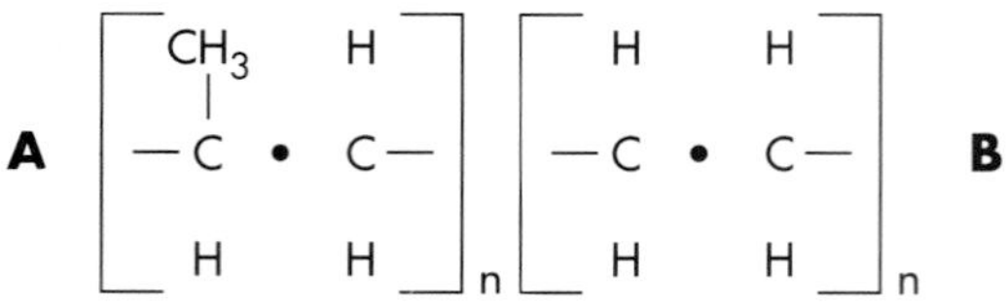

Fig. 14-4. **A,** Polypropylene molecular structure. **B,** Polyethylene molecular structure.

catalyst that controls the position of each monomer unit as it is being polymerized to allow formation of a regular chain structure. Polypropylene is a large molecule, as noted in Figure 14-4**A**. This is necessary since, at low molecular weight, these materials behave like wax and at still lower molecular weight, as an oil or gas. As with all polymers, polypropylene is linked by primary covalent bonding in the main backbone chain.[79] Polypropylene, at temperatures approximately above the freezing point, exists above its Tg, so it tends to be relatively soft and nonbrittle in application. This factor also explains the ability of polypropylene to resist breakage, as well as its flexibility when used in reduced thicknesses. An interesting byproduct of the specific Tg of polypropylene is its seemingly contradictory behavior in cold climates. When increasing and unexpected rates of polypropylene breakage occur in cold weather areas, it is because the polymer is suddenly functioning below its Tg and, as a result, takes on the characteristic hardness and brittleness of methyl methacrylate acrylics and other homogeneous plastics which exist below their Tg. As with polyethylene, polypropylene is a thermoplastic that is heat-formable and -adjustable at approximately 360 to 390°F. The stress-strain curve of polypropylene predicts, however, that expected biomechanical forces produce sufficient stress in the material so as to exceed the yield point and produce plastic behavior and ultimate failure due to plastic deformation (see Fig. 14-2). Polypropylene is typically used in thicknesses ranging from 0.125 to 0.25 in.

Polyethylene

Like polypropylene, polyethylene is also a polyolefin which is synthesized from the monomer ethylene oxide (Fig. 14-4**B**). It is available for orthosis fabrication primarily as Ortholene and Subortholene (Teufel, Stuttgart, Germany). These two versions of polyethylene are similar in many respects, although Subortholene tends to be somewhat lower in toughness and strength, while being easier to thermoform. Like polypropylene, polyethylene exists above its Tg and, as a result, has properties, as well as a stress-strain curve, very similar to those of

polypropylene. Polyethylene differs from polypropylene, however, in that it is a polymer of less density and molecular weight, causing it to have a lower stiffness-to-thickness ratio. This causes polyethylenes to have generally more rapid and severe plastic, or shape, deformation than expected with polypropylene (see Fig. 14-2).

In the cases of both polypropylene and polyethylene, polymerization may take place by methods referred to as either the free radical process or the coordination process. Which polymerization process is used is significant since polyethylene made by the coordination process is virtually unbranched and as a result, is said to have a high degree of crystallinity. Polyolefins that are highly crystalline tend to be mechanically much stronger than those that are not.[79]

TL-2100

Unlike the homogeneous thermoplastic polymers, TL-2100 is a thermoplastic composite. Composites are a family of high-performance materials consisting of a matrix reinforced with a fiber. The combination of resin and fiber results in properties that are quite different in nature than those of either material alone. Among those unique properties is the fact that TL-2100 functions anisotropically, that is, there exist different amounts of bending, for the same force applied, in different directions. Specifically, TL-2100 possesses considerably more longitudinal rigidity than it does torsional rigidity. This is in contrast to the homogeneous thermoplastic polymers, which, owing to the fact that they are homogeneous, display equal rigidity in both of the aforementioned planes and therefore function isotropically to applied stress. In the manufacturing of TL-2100, an acrylic-based thermoplastic resin system is used, reinforced with carbon fiber and combined in a unique, patented sandwich configuration. This allows thermoformability and heat adjustability similar to that of polypropylene. The thermoplastic resin system used in TL-2100 exists below its Tg and, as a result, is typically harder and significantly more rigid than equal thicknesses of the polyolefins. (see Table 14-3). The graphite reinforcement provides stiffness for support and superior strength for durability. Analysis of the stress-strain curve of TL-2100 indicates that this material, in all four available levels of stiffness, functions elastically and does not undergo plastic deformation at any stress level (see Fig. 14-2). It can be predicted, therefore, that, unlike the polyolefins, virtually no creep would be expected to occur in orthotic application with TL-2100. There are four versions of TL-2100 available: Ultrastrength, so

Table 14-4
Standard thicknesses of common orthotic materials

Material	Thickness		
	(in.)	(mL)	(mm)
TL-2100			
Semi-Flexible	0.070	70	1.8
Semi-Rigid	0.090	90	2.3
Rigid	0.110	110	2.8
Ultra	0.110	110	2.8
Polypropylene			
1/8 in.	0.125	125	3.2
3/16 in.	0.188	188	4.8
1/4 in.	0.250	250	6.4
Suborthelene			
3 mm	0.118	118	3.0
4 mm	0.157	157	4.0
5 mm	0.197	197	5.0
Ortholene			
3 mm	0.118	118	3.0
4 mm	0.157	157	4.0
5 mm	0.197	197	5.0

named because it is manufactured with approximately 50% more graphite than the other versions, Rigid, Semi-Rigid, and Semi-Flexible. Thicknesses range from approximately 1.8 to 2.8 mm (Table 14-4).

There are other materials from which foot orthoses are made in addition to those mentioned above. As they do not, for one reason or another, satisfy the entire scope of criteria established to define a functional orthosis, they are not included in this category. As a semifunctional or accommodative foot orthosis, or as additional components to be used in conjunction with a functional orthosis, they do prove effective, however.

Other materials

Closed-cell expanded rubber is manufactured by introducing pressurized nitrogen gas to a rubber matrix. The gas expansion that occurs with curing creates the closed cells which provide the performance features of this product. Available under the product name Spenco (Spenco Medical Corp., Waco, Tex.), this product is effective in absorbing shear and vertical load forces,[65,76,102,110] and is also useful when combined either as a cover or as an extension with a functional orthosis.

Polyurethane foam is an open-celled material, made available as Poron (Rogers Corp., Woodstock, Conn.). It has excellent cushioning properties with regard to vertical load as well as shear.* Both Poron and Spenco are available in sheets of various thicknesses and when combined with a functional

orthosis create an effective combination of functional control as provided by the orthosis, along with a soft surface directly in contact with the foot. The combination of a functional foot orthosis top-covered with materials such as Spenco and Poron effectively addresses the criticism of some authors that "rigid orthotics" are inherently hard and therefore, uncomfortable, while providing the control that can come only from a material sufficiently rigid so as to resist pathogenic ground reaction forces.

Cross-linked polyethylene foam is a closed-cell foam and is manufactured from heat-expanded polyethylene. It is made available under the trade names Aliplast, Nickleplast (both Alimed Inc), Plastazote (BXL Plastics Ltd., ERP Division, Croyden, England), and Pelite (Durr-Fillover, Birmingham, Ala.). Available in different densities, the closed-cell polyethylene foams are very light, but readily compress and undergo rapid and permanent shape deformation. This feature makes this material quite effective as an accommodative material with some short-term shock-absorbing properties.[64,65,86,102,110] This material is frequently used by itself as a foot orthosis in laminates of different densities or as a sulcus or full-length extension on a functional orthosis.

Various cork products made from rubberized cork (rubberized cork [JMS Plastics, Garfield, N.J.] or Korex [Accurate Felt and Gasket Co., Cicero, Ill.]) and thermoplastic cork (Thermocork [JMS Plastics] or Birkocork [Birkenstock Footprint Sandles Inc., Novato, Calif.]) are made from a matrix composed of cork oak. These materials are also effective when used specifically as accomodations, either in conjunction with a standard-length foot orthosis or alone, but unlike the low- and medium-density polyethylene foams, show minimal compression in typically applied loads. These products, like those mentioned above, are available in sheets of various thicknesses.

Viscoelastic polymers are made from polyurethane elastomers and are produced under the product names Sorbothane (Sorbothane, Inc., Kent, Ohio) and Viscolas (Chattanooga Corp., Chattanooga, Tenn.). Their efficacy in absorbing vertical load forces is well documented,* a feature which can indeed be clinically significant in the treatment and prevention of various musculoskeletal conditions.[92] A factor that limits their use, however, is that they are heavy and more difficult to cut than the other accommodative materials. Another limiting factor is the fact that they are virtually impossible to grind.

---

* References 65, 66, 76, 89, 98, 102, 110.

* References 15, 30, 31, 66, 76, 89, 124, 125, 127, 128.

Comparison of materials for functional foot orthoses

It has been noted previously in this chapter that two of the key criteria by which authors qualify materials for functional orthosis fabrication is ease of fabrication and ability to control motion. The principal materials from which the vast majority of functional foot orthoses are made, polypropylene and TL-2100, can be effectively compared and contrasted by analyzing their performance in these two categories, that is, their specific fabrication characteristics and their functional response to imposed loads.

Processing

Both materials thermoform at temperatures ranging from 375 to 390° F. Both are relatively easy to grind, and polypropylene has the particular advantage that the surface of the orthosis shell may be ground, as well as the edges. This is useful, not only when grinding in accommodations, as is often required with a prominent plantar fascia, but also because of the increased surface area that results from surface grinding, as this serves to enhance the adherence of various topcovers. This feature is due to the fact that polypropylene is a homogeneous material. TL-2100 is not amenable to surface grinding, since any compromise of the graphite fibers that would result from grinding either the top or the bottom surface would weaken the overall structure. Edge grinding of TL-2100 is easily performed and in no way compromises the integrity of this material.

Use of extrinsic posts

The use of extrinsic rearfoot posts is significant in the overall rearfoot control achieved through the use of a functional foot orthosis.[14] The materials commonly used for extrinsic posting on functional orthoses include polymethyl methacrylate acrylic for rigid posting and cork or crepe (of various densities) for nonrigid posts. The ability of these posting materials to adhere to the orthosis shell is dissimilar when comparing polypropylene and TL-2100. When formed as an extrinsic post, poly-methyl methacrylate acrylic forms a relatively rigid unit. Its adherence to the polyolefins is through a mechanical bond, and because of the significant dissimilarity of the molecular structure of the two materials and the respective Poisson's ratio of polymethyl methacrylate acrylic and of the polyolefins, post avulsion, post fracture, or orthotic shell failure is almost a certainty. Some facilities have attempted to address this problem through the use of polyolefin extrinsic posts laminated to the orthotic shell. Effectively addressing the problem of post avulsion through the

linking of like molecular structures, polyolefins do not have the impact or abrasion resistance demonstrated by polymethyl methacrylate acrylic and, as such, break down with regard to their prescribed position and motion more rapidly. The process of laminating polyolefin posts to orthotic shells of the same material is also relatively difficult and labor-intensive, compared to the other methods of extrinsic posting available. Thermoplastic cork has also been used by some facilities and has been found to be a fairly effective compromise between the compression compliance required to yield with the polypropylene shell when load is applied and durability. It is more durable than many nonrigid posting materials.

Because of their porous structure, nonrigid posting materials form a fairly effective mechanical bond with polyolefin materials. As previously noted in the case of both rigid and nonrigid posting materials, the effective surface area of the polyolefin materials may be increased by abrading the surface of the orthosis shell, thus enhancing the mechanical bond between the orthosis shell and the post.

In contrast to the polyolefins, TL-2100 forms a chemical bond with acrylic posting materials, since the resin system used in the formulation of TL-2100 is acrylic-based. The advantage of the chemical bond formed is that post avulsion or post fracture is virtually impossible when rigid versions of TL-2100 are used. The disadvantage is that when acrylic posts are utilized with versions of TL-2100 that are designed to provide some degree of flexibility in application (i.e., semiflexible, semirigid), the dissimilarity of Poisson's ratio between the rigid post and the relatively flexible shell will concentrate forces at the interface of those two materials and predispose the orthosis to fracture at that specific point, just distal to the anterior margin of the rearfoot post. For this reason, use of extrinsic acrylic posting with an orthosis shell of any material designed to be relatively flexible in application can result in failure of the device just distal to the rearfoot post, or when an acrylic forefoot post is used, just proximal to the forefoot post, owing to concentration of forces at this point. In contrast to the chemical bond that results from the union of acrylic posting materials and TL-2100, nonrigid posting materials adhere to TL-2100 by means of mechanical bonding.

Thickness

The information in Tables 14-3 and 14-4 indicates that for comparable degrees of stiffness, TL-2100 is 44-56% thinner than polypropylene. This difference can be accounted for by the added strength provided by the graphite reinforcement of TL-2100, as

Table 14-5
Orthotic weight study: shell weight comparison

	Weight (g)*	Thickness (in.)	Rigidity (lb-in.^{2})†
TL-2100 Semi-Flexible	31.2	0.07	70
Polypropylene, 1/8 in.	35.7	0.125	34
Difference (%)	12.6%	44.0%	106.0%
TL-2100 Semi-Rigid	41.6	0.09	185
Polypropylene, 3/16 in.	49.8	0.188	115
Difference (%)	16.5%	52.1%	60.9%
TL-2100 Rigid	52.2	0.11	300
Polypropylene, 1/4 in.	65.2	0.25	273
Difference (%)	19.9%	56.0%	9.9%

* Based on the average weight of a standard men's orthosis fabricated at three podiatry laboratories.
† Based on the product of effective elastic modules and moment of inertia.

well as by the mechanical properties of each material, as previously noted. In a functional environment where added bulk can impede the ability of the patient to wear the prescribed orthosis, such a difference can prove to be significant. Some of this difference can be offset by the fact that an orthosis made from polypropylene can be thinned at its contact points, owing to the fact that it is a homogeneous material.

Weight

As noted in Table 14-5, the difference in weight between comparable stiffnesses of TL-2100 and polypropylene was 4.5 to 13 g, or 12.6% to 19.9%. Specifically, the TL-2100 Semi-Flexible offers a 13% weight savings, yet is twice as rigid as its closest comparable version of polypropylene, 1/8 in. The TL-2100 Semi-Rigid offers a 16% weight savings compared to its closest comparable thickness of polypropylene, 3/16 in., while being 61% stiffer. The closest direct comparison between TL-2100 and polypropylene was that comparing TL-2100 Rigid and 1/4-in. polypropylene. In this comparison, TL-2100 Rigid was 20% lighter than 1/4 in. polypropylene, while measuring 10% more rigid.

Since the data for these weight comparisons were derived from an average of identically sized orthoses made from standard-sized men's and women's casts, it is interesting to note the range in weight in these devices. As noted in Table 14-6, the range in polypropylene, identically prescribed with regard to size, shape, and thickness, was 10.5% to 19% for men's-sized orthoses and 15.3% to 24.7% for women's-sized devices. Since the potential for significant differences in the polypropylene used by orthotic laboratories does indeed exist, due in part

to potential variables in the polymerization process such as degree of crystallinity, molecular purity, and stereoregularity to name a few, this relatively large discrepancy in the weight of seemingly identical polypropylene orthoses is not altogether surprising. By comparison, since TL-2100 is a uniform and standard product, the difference in weights of identically prescribed orthoses made from TL-2100 was 6.5% to 8.0% for men's-sized orthoses and 6.0% to 11.7% for women's devices.

When extrinsically applied posts are used as a part of the fabrication of a functional foot orthosis, most orthotic laboratories utilize either crepe or acrylic. As expected, extrinsic posts also add significantly to the overall weight of the functional orthosis. The data in Table 14-7 indicate that a medium-density crepe adult-sized rearpost adds approximately 5 g to an orthosis, whereas an acrylic post adds 9.4 to 12 g.

The weights of the materials commonly used as either freestanding insoles or as orthotic topcovers are shown in Table 14-8. As noted, when comparing average women's-sized insoles made from Poron, Spenco, and Viscolas, Poron proved approximately 24% lighter than Spenco and 75% lighter than Viscolas. Significant differences are also noted in the two available thickness both of Poron and Spenco.

It can be surmised from these data that the weight of a functional foot orthosis can range from 23.3 g, as in the case of a women's-sized, nonposted orthosis made from TL-2100 Semi-Flexible, to as much as 82 g, as in the case of an acrylic-posted orthosis made from 1/4-in. polypropylene. If topcovers and extension posting or wedging are used in the design and fabrication of the functional orthosis as well, the weight of these various components

Table 14-6
Orthotic weight study: product variation*

Product	Minimum weight (g)	Maximum weight (g)	Difference (%)
Polypropylene			
1/8 in.			
Men's	34.0	38.0	10.5
Women's	26.5	31.3	15.3
3/16 in.			
Men's	44.8	52.8	15.1
Women's	36.1	44.0	18.0
1/4 in.			
Men's	57.0	70.4	19.0
Women's	42.4	56.3	24.7
TL-2100			
Semi-Flexible			
Men's	29.7	32.3	8.0
Women's	23.3	26.4	11.7
Semi-Rigid			
Men's	39.6	43.6	9.2
Women's	30.2	33.6	10.1
Rigid			
Men's	50.6	54.1	6.5
Women's	38.9	41.4	6.0

* The weights were obtained from the fabrication of standard men's- and women's-sized orthoses at three orthotic laboratories.

Table 14-7
Weight study: heel post weights

Material	Category	Average weight (g)*
Crepe	Men's	5.2
	Women's	5.2
Acrylic	Men's	12.0
	Women's	9.4

* The weights were measured from standard men's- and women's-sized orthoses fabricated at three orthotic laboratories.

Table 14-8
Weight comparison of cushioning materials

Material	Weight (g)*
Poron	
1/16 in.	
Men's	12.0
Women's	8.7
1/8 in.	
Men's	22.7
Women's	17.7
Spenco	
1/16 in.	
Men's	18.5
Women's	13.7
1/8 in.	
Men's	29.9
Women's	20.3
Viscolas	
Men's	89.7
Women's	76.9

* Men's weight is based on U.S. insole size D; women's weight, on size B.

must also be taken into consideration. The clinical significance of the weight differences among orthoses of various materials is yet to be conclusively determined, yet studies have indicated that relatively subtle weight differences in orthoses, as well as shoe gear, may not only be perceivable by the patient but may have a measurable impact on athletic performance. Subject sensitivity to relatively subtle differences in orthosis weight was demonstrated in a study by Richie and Olson,[95] in which the average weight difference of only 16 g between 3/16-in. polypropylene and TL-2100 Semi-Flexible was accurately perceived by the study subjects, resulting in a clear preference for the lighter mate-

rial, TL-2100. As previously noted in this chapter, an addition of as little as 100 g per shoe can measurably effect V_{O_2} in the athlete. As a result, these weight comparisons should be considered, as should those of the commonly used insole and topcover materials in the selection process when attempting to predict the physiologic effect on the patient of the final orthosis (see Tables 14-5 to 14-8).

Response to dynamic load

The behavior of a material with respect to its response to loadbearing is a factor, in part, of temperature; the mechanical properties of the material; the speed of loading; direction of loading; amount of creep or permanent set already in the material; and, in the case of functional foot orthoses, the specific location of the imposed stresses as they relate to the orthosis itself. Most important, however, is some quantification of the imposed stresses and how those stresses fall on the stress-strain curve for that particular material. As previously mentioned, if the stress applied to a part does not exceed the yield point for that material, then elastic deformation occurs and that part returns to its original shape. If the applied stress exceeds the yield point, failure occurs, either through fracture for materials functioning elastically or plastic deformation for materials functioning in their inelastic or plastic region. It becomes of critical importance, therefore, to accurately quantify the degree of stress applied to the part, if any accurate prediction is to be made regarding the response of that part to the applied stress. It has been estimated that the ground reaction forces generated during walking are 70% to 200% of body weight, while running results in forces reported to be two to five times body weight.* Estimates of compressive force across the talocrural joint are said to be 3.5 to 5.0 times body weight while walking[91,107,114] and, in some reports, up to 13 times body weight while running.[18] Mann[70] estimates that the average 150-lb person, walking 1 mile, absorbs 63.5 tons on each foot. If this same person runs that mile, the weightbearing absorbed at ground contact increases to 110 tons on each foot. This information alone, however, is of little use in predicting how and to what degree an orthosis is loaded, since key variables, such as specific location of the imposed load on the orthosis; shape, thickness, and composition of the orthosis; and any components attached to the orthosis, are not taken into consideration. In addition, the surface under the orthosis is a critical variable in assessing the actual stress on the orthosis shell. When analyzing the imposed stress on a foot orthosis, it is important to realize that the longer it takes for the velocity of an impacting load to decrease to zero, the slower the deceleration and hence the smaller the forces on that part ($F = M \times A$). Compliant surfaces, whether they be insoles, shoes, surfaces, or the orthosis, can effectively increase

* References 24, 29, 50, 69, 84, 116, 124.

Table 14-9
Percent elongation of tensile specimen for common orthotic materials*

Material	Elongation at failure (%)
TL-2100	
Semi-Flexible	1.1
Semi-Rigid	1.2
Rigid	1.2
Ultra	1.2
Polypropylene	350
Polyethylene	485
Suborthelene	1000
Ortholene	450

* Tests were performed in accordance with the American Society for Testing and Materials D638-87b test.

the time of deceleration and thus significantly reduce impact forces. This assumption is supported by Frederick and co-workers,[47,48] who demonstrated lower V_{O_2} through the use of compliant shoe gear in running.

Any attempts to estimate the forces imposed on a functional foot orthosis must begin with the recognition of those forces imposed by certain pathologic biomechanical disorders (e.g., compensated equinus, compensated forefoot varus) and activities which involve significant impact, acceleration, and deceleration on noncompliant surfaces (e.g., tennis, football, volleyball, basketball). When evaluating all of the aforementioned forces imposed on the orthosis shell, patient body weight is probably the least important factor. It is noted that many commercial facilities, as well as practitioners, use patient body weight as the sole deciding factor in selecting the material from which an orthosis is to be made. When abnormal failure of an orthosis occurs, in my experience it is rare that this is related, to any significant degree, to the weight of the patient.

All of these variables notwithstanding, it is estimated by Anthony[1] that the pressure imposed on an orthosis shell is often in excess of 35 N/mm.[2] This, as well as other supporting data, indicate that, when subjected to the normal loads of running, and under certain biomechanical conditions, walking, polypropylene is forced to perform beyond its relatively low yield point and as a result will undergo plastic deformation and shape deterioration over time.[1,95] In contrast, the linear stress-strain relationship and relatively high yield points of the TL-2100 devices allow them to function well within their elastic range in typical biomechanical applications.[1,58,88] Owing to the propensity for elongation of the molecular structure (Table 14-9), accelerated creep of a polypropylene orthosis is to be expected, a fact that is also apparent in analysis of the stress-strain curve for polypropylene. The opposite is again true with TL-2100, as indicated in Figure 14-3.

The characteristic resistance to breakage of the polyolefins is also readily understood by the plastic response of this material to loads in excess of its yield point. By contrast, TL-2100 fractures with applied loads in excess of its yield point. The use and orientation of carbon fiber in the lamination of TL-2100 products results in a relatively high yield point, which, in turn, results in a proportionally higher resistance to loading in application.

Resilience

Resilience may be defined as the property of a material that allows it to return to its original shape after deflection. Thus, a material is considered to be more resilient than another material if it can spring back into shape more quickly. The properties of a material that allow it to be resilient are its spring rate (K), which is defined by the equation $K = F/$"Δ", where "Δ" is the deformation under the applied load F, and its mass.[123] Materials with high values of stiffness and low mass or weight are invariably more resilient.[121] The importance of resilience or "energy return" has been discussed by numerous authors.[8,49,51,74,109,122] Garrick[51] states that resilience in shoe materials should result in fewer injuries and people running longer and faster. Sims and Cavanagh[109] state that a material that is capable of storing elastic or strain energy and returning it to the body may be able to more than offset the negative effects of its weight and cause a net decrease in V_{O_2}.

As with the stiffness of a material, resilience is a constant that can be easily and objectively measured. Specifically, the modulus of resilience, also referred to as *maximum strain energy*, is determined by the equation Modulus of Resilience = stress (max) squared/Young's modulus, where stress (max) represents the point of maximum stress immediately prior to failure and Young's modulus is a constant for a given material. The Young's modulus for currently available functional orthotic materials is noted in Table 14-10. The data in Table 14-11 represent the results when the modulus of resilience is calculated for these same materials.

It can be said then, that the measurement of resilience actually describes the speed at which a given material returns to its original shape after deflection. When load is applied to any orthosis, a certain degree of deflection will result, with the actual degree of deflection being proportional to the stiffness of the material. The appropriate degree of stiffness that is clinically efficacious is based on the subjective assessment of the clinician and his or her

Table 14-10
Young's modulus for some common orthotic materials*

Material	Young's modulus (10^6 psi)
TL-2100	
Semi-Flexible	3.0
Semi-Rigid	2.3
Rigid	1.7
Ultra	2.2
Polypropylene	0.2

* Tests were performed in accordance with the American Society for Testing and Materials D638-87b test.

Table 14-11
Modulus of resilience for some common orthotic materials*

Material	Modulus of resilience (psi)
TL-2100	
Semi-Flexible	180
Semi-Rigid	160
Rigid	122
Ultra	160
Polypropylene	88
Polyethylene	80

* Tests were performed in accordance with the American Society for Testing and Materials D638-87b test.

determination of the point of optimal balance between normal physiologic motion and excessive or abnormal motion. No matter what degree of stiffness is deemed appropriate for a particular clinical application, however, the advantages of a material that can rapidly rebound to its predeformed shape are evident. When midstance phase deflection of the orthosis occurs, the highly resilient material is able to quickly spring back as the lower extremity moves into the propulsive phase, and is better able to stabilize the foot during propulsion and toe-off. A material that possesses a relatively low modulus of resilience will, on the other hand, be very slow to return to its predeformed state after midstance deflection, and is therefore unable to assist in propulsive phase stabilization or control. If resilience levels are sufficiently low, the orthosis will not even return to its predeformed state by the time of the next stance phase and, therefore, will be limited in its ability to control even midstance motion owing to the degree of deflection that occurred during the prior gait cycle. The data show that TL-2100 has the greatest degree of resilience of the functional orthotic materials currently available,[66] ranging from TL-2100 Rigid at 122 psi to TL-2100 Semi-Flexible, which is 180 psi. Both are significantly more resilient than polypropylene (see Table 14-11).

The ultimate clinical significance of these data remains to be determined by further research and clinical investigation. The concept of "energy return" and "resilience" was, however, never a relevant concept to be analyzed before inherently resilient materials, such as carbon-graphite laminates, were available.[66,95] The high degree of resilience inherent in the TL-2100 devices offers the clinician a new and uniquely efficacious balance between the enhanced patient tolerance found with flexible, compliant materials and the motion control of rigid materials.

Summary

Decades of clinical and laboratory research in the area of lower extremity biomechanics has resulted in the prescribed use of foot orthoses, which have been well documented as efficacious in subjective symptom relief as well as quantitative motion control. Categorizing foot orthoses simply as soft, semirigid, and rigid is, however, an inaccurate, arbitrary, and inappropriate means by which to group the various materials used in the fabrication of foot orthoses and should be discarded. This point is particularly apparent when considering the many prescription and application variables that affect the functional rigidity of the actual orthosis. If orthotic materials are to be categorized accurately, the categorization should be based solely upon their composition (i.e., carbon-graphite composites, plastics, foams, etc.) or their designed function (i.e., functional, semifunctional, accommodative), understanding that the function of a given material or combination of materials depends largely on the prescribed design and composition of the actual orthosis made from the material(s). Of the materials currently available for use in the fabrication of functional foot orthoses, the homogeneous thermoplastics (polyethylene) and polypropylene, and the carbon-graphite thermoplastic composite TL-2100 are the most commonly used and most readily available. Neither material possesses all of the properties that would ideally be available in a functional orthotic material. Polypropylene possesses the desirable property of being virtually impossible to fracture at any degree of imposed stress because it responds in a plastic manner to such stresses and, therefore, may be expected to demonstrate shape deformation over time. TL-2100, on the other hand, can fracture under excessive loads, although the typical stresses imposed in a clinical setting generally fall well below the yield point for this material. TL-2100, however, is uniquely resilient, having the ability to rapidly spring back to its predeformed shape, allowing a potential for compliance and energy return never before possible with homogeneous thermoplastics.

The successful use of functional foot orthoses, of any material, is based upon the shared responsibility of the prescribing clinician and the orthotic laboratory. It is solely the responsibility of the practitioner to accurately assess the biomechanical forces producing the chief complaint, obtain an accurate impression cast, and understand and apply appropriately the many variables involved in prescribing the final orthosis. Additionally, it is the responsibility of the practitioner to make an appropriate choice of material(s) from which the orthosis is to be made based on a sophisticated understanding of how those materials respond to imposed loads, and also to assess as well as orient the expectations of the patient with regard to the expected performance and life expectancy of the patient's orthosis. It is the responsibility of the orthotic laboratory to perform the prescribed cast corrections accurately and fabricate the device accurately and according to the manufacturer's standards. It is only when these standards are strictly adhered to by both clinician and laboratory that the performance of functional foot orthoses in the control of lower extremity motion and relief of related symptoms can be accurately evaluated.

Acknowledgments

William Olson thanks Medical Materials Corp., Allied OSI Laboratory, KLM Laboratory, and Root Functional Orthotic Laboratory for their valuable contributions to the data presented in Chapter 14.

References

1. Anthony R: *The Manufacture and Use of Functional Foot Orthoses,* London, Kargar G, 1991, p 5.
2. Baitch S, Blake R, Senatore J, et al: Analysis of the effectiveness of a rigid veritical orthotic and a rigid twenty-five degree inverted orthotic in controlling subtalar joint pronation in runners, *Phys Ther* 68:801, 1988.
3. Bates BT, James SJ, Ostering LR: Foot function during the support phase of running, *Am J Sports Med* 7:338, 1979.
4. Bates BT, Ostering LR, Mason B: Lower extremity function during the support phase of running. In *Biomechanics,* Vol. 6. Baltimore, University Park Press, 1978, p 31.
5. Bates BT, Ostering LR, Mason B, Functional variability of the lower extremity during the support phase of running, *Med Sci Sports* 11:328, 1979.
6. Bates BT, Ostering LR, Mason B, et al: Foot orthotic devices to modify lower extremity mechanics, *Am J Sports Med* 7:338, 1979.

7. Baxter D: The foot in running and dancing. In Mann RA (ed): *Surgery of the Foot,* St Louis, Mosby–Year Book, 1986.

8. Baxter D: Running injuries. In Jahss M (ed): *Disorders of the Foot and Ankle,* London, WB Saunders, 1991.

9. Benink RJ: The constraint mechanism of the human tarsus: a roentgenological experimental study, *Acta Orthop Scand Suppl* 215:1, 1985.

10. Berg K, Sady S: Oxygen costs of running at submaximal speeds while wearing shoe inserts, *Res Q* 56:86, 1985.

11. Blake RL: Inverted functional orthosis, *J Am Podiatry Assoc* 76:275, 1986.

12. Blake RL, Denton JA: Functional foot orthoses for athletic injuries, *J Am Podiatr Med Assoc* 75:359, 1985.

13. Blake RL, Ferguson H: Foot orthosis for the severe flatfoot in sports, *J Am Podiatr Med Assoc* 81:549, 1991.

14. Blake RB, Ferguson HJ: Effect of extrinsic rearfoot posts on rearfoot motion, *J Am Podiatr Med Assoc* 83:447, 1993.

15. Boulton AJM, Franks CI, Betts RP: Reduction of abnormal foot pressures in diabetic neuropathy using polymer insole material, *Diabetes Care* 7:42, 1984.

16. Brody DM: Running injuries: prevention and management, *Clin Symp* 39:8, 1987.

17. Bunchbinder MR, Napora NJ, Biggs EW: The relationship of abnormal pronation to chondromalacia of the patella in distance runners, *J Am Podiatry Assoc* 69:159, 1979.

18. Burdett RG: Forces predicted at the ankle during running, *Med Sci Sports Exerc* 14:308, 1982.

19. Burkett LN, Kohrt WM, Buchbinder R: Effects of shoes and foot orthotics on Vo_2 and selected frontal plane knee kinematics, *Med Sci Sports Exerc* 17:158, 1985.

20. Campbell G, McLure M, Newell E,: Compressive behavior after simulated service conditions of some foamed materials intended as orthotic shoe insoles, *J Rehabil Res Dev* 21:57, 1984.

21. Campbell G, Newell E, McLure M: Compression testing of foamed plastics and rubbers for use as orthotic shoe insoles, *Prosthet Orthot Int* 6:48, 1982.

22. Campbell JW, Inman VT: Treatment of plantar fasciitis and calcaneal spurs with the UC-BL shoe insert, *Clin Orthop* 103:57, 1974.

23. Campbell KR, Grabiner MD, Hawthorne DL, et al: Three-dimensional kinematic analysis of tibial-calcaneal motions during the support phase of gait; *Med Sci Sports Exerc* 21(suppl):89, 1989.

24. Cappozzo A, Tommaso L, Pedotti A: A general computing method for the analysis of humen locomotion, *J Biomech* 8:307, 1975.

25. Catlin MJ, Dressendorfer, RH: Effect of shoe weight on the energy cost of running, *Med Sci Sports Exerc* 11:80, 1979.

26. Cavanagh PR: The Running Shoe Book. Mountain View, Calif, World Publications, 1981, pp 83, 259.

27. Cavanagh PR, Clark TE, Williams K, et al: An evaluation of the effect of orthotics on force distribution and rearfoot movement during running. Presented at the American Orthopaedic Society for Sports Medicine meeting, Lake Placid, NY, 1978.

28. Cavanagh PR, Edington CJ: What happens to the foot with an in-shoe orthosis? Presented at the Annual Meeting of the American Orthopedic Foot and Ankle Society, Las Vegas, 1989.

29. Cavanagh PR, LaFortune MA: Ground reaction forces in distance running, *J Biomech* 13:397, 1980.

30. Chisin R, Milgrom C, Giladi M, et al: Clinical significance of nonfocal scinitgraphic findings in suspected ibial stress fractures, *Clin Orthop* 220:200, 1987.

31. Cinats J, Reid DC, Haddow JR: A biomechanical evaluation of Sorbothane, *Clin Orthop* 222:281, 1987.

32. Clarke TE, Frederick EC, Hamill CL: The effect of shoe design upon rearfoot control in running, *Med Sci Sports Exerc* 15:376, 1983.

33. Clarke TE, Frederick EC, Hamill CL: The study of rearfoot movement in running. In Frederick EC (ed): *Sports shoes and playing surfaces,* Champaign, Ill, Human Kinetics, 1984.

34. Clarke TE, Frederick EC, Hlavac HF: Effects of a soft orthotic device on rearfoot movement in running, *Podiatr Sports* 1:20, 1983.

35. Clarke TE, LaFortune MA, Williams KR, et al: The relationship between center of pressure location and rearfoot movement in distance running. Presented at the Annual Meeting of the American College of Sports Medicine, Las Vegas, 1980.

36. Clement DB, Taunton JE, Smart GW, et al: A survey of overuse running injuries, *Physician Sports Med* 9:47, 1981.

37. Cook A, Gorman I, Morris J: Evaluation of the neutral position of the subtalar joint, *J Am Podiatr Med Assoc* 78:449, 1988.

38. Cornwall MW, McPoil TG: Effect of rearfoot posts in reducing forefoot forces, *J Am Podiatr Med Assoc* 82:7, 1992.

39. Cureton KJ, Sparling BW, Evans SM,: Effect of experimental alterations in excess weight on aerobic capacity and distance running performance, *Med Sci Sports Exerc* 10:194, 1978.

40. D'Ambrosia R, Douglas R: Orthotics. In D'Ambrosia R, Drez D (eds): *Prevention and treatment of running injuries,* Thorofare, NJ, Charles B Slack, 1982.

41. Donatelli R, Hulbert C, Conaway D, et al: Biomechanical foot orthotics: a retrospective study, *J Orthop Sports Phys Ther* 10:205, 1988.

42. Dress D: Running footware: examination of the training shoe, the foot, and functional orthotic devices, *Am J Sports Med* 8:140, 1980.

43. Eggold J: Orthotics in the prevention of runner's overuse injuries, *Phys Sportsmed* 9:125, 1981.

44. Eng JJ, Pierrynowski MR: Evaluation of soft foot orthotics in the treatment of patellofemoral pain syndrome, *Phys Ther* 73: 62, 1993.

45. Engsberg JR, Andrews JG: Kinematic analysis of the talocaneal/talocrural joint during running support, *Med Sci Sports* Exerc 19:275, 1987.

46. Ferguson H, Raskowsky M, Blake RL, et al: TL-61 versus Rohadur orthoses in heel spur syndrome, *J Am Podiatr Med Assoc* 81:8, 1991.

47. Frederick EC: The energy cost of load carriage on the feet during running. In Norman RW, Wells RP, et al (eds): *Biomechanics* vol 9-B. Champaign, Ill, Human Kinetics, 1987.

48. Frederick EC, Clarke TE, Larson JC, et al: The effects of shoe cushioning on the oxygen demands of running. Nigg B, Kerr B (eds): Biomechanical Aspects of Sports Shoes and Playing Surfaces. Calgary, Alta, Canada, University of Calgary Printing Services, 1983.

49. Frederick EC, Daniels JT, Hayes JW: The effect of shoe weight on the aerobic demands of running. Presented at the World Congress of Sports Medicine, Vienna, Austria, 1982.

50. Frederick EC, Hagy JL, Mann RA: The prediction of vertical impact force during running, *J Biomech* 14:498, 1981.

51. Garrick JG: Personal communication,

52. Gross, ML, Davlin LB, Evanski PM: Effectiveness of orthotic shoe inserts in the long-distance runner, *Am J Sports Med* 19:409, 1991.

53. Gross ML, Napoli RC: Treatment of lower extremity Injuries with orthotic shoe inserts, *Sports Med* 15:66, 1993.

54. Hayes J, Smith L, Santopietro F: The effects of orthotics on the aerobic demands of running, *Med Sci Sports Exerc* 15:169, 1983.

55. Hice GA, Kendrick Z, Weeber K, et al: The effect of foot orthoses on oxygen consumption while cycling, *J Am Podiatr Med Assoc* 75:513, 1985.

56. Hicks JH: The mechanics of the foot: I. The joints, *J Anat* 87:345–357, 1953.

57. James SI, Bates BT, Osternig, LR: Injuries to runners, *Am J Sports Med* 6:40, 1978.

58. Jensen A, Chenoweth HH: *Applied Strength of Materials*, ed 3, New York, McGraw-Hill, 1975.

59. Jones RL: The human foot: an experimental study of its mechanics, and the role of its muscles and ligaments in the support of the arch, *Am J Anat* 68:1, 1941.

60. Jones RL: The functional significance of the declination of the axis of the subtalar joint, *Anat Rec* 93:151, 1945.

61. Kaufman HS: An introduction to polymer science. In *Modern Plastics Encyclopedia*, vol 45. New York, McGraw Hill, 1968, p 24.

62. Kirby KA: Methods for determination of positional variations in the subtalar joint axis, *J Am Podiatr Med Assoc* 77:117, 1987.

63. Kirby KA: The medial heel skive technique, *J Am Podiatr Med Assoc* 82:4, 1992.

64. Kuncir EJ, Wirta RW, Goldbranson FL: Load-bearing characteristics of polyethylene foam: an examination of structural and compression properties, *J Rehabil Res Dev* 27:229, 1990.

65. Leber C, Evanski PM: A comparison of shoe insole materials in plantar pressure relief, *Prosthet Orthot Int* 10:135, 1986.

66. Lewis G, Tan T, Shiue YS: Characterization of the performance of shoe insert materials, *J Am Podiatr Med Assoc* 81:418, 1991.

67. Lockard MS: Foot orthoses, *Phys Ther* 68:1866, 1988.

68. Lundeen, RO: Polysectional triaxial posting, *J Am Podiatry Assoc* 78:55, 1988.

69. Lutter LD: Foot related knee problems in the long distance runner, *Foot Ankle* 1:112, 1980.

70. Mann RA: Biomechanics of running. In *AAOS Symposium on the Foot and Leg in Running Sports*, St Louis, Mosby–Year Book, 1982.

71. Mann RA: In Mann RA, editor: *Surgery of the Foot*, St Louis, Mosby–Year Book, 1986.

72. McCulloch MU, Brunt D, Vander Linden D: The effect of foot orthotics and gait velocity on lower limb kinimatics and temporal events of stance, *J Orthop Sports Phys Ther* 17:2, 1993.

73. McKenzie DC, Clement DB, Taunton JE: Running shoes, orthotics and injuries, *Sports Med* 2:334, 1985.

74. McNeill R: The spring in your step, *New Sci* 114:42, 1987.

75. McPoil TG, Cornwall MW: Rigid versus soft orthoses, *J Am Podiatr Med Assoc* 81:638, 1991.

76. McPoil TG, Cornwall MW: Effect of insole material on force and plantar pressures during walking, *J Am Podiatr Med Assoc* 82:412, 1992.

77. Meyers MJ, Steudel K: Effect of limb mass and its distribution on the energetic cost of running, *J Exp Biol* 116:363, 1985.

78. Moraros J, Hodge W: Orthotic survey preliminary results, *J Am Podiatr Med Assoc* 83:139, 1993.

79. Morrison RF, Boyd RN: *Organic chemistry*, Allyn Boston, & Bacon, 1973, pp 1030, 1040.

80. Moskowitz R, Howell D, Goldberg M, et al, editors: *Osteoarthritis Diagnosis and Management*, ed 2. Philadelphia, WB Saunders, 1984.

81. Murphy P: Orthoses: not the sole solution for running ailments, *Phys Sportsmed* 14:164, 1986.

82. Nigg BM, Denoth J, Luethi S, et al: Methodological aspects of sport shoe and sport floor analysis. Presented at the International Congress of Biomechanics, Nagoya, Japan, 1981.

83. Novick A, Stone J, Birke JA et al: Reduction of plantar pressure with the rigid relief orthosis. *J Am Podiatr Med Assoc* 83:115, 1993.

84. Nuber GW: Biomechanics of the foot and ankle during gait. In Yocum L, editor: *Clinics in sports medicine*, Philadelphia, WB Saunders, 1988.

85. Olson WR: Orthoses: an analysis of their component materials, *J Am Podiatr Med Assoc* 78:203, 1988.

86. Orders C: A comparison in medium and low density Plastazote in the fabrication of insole, *Can J Occup Ther* 45:17, 1977.

87. Otman S, Basgoze O, Gokce-Kutsal Y: Energy cast of running with flat feet, *Prosthet Orthet Int* 12:93, 1988.

88. Popov EP: *Mechanics of Materials*, Englewood Cliffs, NJ, Prentice-Hall, 1976.

89. Pratt DJ, Rees PH, Rodgers C: Assessment of some shock absorbing insoles, *Prosthet Orthet Int* 10:43, 1986.

90. Preston ET: Flat foot deformity, *Am Fam Physician* 9:143, 1974.

91. Procter P, Paul JP: Ankle joint biomechanics, *J Biomech* 15:627, 1982.

92. Radin EL, Parker HS, Pugh JW, et al: Response of joints to impact loading. III. Relationship between tabecular microfractures and cartilage degeneration, *J Biomech* 1:51, 1973.

93. Reed JK, Theriot SM: Orthotic devices, shoes and modifications. In Hunt CG, editor: *Physical therapy of the foot and ankle*, New York, Churchill Livingstone, 1988.

94. Reinschmidt C, Stacoff A, Stussi E: Heel movement within a court shoe, *Med Sci Sports Exerc* 24:1390, 1992.

95. Richie DH, Olson, WR: Orthoses for athletic overuse injuries. *J Am Pediatr Med Assoc* 83:492, 1993.

96. Rodgers MM, LeVeau BF: Effectiveness of foot orthotic devices used to modify pronation in runners, *J Orthop Sports Phys Ther* 4:86, 1982.

97. Rome K: Behavior of orthotic materials in chiropody, *J Am Podiatr Med Assoc* 80:471, 1990.

98. Rome K: A study of the properties of materials used in podiatry, *J Am Podiatr Med Assoc* 81:73, 1991.

99. Root ML, Orien WP, Weed JH, et al: *Biomechanical Examination of the Foot*, Los Angeles, Clinical Biomechanics Corp, 1971.

100. Rose GK: Correction of the pronated foot, *J Bone Joint Surg [Br]* 44:642, 1962.

101. Roy S, Irvin R: *Sports Medicine, Prevention, Evaluation, Management and Rehabilitation*, Prentice-Hall, Englewood Cliffs, NJ, 1983.

102. Sanfilippo, PB, Stess RM, Moss KM: Dynamic plantar pressure analysis, *J Am Podiatr Med Assoc* 82:507, 1992.

103. Santoro JP, Cachia VV, Tilley GE, et al: Effect of the orthosis on performance in alpine skiing, *J Am Podiatr Med Assoc* 79:39, 1989.

104. Schuster ON: *Foot orthopedics*, New York, Marbridge, 1927, p 198.

105. Schuster, RO: A history of orthopedics in podiatry, *J Am Podiatry Med Assoc* 64:332, 1974.

106. Schwartz R: Foot orthoses and materials. In Jahss M, editor: *Disorders of the foot and ankle*, London, W.B. Saunders, 1991.

107. Seireg A, Arvikar RJ: The prediction of muscular load sharing and joint forces in the lower extremities during walking, *J Biomech* 8:89, 1975.

108. Sims DS: The effect of a balanced foot orthosis on muscle function and foot pronation in compensated forefoot varus, master's thesis, University of Iowa, Iowa City, 1983.

109. Sims, DS, Cavanagh, PR: Selected foot mechanics related to the prescription of foot orthoses. In Jahss M (ed): *Disorders of the foot and ankle*, London, WB Saunders, 1991.

110. Smith L, Plehive W, McGill M: Foot bearing pressure in patients with unilateral diabetic foot ulcers, *Diabetic Med* 6:573, 1989.

111. Smith LS, Clarke TE, Hamill CL, et al: The effects of soft and

semi-rigid orthoses upon rearfoot movement in running, *J Am Podiatr Med Assoc* 76:227, 1986.

112. Soutas-Little RW, Beavis GC, Verstraete MC, et al: Analysis of foot motion during running using a joint co-ordinate system, *Med Sci Sports Exerc* 19:285, 1987.

113. Stacoff A, Reinschmidt C, Stussi E: The movement of the heel within a running shoe, *Med Sci Sports Exerc* 24:695, 1992.

114. Stauffer RN, Chao EYS, Brewster RC: Force and motion analysis of the normal, diseased and prosthetic ankle joint, *Clin Orthop* 127:189, 1977.

115. Stipe P: The effects of orthotics on rearfoot movement in running. *Nike Res Newsletter* 2:no. 3, 1983.

116. Subotnick SI: Orthotic foot control and the overuse syndrome, *Phys Sportsmed* 3:75, 1975.

117. Subotnick SI: The abuses of orthotic devices, *J Am Podiatry Assoc* 65:1025, 1975.

118. Subotnick SI: Foot orthoses: an update. *Phys Sportsmed* 11:103, 1983.

119. Taunton JE, Clement DB, Smart GW, et al: A triplanar electrogoniometric investigation of running mechanics in runners with compesatory overpronation, *Can J Appl Sport Sci* 10:104, 1985.

120. Thompson JA, Jennings MB, Hodge W: Orthotic therapy in the management of osteoarthritis, *J Am Podiatr Med Assoc* 82:136, 1992.

121. Tue FS, Morse IE, Hinkle RT: *Mechanical vibrations*, ed 2. Boston, Allyn & Bacon, 1981.

122. Turnbull A: The race for a better running shoe. *New Sci* 123:42, 1989.

123. van Langelaan EJ: A kinematical analysis of the tarsal joints, *Acta Orthop Scand Suppl* 54:1, 1983.

124. Vierok RK: *Vibration Analysis*, ed 2. San Francisco, WH Freeman, 1981.

125. Voloshin AS: Shock absorption during running and walking. *J Am Podiatr Med Assoc* 78:295, 1988.

126. Voloshin AS, Wosk J: In-vivo study of low back pain and shock absorbtion in human locomotor system, *J Biomech* 15:21, 1982.

127. Whitman R: The importance of positive suport in the curative treatment of weak feet and a comparison of the means employed to assure it, *Am J Orthop Surg* 11:215, 1913.

128. Wosk J, Voloshin AS: Wave attenuation in skeletons of young healthy persons, *J Biomech* 14:216, 1981.

129. Wosk J, Voloshin AS: Low back pain; conservative treatment with artificial shock absorbers, *Arch Phys Med Rehabil* 66:145, 1985.

troubleshooting functional foot orthoses

Kevin A. Kirby, DPM

Negative casting

Positive cast preparation

Orthosis fabrication and material selection

Rearfoot posts

Shoe problems

**Common orthosis problems and their
  solutions**
  Heel slippage
  Plantar fascial irritation
  Heel cup irritation
  Lateral orthosis edge irritation
  Anterior orthosis irritation
  Dorsal first metatarsophalangeal joint pain
  Fifth metatarsal head pain

Summary

The functional foot orthosis is a device that is placed in a patient's shoe to alleviate mechanically related pathologic conditions of the lower extremity. Functional foot orthoses are constructed from a cast or from a three-dimensional (3-D) digitized image of the foot, which ensures that the orthosis is congruent with the plantar surface of the foot of the patient.

Functional foot orthoses are a design variant of the Root functional orthosis. The Root functional orthosis originated in the late 1950s with the podiatrist Merton Root as a thermoplastic foot orthosis to replace the less hygienic and less durable cork and leather orthoses of that era.[9] Today, the functional foot orthosis is the standard used within the podiatric medical community for the treatment of mechanical problems in the feet and lower extremitites.

It must be understood that this chapter only addresses true prescription foot orthoses that are made from a plaster cast or from 3-D digitized images of the foot. Foot orthoses made from foam bed impressions, footprints on inkmats, or tracings of the foot cannot be considered true functional foot orthoses since these foot-modeling methods are not sufficiently accurate to reproduce the plantar form of a foot. In addition, over-the-counter or generic foot orthoses are not discussed because they are not congruent with the multitude of individual plantar foot shapes seen within the general population. Excellent congruence of the orthosis to the foot is one of the hallmarks of a true functional foot orthosis.

Practitioners must possess the following qualities to be effective at troubleshooting foot orthoses:

1. The practitioner must have a detailed understanding of the fabrication of the foot orthosis from start to finish. He or she must realize how errors in negative casting and positive cast preparation affect the shape of the orthosis.
2. The practitioner must understand how the different types of orthotic materials and different types of orthosis construction can affect the final fit and function of the orthosis.
3. The practitioner must understand how different shoe designs can both help and hinder orthosis fit and function.
4. Most important, the practitioner must understand the biomechanics of the lower extremity; without this basic knowledge, the prescription for the foot orthosis has no foundation.

Because the practitioner must be proficient at many subjects to troubleshoot orthoses effectively, this chapter is divided into sections dealing with orthosis fabrication, orthosis materials, and orthosis-shoe interactions. In addition, more advanced biomechanical specifics are discussed. Finally, the last section is devoted to practical solutions for common orthotic problems that are seen daily in a busy podiatric biomechanical practice.

Negative casting

The first step in the fabrication of a foot orthosis is to ensure that an accurate cast or image has been made of the foot in a nonweightbearing position. The preferred technique for casting the foot is the neutral suspension casting method in which the subtalar joint is placed in the neutral position with the longitudinal and oblique axes of the midtarsal joint held in their maximally pronated positions.[10]

Errors in positioning the foot during negative casting can greatly affect the resultant orthosis. The most common negative casting error is supination of the longitudinal midtarsal joint (LMTJ) away from its maximally pronated position. Causes for this error include the patient contracting the anterior tibial muscle during casting or the practitioner grasping the digits of the foot too far medially during casting. Preferably, only the fourth and fifth digits should be grasped during negative casting.[10]

A negative cast that has the LMTJ supinated will have less medial arch height and more forefoot varus deformity or less forefoot valgus deformity than an appropriate negative cast would have (Fig. 15-1). Orthoses fabricated over casts with supinated LMTJs will often cause discomfort plantar to the distal aspect of the first metatarsal shaft owing to the increased forefoot varus correction in the orthosis. Patients will also demonstrate a greater tendency toward developing lateral ankle instability, functional hallux limitus, and hallux valgus deformities.

Other common negative casting errors include holding the foot so that the oblique midtarsal joint (OMTJ) is supinated away from its maximally pronated position. The most likely cause of this error is that the practitioner did not exert enough superiorly directed loading force on the fourth and fifth digits during casting. With a supinated OMTJ, the forefoot is not fully dorsiflexed on the rearfoot. The result is a cast with an abrupt sagittal plane angulation plantar to the calcaneocuboid joint in the lateral longitudinal arch of the cast. Transverse skin wrinkles across the midtarsal joint area of the interior of the cast may also result from OMTJ supination during casting. The patient will commonly experience pain and irritation transversely across the midtarsal joint (MTJ) area of the ortho-

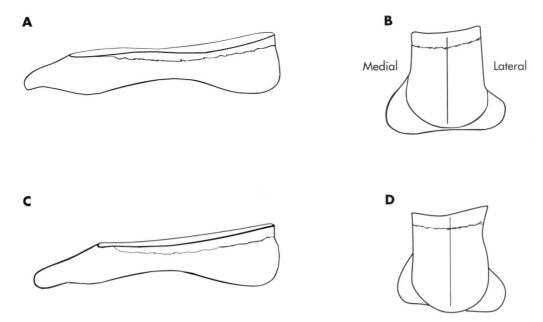

Fig. 15-1. 1A and B, The shape of a normal neutral suspension negative plaster cast of a right foot from the medial (**A**) and posterior (**B**) aspects. **C** and **D,** The same views of another negative cast taken with the longitudinal midtarsal joint supinated. Note the decrease in medial-longitudinal arch height (**C**) and the more inverted position of the forefoot (**D**).

sis.[10] This pain is generally felt in the first few steps with the orthosis inside the shoe.

One other common negative casting error is that the subtalar joint (STJ) may be held in a position that is pronated away from the neutral position. The result is a cast with a more flattened contour through the MTJ area and either greater forefoot valgus or less forefoot varus than would be present in an appropriate cast.[10] Orthoses fabricated from casts with a pronated STJ will be unable to relieve symptoms related to abnormal pronation of the STJ during weightbearing since they do not exert sufficient force on the foot at the medial midtarsal joint area.

Positive cast preparation

The positive cast is made by pouring plaster of Paris into the negative cast, then stripping away the negative cast plaster splints once the positive cast has hardened. From this point the anterior platform, lateral expansion, and medial expansion are added to the positive cast with additional plaster to prepare the cast for thermoforming of the orthosis plate material over the cast (Fig. 15-2).

It is beyond the scope of this chapter to detail all of the variables that go into the construction of the positive cast. However, a few of the more common errors of positive cast construction are described here to emphasize the importance of proper positive

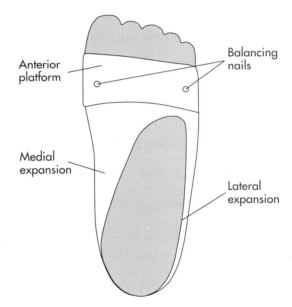

Fig. 15-2. A correctly fabricated positive cast should include balancing nails to place the cast in the proper frontal plane position, an anterior platform to provide for a horizontal plane for the anterior orthotic edge, and medial and lateral expansions to allow for soft tissue displacement of the foot on the orthosis.

cast construction in the fabrication of an appropriately fitting and trouble-free foot orthosis.

First, the physician should have the orthotic laboratory return the positive casts with the ortho-

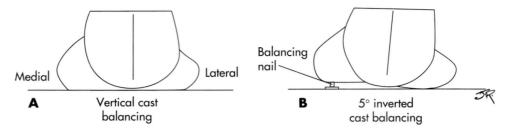

Fig. 15-3. **A,** A positive cast that is balanced in a vertical position has its heel bisection perpendicular to the ground. **B,** When the positive cast needs to be balanced 5 degrees inverted, the nail driven into the first metatarsal head portion of the cast protrudes more than in a vertically balanced cast.

sis. The positive casts are inspected to guarantee that the construction prescribed and the patient's foot shape have been incorporated properly into the casts. At the time of dispensing it is also important that the orthotic plates are compared with the positive casts to ensure that accurate thermoforming of the orthotic material to the cast has been achieved. Any significant incongruence between the orthosis and positive cast shapes requires that the orthosis and cast be returned to the laboratory for refabrication.

It is of prime importance that the positive cast is balanced in the proper frontal plane position so that the proper medial longitudinal arch height and forefoot correction is achieved. "Balancing of the positive cast" refers to driving nails a variable distance into the first and fifth metatarsal head areas of the cast to tilt the cast into an inverted, perpendicular, or everted position. For example, if the cast is balanced 5 degrees inverted, the heel bisection of the resultant positive cast will be 5 degrees inverted when laid on a flat surface (Fig. 15-3).

Balancing a cast in an inverted position tends to make an orthosis that has a different shape than an orthosis made over a vertically balanced positive cast. Inverted orthoses have higher medial-longitudinal arch heights, less forefoot valgus correction (or more forefoot varus correction), and an increased varus shape in the heel cup compared to vertically balanced orthoses. In general, these changes in the shape of the inverted orthosis increase the ability of the orthosis to control excessive pronation.

Because of the increased forefoot varus correction and increased medial-longitudinal arch height, orthoses fabricated from inverted casts have a tendency to irritate the medial band of the plantar fascia. This is one of the most common causes of medial arch pain with orthoses.[6]

Inverted orthoses, since they increase the supination torque on the STJ during weightbearing, also have an increased tendency to cause lateral ankle instability. It is crucial that the prescribing practi-

tioner understand that, in general, the more an orthosis controls pronation, the more likely that orthosis is to cause inversion ankle sprains.[6]

Balancing the cast in an everted position has opposite effects to those seen after balancing the cast in an inverted position. Everted orthoses have lower medial-longitudinal arch heights, more forefoot valgus correction (or less forefoot varus correction), and an increased valgus shape in the heel cup. In general, orthoses made from everted casts lack the ability to control excessive pronation of the STJ but may very well become comfortable arch supports for patients.

Another common positive cast error is the addition of an excessive thickness of medial expansion plaster to the positive cast (Fig. 15-4). This error results in the orthosis being fabricated with a lower medial-longitudinal arch height than normal. Unfortunately, many orthotic laboratories add excessive medial expansion plaster to positive casts because this decreases the chance of medial arch irritation. However, the decreased medial-longitudinal arch height also greatly reduces the ability of the orthosis to control excessive pronation and therefore the ability of the orthosis to relieve pronation-related symptoms.

In regard to proper medial-longitudinal arch height in prescription foot orthoses, it is better to err on the side of a higher medial-longitudinal arch for patients with pronation-related symptoms, since higher medial arches control pronation motion better than lower medial arches. The negative aspect in fabricating orthoses slightly higher in the medial-longitudinal arch is that these orthoses have an increased tendency to cause medial-longitudinal arch irritation. This is not a problem provided the practitioner has basic mechanical skills and the proper equipment, such as an electric drum grinder, to make adjustments to the orthoses.

There are many patients that will benefit in comfort and symptomatic relief with orthoses made with higher medial-longitudinal arch heights. Again, there will be a slight increase in the number

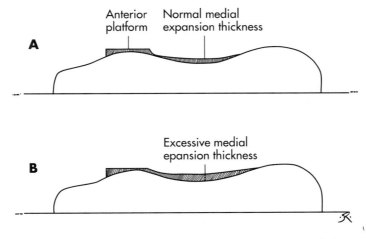

Fig. 15-4. A and B The medial aspect of two positive casts. When excessive medial expansion plaster is added to the positive cast **(B),** a lower-than-normal medial-longitudinal arch height is created.

of complaints and a slightly longer adjustment period. The practitioner must decide whether the added patient benefit of increasing the arch height is worth the complaints.

Orthosis fabrication and material selection

Most prescription foot orthoses are fabricated by thermoforming a heat-moldable material over the positive cast of the foot. After thermoforming has been accomplished, the orthotic plate is cut and ground so that it fits into the shoe properly and does not irritate the patient's foot. Rearfoot or forefoot posting, or both, may be added to the orthotic plate at this point. Finally, a topcover may be added to the plate along with a forefoot extension and accommodative padding to finish the orthosis.

Many modifications may be made in the shape and function of the orthosis to allow a true prescription foot orthosis to be fashioned. These modifications may include, but are not limited to, making positive cast modifications, using different orthotic shell materials, different materials for rearfoot and forefoot posting, and different types of forefoot extensions, accommodative padding, and topcovers. It is beyond the scope of this chapter to list all of the variables involved in orthosis design, but some of the more common problems will be outlined here.

One of the most common problems is that the foot orthosis is not made wide enough anteriorly to allow a snug fit inside the shoe. An ideal orthosis width is such that the anterior edge of the orthosis sits flat on top of the insole of the shoe and just touches the medial and lateral edges of the upper (Fig. 15-5A). This width ensures that the orthosis sits flat and does not migrate inside the shoe.

Unfortunately, since most orthoses are made to be

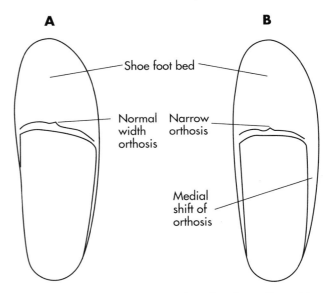

Fig. 15-5. A foot orthosis should just fit within the confines of the foot bed of the shoe **(A).** If the orthosis is too narrow **(B)** it will shift medially within the shoe, which can lead to lateral orthosis edge irritation and decreased control of foot pronation.

worn in a variety of shoes, transverse plane migration of the orthosis is a relatively common cause of irritation. The orthosis will nearly always slide medially because the medial longitudinal arch flattening seen with closed kinetic chain STJ pronation causes a medially directed shearing force on the orthosis. If the orthosis does not fit snugly it will generally move medially and may also internally rotate inside the shoe (Fig. 15-5**B**).

The main problem seen with the orthosis shifting medially is that there is a decreased ability of the orthosis to control abnormal pronation. The foot

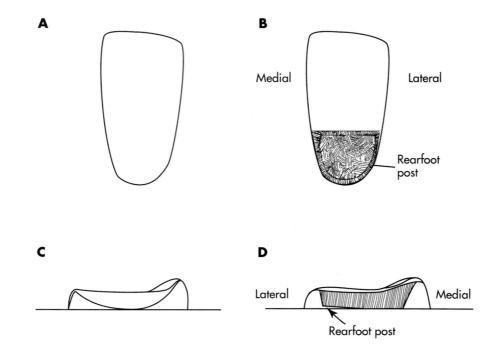

Fig. 15-6. **A** and **B,** The appearance of the inferior surface of foot orthoses with **(B)** and without **(A)** a rearfoot post. **C** and **D,** The same orthoses from the posterior view. Rearfoot posts are important to control excessive frontal plane rotation of the orthosis.

comes to rest in a relatively more lateral position on the orthosis, which makes the medial-longitudinal arch height of the orthosis effectively lower. This medial migration may also cause the lateral edge of the orthosis to dig into the plantar fifth metatarsal region of the foot, causing irritation and pain. To correct this problem, a wider orthosis must be made or a medial buttress pad must be attached to the medial edge of the orthosis.

Another common problem is that the material used in the orthosis is too flexible to adequately control pronation of the foot during weightbearing. Many podiatrists use thin or flexible thermoplastic materials for obese patients and in patients who undergo extreme medial-longitudinal arch collapse during gait. These patients generally experience little relief of their pronation-related symptoms with more flexible orthoses because flexible orthoses collapse under their weight and provide little control of foot pronation. More rigid foot orthoses greatly aid in controlling the pronation-related symptoms in these patients.

Another common problem is that the orthoses are not ordered with the extra features that would aid in the patient's recovery. For example, patients with capsulitis in the second metatarsophalangeal joint (MPJ) often only partially improve with foot orthoses that extend only to the metatarsal necks and lack forefoot extensions or metatarsal pads. The addition of an 1/8-in. rubberized cork forefoot extension to accommodate the second metatarsal head, along with the addition of a metatarsal pad at the distal-superior edge of the orthosis, is much more effective in treating second MPJ capsulitis than an orthosis that is made of a thermoplastic shell extending only to the metatarsal necks.

Problems such as the lack of forefoot extensions and other variations in design probably represent the most difficult troubleshooting problems. These problems are difficult to detect and correct since they are mostly due either to the practitioner attempting to limit expenses or not having the knowledge or experience with the various modification techniques to be able to design the most effective device. The only reasonable method by which to troubleshoot these problems is for the prescribing clinician to consult with the orthotic laboratory or with a colleague who has more experience.

Rearfoot posts

Rearfoot posts greatly increase the stiffness of the orthotic plate and increase the frontal plane stability of the foot on the ground. Therefore, orthoses with rearfoot posts are nearly always better at relieving symptoms related to excessive pronation or supination forces during weightbearing[4] (Fig. 15-6). For

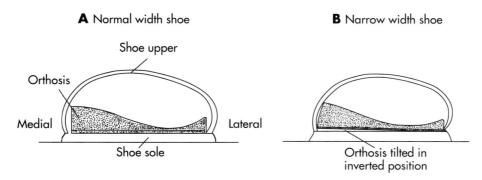

A Normal width shoe

Shoe upper

Orthosis

Medial

Lateral

Shoe sole

B Narrow width shoe

Orthosis tilted in inverted position

Fig. 15-7. A, A frontal plane sectional view through a shoe with an orthosis shows that an orthosis should fit so that it rests flat on the insole or foot bed of the shoe. **B,** The same orthosis placed in a more narrow shoe will become tilted into either an inverted or everted position because it can no longer sit flat.

this reason, rearfoot posts are used with the vast majority of foot orthoses. The simple addition of rearfoot posts to a pair of unposted orthoses often results in excellent resolution of mechanically related symptoms.

Rearfoot posts may be made of either firm or soft materials. In general, the firmer the material, the more durable the rearfoot post, and the better it is at resisting frontal plane motion of the orthosis inside the shoe. The rearfoot post may be constructed so that it is flat and parallel to the anterior orthosis edge (i.e., a flat rearfoot post) or it may be shaped so that the medial and lateral aspects of its plantar surface are at different frontal plane angles (i.e., a rearfoot post with motion). The most common rearfoot post construction is one in which the medial surface of the post is parallel to the anterior orthosis edge and the lateral surface is 4 degrees everted to the anterior orthosis edge. This type of rearfoot post is known as a 4-degree varus rearfoot post with 4 degrees of motion.

Rearfoot posts made of firmer materials and with little motion built into them are efficient at resisting STJ pronation and supination. This is especially the case if the shoe sole is also made of a firm material. Unfortunately, patients may complain of lateral knee pain, hip pain, or low back pain if the rearfoot post–shoe sole combination does not permit adequate STJ pronation when the foot contacts the ground during weightbearing.

On the other hand, if the rearfoot post is made of a relatively soft material, with a large degree of motion, or is used in a shoe that has a soft sole, there is increased likelihood that the orthosis-shoe combination will not adequately resist STJ pronation or supination. The result is that the patient's pronation- or supination-related symptoms are not resolved.

It is crucial that the practitioner realize that the composition and construction of the rearfoot post

has a great effect on the function of the orthosis inside the shoe. The rearfoot post must be factored into every clinical decision.

Shoe problems

The interaction of the shoe with the orthosis and the shoe with the foot is by far the most important consideration in troubleshooting orthotic problems. In order for the foot orthosis to work effectively, the shoe must have the following design characteristics.

First, as mentioned earlier, the shoe insole must be broad enough throughout its length so that the orthosis sits flat on top of the insole. If the shoe insole is too narrow, the orthosis will become tilted inside the shoe which will greatly affect orthosis comfort and function (Fig. 15-7). If the shoe insole is too wide, the orthosis will shift medially or laterally, increasing the chances of orthosis irritation (see Fig. 15-5).

Next, the insole of the shoe must be flat enough throughout its length so that the orthosis rests on a horizontal surface in the areas of both the rearfoot post and the anterior edges of the orthosis. Unfortunately, many recent athletic shoes have incorporated an integrated contoured foot bed within their designs. These shoes with contoured foot beds generally are made so that the heel area of the sole is concave while the medial arch area of the sole is convex. This contoured foot bed shape may interfere with proper orthosis fit because the orthosis will not have a flat, horizontal surface to lie on. The result is that the patient feels uncomfortable owing to the abnormal inverted or everted position of the orthosis.

The shoe must also have enough room to allow the foot to fit comfortably within it. Most lace-up shoes, including athletic shoes, walking shoes, and men's Oxfords have adequate room to accommo-

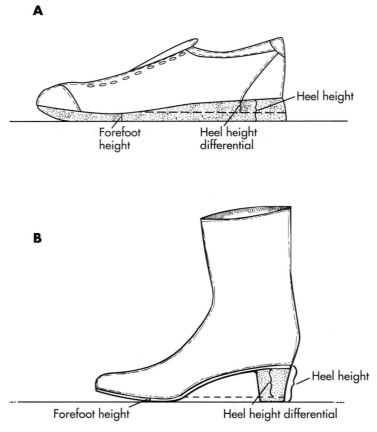

Fig. 15-8. The heel height differential of a shoe is the thickness of the heel minus the thickness of the forefoot of the shoe. Running shoes typically have a heel height differential of 3/8 in. **(A)** and cowboy boots typically have a heel height differential of at least 1-1/2 in. **(B).**

date the foot and the orthosis comfortably. Shoes with removable insoles work very well with orthoses since the extra room created by removal of the insole significantly improves the ability of the foot to coexist comfortably with the orthosis.

Unfortunately, many women's dress shoes are so narrow in the toe box and vamp area that any type of orthotic device added to the shoe increases the pressure of the vamp on the toes and forefoot. In addition, slip-on shoes, such as dress pumps, tend to cause heel slippage when orthoses are worn. Even the thinnest of orthoses may cause heel slippage in dress pumps.

The sole is also an important consideration when foot orthoses are used in treating the patient. In general, if the shoe has a hard sole, or midsole, then the shoe will be better at working with the orthosis to control foot pronation. However, it will be less effective in providing shock absorption. If, on the other hand, the shoe has a soft sole, then the shoe will be an effective shock absorber but poor at working with the orthosis to control foot pronation.

The major exception to this generalization is that heavy people who run or jog for exercise may actually experience less shock absorption from shoes with soft midsoles than from shoes with a firmer midsole since heavy people can actually "bottom out" the cushioning of these shoes.[8]

As an analogy, the shoe sole can be thought to work like a spring. If the spring is loaded within its working range, then for every pound added, further compression of the spring occurs. This displacement caused by the spring compression allows shock absorption. However, if the spring is loaded past its working range so that the coils of the spring start to touch one another, increasing loads on the spring will no longer compress the spring. In this scenario, the lack of compression allows no shock absorption. Therefore, shoe soles need to be tailored to the weight of the patient if the shoe is to provide maximal shock absorption.

Another important facet of shoe design that affects orthosis function is the *heel height differential* of the shoe. The heel height differential is the difference in thickness of the shoe sole under the heel compared to the thickness of the sole under the metatarsal heads.[2] Most running shoes have a heel height differential on the order of 3/8 in. Cowboy-style boots have a heel height differential of about 1.5 to 2.0 in. (Fig. 15-8).

Owing to their more curved design, shoes with increased heel height differentials are more likely to cause the orthosis to rock on top of the shank of the shoe. To test whether the orthosis is seated appropriately on top of the shoe insole the orthosis must first be placed within the shoe. When manual pressure is placed on top of the center of the heel cup area, the front edge of the orthosis should remain in place touching the insole on the forefoot of the shoe (Fig. 15-9). If the anterior edge of the orthosis lifts up off of the insole when the heel cup is manually pressed down, this indicates that the plantar surface of the orthosis is resting on a high spot on the shank somewhere between the heel cup and the anterior edge of the shoe.

The area on the orthosis that most commonly causes rocking on the shank is just plantar to the base, or styloid process, of the fifth metatarsal. If the orthosis is fabricated with a filler material plantar to the arch area, then some of the filler material in the plantar-lateral and plantar-medial arch should be ground out so that the orthosis does not hit a high point midway on the shank (see Fig. 15-9). If, however, the orthosis does not have filler material in the medial arch and is made with a shell material such as polypropylene, polyethylene, or an acrylic, grinding of the shell material itself may need to be performed. Since grinding of a graphite composite orthosis is not recommended, either the shoe or the orthosis may need to be changed or replaced.

Another method to correct rocking of the orthosis over the shank is to heat the orthosis in the midtarsal area with a heat gun and bend the orthosis to form a higher arch shape. The orthosis needs to be heated in the MTJ area and is bent just enough to allow it to rest on the shank of the shoe without rocking. It must be remembered that spot heating of orthoses is a last resort since improper spot heating can permanently deform the orthosis into a shape that is intolerable and possibly harmful for the patient. Nevertheless, many orthotic laboratories and podiatrists use spot heating with good results.

The heel height differential of the shoe will also, by itself, affect the overall function of the foot on the orthosis. For example, an increased heel height differential tends to cause decreased tension in the Achilles tendon during weightbearing owing to the more plantarflexed position of the ankle in these higher-heeled shoes. Decreased tension in the Achilles tendon can cause dramatic differences in the function of the STJ and MTJ.[2]

Patients with increased tension in the Achilles tendon (e.g., gastrocnemius or soleus equinus de-

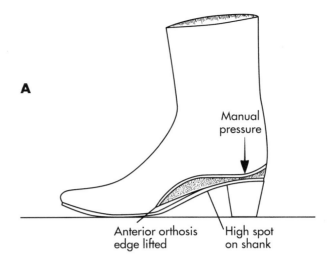

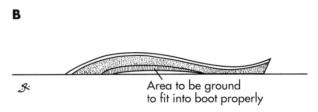

Fig. 15-9. Shoes with high heel height differentials typically have an increased curve within the shank which can create rocking of the orthosis. If manual pressure is applied to the heel cup and the anterior edge of the orthosis lifts from the sole, rocking of the orthosis will occur during gait **(A)**. The *arrow* in **B** indicates the point on the orthosis which needs to be ground down in order to fit properly over the shank.

formities) tend to have greater magnitudes of pronation moment across the OMTJ and STJ than patients with decreased Achilles tendon tension. Equinus deformities tend to cause rapidly increasing magnitudes of pronation moment across the OMTJ from the time of early midstance to late midstance. The increased moment across the OMTJ during late midstance is caused by the increased tension in the Achilles tendon caused by plantarflexing the rearfoot on the forefoot (Fig. 15-10).

Because of the increased pronation moment with increased Achilles tendon tension, shoes with different heel height differentials affect the amount of OMTJ and STJ pronation moment acting on the foot in different shoes. Shoes with increased heel height differentials tend to cause the foot to have decreased OMTJ and STJ pronation moment during weightbearing owing to the decreased tension in the Achilles tendon (see Fig. 15-10). Shoes with decreased heel height differentials tend to cause the foot to have increased OMTJ and STJ pronation moment due to the increased tension in the Achilles tendon.[2]

For example, if a person with a gastrocnemius

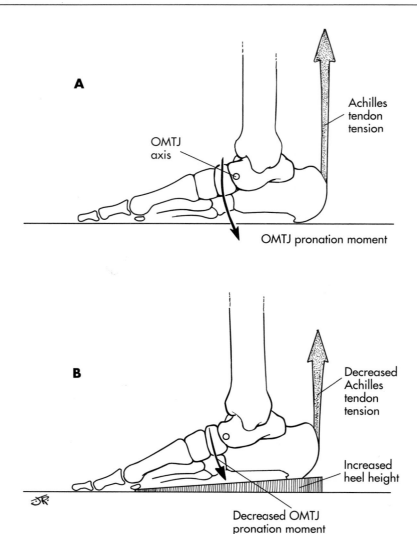

A, OMTJ axis
Achilles tendon tension
OMTJ pronation moment

B, Decreased Achilles tendon tension
Increased heel height
Decreased OMTJ pronation moment

Fig. 15-10. A, During closed kinetic chain walking, increased tension in the Achilles tendon causes a pronation moment across the oblique midtarsal joint *(OMTJ)* which increases the tendency toward medial arch flattening during gait. **B,** Adding a heel lift to a shoe decreases tension in the Achilles tendon, thereby decreasing the pronation moment on the OMTJ and the tendency for medial arch flattening.

equinus deformity walks in a shoe with a flat sole (i.e., no heel height differential) he or she will most commonly have significant pronation moment across the OMTJ and STJ during the latter half of midstance. If, however, this same person now walks in a shoe with a half-inch heel height differential, the OMTJ and STJ pronation moment will be decreased and less pronation will occur in that foot during weightbearing.

An appreciation of these interactions is important in understanding how shoes with different heel height differentials affect the comfort of the patient wearing an orthosis. In general, low-heeled shoes tend to cause the medial arch of the foot to flatten more forcefully during gait because of the increased OMTJ and STJ pronation moment that occurs in

these shoes. If an orthosis is worn in a low-heeled shoe there is increased likelihood that there will be medial arch irritation due to the medial arch of the foot being flattened harder on top of the orthosis. Adding a 1/8- or 1/4-in. heel lift underneath the rearfoot post will often eliminate medial plantar arch pain because of the decreased tension in the Achilles tendon.

Because of the very important role that Achilles tendon tension has on foot function inside a shoe with an orthosis, all orthotic and shoe design factors must be taken into consideration when analyzing the effects of the Achilles tendon on the force of medial arch flattening. It is not only the heel height differential of the shoe that is important, but also the thickness of the heel contact point of the orthosis

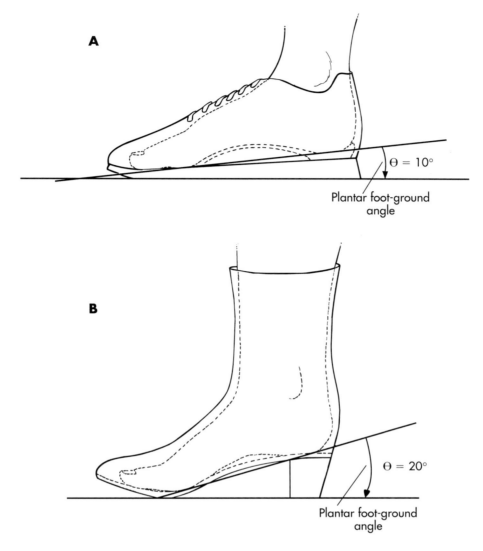

Fig. 15-11. The *plantar foot-ground angle* is the angle formed by the plantar surface of the heel and the plantar surface of the metatarsal heads. **A,** A running shoe with an orthosis has a higher plantar foot-ground angle than a running shoe with no orthosis. **B,** Cowboy boots have fairly large plantar foot-ground angles.

and whether any heel lifts have been added underneath one or both of the orthoses. In other words, the actual slope of the foot from the plantar surface of the calcaneus to the plantar surface of the metatarsal heads in relation to the ground is the determining factor as to whether tension in the Achilles tendon will be increased or decreased during gait. This angle of the plantar surface of the foot to the ground may be named the *plantar foot-ground angle* (Fig. 15-11).

The plantar foot-ground angle is determined by a line drawn from the most plantar aspect of the calcaneus to the plantar aspect of the metatarsal heads in relation to the weightbearing surface. Positive plantar foot-ground angles mean that the heel is higher than the forefoot inside the shoe. Negative plantar foot-ground angles mean that the heel is lower than the forefoot inside the shoe.

The plantar foot-ground angle is similar to the heel height differential of the shoe but is expressed as an angular relationship and incorporates any increases in heel height which heel lifts or orthoses provide. In other words, the plantar foot-ground angle is increased by shoes with increased heel height differentials, by orthoses with thicker heel contact points, and by heel lifts. The plantar foot-ground angle is decreased by shoes with decreased heel height differentials, by orthoses with thinner heel contact points, and by orthoses with thick padding under the metatarsal heads. The plantar

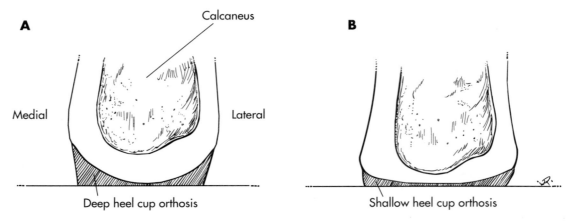

Fig. 15-12. Orthoses with deep heel cups **(A)** raise the calcaneus more than orthoses with shallow heel cups **(B)** due to the increased plantar fat pad which the deep heel cup gathers plantar to the calcaneus. This is one of the reasons why deep heel cup orthoses tend to create more heel slippage than shallow heel cup orthoses.

foot-ground angle is the most important factor in determining the tension in the Achilles tendon during gait and is therefore important to consider when troubleshooting an orthosis problem.

Common orthosis problems and their solutions

Heel slippage

The most common problem with foot orthoses is that they often cause the heel of the foot to lift partially out of the shoe during the propulsive phase of gait. This slippage can be affected by many design factors of the shoe and the orthosis. The most frequent cause is the thickness of the heel contact point of the orthosis. Any material that is placed under the heel increases the likelihood of slippage. Heel lifts, accommodative padding in the heel seat area, topcovers, and some types of rearfoot posts raise the calcaneus inside the shoe.

Any orthotic modification that raises the heel significantly inside the shoe decreases the congruence of the posterior calcaneus with the posterior heel counter. For example, orthoses with deeper heel cups or heel cups with a smaller radius of curvature increase the tendency toward heel slippage because they gather more plantar calcaneal fat pad underneath the calcaneus and raise the calcaneus within the shoe (Fig. 15-12).

Heel slippage is also caused by an orthosis that shifts the foot more anteriorly inside the shoe because of the decrease in frictional force and congruence between the posterior calcaneus and heel counter (Fig. 15-13). Deep heel cup orthoses may shift the foot more anteriorly within the shoe owing to the larger posterior lip on the orthosis.[7] The larger posterior heel cup lip pushes the foot

anteriorly inside the shoe, which prevents the posterior calcaneus from fitting snugly against the posterior heel counter.

Shoes that have short heel counters or shoes that have flat posterior heel counters also have a greater tendency to create heel slippage with orthoses. A taller and more curved posterior heel counter has a better ability to "grab" the posterior calcaneus.

Shoes that have laces or buckled straps that extend proximally on the dorsal aspect of the foot close to the ankle joint are much less likely to cause heel slippage than shoes with shorter closure systems that only extend, for example, to the midfoot. Shoes that have closure systems that extend proximally toward the ankle have a much longer area of snug contact on the dorsal aspect of the foot (Fig. 15-14). This increased area of dorsal contact with the foot increases the likelihood that the rearfoot portion of the shoe will rise off the ground with the foot at heel-off and thus prevent heel slippage. Slip-on shoes such as men's loafers and women's pumps have an increased tendency toward heel slippage when orthoses are worn since they do not contact the dorsal foot proximally enough to maintain a snug fit to the foot at heel-off (see Fig. 15-14).

Shoes with stiff soles also tend to cause increased heel slippage since these shoes are not as flexible at the forefoot. When the calcaneus leaves the ground at heel-off, the heel tends to stay on the ground. In addition, shoes with less "toe rocker" than normal ("less toe rocker" means that the distal sole of the shoe is almost flat on the ground) tend also to cause more heel slippage since more sole flexion is required in these shoes during propulsion, thereby increasing the tendency toward slippage.

There are many different measures that may be used to alleviate heel slippage when orthoses are

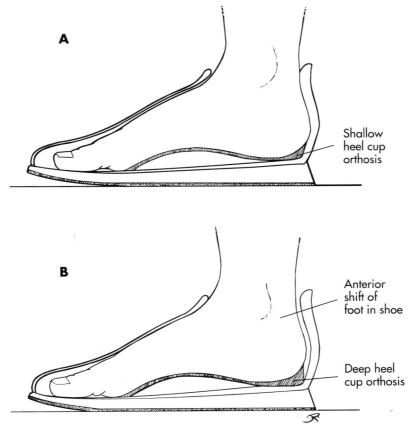

Fig. 15-13. A, Shallow heel cup orthoses have shallow posterior lips which fit well into most shoes. **B,** Deep heel cup orthoses have large posterior lips which may force the foot more anteriorly inside the shoe and lead to increased tendency toward heel slippage.

worn inside shoes. First, a tongue pad made of 1/8 -in. adhesive felt may be placed on the tongue of the shoe. The tongue pad places a force on the foot in a posterior direction which makes the posterior calcaneus fit more snugly against the posterior heel counter. This often greatly helps in preventing heel slippage.

The shoe should be laced up as high toward the ankle as possible. This may mean showing the patient how to use shoelace holes that have not been used before or even having new holes added farther up toward the ankle. Of course, if the shoe is not the style of shoe that can be used with orthoses, a different style should be recommended to the patient.

If the heel area of the orthosis is too thick, it may be necessary to remove topcovers or heel accommodations or insoles from underneath the orthosis. Many types of orthoses may be thinned under the plantar heel area by grinding at the heel contact point. Most thermoplastics may be ground to within 1-mm thickness under the heel contact point or may even be ground so that there is an actual hole in the

plantar heel seat of the orthosis, which may allow the calcaneus to sit lower in the shoe and lessen the heel slippage problem. Grinding down the heel cup height of the orthosis also alleviates some heel slippage since it allows the orthosis to rest in a more posterior position inside the shoe, which allows, in turn, for the calcaneus to fit more snugly against the posterior heel counter.

In general, however, it is recommended that the patient make the effort to purchase new shoes before the orthosis is modified. Shoe design is the culprit in causing much of the heel slippage seen with orthoses. If this is discussed with the patient before the patient is cast for the orthoses, the patient will be anticipating a new shoe purchase at the time of orthosis dispensing.

Plantar fascial irritation

The most common area for medial arch pain in the foot with orthoses is the medial band of the plantar fascia. The medial band originates at the medial calcaneal tubercle and inserts onto the medial and lateral sesamoids of the proximal phalanx of the

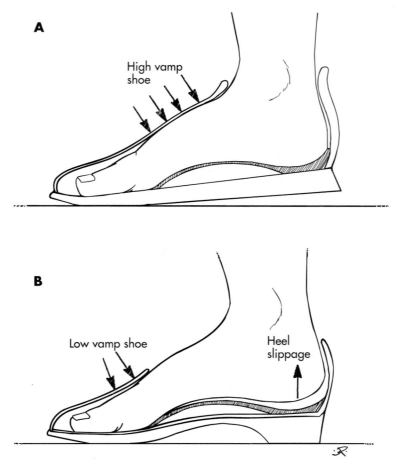

Fig. 15-14. Shoes with a vamp that extends proximally close to the ankle **(A)** cause less heel slippage than shoes with a lower-cut vamp **(B)** because of the larger surface area in contact with the foot at the time of heel lift.

hallux and ultimately into the base of the proximal phalanx of the hallux. The tension in the medial band increases considerably during weightbearing because of the loading of the first ray secondary to ground reaction force. This causes a marked bow-stringing of the medial band in a plantar direction away from the foot, especially in feet with normal to higher-than-normal medial-longitudinal arch heights.

Since negative casting of the foot is accomplished with no loading force on the first metatarsal, the medial band of the plantar fascia is not placed under tension during casting for functional foot orthoses. Because the medial band of the plantar fascia is not under tension, the orthosis made from this cast will commonly cause irritation where the plantar fascia protrudes significantly on the plantar foot during weightbearing.[1]

Another factor that influences plantar fascial irritation is the medial-longitudinal arch height of the orthosis. Medial-longitudinal arch height is increased when the positive cast is balanced in an inverted position, when the positive cast has less-than-normal medial expansion plaster added, and when extra forefoot varus posting is added. Often plantar fascial irritation can be lessened by grinding the medial-plantar aspect of the rearfoot post and the plantar-anterior edge of the orthosis to evert the orthosis and lower the medial-longitudinal arch height.

The best solution for plantar fascial irritation, however, is to have a *plantar fascial accommodation* placed in the orthosis. This is done by either grinding a shallow furrow on the dorsal surface of an existing orthosis or by adding a slightly raised ridge of plaster on the medial arch area of the positive cast (Fig. 15-15). The plantar fascial accommodation should be located on the orthosis in a line from the medial calcaneal tubercle to the first metatarsal head since this is the anatomical location of the medial band of the plantar fascia.

If it is noted during clinical examination that, with simultaneous first metatarsal head loading and hallux dorsiflexion to 20 degrees, the plantar fascia

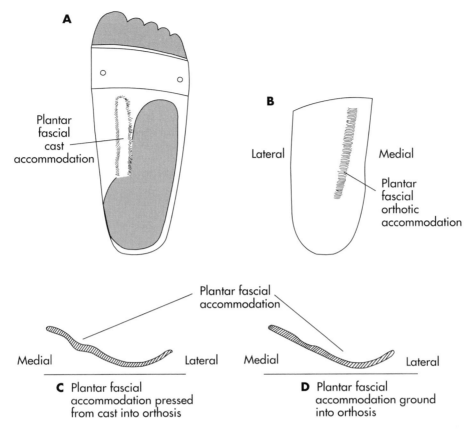

Fig. 15-15. A plantar fascial accommodation may be added to the positive cast **(A)** or it may be ground into the orthosis after it has been molded over the cast **(B).** A frontal plane section through an orthosis with a plantar fascial accommodation molded over a cast **(C)** shows that it has more potential for deep plantar fascial accommodation because the depth of a plantar fascial accommodation that is ground into the orthosis plate **(D)** is limited to the thickness of the plate.

bowstrings away from the foot by 3 mm or more, then a plantar fascial accommodation should be included in the orthosis prescription. The practitioner orders the depth of the plantar fascial accommodation in millimeters, with 3 mm being the average accommodation. Since grinding into the orthosis to make a plantar fascial accommodation is limited to the thickness of the orthotic material itself, it is almost always better to have the positive cast modified to include the accommodation than to grind in the accommodation after the orthosis is fabricated[1] (see Fig. 15-15). Both methods of accommodating the plantar fascia are effective in treating this annoying but common foot problem.

Heel cup irritation

The heel cup of the orthosis can be made in a variety of heights. Increased heel cup heights are excellent in the treatment of excessively pronated feet which require stabilization of eversion motion of the calcaneus. Decreased heel cup heights are often used when shoes with narrow heel seats are worn.

In order for the heel cup to be nonirritating to the tissues of the heel, the heel must be positioned congruent with the heel cup of the orthosis. To achieve this, the heel cup must fit within the shoe so that it is not shifted in relation to the plantar heel of the foot.

If lateral heel irritation occurs, then most likely the heel cup is resting too far medial within the shoe.[5] In order to determine the cause of the heel irritation, the position of the orthosis heel cup within the shoe must first be checked. If the lateral heel cup does not rest flush against the lateral heel counter, the heel cup may need to be reshaped until it is congruent with the lateral heel counter.

Often, the plantar aspect of the lateral rearfoot post may abut against the lateral heel counter, preventing the lateral heel cup edge from resting flush against the lateral aspect of the heel counter. This problem may be solved by grinding the lateral surface of the rearfoot post so that it does not protrude as far laterally as previously (Fig. 15-16). Lateral flares on rearfoot posts increase the tendency

A

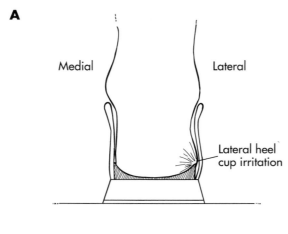

Medial   Lateral

Lateral heel cup irritation

B

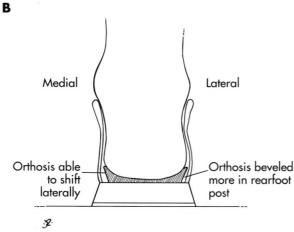

Medial   Lateral

Orthosis able to shift laterally   Orthosis beveled more in rearfoot post

Fig. 15-16. A, If the lateral aspect of the rearfoot post of the orthosis is ground so that there is only a slight bevel, the lateral heel cup of the orthosis may not be able to rest flush against the lateral heel counter, which may lead to lateral heel irritation. **B,** This problem may be solved by grinding more bevel into the lateral rearfoot post.

toward lateral heel cup irritation for this reason, since the plantar aspect of the lateral flare often prevents the lateral heel cup edge from resting flush against the lateral heel counter.

If other adjustments to the orthosis fail, a strip of one-eighth-inch adhesive felt is added to the medial surface of the rearfoot post of the orthosis as a shim to displace the posterior half of the orthosis laterally (Fig. 15-17). Sometimes, as much as 1/4 in. of adhesive felt must be placed on the medial rearfoot post to reduce or eliminate lateral heel cup irritation. If this shim is successful after a few weeks of trial fitting, a more durable shim material, such as 1/8-in. rubberized cork, may be glued as a permanent addition.[5]

Medial heel cup irritation is caused by the same factors that cause lateral heel cup irritation, but on the opposite side of the orthosis. To resolve this problem, the medial aspect of the rearfoot post is ground so that it does not protrude as far medially as before. In addition, medial rearfoot post flares increase the tendency toward medial heel cup irritation. If grinding of the heel cup or rearfoot post is unsuccessful or unnecessary, a shim may be added to the lateral aspect of the rearfoot post to displace the orthosis medially inside the shoe.

Posterior heel cup irritation is most commonly caused by anterior migration of the orthosis inside the shoe, which results in the posterior lip of the heel cup not fitting flush against the heel counter (Fig. 15-18). The use of deep heel cups is a very common cause of anterior migration of the orthosis. Increasing the depth of the heel cup increases the medial, lateral, and posterior width of the cup (i.e., the overall area of the cup). The increase in width increases the tendency for the heel cup to not fit congruently within the posterior heel counter. Therefore, an orthosis with a deeper heel cup has a greater chance of causing posterior heel irritation because of its greater width.[7]

To correct posterior heel irritation in an orthosis with a wide or deep heel cup, either the shoe must be changed or the orthosis heel cup must be narrowed or lowered, or both. If the shoes cannot be changed, the heel cup height of the orthosis must be lowered so that the heel cup fits flush against the posterior heel counter. This modification is easy to perform in the office with an electric drum grinder.

Anterior migration of the orthosis may also be caused by irregularities in the shape of the sole of the shoe. Ideally, the orthosis should sit on a flat heel seat of the insole so that it is not pushed anteriorly by a sloping surface in the insole. Many modern walking and athletic shoes have insoles or sock liners with curved posterior heel cups that cause the orthosis to be pushed anteriorly inside the shoe, which, again, leads to posterior heel cup irritation (Fig. 15-19). In order for the orthosis to rest flush against the posterior heel counter in these, either the sock liner must be removed completely or the curved portion of the sock liner must be trimmed from the heel cup of the sock liner.

Lateral orthosis edge irritation

The lateral edge of the orthosis can irritate the foot for a variety of reasons. Improper orthosis construction accounts for a small number of these cases. The majority of cases of irritation from the lateral border of the orthosis are caused by improper fit of the orthosis inside the shoe.

Lateral orthosis edge irritation is most frequently seen at the styloid process or base of the fifth metatarsal. Assuming that the orthosis is constructed properly with no vertical or sharp lateral

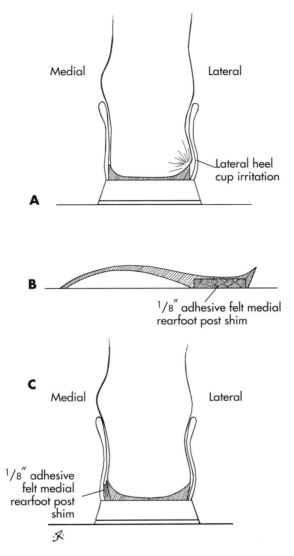

Fig. 15-17. If lateral heel cup irritation is caused by the lateral heel cup of the orthosis not resting flush against the lateral heel counter **(A)**, it is often helpful to add a strip of 1/8-in. adhesive felt on the medial aspect of the rearfoot post **(B)** to act as a shim. The shim invariably improves or eliminates the irritation by shifting the heel cup laterally **(C)**.

borders in the area of the styloid process, the most common cause of lateral edge irritation is medial migration or internal rotation of the orthosis inside the shoe (see Fig. 15-5).

As mentioned earlier, the orthosis should fit inside the shoe so that its medial and lateral edges lightly touch the lateral and medial upper of the shoe. This slightly snug fit prevents the orthosis from shifting medially.

If the orthosis has shifted medially the lateral edge of the orthosis will gap away from the lateral upper (see Fig. 15-5). The patient's foot will then rest in a relatively more lateral position on the orthosis. This causes the lateral edge of the orthosis to dig into the foot, especially at the styloid process of the fifth

metatarsal, leading to irritation of the lateral border of the foot.

Orthoses made for children have an increased incidence of lateral edge irritation because the orthosis is used in shoes that are increasingly longer and wider to accommodate foot growth. Therefore, children's orthoses should be made as wide as their current shoes to reduce the chance of lateral edge irritation as the foot grows.

To eliminate the lateral edge irritation caused by improper orthosis fit, the orthosis must be refabricated to a wider dimension or the existing orthosis must be modified. The easiest way to eliminate medial migration of a relatively narrow orthosis is to place a medial shim at the anterior aspect of the

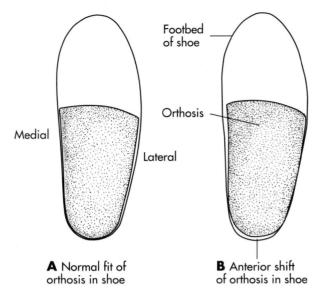

A Normal fit of orthosis in shoe

B Anterior shift of orthosis in shoe

Fig. 15-18. A, An orthosis should rest inside the foot bed of the shoe so that the posterior margin of the heel cup is flush against the posterior heel counter. **B,** If the orthosis is shifted anteriorly inside the shoe, posterior heel cup irritation is likely.

medial arch of the orthosis. A 1 × 2 in. piece of 1/4 in. rubberized cork is cemented to the plantar aspect of the medial arch so that it protrudes to the medial upper of the shoe (Christopher Smith, D.P.M., personal communication, 1982). The shim repositions the anterior half of the orthosis more laterally, which alleviates the lateral orthosis irritation (Fig. 15-20).

If, however, the narrow orthosis is also placed in a narrower shoe, then a shim should not be added to the orthosis but to the shoe itself. In this case, layers of adhesive felt can be added to the medial aspect of the inside upper so that the orthosis is repositioned back into a more lateral position. In either case, whether the shim is added to the orthosis or to the shoe, lateral edge irritation is routinely alleviated with these modifications.

Anterior orthosis irritation

The shell of a foot orthosis should normally be constructed so that the anterior edge of the orthosis ends just proximal to the metatarsal heads. The anterior edge of the orthosis should also rest flat on

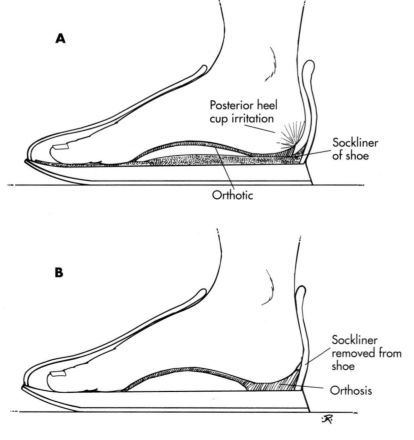

Fig. 15-19. A, Shoes that have molded sock liners (insoles) create orthosis fit problems because the posterior lip of the heel cup of the sock liner will wedge the orthosis anteriorly leading to posterior heel cup irritation. **B,** Removal or modification of the sock liner will correct this problem.

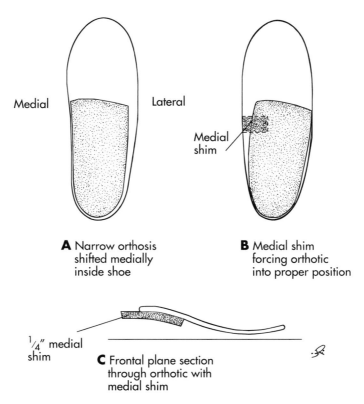

Medial   Lateral

Medial
shim

A Narrow orthosis
shifted medially
inside shoe

B Medial shim
forcing orthotic
into proper position

1/4" medial
shim

C Frontal plane section
through orthotic with
medial shim

Fig. 15-20. **A–C,** Since an orthosis that is too narrow will tend to shift medially, possibly causing lateral orthosis edge irritation or poor control of foot pronation **(A)**, a medial shim of rubberized cork is helpful in preventing this **(B).** The medial shim should adhere to the plantar aspect of the medial longitudinal arch of the orthosis so that it protrudes to contact the medial aspect of the upper **(C).**

the insole, not tilted into an inverted or everted position.

The most common reason for anterior orthosis edge irritation is an orthosis that is too long. In this instance the plantar metatarsal heads actually rest on the anterior edge of the orthosis, which leads to discomfort during extended weightbearing (Fig. 15-21). Obviously, the remedy for an orthosis that is too long is to shorten it, taking care to skive the anterior edge normally so that there is no dorsal prominence at the anterior edge.

The entire width of the anterior edge of the orthosis needs to rest flush against the insole of the shoe, otherwise a part of the anterior edge will gap away from the shoe insole, possibly causing discomfort. In addition, shoes with thick or prominent arch supports will often cause the medial aspect of the anterior edge to be elevated within the shoe, which commonly causes irritation just proximal to the first and second metatarsal heads. Orthoses that are too wide may rest either in an inverted or everted position within the shoe since their medial or lateral anterior edge, or both edges, will actually rest on the upper rather than on the insole (see Fig. 15-7).

Intrinsic or extrinsic forefoot varus or valgus posting may also cause anterior orthosis edge discomfort. Large amounts of forefoot varus posting create an abrupt slope at the anterior aspect of the medial-longitudinal arch of the orthosis. This may cause irritation to the foot approximately 1 cm posterior to the medial-anterior edge. Excessive forefoot valgus posting creates an abrupt slope at the anterior aspect of the lateral orthosis, which may cause irritation to the foot about 1 cm posterior to the lateral-anterior orthosis edge. It may be necessary to reduce the amount of intrinsic or extrinsic forefoot posting in the orthosis if the irritation at the anterior edge cannot be solved by other means.

Dorsal first metatarsophalangeal joint pain

If a patient complains of pain in the dorsal aspect of the first MPJ with foot orthoses, it can be assumed that the normal mechanics of the first MPJ has been altered unfavorably by the orthosis. The most common cause of MPJ pain is increased loading force by either the ground or the orthosis.

A Morton's extension in the forefoot often causes dorsal first MPJ pain due to the increased loading force it creates at the firt metatarsal head during gait.

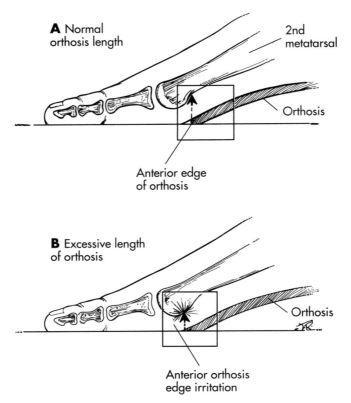

A Normal orthosis length

2nd metatarsal

Orthosis

Anterior edge of orthosis

B Excessive length of orthosis

Orthosis

Anterior orthosis edge irritation

Fig. 15-21. A, An ideal length for a foot orthosis exists when the anterior edge of the orthosis is adjacent to the neck of the metatarsals. **B,** Orthoses that are too long can create metatarsal head irritation since the metatarsal head will rest on the anterior edge of the orthosis during weightbearing.

A Morton's extension is a raised area at the first MPJ area of the forefoot extension of the orthosis, which effectively increases the ground reactive force under the first metatarsal head (Fig. 15-22). Increased dorsiflexion force on the first metatarsal head during gait may prevent the first metatarsal from plantarflexing normally during the propulsive phase. This prevents normal hallux dorsiflexion and leads to increased interosseous compression forces at the dorsal margins of the first MPJ. The increased interosseous compression forces between the dorsal base of the proximal phalanx of the hallux and the dorsal head of the first metatarsal can lead to pain and tenderness of the dorsal first MPJ (see Fig. 15-22). The greater the thickness of the extension, the greater the likelihood of first MPJ pain.

Any orthosis modification that tends to cause an increased loading force on the distal first metatarsal may lead to dorsal first MPJ pain. Modifications such as increased forefoot varus posting and forefoot varus extensions on the orthosis may also lead to first MPJ pain due to the increased loading force that is placed on the first metatarsal during weightbearing. In addition, errors in negative casting of the foot may lead to an orthosis that causes dorsal first

MPJ pain. If the LMTJ axis is supinated during casting, the resultant orthosis will have increased forefoot varus (or decreased forefoot valgus) correction built into it, which may cause dorsal first MPJ pain.

It is important that dorsal first MPJ pain be dealt with promptly or more serious problems will arise. The biomechanical factors that lead to dorsal first MPJ pain may also lead to development of dorsal exostoses at the first metatarsal head, and to hallux limitus and hallux abducto valgus deformities. If dorsal first MPJ pain or tenderness cannot be resolved promptly by orthosis modification, use of the orthosis should be discontinued.

Fifth metatarsal head pain

The fifth metatarsal head commonly becomes irritated by increased varus support by the foot orthosis. Orthosis modifications such as balancing the orthosis inverted and placing increased forefoot varus correction into the orthosis tends to place an inversion force on the forefoot, which can lead to either plantar fifth metatarsal head pain, a painful plantar tyloma at the fifth metatarsal head, or an aggravation of a preexisting tailor's bunion deformity.

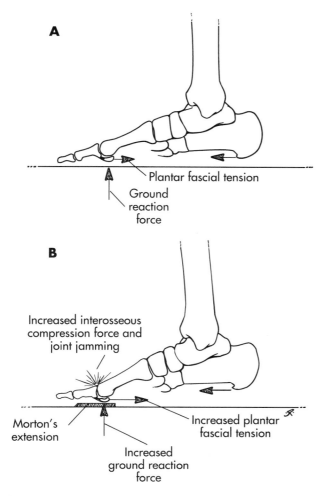

Fig. 15-22. A, Ground reaction forces on the first metatarsal tend to increase tension in the medial band of the plantar fascia which attaches to the base of the proximal phalanx of the hallux. **B,** Increased forefoot extension padding in the orthosis plantar to the first metatarsal head, as in a Morton's extension, creates increased plantar fascial tension and may lead to joint jamming in the dorsal first metatarsophalangeal joint during the early propulsive phase of gait.

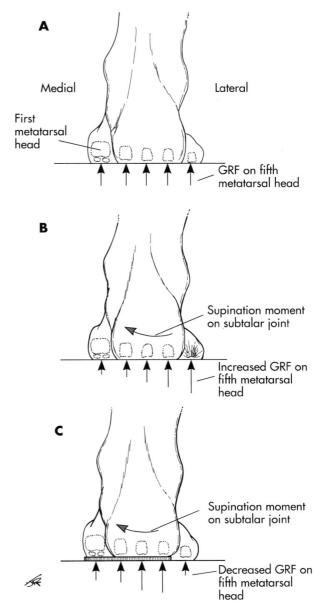

Fig. 15-23. A, Normally, the ground reaction force *(GRF)* on the plantar metatarsal heads is distributed fairly equally during standing. **B,** If increased supination moment is then placed on the foot, as by an inverted orthosis, the medial metatarsal heads have decreased GRF and the lateral metatarsal heads have increased GRF, which can lead to irritation, especially of the fifth metatarsal head. **C,** Fifth metatarsal head pain can be eliminated in this situation by adding an accommodative pad to the forefoot extension to decrease the GRF, specifically to the fifth metatarsal head.

Increased varus support by the orthosis causes increased inversion force on the forefoot which in turn causes decreased ground reactive force on the medial metatarsal heads and increased ground reactive force on the lateral metatarsal heads (Fig. 15-23**A** and **B**). The latter is generally greatest at the fifth metatarsal head since it is the most lateral of the metatarsal heads. However, if the fifth metatarsal has an abnormally large dorsiflexion range of motion the fourth metatarsal may receive the greatest increase in ground reactive force and become symptomatic.

If fifth metatarsal pain or plantar callus does occur, the best solution is to reduce the degree of forefoot varus correction in the orthosis. By reducing the degree of forefoot varus correction, the ground reactive force is decreased plantar to the fifth metatarsal head and the symptoms should be alleviated. One other modification that may be utilized if there is a critical need to maintain varus support is to add a fifth metatarsal head accommodation of 1/8-in. rubberized cork as a forefoot extension (Fig. 15-23**C**). The extension reduces the ground reactive force under the fifth metatarsal head sufficiently to relieve the symptoms or hyperkeratotic lesion.[3]

Summary

Troubleshooting foot orthoses requires that the practitioner have a thorough understanding of the biomechanics of the lower extremity and a detailed knowledge of the process involved in construction of the foot orthosis. From the biomechanical examination and negative casting of the foot to the resultant foot orthosis, the practitioner must use painstaking care to insure that the correct orthosis has been fabricated.

If problems result, such as irritation or continuing discomfort, decisions must be made as to what modifications will improve the situation. These may entail simple modifications such as adding a heel lift or be more complicated, such as regrinding the foot orthosis to fit the shoe properly. Whatever method is used to bring about an improvement in comfort and function, the benefit to the patient is nearly always immense.

The orthosis that improves function but is uncomfortable to wear is useless because it will not be worn. The orthosis that is comfortable to wear but does not improve function is harmful because it does not treat the problem. The foot orthosis that both improves foot function *and* is comfortable is a remarkable device which can positively and dramatically alter the course of a patient's life.

References

1. Kirby KA: Troubleshooting medial arch irritation in orthoses. Precision Intricast Newsletter, November 1986, pp 1-3.
2. Kirby KA: Effect of heel height differential in shoes on orthosis function. Precision Intricast Newsletter, March 1987, pp 1-3.
3. Kirby KA: Etiology and treatment of plantar fifth metatarsal head lesions. Precision Intricast Newsletter, April 1988, pp 1-3.
4. Kirby KA: Effects of rearfoot posts on foot orthoses. Precision Intricast Newsletter, May 1988, pp 1-3.
5. Kirby KA: Heel cup irritation in foot orthoses. Precision Intricast Newsletter, April 1989, pp 1-3.
6. Kirby KA: Inverting orthoses. Precision Intricast Newsletter, September 1991, pp 1-2.
7. Kirby KA: Effect of orthosis heel cup height on orthosis-shoe fit. Precision Intricast Newsletter, August 1993, pp 1-2.
8. Nigg BM, editor: *Biomechanics of running shoes*. Champaign, Ill, Human Kinetics, 1986.
9. Root ML: How was the Root functional orthotic developed? Podiatry Arts Laboratory Newsletter, Fall, 1981, pp. 1-4.
10. Root ML, Weed JH, Orien WP: *Neutral position casting techniques*. Los Angeles, Clinical Biomechanics Corp, 1978.

utilizing footwear as a therapeutic modality

Notty Bumbo, Pedorthist

A brief history of shoes
Shoe designs and styles
   Closure systems
   Shoe fit
Shoe construction and styles: an overview
Shoe therapy
   Upper modifications
      Stretching
      Padding
   External modifications
      Limb length discrepancy and lift therapy
      Rocker soles
      SACH heels
      Thomas heel
      Footwear considerations for orthotic therapy
      The pedorthist-utilizing the experts
The shoe as a "functional" orthosis:
Summary

The patients a practitioner sees throughout his or her practice will have one thing in common—they will all be wearing shoes. With the possible exception of certain tropical climates, all feet come clad. Whether in leather, rubber, fabric, or synthetic materials, and in more styles and types than can be counted, patients' feet will enter encased and leave the same way. Some of these shoes will be new; most will be old. Some of them will fit properly; most of them will not. Some of them will be practical; most will not. Some of these shoes will complement the care a doctor gives to the patient; most of these shoes will not.

Whatever the case may be, footwear has a direct impact on the outcome of care related to nearly every pathologic or pathomechanical presentation. Footwear may have contributed to the existing problem, may contribute to the continuation of the problem, may hinder the resolution of the initial problem or its sequelae, or if the clinician is particularly fortunate, assist in the treatment plan. Since each foot treated will return to the shoe environment after treatment or surgery, practitioners will do well to be informed about footwear, its relationship to various abnormalities and pathomechanics, its ability to assist with resolutions or improvements to the complaint, and especially to assist with the prevention of reoccurrence.

The goal of this chapter is to assist the foot care specialist in developing a background on basic shoe styles and construction, aspects of shoe therapy via shoe modifications, recommendations for treatment related to most pathomechanical and trauma-related foot problems, as well as the relationship of shoe style and function to the dispensing, prescribing, and functioning of foot orthoses, both functional and accommodative. There is also discussion of some common foot ailments that can be linked to choice of shoe styles and fit. While there continues to be some debate about this particular topic, it will become clear that there is indeed some causal relationship between feet and the shoes that encase those feet.

A brief history of shoes

Humans have worn some form of covering over their feet for thousands of years. A recent find of a frozen man in the mountains separating Italy and Austria revealed the remarkably intact remains of a hunter complete with an intact pair of fur moccasins. Humans have long worn foot coverings for a number of fairly obvious reasons: to protect themselves from the environment, as an aspect of fashion and status, as a sexual signal,[8] as an aid to functioning in various sports and work endeavors, and

to assist ambulation when there is impaired mechanical function of gait.

The first great leap forward in shoe design was originated by the Persians, who added heels to their sandals. This elevated them off the hot desert during long journeys and military campaigns. Another improvement is attributed to St. Clement. When St. Clement was on a long journey, he became footsore. He gathered tufts of wool from along the path where sheep had passed and placed them in the sandals under his feet. After wearing this wool for some time, St. Clement noticed that the tufts had entwined and had matted into a rudimentary foot bed. Wool felt is still used today as foot padding.

While footwear styles continued to develop over the next 2,000 years, it was not until America's Civil War that the next major development in footwear took place. Until the mid-19th century, all shoes were made to fit on either foot. This type of shoe is known today as a straight-last shoe. In the 1850s, shoemakers who were supplying shoes for the Union army developed the first rights and lefts, a concept that did not catch on with the general public until another 30 or 40 years had elapsed.[5]

Another concept in shoe design was not developed until early in the 20th century. Widths were an aspect of shoemaking that was largely left to the discretion of the various shoe producers and their designers. Although the first "grading" system to include widths was introduced as early as 1848, it did not become a standard feature in shoes until 1900. Even then, there was no true consensus on shoe sizes and widths. Today, there are at least four competing systems in use in North America and Europe.

While this is a very scanty history of a very significant subject, it should be noted that the complexity of footwear styles available to consumers today is the result of centuries of style development coupled with modern materials science and an increasingly sophisticated knowledge of biomechanics of the human foot and gait. This combination of knowledge has brought footwear design to new heights, enabling athletes to break records in all sports, to assist with the protection of the feet of workers in many demanding and dangerous occupations, and contributing to the improvement of foot health for all people.

The human foot is the foundation of the species. Below the foot, and therefore the true foundation, is the shoe. Shoes are subject to an amazing amount of abuse, and must be designed to withstand wear and tear on a daily basis. No other article of clothing that we wear is subject to nearly as much abuse, while being expected to perform just as well day after day. The materials and designs of shoes must be capable

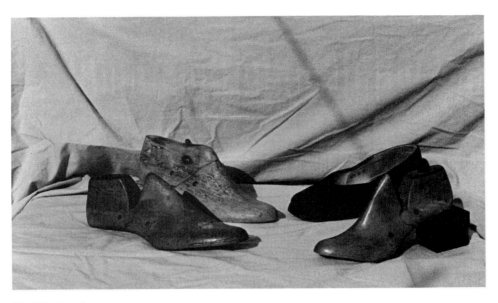

Fig. 16-1. Shoe lasts.

of withstanding constant moisture, abrasion, exposure to acids from foot perspiration, repeated bending and flexing, exposure to weather and terrain of all kinds, and still come up smelling like a rose. On top of all this, we insist that shoes be affordable.

Shoe designs and styles

Closure systems

Most shoe styles are defined by their method of closure. Closure systems include laces, hooks, hook-and-loop materials, slip-on or pull-on pumps or boots, buckles, and clamping systems (ski boots). A style can be a pump, yet still have straps and buckles. A shoe style can have more than one closure system, or even be made to resemble a different closure system than the one used in the actual design. The aesthetic design of a shoe, while primarily market-driven, must still be based on some type of closure system. After all, once the shoe is on the foot, it has to be kept in place.

Shoe fit

Besides having an adequate closure system, a shoe must fit. While this seems to be an obvious idea, this is not as easy for the consumer to achieve as one would expect. While shoe fit is predicated on dynamic structural volume and the bony proportions of the foot, shoe manufacturers are often more concerned with sales and what is being developed for the next season than with making shoes to fit every type and size of foot. If a person happens to

have a foot size that falls in the middle areas of the size spectrum, that person has little trouble finding good fit, comfort, and style.

If, however, a person has a very wide or very narrow foot, or a very long or very short foot, that person is going to have a very difficult time finding shoes that fit, style not even being a consideration at that point. Not too many years ago, shoes were made available in a very wide array of sizes and widths by nearly every manufacturer. One could even quite easily find combination-last shoes, which were wider in the forefoot than in the heel. (The *last* is the form that a shoe is made over, which imparts the shape and size to the shoe. Last also refers to the inside volume of the shoe itself (Fig. 16-1). Today, however, most shoes are available only in narrows and mediums, and only occasionally, wides. These are not terms that are based on some set standard, but rather on the individual designer's ideas of these terms. It is not far from the mark to say that shoe design has gone backward in recent years, when one looks at the concept of shoe fit. Fit is perhaps the most important aspect of a shoe, from the perspective of comfort, function, and foot health. If a shoe fits improperly, it can contribute to something as mild as corns and calluses, or to something as extreme as ulceration in the diabetic patient, sometimes leading to amputation. However, making a shoe fit is not an easy task, nor is there much agreement within the shoe manufacturing community on the best approach to achieving proper fit.

A shoe is expected to fit well in the heel, without slipping, but also without extreme pinching. The instep must also be held snugly while allowing proper motion during gait. The forefoot must be allowed to move properly, especially during toe-off, but not so much as to promote lateral and retrograde instability during midstance. The shoe must achieve all of this by being flexible enough to allow proper motion, yet durable enough to maintain its shape. For all of this to happen successfully, the combinations of materials, closure systems, style, and method of construction must all work together. If even one of these components is not properly suited to the combined elements, the shoe will either not fit, or it will not function as it was originally intended.

One example of improper shoe fit can be seen in patients with medium-to-severe bunion deformities. While it can be argued that poor fit or even high heels can contribute to bunion deformity in the first place, there is no doubt that, subsequent to the formation of the deformity, improper shoe fit is more the rule than the exception. In order to find shoes that do not feel too tight across the ball of the foot, this patient will buy a wider shoe than he or she really needs. Because combination-last shoes are difficult to find today, such a patient will often be forced to wear a shoe that slips in the heel. The proper approach for this problem is to purchase shoes that fit correctly in the heel, and to stretch the forefoot of the shoe. Most leather-upper shoes can be adequately stretched at a local shoe repair shop. This results in a shoe that will fit the entire foot, not just a part of the foot.

Another important aspect of shoe fit is the proper measurement for length. While overall length, from heel to toe, is important, the length from heel to ball is the most important measurement for shoe fit. This is because a shoe is designed to "break," or flex best across the dorsum of the metatarsophalangeal parabola. If the shoe is fitted improperly from heel to ball, the vamp, or forepart of the shoe, will not flex with the natural flex of the metatarsals during the propulsive phase of gait, and may actually flex *against* the foot. In some shoe styles, this can even result in a "double" flex, which could have serious consequences in patients with insensitive feet.

Perhaps the most frustrating fit-related problem occurs with patients who wear high-heeled shoes. These may be either men or women, because we must include many types of men's footwear in the high-heel category. This includes western boots, linemans' boots, and many fashion styles that utilize a more elevated heel. While women present with foot problems related to or exacerbated by high-heeled shoes more frequently than men, the same types of problems appear in both groups.

What makes a high-heeled shoe, especially a slip-on style or pump, fit the foot is a set of factors that must be present, yet whose presence is the cause of many foot and gait problems. Because the foot is essentially on a slope, and involved in forward momentum on that slope, such shoes must be narrower in the toes and ball of the shoe, simply to prevent the foot from sliding down the hill. The effect of this tightness is to pinch the metatarsals and digits together and impinge on the foot's natural functioning, especially during toe-off. Because this type of footwear is so snug, such heat- and moisture-related foot problems as fungal and bacterial infections, calluses, ingrown nails, and verrucae are likely to develop much more readily.

The other factor that assists in high-heeled shoes staying on the feet is something known as "bite." This refers to the topline of the shoe or boot (Fig. 16-2). The topline is designed to fit the foot very tightly, essentially compressing soft tissue to establish a good grip on the heel of the foot and prevent the foot from slipping out of the shoe with every step at toe-off. The topline is, in essence, the closure system in the slip-on style of footwear.

It is a common problem to encounter the female patient who insists that she can only wear high-heeled shoes, that low-heeled shoes cause her pain. This is usually a patient who has worn high-heeled footwear most of her life. Such a history can easily contribute to the development of an acquired equinus. In such cases, palliative care may be the best option available. The effectiveness of foot appliances in such cases is marginal, because the compromises that are necessary to achieve good fit in the shoe render the resultant orthoses less than functional in design. This is also true because of the overall equinus position of the foot in such footwear.

Shoe construction and styles: an overview

While there are many different styles of footwear on the market today, there are only a handful of actual construction techniques. This topic is important to the podiatric practitioner because while styles change, construction techniques are only refined, never discarded. If the clinician knows how to inform the patient regarding acceptable footwear that will aid with foot health and work most effectively with prescribed orthoses, overall patient compliance will improve significantly.

Shoe construction styles are based on one or several of three key approaches. Shoes are made up of parts, usually of a variety of materials, in any given style of footwear. Because these various materials are usually of different composition, strengths, elasticity, and chemical makeup, these parts may require several techniques to hold all the parts together. Thus, sewing, stitching, cementing,

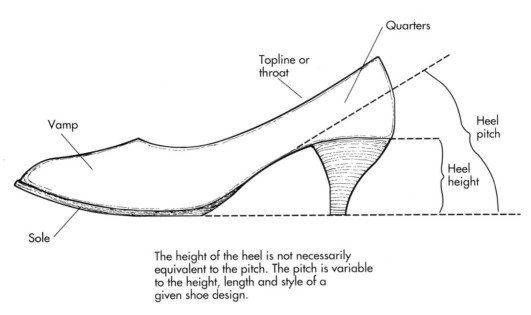

Woman's Pump
(It is the closure style which
defines a pump, not the heel height)

Quarters

Topline or
throat

Vamp

Heel
pitch

Heel
height

Sole

The height of the heel is not necessarily
equivalent to the pitch. The pitch is variable
to the height, length and style of a
given shoe design.

Fig. 16-2. Woman's pump.

or injection-molding are the primary methods of holding footwear together. This is not all there is to it, however. Today, some forms of cement construction techniques account for more than 50% of all footwear produced in the world. Nearly all athletic shoes use a combination of stitching of uppers and cementing of sole and midsole (Fig. 16-3). Most casual and many dress-style shoes also use this combination of techniques. And while many shoe soles are injection-molded before being attached to the upper of a shoe, even these types of footwear must use some form of adhesion to bond the two parts together. Injection-molding is also used in making waterproof boots, beach footwear, specialty fashion shoes, specialty work footwear, and other types of shoes that require a very "designed" sole. There are very few shoe designs that rely only on cement construction techniques, at least for upper construction.

Of greatest importance to the practitioner is the ability to direct a patient to shoe types that fit well and are able to move with the patient's foot in such a manner as to assist that foot with its daily activities. A high-heeled boot designed for a lineman will hardly be of use to a salesperson standing and walking on flat, hard floors all day. So a shoe should not only fit the foot, but the task as well. What follows is an outline of general shoe construc-

tion types, and their various parts (Figs. 16-2, 16-3, and 16-4).

As can be seen in the figures, there are many parts to even the simplest shoe design. Even when these basic design ideas are radically changed, they remain true to several basic concepts: the toe box and the heel counter of the shoe must function to maintain the shape of the shoe while enhancing support of the foot within; the closure system must serve to hold the shoe on the foot during any activity, without hindering natural movement; the materials used in a given design must function together and maintain their durability during continuous use and under a wide range of environmental conditions, both internal and external.

Shoe therapy

Shoe therapy is the term used to describe any alteration to an existing shoe design for the purpose of accommodating or altering the functionality of a shoe in response to a pathologic or pathomechanical problem in the foot. Shoe therapy can be something as simple as a tongue pad, or as radical as a lift and brace attachment. If the practitioner is to properly prescribe for therapeutic alterations, a grounding in terminology and approach is essential. While most shoe modifications should be performed by trained

Standard Man's Shoe Construction
(Most styles are variations of this theme.)
Separate sole and heel style

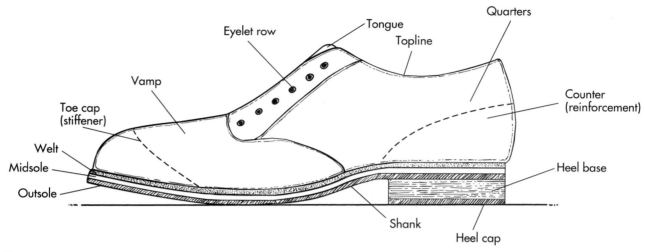

Fig. 16-3. Standard men's shoe construction.

Wedge-style Sole Design

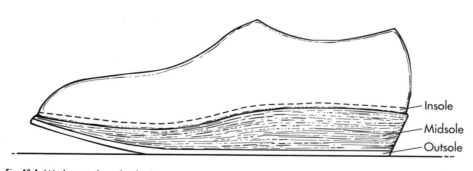

Fig. 16-4. Wedge-style sole design.

pedorthists or orthotists, some modifications, such as paddings, lacing patterns, and even spot-stretching, can be performed quite simply by the practitioner in the office.

This section describes the most frequently employed shoe modifications, the purpose for and technique of application, and the shoe types best suited to such modifications. The section is presented in two parts—upper modifications and bottom modifications. The materials used and the construction style employed must both be considered when examining a patient's footwear to determine its applicability for use either with foot orthoses or with other types of shoe therapy. A shoe can appear to have a sole that can be separated from

the shoe for the inclusion of a lift, but it may be a very artfully designed injection-molded sole, and therefore impractical for such use. It must again be emphasized that shoe designs change so frequently that it is not practical to list by brand or style what shoes should be recommended for what therapy. There are, however, some general guidelines:

1. In wedge-sole design shoes, the outsole layer should be clearly a separate piece of material. If the separation between the outsole and the midsole is indented, then the shoe may be appropriate for bottom modification. If, however, the separation appears

"Depth" Style Shoe

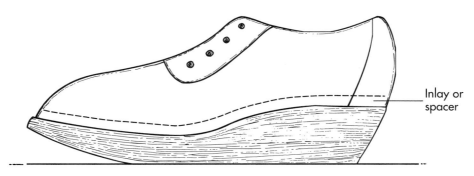

Inlay or spacer

Fig. 16-5. Depth-style shoe.

to be a seam, then that shoe is most likely an injection-molded sole.

2. With children's footwear, especially where the attachment of a night splint is required, a rubber-soled shoe is a poor choice. Try to use a leather-soled shoe, instead. Also, be sure such shoes have a firm counter, with a long medial counter offering the best support.

3. With athletic footwear, avoid all the air- and gel-type shoes if the need is for lifts or rocker sole modifications. These shoes, especially the multilayered sole styles, cannot be readily adapted for these purposes.

4. For those patients who require more room in their shoes for extra-bulky orthoses, or to accommodate fluctuating edema, there is a style of shoe known as the depth shoe (Fig. 16-5). These shoes are available from several companies.* A depth shoe is designed on a deeper last than nondepth shoe styles, and includes a removable layer of material. This layer may be between 1/8 and 3/16 in. in thickness. Removing this layer allows more room in the shoe for necessary therapeutic alterations. While many athletic shoes available today have a removable foot bed, most of these shoes are not truly depth shoes, because the foot bed is added after the shoe is completed and is usually soft enough to present little interference with normal fit.

---

* P.W. Minor Shoe Co., Batavia, New York; Drew Shoes, Lancaster, Ohio; Alden Shoe Co, Middleboro, Massachusetts. These are just a few sources; depth shoes are usually available through a local pedorthist and through some orthotic and prosthetic facilities.

Upper modifications
Stretching

One of the advantages of using leather to make shoes is that leather not only conforms to the foot through the course of normal wear, but can also be force-conformed by stretching. Shoe repair shops have been stretching shoes for as long as shoes have been worn. Many practitioners have kept a variety of shoe-stretching tools in their office to perform immediate adjustments to their patients' shoes (Fig. 16-6). While this may seem an old-fashioned idea to many modern practitioners, shoe stretching, especially spot-stretching, can be of great benefit to both practitioner and patient.

Perhaps the most regular foot complaints a practitioner encounters are bunions and hammer toes. While the treatment plan might eventually involve surgical intervention, immediate comfort is what most concerns the patient. While removal of corns and calluses provides some relief, that relief can be significantly improved with spot-stretching of the shoe over the affected area. Spot-stretching is done with a tool known as a ball-and-ring stretcher, available from several podiatric supply houses, and from most shoe manufacturing companies, which can be found under that heading in most telephone books. A ball-and-ring stretcher is used in conjunction with a liberal application of stretching fluid, which is merely a fifty-fifty mix of rubbing alcohol and water. The ball portion of the tool is placed inside the shoe at the desired location, with the ring on the outside of the shoe. Stretching can be either pinpoint, or the stretcher can be "walked" around the area to create a more diffuse stretch.

With a shoe that has a leather upper, stretching is quite simple. The only area of concern is discoloration. This can be minimized by applying the stretching fluid well beyond the area to be stretched.

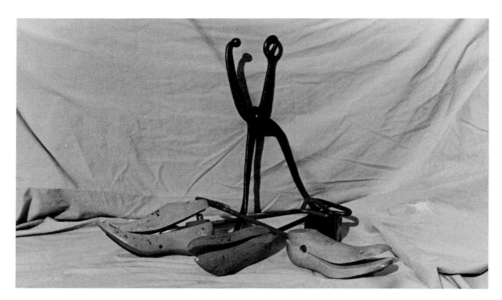

Fig. 16-6. Shoe stretchers.

The real problem occurs with shoes made of manmade pseudoleathers or fabrics. Some of the pseudoleathers can accept a minor amount of stretching, but they may return to their original size over a short time. Fabric uppers should not be stretched, as they do not have enough elasticity and can be damaged by the effort. Remember also that any stretching is improved by increasing the amount of time the shoe is kept on the stretcher.

Another type of stretching is used to actually increase the width, and to a lesser degree, the length, of a patient's footwear. There are two types of tools used for this modification. One is the traditional shoe stretcher (see Fig. 16-6). This tool comes in various configurations; some are used to stretch the forepart width at the toe, some at the ball. Other types of stretchers are used to stretch the vamp of the shoe at the instep; another is used to raise the overall height of the toe box. Again, these tools take up little room in the practitioner's office, and can make an immediate difference for a patient who needs to have shoe pressure relieved to complement the primary treatment.

The other tool used for general shoe stretching is called a Eupidus stretcher, and can be found in most shoe repair, pedorthic, and orthotic facilities. This tool has the advantage of greater leverage in the stretching of a shoe. When trying to stretch a shoe that is constructed of fairly thick leather that needs a great increase in size, or a shoe that requires a permanent stretch, this tool is essential. The practitioner should define the area to be stretched by putting a piece of masking tape over the area or with an accurate description in the prescription.

Stretching shoes may seem an old-fashioned idea, but the effect on the patient is immediate, and usually decreases the frequency of visits for palliative care.

Padding

In-shoe padding is the oldest form of shoe therapy.[1] Indeed, it may be the oldest form of foot care. It is a common idea that if something hurts on the foot, some type of pad will reduce the pressure. There are many different types of pads for alleviating pain and pressure in the foot, but this section focuses on the primary types. While there are many padding techniques for a bunion, for example, they are mostly variations on a theme, and are covered elsewhere in this book.

Metatarsal pads. Metatarsal pads are also referred to as met pads, met cookies, and neuroma pads. While the purpose of a neuroma pad is different from that of a standard met pad, the general shape and placement are similar (Fig. 16-7). Metatarsal pads are used to support the metatarsal shafts, especially shafts 2, 3, and 4. They might be used to relieve pressure on one or all of these metatarsophalangeal joints, or to take some weightbearing away from the first or fifth metatarsophalangeal joint. Metatarsal pads are available in prefabricated styles, either lefts or rights, or universal, and come in soft, medium, and hard, sized from small to extra-large. They are available through most podiatric supply houses. Metatarsal pads can also be readily fabricated from adhesive-backed felt in the office. A skiving knife is of great assistance in skiving the thickness of the pad into its proper shape. The

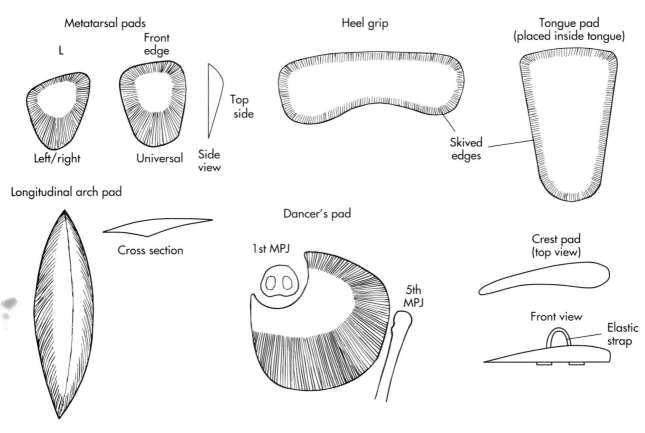

Metatarsal pads
L
Front edge
Left/right   Universal   Side view   Top side

Heel grip

Tongue pad
(placed inside tongue)
Skived edges

Longitudinal arch pad
Cross section

Dancer's pad
1st MPJ   5th MPJ

Crest pad
(top view)

Front view   Elastic strap

Fig. 16-7. Shoe therapy pads.

difference between a standard metatarsal pad and a neuroma pad is size, and to a lesser degree, placement. A metatarsal pad is usually employed to relieve pressure in a diffused manner, over a larger area. The neuroma pad is smaller, and more specific, being placed between the two metatarsal shafts, where the neuroma is located. The purpose here is more to separate the metatarsophalangeal joints than to lift them, in order to relieve pressure on the neuroma. The overall shape, however, is the same for both types of pads.

Tongue pads. A tongue pad can be made of adhesive-backed felt in the office. This pad is perhaps the least used yet the most effective pad to relieve anterior shoe pressure and heel slippage due to a combination-type foot (narrow heel, wide forefoot) and when "pocketed," to relieve dorsal "pump bump" pressure. Obviously, a tongue pad can only be used in footwear that has a tongue, though it can be used with some success in pull-on style boots, as well. The placement of the tongue pad is obvious. The thickness of the pad is determined by the amount of space available when the shoe is examined, but generally 1/8 to 1/4 in. is best.

The application of a tongue pad to prevent heel slippage is very effective. It functions by holding the foot farther back in the shoe, thereby keeping the ball of the foot in the widest part of the shoe, and the heel snug against the counter of the shoe. Since many heel blisters, Achilles tendon irritations, and retrocalcaneal bursae may be caused, or at least exacerbated by heel slippage, this is an effective technique for reducing this area of irritation.

The tongue pad can also be used to relieve pressure on the dorsum of the foot, such as that precipitated by a pump bump. By simply cutting a "window" in the pad in the proper location, pressure is diverted around the bump instead of directly on the site. Relief is usually immediate for the patient (see Fig. 16-7).

Dancer's pad. A dancer's pad is a combination of metatarsal pad and a aperture pad. It serves to support metatarsal shafts 1 to 4 and the second metatarsophalangeal joint, in order to relieve excess pressure at the first metatarsophalangeal joint. This pad can be made of felt, Poron (Rogers-Woodstock, CT), or Korex (cork and rubber) (Accurate Felt and Gasket Co., Cicero, IL), and is sometimes used in conjunction with a custom foot orthosis. The pad retains its full thickness around the first metatarsophalangeal joint, and is skived away at all other edges (see Fig. 16-7).

Crest pad. The crest pad is used when one or several digits of a patient's foot are in moderate contracture, and are becoming irritated on the distal end of the digit owing to excessive prehensile action. The crest pad (see Fig. 16-7) has a strap that is worn over the third toe to maintain the pad in the proper location during gait. A custom crest pad can also be incorporated into the distal extension of a custom foot orthosis. When requesting a crest pad from the orthotic laboratory, be sure to include a weightbearing tracing, following the digital inner spaces with the pen. This enables accurate placement of the pad by the laboratory. Reliance on the negative cast for this placement can lead to incorrect positioning, as the plaster can significantly distort the sulcus position, as well as the true depth of the sulcus. Prefabricated crest pads are usually available through podiatric supply houses, and in some drugstore foot care products displays.

Longitudinal arch pads. This type of pad is also referred to as a "cookie" by some practitioners. It is available in a wide variety of prefabricated styles, and in a number of materials. While arch pads can be made from felt quite easily, the low cost and wide availability of this type of pad are such that stocking a variety of sizes and densities of prefabricated arch pads is more efficient. While some rather exotic shapes are available, the type shown in Figure 16-7 is a standard shape, which works quite well for the majority of applications. Longitudinal arch pads can be used with or without a custom foot orthosis. Use with a custom device is usually as an adjustment to the original orthosis.

Heel grip, or counter pad. This is another type of pad that can be used in response to a complaint of heel slippage. Made of adhesive-backed felt, and available as a prefabricated item, it is used in the back of the shoe, just below the posterior topline. It is best to skive the center of the pad much thinner that the two "wings," to prevent excess pressure on the Achilles tendon (see Fig. 16-7).

Morton's extension and reverse Morton's extension. The first ray is subject to a variety of positional and pathomechanical abnormalities. The foot that displays a plantarflexed first ray, or a significant forefoot valgus angulation, is not always adequately controlled by a standard functional foot orthosis. Since the pathomechanics of this type of foot occurs during late midstance, heel-off, and finally the toe-off phases of gait, it is often beneficial to provide additional correction distal to the orthosis if the mechanical problem is to be alleviated. The same holds true for a short first ray, a hypermobile first ray, and for a metatarsus primus elevatus. In these latter problems, the first ray is either not contacting

the ground at the proper moment, thereby increasing pressure on the second or third metatarsophalangeal joint or it is not stabilizing the medial column at all, leading in some instances to excessive late midstance pronation, with subsequent problems.

A Morton's extension can be incorporated into the shoe directly, as an adjunct to a longitudinal arch pad, or incorporated into the custom foot orthosis as an extension distal to the device itself. Korex, Poron, or a similar material is used, with the firmer materials producing the best mechanical advantage, as well as increased durability. In the case of a hallux rigidus, the application of a short Morton's extension, ending at the sulcus, can greatly reduce dorsiflexion force on the hallux, allowing the hallux to clear the ground during toe-off while minimizing motion (Fig. 16-8).

A reverse Morton's extension is used when treating a foot with a plantarflexed first ray, a forefoot valgus deformity, or in the mechanical treatment of sesamoiditis. This type of pad is simply an extension to the custom foot orthosis, applied plantar to the second through fifth metatarsophalangeal joints, and usually made from a firm extension material, such as Korex, or Nickleplast (Alimed, Inc., Dedham, MA).

Heel spur pads. Heel spur pads (donuts, U-pads) are used to relieve weightbearing pressure in the center of the plantar calcaneus, usually in response to an actual spur, but also in the diagnosis of heel spur syndrome. These pads are configured in one of three ways: (1) as a simple heel pad, (2) as a "donut," with a hole cut in the center, or as a U-shaped pad (Fig. 16-8). The U-shaped pad is most useful in response to a combination of heel spur syndrome and mild plantar fasciitis. The donut pad is best in the presence of an actual bony spur.

Heel spur pads can be used directly in the shoe, or in conjunction with a custom foot orthosis. Either firm- or soft-density materials can be used, but the choice should be made based on the patient's weight, as softer materials are less likely to be adequate when used on a heavier patient.

Cuboid pad. The cuboid pad is usually used in response to a chronically subluxing cuboid. The pad is best made of felt or Korex, and is placed beneath the calcaneocuboid joint. This is usually a small pad, not more than 3/16 in. in thickness. It usually requires some adjustment before both size and placement are correct. Cuboid pads are always custom-made.

In-shoe padding clearly encompasses a wider variety of styles than covered here, but most are simply variations on the various pads discussed

Morton's extension   Reverse Morton's extension

Heel spur "donut"   U-pad

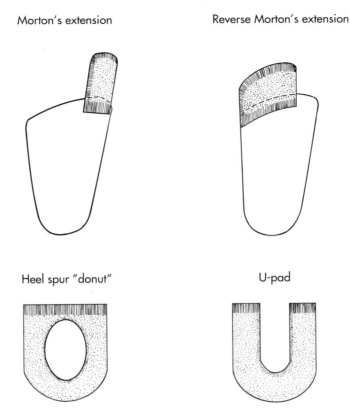

Fig. 16-8. Morton's extension, reverse Morton's extension, heel spur pad.

above. There will always be circumstances where any one of these pads needs to be modified for a specific purpose, and all of these pads can be made of any material that the practitioner chooses. The most important principle to remember regarding materials used in padding is that the amount of pressure relieved by the pad is based on the weight of the patient, the location of the pad, and the firmness of the material used.

In-shoe accommodations. While most lesions and spurs can be adequately accommodated either through the application of in-shoe padding, or with prescription foot appliances, some lesions and spurs can be extreme in both size and sensitivity. With an acute calcaneal spur or a rigidly plantarflexed first ray, it is sometimes necessary to create a pocket, or aperture, within the shoe itself. This can easily be accomplished with the judicious use of a cable-style drill with a cutting bit. Most shoe styles lend themselves to this technique, with the exception of thin-soled dress-style shoes and women's high-heeled styles (Fig. 16-9).

External modifications

The sole of the shoe should be thought of as the primary interface between the upright human body and the ground on which it treads. The balance of

that sole, and by extension, the balance of the insole of the shoe, or the prescription foot orthosis inside the shoe, all work together to support, cushion, and control the foot during gait. If any of these components are out of alignment with the neutral position of the foot in any of the phases of gait, the foot and its proper function will be compromised to varying degrees. With this in mind, it should be obvious that the most perfectly cast and manufactured foot orthosis will fail to some degree if it is placed in a shoe that is unbalanced, whether due to wear and compression of sole and midsole materials, or to a flaw in the original manufacturing.

When the patient presents with more serious foot complaints than maintaining a neutral position, however, the shoe-foot interface often requires more radical modification. In the event of such situations as limb length inequality, subtalar fusion, hallux rigidus, acute diabetic neuropathy, and a number of other significant pathologic and pathomechanical presentations, the patient's footwear may provide the practitioner with the ideal vehicle for ongoing conservative treatment and prevention, as well as assisting the patient with restoring his or her comfort level to normal or near normal. In this section, the practitioner will gain an appreciation of the various types of modifications that can be

In-shoe Accommodations

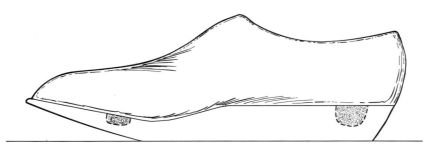

Fig. 16-9. In-shoe accommodations.

applied to the bottom of the patient's shoe to assist with the proposed treatment plan. Keep in mind that certain shoe styles lend themselves readily to modifications, and that the practitioner may have an uphill struggle to convince some patients that function and comfort need to be placed before fashion.

Limb length discrepancy and lift therapy

Perhaps the most common shoe modification performed is the shoe lift in response to limb length inequality. While the majority of length discrepancies can be treated with an in-shoe lift, often in combination with custom orthoses, there is a distinct limitation to the amount of lift that can be placed inside a shoe. Generally, 1/4 in. is the maximum thickness of in-shoe lifts, though some shoes might accommodate up to 3/16 in. without causing heel slippage. Some styles, such as pumps, both low- and high-heeled styles, can seldom accommodate any lift at all, though there is a technique that can be used with limited success in high-heeled shoes.

Limb length inequality has many causes, though the practitioner is seldom called upon to treat the original cause. More frequently, the practitioner is asked to respond to the compensations related to the original cause of the discrepancy. Having a grasp of some of the compensatory complexes will assist the practitioner with developing the treatment plan. While there are some proven surgical techniques available for treatment of limb length inequality, this chapter focuses on the mechanical forms of treatment. First, however, an overview of methods of compensation and a brief look at gait evaluation and limb measurement techniques are presented.

Four levels of compensation. The human body is essentially bilateral in structural design. While there are some differences left and right, the mechanical function of the body, in gait and in stance, works best when both halves of the body work in a balanced, symmetric manner. When this balance is disrupted, the body adjusts with two primary end goals. First, the inner ear must maintain its level position, or the body develops acute symptoms of vertigo, which is essentially an intolerable condition. Second, the visual horizon line must remain at its normal level. Note that both of these goals are related to the balance of the head, seemingly far removed from the feet. Yet if the feet are the primary foundation for the body, then the head is the roof, so to speak. And if the foundation is out of "plumb," either the roof must tilt in response, or the intervening structure must shift to compensate for the imbalance in the foundation.

There are four distinct levels of compensation in the human body in response to limb length inequality. The primary level of compensation is in the feet themselves. When a child begins to walk, compensation begins as well. And if an adult, subsequent to trauma, develops a limb length discrepancy (LLD) compensation begins shortly thereafter. The body always attempts to achieve the easiest route available for compensation. If the LLD is minor, for example, 1/4 in., compensation initially takes the form of an early heel-off on the short side. In many instances, this manifestation is accompanied by excessive pronation of the longer limb. When a practitioner evaluates a patient who presents with a "windswept" type of gait, that is, one side pronated, and the other side supinated, there is a high likelihood of an LLD. The danger here is the tendency to consider only the more pronated foot, as that is the foot most likely demonstrating symptoms. If only the pronated foot is treated, the practitioner may simply be interrupting one half of the compensatory chain, thereby lengthening the longer limb, and creating further pathologic changes. Even in the case of a functional LLD, contrasted with an anatomical LLD, the compensatory process is identical. It is important that the practitioner recognize that while there is a difference between the two types of LLD, the mechanical considerations for treatment are closely linked.

The secondary level of compensation occurs in the knees and hips. Hyperextension and hyperflexion are attempts by the body to lengthen the short limb or to shorten the long limb. While these types of compensation are more physically demanding than any other types of compensation, these manifestations are not rare. The more common type of secondary compensation is demonstrated as an elevated hip on the long side. If left untreated beyond the secondary level, LLD very readily develops tertiary compensations.

Tertiary compensation always contains one or several components of the primary and secondary levels, as well as pathomechanical manifestations within the torso, from the pelvis to the shoulders. Scoliotic and lordotic changes are nearly always present. Tertiary level compensations are demonstrated in gait in the most striking of all levels. A marked shoulder drop, nearly always on the long limb side, will be apparent, usually accompanied by a difference in the length and path of travel of arm swing. Because the shorter limb has a shorter stride length, the offset swing of the arms will also be asymmetrical. There will often be an obvious bounce to the head at one side of gait. Minor to severe scoliotic changes can be palpated along the spinal column. The patient often complains of back and knee problems, although this information may require a bit of creative questioning. This is because most people come to think of the various aches and pains associated with LLD as "just the way their body is," and fail to volunteer the information unless the matter is pursued by the examiner.

The final level of compensation is the quaternary level, and refers to compensations in the neck and head. This is the most difficult level for the body to compensate, but it is not a rare occurrence. A pronounced head tilt, a possible history of temporomandibular joint problems, and severe chronic headaches unexplainable by other examinations may all be linked to a long-standing, untreated LLD. If a patient presents with quaternary compensations, it is usually an older patient, or a younger patient with marked ligamentous laxity.

All levels of compensation are affected by a number of variable factors. Ligamentous laxity contributes to more extreme, and more levels of compensation than will be found in the patient with normal ligamentous tone. Age is an obvious factor, though less pertinent than the time between onset of the LLD and the initiation of treatment. If a patient has recently lost a 1/2-in. length to the femur as the result of a skiing accident, treatment can begin immediately, with no fear of disrupting the compensation cycle.

It is important that the practitioner act conservatively when considering a treatment approach for LLD. If the discrepancy is significant, of long standing, or significantly compensated, or if the compensatory process has itself created other trauma, one must proceed with caution. While there are formulas available to assist the practitioner with assessment,[4] such formulas should only be seen as guidelines, not as rules. This is because each patient seems to compensate in a somewhat unique pattern, making it very difficult to apply rigid rules to assessment and treatment. The general rule, however, is to examine all the factors in relationship to the general health and age of the patient. The longer-standing the untreated LLD, the longer it will take to successfully alter the compensations, and usually with varying degrees of success. If the practitioner proceeds too quickly with the leveling process, there is sure to be some trauma induced, from mild back pain, to severe, even crippling, outcomes.

As an example, consider the case of this 58-year-old woman, mildly overweight, mother of three children, who presents with a true 5/8-in. anatomic LLD. Clinical examination displays all four levels of compensation, with a distinct lordotic curve. The patient's primary complaint is sinus tarsi pain on the left foot, medial knee pain on the left side, and chronic back pain across her lower back. History reveals no evidence of trauma, not even a long bone fracture as might occur in childhood. Subsequent examination reveals an acute anterior-group muscle weakness on the left lower limb. These symptoms, taken in conjunction with the patient's age, might suggest a mild case of poliomyelitis or may be incidental to a congenital limb shortening. In either case, this patient has developed significant compensation.

With the amount of discrepancy presenting in this case the practitioner should proceed with the application of lift therapy very conservatively. A 1/8-in. lift applied to the inside of the left shoe would be an ideal start, with the same instructions given to the patient as those given for breaking in custom foot orthoses. In especially severe forms of spinal compensation related to LLD, back therapy will assist the patient with the transition through the reversal of the compensatory process. This amount of lift should be maintained in this particular case for at least 6 to 8 months, but at a minimum until the patient has thoroughly adapted to the lift. The lift should be increased in height at no greater than 1/8-in. increments, with sufficient time between increases to allow the compensation cycle time to reverse. It may not be possible for this patient to attain complete leveling, owing to her age, the duration of the LLD, and other health-related factors.

Measurement and assessment. It should be apparent by now that this is not a straightforward topic. There are many factors to be taken into account for the proper assessment of LLD, and to determine the proper path for treatment. Some patients do not respond positively to lift therapy at all, while others experience significant improvement. Another thing that makes LLD a difficult assessment to quantify is that measurement techniques are conflicting and difficult, at best, to reproduce.

There are at least a half-dozen techniques for measuring limb length, and all of them are fraught with problems.[2,6] Arguments have been raised to support supine measurement, standing measurement, and seated measurement. Factors such as compensatory contractures, circumferential differences of the thigh, the type of tape measure used, and particularly, the accuracy of locating fixed anatomic reference points all make accurate measurement of LLD difficult at best. While other chapters have covered these different techniques in detail, as well as the pros and cons of each technique, the practitioner has one technique that produces more than adequate results for assessment. This is the block method of assessment.

Because the treatment of LLD involves the whole body of the patient, the patient is usually able to provide the practitioner with near-immediate feedback to changes induced by the application of a lift. Practitioners should keep in their office a set of blocks of various thicknesses, 1/8, 3/16, 1/4, and 1/2 in., with at least a few of each thickness. These blocks are made of wood or plastic, somewhat longer and wider than a large men's-size shoe. The blocks are placed under the patient's shoe and increased in layers until the patient reports that the difference is both notable and still comfortable. Another way to use the block technique is to use different thicknesses of Korex taped to the shoe with masking tape. This enables both the practitioner and the patient to assess the proposed amount of lift in actual use. While the block technique has the seeming disadvantage of imprecision, it does produce consistently workable results.

External lift application. Any lift greater than 1/4 in. should be applied to the outsole of the patient's shoe. While a wedge-style sole design is the ideal vehicle for a shoe lift, separate sole and heel styles are often used in lift therapy with great success. The use of lift therapy with a high-heeled shoe is problematic, though one technique will allow a limited application of a lift to a high-heeled shoe. If, for example, the patient presents with a 3/8-in. LLD, with the right side being the short side, at least 1/4 in. of that amount could be safely removed from the heel of the left shoe. This would leave only 1/8 in. to account for, which can be added to the heel of the right shoe, or, in some types of shoes, to the inside of the right shoe. The result is identical to adding the entire amount to the right shoe, yet it is less noticeable and causes less disruption to the pitch of the shoe.

There is also an upper limit to the amount of lift that can be added to the heel without an accompanying sole lift. Generally, anything greater than a 1/2-in. in heel lift should be accompanied by a sole lift not less than one-half the thickness of the heel lift. In the presence of an LLD accompanied by a fixed equinus deformity, this rule would be modified appropriately. Also, this rule would not apply in the presence of an ankle or digital fusion, as the proper pitch of the foot must be maintained.[3] Table 16-1 gives a brief example of heel lift–sole lift correlations. It should be regarded as a general guide, not a firm rule.

Several things will be noted in the recommendations presented in Table 16-1. Every attempt should be made to maintain as normal a pitch as possible, keeping the opposite shoe in mind as a guide. Also, the amount that the sole lift tapers up to the toe is fairly consistent, despite differing amounts of sole lift being applied. This is to allow the shoe to assist in toe-off. As more lift is applied to a shoe, the stiffer and higher that shoe becomes. The traditional method of applying lifts did not take this into account, which resulted in a steppage gait in those patients with larger amounts of required lift. By using a rocker sole design with full shoe lifts, normal or near-normal gait patterns can be attained. Rocker sole design is covered in greater depth later in this chapter.

The materials used for lift application should be lightweight yet firm. There are a number of ethyl vinyl acetate (EVA)-based materials that are used for the application of midsoles in the pedorthic and shoe repair industries that are ideal for lifts. In extreme lifts, 2 in. or more, it is advisable that the technician cut out the center of the first few layers of the lift material (Fig. 16-10). By hollowing out the center in this manner, additional weight reductions can be achieved in the final product. The lighter the modified shoe, the less the energy expenditure required by the patient. Ideally, the modified shoe should not weigh more than twice the unmodified shoe weight. More traditional materials for lifts include cork blocks, and sometimes, balsa wood. However, these materials require covering with a leather that matches the color of the shoe. This technique is practiced by few craftsmen today.

**Shoe Lift
(cut-away view)**

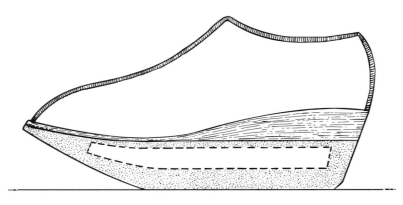

Hollowed center for weight reduction

Fig. 16-10. Shoe lift (cutaway view).

Table 16-1
Shoe lift chart

Heel lift	Sole lift	Taper to toe
1/2″	1/4″	0″
5/8″	3/8″	1/8″
3/4″	1/2″	1/8″
1″	5/8″	1/8″
1-1/4″	3/4″	3/16″
1-1/2″	1″	3/16″
2″	1-1/2″	1/4″

When writing a prescription for a shoe lift, it is important to be clear about three points: (1) the side on which the lift will be applied, (2) the extent of the discrepancy versus the amount of lift required at this time, and (3) whether to maintain a given pitch between the rearfoot and the forefoot. The technician will make material and construction determinations as they relate to the style of shoe to be modified. It should be emphasized again that a proper break-in period is crucial to the success of the treatment plan, except in immediate post-trauma-induced LLD.

For example, a patient with an LLD of 1/2 in., of 10 years' duration, untreated, is treated initially with a 1/8-in. to 3/16-in. inside shoe lift for a minimum of 6 months before any additional lift is added. This time scale will be modified by the pertinent factors: age, degree of compensation, activity level, accompanying abnormalities, patient acceptance, and the use of body work to assist in the reversal of compensatory mechanisms. Subsequent additions to the lift will be in similar amounts,

though the time frame depends on the rate of reversal of all compensatory levels. It is not clinically possible to establish strict guidelines regarding this subject. The practitioner must exercise his or her judgment based on the patient's response over time.

Of special interest is the patient who is diabetic, with attendant neuropathic changes, who also presents with the symptoms of an LLD. A significant number of diabetic ulcers are precipitated by excessive pressure unilaterally, and there is some reason to suspect that LLD plays a role in this. LLD may also play a role in the development of Charcot's joint in many neuropathic patients. While there are few studies available on this subject, observation seems to support some clinical correlation. At the least, the practitioner should routinely examine diabetic and other neuropathic patients for an LLD, if only to take preventive measures well before a likely ulceration occurs. By equalizing weightbearing in such patients, the probability of tissue breakdown is significantly reduced. This type of patient also benefits greatly from another shoe modification that is usually applied bilaterally—the rocker sole.

Rocker soles

A rocker sole modification is used for any type of pathologic or pathomechanical condition that either limits normal movement of the ankle, metatarsal, or metatarsophalangeal joints, or in situations where it is desirable to limit such motion. A rocker sole achieves both of these by being a dynamic lever that assists with the normal movement of the lower extremity during gait, and by preventing the shoe's sole from flexing during all phases of gait. The two conditions that must be present for a rocker sole design to be successful are a sole that is raised

Rocker-sole Modification
Side View

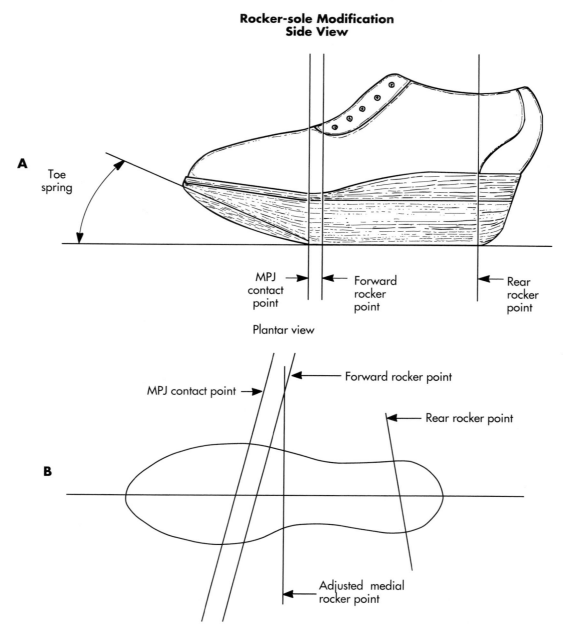

Fig. 16-11. **A** and **B,** Rocker sole modification.

sufficiently to induce the required stiffening of the sole, and the correct placement of the rear and forward rocker points (Fig. 16-11A).

While there are a number of ready-made shoes on the market that claim to have a rocker sole design incorporated in the sole of the shoe, none of these shoes has the rocker point in the correct location, that is, proximal to the metatarsophalangeal joint contact point, and parallel to the arc of the joint. Proper placement of the rocker point allows the foot to begin the toe-off phase of gait prior to the normal moment, preventing the foot from flexing at the time it would usually do so. This assists the foot

with forward propulsion into the swing phase.

Similarly, the rear rocker point acts to assist in decelerating the limb during heel-strike, and preventing abrupt plantarflexion "slap" into full foot loading. This also acts to reduce shock significantly. The placement of the rear rocker point is as crucial as the forward rocker point. It should always extend to a point across the middle of the widest part of the heel of the shoe, and should be angled outward toward the lateral corner of the heel (Fig. 16-11B).

Some variations of the forward rocker angle can improve forward travel of the leg during toe-off in those patients who present with a marked abducted

SACH Heel Modification

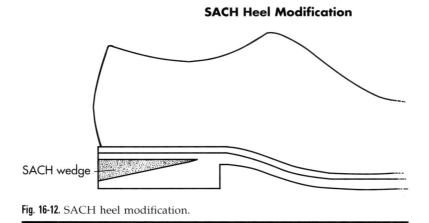

SACH wedge

Fig. 16-12. SACH heel modification.

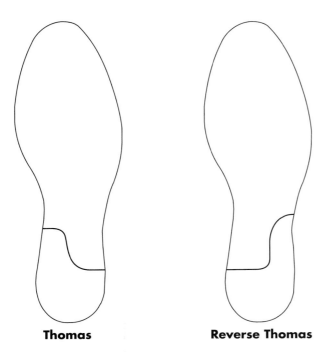

Thomas   **Reverse Thomas**

Fig. 16-13. Thomas and reverse Thomas heel.

stance. By leaving the lateral end of the rocker point line alone and moving the medial end of the line proximally, the rocker line can be shifted closer to perpendicular to the line of progression. This modification can greatly reduce medial knee strain in this type of patient.

Rocker soles should always be bilateral, unless a rocker sole is being applied along with a shoe lift, which enables an external lift to mimic normal limb movement in gait. The materials used for rocker soles are essentially the same as for external lifts. Both light weight and firmness are important.

Rocker sole modification has applications in the treatment of patients who have diabetic neuropathy, as noted in numerous studies with Hansen's disease

patients, who also present with neuropathy.[7] The rocker sole functions to reduce flexion of the metatarsophalangeal joints during gait, and reduce heel shock at heel-strike. Used in conjunction with a custom-molded accommodative insert, the possibility of plantar ulceration can be minimized. Depth-style shoes (see Fig. 16-5) are highly recommended for this combined treatment approach.

Because rocker sole modification assists the lower limb so effectively in gait, it has applications in the mechanical treatment of patients with triple arthrodesis, postcerebrovascular accident, multiple sclerosis, and other conditions that create a weakness or loss of the anterior muscle groups. Rocker soles are an improvement on another modification called metatarsal bars, or rocker bars. These modifications are less effective than rocker soles, because they only apply force proximal to the metatarsophalangeal joints, and often cause severe deformation of the sole of the shoe over a brief time. The only caution on the use of rocker soles is that the patient may become laterally unstable on open ground. On the majority of urban surfaces, however, this is not a problem.

SACH heels

When the practitioner is confronted with a patient who displays an extreme shock-absorption problem, such as an acute synovitis in the subtalar joint, functional foot orthoses are not always enough to attenuate shock at heel-strike. The application of a SACH heel to the midsole of the patient's shoe acts as an extrinsic shock absorber (Fig. 16-12). The SACH insert is made from a high-density foam rubber wedge that is inserted into the posterior midsole of the shoe. This allows the more durable outsole to prevent wear, while the SACH heel absorbs shock and rebounds immediately for the next heel-strike. The SACH heel is often used in conjunction with short-leg braces, and can replace some lost rotational movement of the limb on the foot when such torque is lost due to fusion or trauma.

Thomas heel

A Thomas heel is used on shoes that have a separate sole and heel construction style. This type of modification acts to increase medial support and stability in cases of extreme pes planus. Thomas heels are an excellent adjunct to functional foot orthoses with this foot type, as they greatly reduce medial shoe breakdown. A reverse Thomas heel extends lateral-distal, when more lateral stability is desired (Fig. 16-13).

Footwear considerations for orthotic therapy

Functional and accommodative orthoses are a significant treatment modality for pathomechanical disorders. Every practitioner encounters problems with the footwear choices presented by their patients when trying to fit foot orthoses into their shoes. Some shoes, particularly dress styles, have hardly enough room for the foot, and make fitting orthoses into such shoes very difficult. The compromise is usually to reduce functional control in favor of fit. Some practitioners refuse to prescribe orthoses unless the patient is willing to change his or her shoe styles to one more appropriate to orthotic therapy. Not every practitioner is willing to be so insistent, however, and often seeks alternatives.

One alternative is to ask the orthotic laboratory to grind the orthosis thin at the contact point. This technique works quite well with such materials as polypropylene or accommodative devices, but is contraindicated with acrylic or composite materials. Composite orthotic materials are already very thin, but the thickness of the material is only one aspect of the problem. The depth of the heel cup contributes to heel slippage more than the thickness of the device. By reducing the heel cup height, fit can be significantly improved.

Another issue related to proper orthotic function is the lateral and medial stability of the shoe. If a shoe has little or no counter stiffness, the orthosis will gradually shift off the center of the heel of the shoe. This shift will contribute to accelerated shoe breakdown, thereby reducing orthotic effectiveness over time. Footwear with a sturdy counter will improve the long-term outcome of orthotic therapy.

Finally, the pitch of the shoe and the pitch, or elevator, of the rear post on the orthosis must align. If the shoe pitch is less or greater than that of the orthosis, the device will either rock over the "high" point of the shank of the shoe, or it will seat with little or no contact at the anterior aspect of the rear post. This leads, in some instances, to the feeling that the orthosis is too high in the arch. If the pitch of both components is similar, orthotic therapy will have a more successful outcome.

The pedorthist: utilizing the experts

The full range of shoe modifications with therapeutic application is a broad subject. While this chapter has introduced the most frequently employed modifications, the practitioner should be aware that there are other techniques available to assist their patients with foot complaints using the shoe as a treatment modality. While some of these techniques can be applied adequately at local shoe repair facilities, the pedorthist is the best-trained professional to handle shoe therapy prescriptions. Most pedorthists carry selections of depth and comfort shoes in their inventory, and all pedorthists are trained to work with the practitioner in a team approach.

The shoe as a "functional" orthosis: Summary

Patients come to a practitioner seeking comfort. While acute trauma, disease processes, or pathomechanical abnormalities might appear to be of greater import than the simple desire for comfort, that desire is basic to every patient. If the practitioner has knowledge of all the necessary tools that might assist patients with the reestablishment of comfort, that practitioner will effectively fulfill his or her task. Footwear, with the proper combination of fit, style, and when necessary, therapeutic modifications, becomes a functional adjunct to the chosen treatment plan. Shoes are expected to function with, not against, the patient's foot. Because the shoe can act to support, protect, and modify function, and thus affect the entire body, footwear used as a therapeutic modality should be viewed as functional orthoses in their own right. By making use of this modality when the need arises, the practitioner can broaden the treatment choices dramatically.

References

1. Brachman P: *Shoe therapy*, Chicago, 1979, Illinois College of Podiatric Medicine Press.
2. Eichler J: Methodological errors in documenting leg length and leg length discrepancies. Trans from *Der Orthopäde*, vol 1, 1972, Springer-Verlag, pp 14-20.
3. Greenman P: Lift therapy: use and abuse, *JAOA*, 79:63-75, 1979.
4. Heilig D: Principals of lift therapy, *JAOA*, 77:89-95, 1978.
5. *Historical highlights of American lastmaking and American shoemaking*, New York, 1982, Sterling Last.
6. Morscher E, Figner G: Measurement of leg length. Trans from *Der Orthopäde*, vol 1, 1972, Springer-Verlag, pp 9–13.
7. Nawoczenski D, Birke J, Coleman W: Effect of rocker sole design on plantar forefoot pressures, *J Am Podiatr Med Assoc* 78:455–460, 1988.
8. Rossi W: *The sex life of the foot and shoe*, ed 2, Melbourne, Fla, 1992, Krieger.

padding and taping techniques

Stephen C. White, DPM

History

Palliative padding and strapping
    Purpose
    Materials

Padding and strapping techniques
    The Low Dye strap
    Gibney or basket weave strap
    The J strap and reverse J strap
    Digital strap for fracture or sprain
    The buddy splint for fracture or sprain
    Hallux fracture or sprain
    Skiving accessories
    Padding materials

Pads, shields, and slings
    Plantar pads
    Removable Elastoplast pad
    Digital pads or shields

Summary

History

The care and treatment of the human foot has a long and varied history. In biblical references the height of hospitality to the weary-footed traveler or guest was to wash and anoint his feet. During the crusades of the Middle Ages the pilgrims of Europe walked for weeks and months in the hopes of reaching their goal, the Holy Land. Weary-footed and victimized by enterprising townsmen along the way, we can only imagine the condition of their health and, in particular, their feet.

The more charitable members of society established the hospice whose purpose was the pilgrim's medical care, such as it was, including care of the pilgrim's feet. These hospices were the forerunner of the hospital.

The Middle Ages, particularly in Europe, witnessed untold ignorance, superstition, and lack of, among other things, medical knowledge. The blacksmith was held in high esteem owing to his reputation for casting out spells and curing disease, and was resorted to when broken bones needed repair. The physician, in most cases, was a charlatan who refused to dirty his hands and reputation with the demeaning occupation of surgery. Surgery was referred to the barbers, hence the "barber surgeons" of the Middle Ages. This practice continued into the 18th century.

It was at this time that the care of the foot emerged as a profession or speciality, particularly in England. In 1818 a third edition of a treatise "The Art of Preserving the Feet" was published in London. The author, Henry Colburn, suggested in his preface that the profession should be known as "chiropody" to distinguish it from the untrained persons who had usurped the profession of foot care and were calling themselves "podologists."

William Ernest Henley (1849–1903) on more than one occasion underwent agonizing and unsuccessful surgical procedures on his feet. One may wonder if these surgical onslaughts influenced the thoughts expressed in the first two stanzas of his "Invictus."

Out of the night that covers me,
Black as the pit from pole to pole,
I thank what ever gods there be
For my unconquerable soul.
In the fell clutch of circumstance
I have not winced nor cried aloud.
Under bludgeoning of chance
My head is bloody but unbowed.[3]

Palliative padding and strapping

Occupation; sports; ill-fitting shoes; weightbearing abnormalities, congenital or acquired; trauma; neuropathies; circulatory diseases; and a host of other problems contribute to various debilitating assaults upon the human foot.

In many cases a change of footwear, biomechanical evaluation with orthoses, or surgical procedures with or without orthotic follow-up are the treatment of choice. There are, however, instances when these methods are not entirely successful or indicated. The aged, reluctant, or compromised patient is not always a candidate for treatment or procedures that otherwise would be successful. Such patients with chronic or acute conditions require periodic care and attention in order that they may have useful and pain-free ambulatory activities. These patients should not be ignored, left to the questionable administrations of the pedicurist or to the innumerable and often harmful proprietary devices and medications that are available. Proper, adequate, surgical, biomechanical, and palliative care results in a happy, appreciative, and more active member of the community.

Purpose

The primary purpose of padding is to shield or protect mild, acute, or chronic pathologic areas of the foot. These disorders include trauma, surgical sites, infections, abscesses, ulcers, exostoses, and hyperkeratotic lesions with their sequelae.

Hyperkeratotic lesions, such as the corn or callus, and in particular the enucleated lesion, are inert and insensitive tissue. The sequelae, however, may be considered the result of the tissue response to the hyperkeratotic lesion as a foreign body with the consequent classic foreign body reaction.

Unattended, the mild to painfully inflamed tissue underlying a hyperkeratosis will progress and break down into an abscess, ulcer, pressure necrosis, sinus abscess, and ultimately an infection of skin and bone. In the compromised patient these conditions may progress to more tragic results.

It is important to keep in mind that the bone underlying keratoses is stimulated to reproduce, resulting in exostoses such as bunions, enlarged condyles, and metatarsal and phalangeal heads. Bone malformations, congenital or acquired, with their excrescences and pathologic changes, will, along with surgical and biomechanical approaches, require palliative podiatric shielding and medications.

Materials

Adhesive tape

Adhesive tape is manufactured using various materials such as fabric, plastic, and cellulose. Tape is mainly white or flesh-colored. In instances where adhesive tape will show above footwear or through hosiery, flesh-colored adhesive tape is more desirable. The most common widths used in podiatry are 1/4 to 3 in.

Adhesive tape is placed on the spool using machinery that allows the tape to unroll freely with an even tension. Using the fingers as spindles is a comfortable method of shifting the roll of tape from finger to finger. This method eliminates squeezing and deforming a roll of adhesive tape. Adhesive tape is shipped by the manufacturer with the spools on spindles in order to keep the tape resting on the fabric rim. A roll of adhesive should always rest on its flat side to prevent the development of a flat area on the rim. To crush or squeeze and deform a roll of adhesive tape causes the adhesive surface to adhere to the adjacent fabric, creates irregular flat areas, and gives an unattractive appearance to the roll. The loss of even tension and the awkwardness of using such a roll of adhesive tape will reflect on the adeptness of the practitioner.

The purpose of adhesive taping is to produce complete or partial immobilization, and as a rest strap for joints, muscles, tendons, and ligaments.

In preparing the skin for taping, the skin is cleaned with alcohol, hair is covered or shaved, and a pretape cover (optional), and skin adherent are applied. Some patients may be allergic to the latter.

Contraindications to skin taping are allergies, skin lesions (e.g., dermatitis, fungi, psoriasis, trauma), fragile skin, ischemic skin, and varicosities in the area to be taped.

Perforated adhesive. The purpose of fine perforations in adhesive tape is to minimize skin maceration. This, of course, is questionable. Perforated tape has a weaker tensile strength and is not always adequate for strapping.

Micropore adhesive (3M Health Care). Micropore is a cellulose tape and is commonly referred to as "paper tape." Micropore adhesive tape is available in white and flesh color. Micropore adhesive is relatively nonallergenic, results in little or no skin maceration, withstands soap and water, adheres well, has less bulk than other adhesives, and breaks freely with the fingers. A disadvantage is that it is inadequate for tension strapping.

Padding and strapping techniques
The Low Dye strap

The Low Dye strap, devised by Ralph Dye,[2] is essentially a rest strap at the medial-plantar aspect of the metatarsal, tarsal, and tarsal joints of the foot. The Low Dye strap is a therapeutic strap, which, like other straps, will benefit fasciitis, periostitis, and stress and strain of the muscles, ligaments, and joints of the foot.

Over a period of years, the Low Dye has evolved and been modified in its application and uses. For example, the addition of a longitudinal arch pad and heel-to-ball strip of moleskin produces effective immobilization of the subtalar joint. The Low Dye may, at times, make an excellent flexible cast along with a postoperative shoe for hairline fractures of the shaft of the fifth metatarsal when a more cumbersome cast is not wanted.

The Low Dye strap with or without padding is effective in evaluating biomechanical methods prior to follow-up orthotic therapy. It may, therefore, at times be considered a type of trial-and-error temporary orthosis. It will also give the patient an understanding of and confidence in what is being attempted and contemplated for future orthotic therapy.

Application

1. The skin is inspected for contraindications to adhesive tape.
2. The skin is cleaned with alcohol.
3. Skin adherent is applied. The skin adherent may be a specific skin adherent or compound tincture of benzoin. Compound tincture of benzoin may, at times, be the adherent of choice. It does not, however, have the adherent qualities of the various specific pretape adherents. Skin adherents are available in pint-sized bottles and may be decanted into smaller containers and applied to the skin with cotton-tipped applicators. Skin adherents in spray containers may suffice for locker rooms and such, but present a problem in an office setting. Skin adherent is applied to the medial and lateral sides of the foot from proximal to the first and fifth metatarsal heads to the medial and lateral aspects of the heel. It is not necessary to apply skin adherent to the plantar surface of the foot.
4. The subtalar joint is locked, that is, placed in neutral position. The patient is asked to hold this position but not in a rigid manner. Frequent reminders may be necessary.
5. Heel lock strips are applied (Fig. 17-1). A 1-in. strip of adhesive tape is applied from lateral to medial, beginning immediately proximal to the fifth metatarsal head, keeping the lower edge of the tape along the lateral plantar junction. If the lateral side is applied too low on the foot it will wrinkle at the heel and be too low along the medial side. The tape is continued around the heel at the same level, medially along the longitudinal arch. Under moderate tension, the

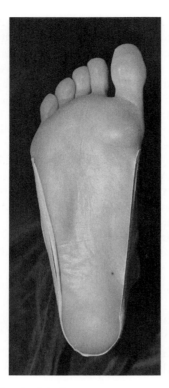

Fig. 17-1. Low Dye heel locks.

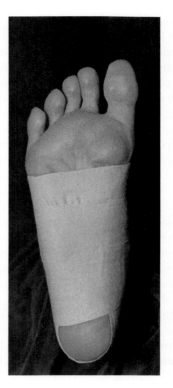

Fig. 17-2. Low Dye plantar straps.

medial side is anchored immediately proximal to the head of the first metatarsal. If the medial longitudinal arch strips are nicked in order to have them conform to the arch, the tension and therapeutic benefits of the heel locks are lost. The heel lock strips should fit and adhere to the medial foot contours without being nicked or cut.

Care should be taken not to place the lateral and medial ends of the heel locks over the articulations of the first and fifth metatarsophalangeal joints. To do so will restrict the normal motions of these joints. The extensor digitorum longus tendon should also be avoided.

Just prior to anchoring the end of the medial side, the forefoot is adducted or the head of the first metatarsal plantarflexed. If the hallux is in a pronounced dorsiflexed position prior to anchoring the medial end, it should be slightly plantarflexed. This will prevent uncomfortable tension on the skin when the foot attempts to elongate on weightbearing.

6. Plantar straps are applied (Fig. 17-2). The plantar surface of the foot should be checked for wrinkles or folds when the foot is squeezed from side to side. Folds or wrinkles under the plantar straps may

result in painful pinching and inflammation. Gauze or absorbent cotton should be placed along the folds prior to the application of the plantar straps. Although pretape covering may address this problem, it tends to reduce the desired strap tension.

Adhesive strips 1-1/2 to 2 in. wide are then applied to the plantar surface from lateral to medial. Plantar straps may be placed from heel to ball, for example, from proximal to distal, or vice versa. The constant, however, is that the distal plantar strap has the least tension. This is necessary to ensure that flexion of the metatarsophalangeal joints is not limited. Tension is increased proximally with the most tension on the last or most proximal strip. If the plantar straps are started at the heel, the tension decreases as one proceeds distally.

The plantar straps are begun approximately 1/4 to 1/2 in. above the lateral heel lock and continued under the foot, keeping the strap at right angles to the foot. The tension is increased as one proceeds up the plantar-medial aspect of the foot, ending approximately 1/4 to 1/2 in. above the medial heel lock. The distal plantar strap should be immediately proximal to the first and fifth metatarsal heads. The proximal plantar strap may end at the calcaneus or cover the entire heel.

As a rule, three 2-in. plantar straps are adequate for the average foot. Additional strips may be necessary for longer feet. To provide effective strength to the strap, the plantar straps should overlap by approximately one-half their widths. An overlapping additional middle strap may be necessary for a heavy person or a very broad foot.

The Low Dye strap adheres to the foot by virtue of the amount of adhesive tape along the medial and lateral borders of the foot, that is, the heel lock strips. Additional adhesive surface area to the skin is gained when the plantar straps are placed slightly above the heel locks.

A neat professional appearance is given to the strap as well as additional adhesive contact when the medial and lateral anchor straps are applied over the upper edges of the plantar straps. The anchor straps may be medial and lateral or a continuous strap around the heel to the medial and lateral sides. The anchor strap does not require tension and is not therapeutic. The ends of the anchor straps should be rounded to prevent corners from curling and sticking to stockings.

To ensure that the medial and lateral sides of the strap adhere to the foot, particularly the broad-splaying foot or the active patient, a 2-in. adhesive strip is placed over the dorsum of the foot at the midlongitudinal arch extending down both sides of the foot to just below the anchor straps. A piece of 2- × 2-inch gauze or upturned piece of adhesive tape under the dorsal strip will prevent irritation to the skin on the dorsum of the foot. The dorsal strip should be loose enough that it does not wrinkle when the foot is loaded. The dorsal strip should be placed over the anchor straps, thus allowing the patient to loosen or remove it if necessary without disturbing the rest of the Low Dye.

The patient should be asked to stand and be checked for excessive tightness of the strap, particularly proximal to the first and fifth metatarsal heads. To ease or release excess tension, all layers of the adhesive tape are grasped at the metatarsal heads and the skin is gently pushed away from the adhesive tape. In doing so one will feel the release of tension on the skin. The adhesive is placed back on the skin without tension. The plantar medial tension of the strap should not be disturbed unless necessary.

To prevent the strap from sticking to stockings, paraffin wax or talcum powder should be applied. It is believed that paraffin will waterproof the adhesive tape and it may do so minimally. For hygienic reasons and professional appearances, a previously used piece of paraffin should be avoided. Patient reaction and contamination are to be considered. Patients are more likely to have talcum or foot powder at home and should be advised to powder the strap before putting their hose on.

The Low Dye strap is effective for approximately 4 or 5 days, after which the strap becomes loose. With the effective use of skin adherent, the strap will survive a short period of bathing each day. The strap will dry if the patient allows a short time to elapse between bathing and dressing. The patient should be instructed to remove the strap immediately if there is discomfort, that is, tightness, itching, or burning. The strap should be removed and the foot bathed several hours before application of a follow-up strap.

If a pad is used in conjunction with the Low Dye it should be placed over the Low Dye and strapped to it. To place a pad under the Low Dye will effectively reduce the desired tension of the strap (Fig. 17-3).

Gibney or basket weave strap

The Gibney or basket weave strap (Fig. 17-4) is used in various injuries to ligaments and tendons of the ankle. It allows dorsiflexion and plantarflexion but limits inversion and eversion of the ankle.[5]

After cleaning and preparing the skin, the foot is held in a neutral position 90 degrees to the leg or slightly plantarflexed. One-inch adhesive tape is used. The first vertical strip is placed next to the Achilles tendon approximately 5 to 6 in. above the medial malleolus, and continued down the leg, under the heel, and up the lateral side to a length equal to the medial side. A second horizontal strip is applied starting proximal to the fifth metatarsal head around the heel to proximal to the first metatarsal head. The process is repeated overlapping the strips by approximately 1/4 to 1/2 in. The closer the overlap, the firmer and more supportive the strap. The number of strips will be determined by the size of the foot and ankle. The appearance is that of a basket weave. The strap is sometimes referred to as a flexible cast. With the advent of air casts, the Gibney is not used as frequently as in the past.

For mild ankle sprains the Gibney may be placed on the foot and ankle from distal to proximal.

The J strap and reverse J strap

The J strap limits eversion of the calcaneus. The reverse J strap limits inversion of the calcaneus.

One-half to 2-in. adhesive tape is used. The J strap is started immediately below the lateral malleolus, downward and under the heel, and upward along

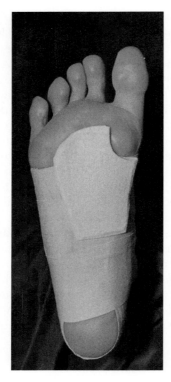

Fig. 17-3. Plantar pad applied over Low Dye.

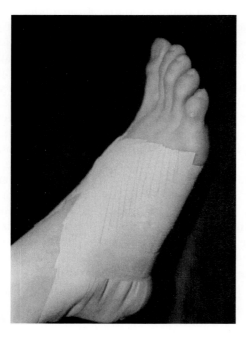

Fig. 17-4. Basket weave ankle strap.

the medial aspect of the leg. The reverse J strap is applied immediately below the medial malleolus downward and under the heel, and then up the lateral leg.

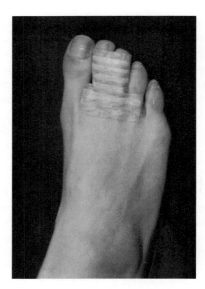

Fig. 17-5. Buddy splint or flexible cast for fractured or sprained toe.

Digital strap for fracture or sprain

This strap consists of overlapping strips of 1/4- to 1/2-in. adhesive tape. The strap is begun at the plantar base of the toe, bringing the ends to overlap and anchor on the dorsum. Additional strips are added continuing distally, overlapping approximately one-half the previous strip. This overlapping ensures a firm supportive strap.

An adjacent toe may be used to act as a splint. If an adjacent toe is used, the interdigital skin should be cleaned and a small piece of gauze placed between the toes to prevent chafing.

The buddy splint for fracture or sprain

This strap uses an adjacent toe as a splint (Fig. 17-5). The interdigital spaces are cleaned and a small piece of gauze is placed between the toes. Skin adherent is applied dorsally at the base of the toes to the metatarsophalangeal areas. An appropriate adjacent toe is chosen and the taping is begun at the distal end of the toes using 1/2-in. adhesive strips. The adhesive strips are placed over the dorsum of the toes and carried downward between the toes with a minimum of tension, not necessarily encircling the toes completely. The overlaps should be approximately 1/8 in. apart to ensure firmness. The strips are continued to the toe webs. Two or three additional strips are continued proximally to the metatarsophalangeal joints to anchor the strap to the dorsum of the foot.

Coban (3M Corp.) as well as various adhesives, may be used for this splint. One-half-inch Micropore adhesive ensures less maceration, bulk, and withstands bathing. The splint should be changed every

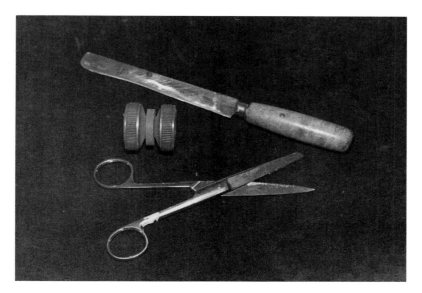

Fig. 17-6. Skiving knife, sharpening wheel, and Miltex felt and moleskin scissors.

7 to 10 days. The patient should be able to wear a shoe.

Hallux fracture or sprain

A spica strap may be adequate for a hallux fracture or sprain. The buddy splint does not lend itself well to this situation. Prefabricated splints are available and are contoured to the toe. A tongue blade makes an effective hallux splint. The tongue blade is placed along the medial aspect of the hallux and first metatarsal. Absorbent cotton filler is placed between the splint and the foot distal to the first metatarsal head along the shaft of the proximal phalanx and along the first metatarsal shaft proximal to the metatarsal head. This provides a level support for the tongue blade along the medial side of the foot. The tongue blade is strapped to the foot and a postoperative shoe is used.

Skiving accessories

The purpose of skiving is for the comfort of the patient, to eliminate the sharp right-angled edge of the padding material and for a professional appearance of the completed pad. Accessories for skiving are the sharpening wheel, scissors, and the skiving knife (Fig. 17–6).

Grinding wheel

The grinding wheel is used for firm materials such as cork, sponge rubber, PPT (Langer Biomechanics Group, Inc.) Plastazote (JMS Plastics) and leather.

Scissors

Various materials used in padding and strapping require special scissors designed for cutting and skiving. Many types of scissors are available. Not all types are adequate. Felt and moleskin scissors such as the Miltex (Miltex Instrument Co.) are recommended. Felt and moleskin scissors are serrated along the broad, blunt-ended blade. The serrated blade facilitates feeding materials through the scissors. A loose play at the hinge of the scissors may be noted and is desirable. It is advisable not to attempt to tighten the hinge. To do so may misalign the blades. Using small and lightweight scissors for cutting thick materials (such as felt) may result in springing the hinge and rendering the scissors useless. Materials, such as felt and PPT, up to approximately 1/4 in. thick, can be skived with little difficulty using the serrated scissors. Scissors should be angled to the left or right to accomplish a skive. To achieve a smooth-appearing skive with scissors, one makes a continuous cut rather than short snipping cuts. Short, interrupted cuts give an irregular, scalloped, and unprofessional appearance to the skive. When cutting padding material, the cut is made well back into the scissors blades.

Adhesive material will, from time to time, adhere to scissors blades, making efficient use of the scissors difficult and awkward. This problem may be prevented by occasionally applying paraffin, petroleum jelly (Vaseline), cream, ointment, or lotion to the blades. With the exception of paraffin, these products will also loosen and remove adhesive from the scissors blades.

Skiving knife

Skiving knives are available from podiatry supply houses. They are of a rather poor-quality carbon steel, lose their cutting edge rapidly, and require constant sharpening. Various stones are available for sharpening. Skiving knives are primarily for skiving felt and to a lesser degree other materials such as PPT and Plastazote. Various thicknesses of felt can be skived. The skived edge may vary from a fraction of an inch to several inches. The felt or material to be skived should be placed on a hard surface and held firmly in place. A long gliding motion rather than short jerky motions should be used, allowing the sharp knife to cut effortlessly, without force or pressure, through the felt until the knife hits the underlying surface. This provides an acceptable feathered edge and professional appearance to the pad.

Basic rule for skiving

If, for example, a metatarsal pad of 1/4-in. felt is used, the skive would be approximately equal to the thickness of the pad, that is, 1/4 in. along the medial, distal, and lateral borders of the pad, and two to three times the thickness, that is, 1/2 to 3/4 in. at the proximal end or base of the pad. The 1/4-in. skive can be accomplished with scissors as well as with the skiving knife. To skive with scissors the scissors should be angled to the right or left and the cutting done well back into the blades. To avoid a fluted or scalloped appearance to a scissors skive, the scissors cut should be continuous rather than snipped or interrupted.

Padding materials

Materials frequently used for padding include felt, PPT, sponge rubber, foam rubber, Plastazote, and Spenco (Rubitex Corp.) cork. These materials are available from manufacturers and supply houses in bulk sheets and prefabricated pads. Prefabricated pads or pads fabricated in the office may be used, in some instances, directly on the foot. They may be placed over or under the stocking lining of a shoe, incorporated into the construction of an orthosis, or added to a cushion innersole or to the removable innersole of a shoe. The foot impressions and markings in the shoe or on the various innersole materials aid in the correct and effective placement of a pad.

Felt

Felt, adhesive and nonadhesive, is available in various thicknesses, usually 1/16, 1/8, and 1/4 in. Felt is manufactured using varying amounts of wool and cotton. The higher the cotton content, the firmer or harder the felt will be, and it will bottom out or pack less than a felt with a high wool content. The better-grade felts have a higher wool content, are softer, and make a more comfortable pad. The higher-grade felts are also superior for digital pads and other pads that are placed directly onto the foot.

To maintain a desired thickness, additional layers of felt may be added as packing occurs, as with weightbearing pads. Layers are easily spliced or pulled apart to make a thinner thickness of felt.

PPT

PPT is used extensively in podiatric pads and orthoses. It is available in various thicknesses, in bulk sheets, prefabricated pads, and orthoses. An advantage of PPT is that its open cell structure permits air to pass into and out of the material, it remains cool, and does not bottom out. PPT is an excellent shock absorber and lends itself well to skiving with scissors and the grinding wheel.

Sponge rubber

Sponge rubber pads are available primarily as metatarsal and longitudinal arch pads. They vary from soft to hard. The firm-to-hard type may be adjusted on the grinding wheel. Sponge rubber maintains its form for long periods of time, but the softer type tends to deteriorate with time and wear. With the advent of newer materials, sponge rubber is not used as extensively as in the past. Sponge rubber metatarsal buttons are used by shoe manufacturers. Some heel lifts and prefabricated orthoses utilize sponge rubber.

Cork

Cork, or Korex, is manufactured from ground cork, wood flour, and latex rubber. It is firm to hard and grindable. Cork is excellent for internal shoe modifications and orthoses.

Foam rubber

Foam rubber is a soft cellular material available in various thicknesses, adhesive or nonadhesive, in bulk sheets, and as prefabricated pads. Foam rubber is used in the manufacture of over-the-counter orthoses, heel cushions, and interdigital pads. Foam rubber compresses and deteriorates rapidly and is therefore not an effective weightbearing or shielding material. Foam rubber is well tolerated for interdigital padding and when used as a shield in conjunction with Rolofoam, that is, bunion shields, etc.

Plastazote

Plastazote is a polyethylene foam and is available in various thicknesses and densities. It is used as a cushion material and is frequently laminated to other materials such as PPT. Plastazote is lightweight, nontoxic, and moldable. Although Plastazote tends to bottom out, its moldable qualities aid in determining excessive weightbearing areas that require accommodative pads, that is, felt or PPT.

Spenco

Spenco is neoprene infused with nitrogen to form a cushioning sponge. Spenco is available in bulk sheets and prefabricated innersoles and orthoses. Thicknesses are 1/8 and 1/4 in. Spenco was developed to reduce callus and blister formation during athletic activities. Along with its cushioning qualities, there is a torsion component as well—that is, absorption of horizontal and vertical forces.

Spenco is covered with a multistretch nylon. After some wear the nylon will show color change as well as impressions at points of excessive weightbearing. These areas of fabric wear and compression will aid in placing additional accommodative padding. Spenco innersoles are superior to foam rubber innersoles owing to their inherent torsion quality and their resistance for compressing or deteriorating as rapidly.

Spenco skin care

Spenco Skin Care is a synthetic "biosoft polymer." It is designed to help absorb pressure and reduce friction. It has a soft gelatin texture, is washable, and can be sterilized. It seems to be an excellent posterior heel padding for bedridden patients as well as a shielding medium. Additionally, it is capable of preventing chafing and friction from casts, protheses, and so forth.

Pads, shields, and slings
Plantar pads

Pads commonly used for the plantar aspect of the foot are:

1. Metatarsal or short metatarsal pad. This is also referred to as a metatarsal bar or metatarsal button.
2. Long arch or medial arch pad, or Mayo pad.
3. Long metatarsal pad.
4. Modifications of the basic metatarsal pad.
5. Heel pad.
6. Cuboid pad.

Metatarsal pad

The purpose of the metatarsal pad is to transfer weightbearing proximally from the second, third, and fourth metatarsal heads. Weightbearing is transferred to the metatarsal shafts. The basic metatarsal pad comes in many shapes, sizes, thicknesses, and materials.

In most cases, the metatarsal pad should not be placed under the metatarsal heads. A close scrutiny of metatarsal pad illustrations in texts and catalogues shows that they are designed to be placed between the first and fifth metatarsal heads (Fig. 17-7). The metatarsal pad should *not* be placed under the first and fifth metatarsal heads. To do so may create an uncomfortable upward thrust to the

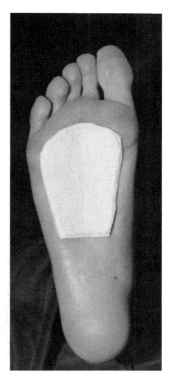

Fig. 17-7. Basic metatarsal pad, placed between first and fifth metatarsal heads.

metatarsal heads and sesamoids, as well as the metatarsophalangeal joints. An exception, of course, is Morton's extension which is intended to increase weightbearing at the first metatarsal head when there is a hypermobile first metatarsal.

When properly placed between the first and fifth metatarsal heads the metatarsal pad should more or less automatically fall immediately proximal to the second, third, and fourth metatarsal heads and plantar to the metatarsal shafts. Care should be taken that the pad does not extend proximally to the metatarsotarsal articulations, creating an uncomfortable pressure on these joints. Careful skiving of two to three times the thickness of the proximal end of the pad will avoid this problem. Prefabricated pads may be utilized effectively. The distal skived edge may be placed close to and under the metatarsal heads to ensure that the unskived thicker part of the pad is immediately proximal to the heads. Owing to the anatomical configuration of the metatarsal, many pads are rhomboid in shape. The pad is wider distally, higher on the medial-distal border, and slopes laterally toward the fifth metatarsal head. The pad then becomes narrower proximally at the second, third, and fourth metatarsal shafts.

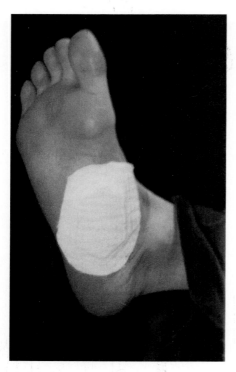

Fig. 17-8. Long arch or Mayo pad.

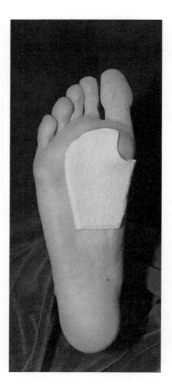

Fig. 17-9. Metatarsal pad with sesamoid accommodation.

Medial or long arch pad

This pad is also referred to as the Mayo pad (Fig. 17-8). It is an oval pad placed along the medial-plantar aspect of the foot from approximately the calcaneus to the first metatarsal head and extending under the longitudinal arch in the plantar direction. The long arch pad may be fabricated from felt. It is also available commercially, prefabricated from felt, PPT, and sponge rubber. Long arch pads are generally available in three sizes to accommodate the height and length of the longitudinal arch. The long arch pad has wide, sloping, skived edges. It supports the medial-plantar aspect of the foot and creates weightbearing in the area of the longitudinal arch. Many patients find it to be a comfortable filler between the foot and the shank of the shoe. The long arch pad may be modified with a medial-plantar accommodative cut for lesions or exostoses at the level of the navicular.

Long metatarsal pad

The long metatarsal pad is a combination of the short metatarsal pad and the long arch pad. One might consider this pad with its distal metatarsal arch buildup and the longitudinal arch medial flange as the basic orthosis. The long metatarsal pad is skived approximately once its thickness along the lateral, distal, and distal one third of the medial borders and two to three times its thickness along the medial flange and proximal end.

The long metatarsal pad is not usually prefabricated but can be fabricated from felt. It can also be fabricated from its prefabricated metatarsal pad and long arch pad components. The long metatarsal pad can be used for shoe padding or incorporated into an orthosis. Many molded orthoses utilize this concept.

Plantar accommodative pads

The purpose of plantar accommodative pads is to reduce or eliminate weightbearing on lesions such as wounds, abscesses, ulcers, areas of pressure necrosis, intractable hyperkeratoses, exostoses, etc. This is accomplished by attempting to transfer weightbearing temporarily or permanently to non-weightbearing areas or to increase weightbearing to adjoining parts. Plantar accommodative pads include (1) a modification of the basic metatarsal pad, (2) plantar heel pads, (3) plantar-medial and lateral pads to accommodate lesions, etc. at the talonavicular and styloid process of the fifth metatarsal, and (4) a plantar heel-to-toe cushion with aperture.[6]

Modification of the basic metatarsal pad

The modified accommodative metatarsal pad reduces or eliminates weightbearing primarily on a metatarsal head or heads by transferring weightbearing from the head to the shaft of the same and or other metatarsals. This requires a careful consideration of the osseous anatomy involved.

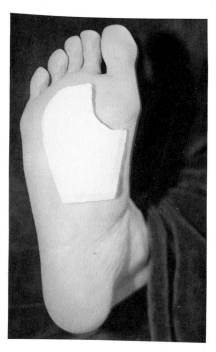

Fig. 17-10. Sesamoid pad with too large an accommodative cut.

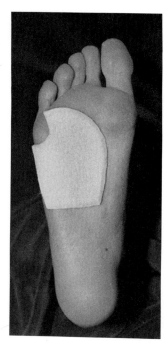

Fig. 17-11. Metatarsal pad with fifth metatarsal head accommodation.

The section of the pad that is cut away is referred to as the accommodation. Podiatric accommodative padding was used more frequently in the past. The aperture pad is used more frequently today.

Sesamoid or first metatarsal head accommodation. In fashioning the accommodation for the sesamoids or first metatarsal head, the size and shape of the sesamoids and metatarsal head must be considered.

A small circular cut large enough to accommodate the head is made at the distal medial corner of the metatarsal pad (Fig. 17-9). Too large or too sloping a cut will allow the sesamoids and head to bear excessive weight (Fig. 17-10). In placing the sesamoid pad it is moved medially so that the medial edge of the pad is proximal to the metatarsal head and runs plantar to the shaft of the first metatarsal. The sesamoid or first metatarsal accommodative pad, therefore, will be plantar to and bear weight along four metatarsal shafts, whereas the basic metatarsal pad will support three metatarsal shafts.

A sesamoid pad may also consist of a narrow strip with a crescent cut at the distal end to accommodate the first metatarsal head or sesamoids. It is placed plantar to the shaft of the first metatarsal. This smaller version of the sesamoid pad may be preferred in a pump or added to an orthosis or innersole when a larger pad is not required. The sesamoid pad is effective in the treatment of sesamoiditis, intractable hyperkeratosis, and open lesions plantar to the first metatarsal head.

The term "dancer's pad" does not indicate the anatomical area of the foot involved and should not be used.

Fifth metatarsal head accommodation. The fifth metatarsal head accommodation is made using a small circular cut at the distal lateral corner of the metatarsal pad (Fig. 17-11). The cut should be no larger than is necessary to accommodate the fifth metatarsal head and the lesion involved. The pad is moved laterally so that the lateral border is plantar to the fifth metatarsal shaft, extending medially and plantar to the shafts of the second, third, and fourth metatarsals. A smaller and narrower version with a distal crescent cut may be used. It is placed plantar to the fifth metatarsal shaft avoiding the styloid process.

First and fifth metatarsal head accommodation. The purpose of this pad is to relieve or eliminate weightbearing on the first and fifth metatarsal heads (Fig. 17-12). The metatarsal pad at its distal end must be the full width of the five metatarsal heads and narrowed proximally along the medial and lateral borders. Accommodative cuts are made first for the first metatarsal head and then for the fifth metatarsal head. The fifth metatarsal head cut should be at a slight angle and proximal to the first. This pad creates weightbearing on all five metatarsal shafts. The skiving and proximal narrowing of the pad along the medial and lateral borders determine just how

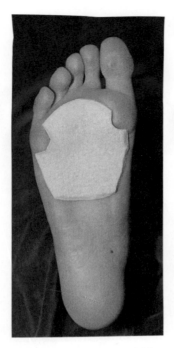

Fig. 17-12. Metatarsal pad with first and fifth metatarsal head accommodation.

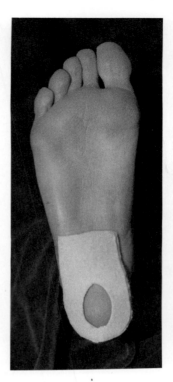

Fig. 17-13. Heel pad with aperture.

much weightbearing will be placed on the first and fifth shafts.

Accommodative cuts for one or more metatarsal heads. Accommodative cuts may be made for any one metatarsal head or any combination of metatarsal heads 2, 3, and 4. The sesamoid or fifth head accommodative pads may also include additional accommodative cuts.

Heel pads

Heel pads are available prefabricated or may be fabricated from PPT, felt, cork, sponge rubber, etc. Materials that bottom out or deteriorate rapidly are not effective for heel pads. The purpose of the basic heel pad is to cushion or elevate the heel in the shoe. This may be necessary to alleviate apophysitis or irritation to the posterior heel and Achilles tendon. Accommodative cuts at the medial, lateral, and posterior borders of the heel pad eliminate weightbearing at the site of plantar heel lesions, such as hyperkeratoses, ulcers, wounds, etc. Heel pads for calcaneal spurs or syndrome are (1) the aperture pad, (2) horseshoe pad, and (3) cobra or J pad.[4]

Aperture pad. The aperture pad is a modification of the basic heel pad (Fig. 17-13). An aperture is cut in the center of the pad. The aperture and distal end of the pad are skived dorsally. If the scissors are held at an angle while the aperture is being cut, the result will be a skived aperture.

Horseshoe pad. The horseshoe pad is a modification of the aperture pad (Fig. 17-14). The center distal portion of the pad is eliminated resulting in a U- or horseshoe-shaped pad. The pad is approximately 1/2 to 3/4 in. wide. The distal ends and the inner edge of the U are skived.

Cobra or J pad. The cobra or J pad is a modification of the horseshoe pad (Fig. 17-15). The medial arm of the U is carried distally and medially as a flange under the longitudinal arch.

Purpose. The purpose of the calcaneal spur heel pad is to transfer weightbearing to the periphery of the heel. This in turn reduces weightbearing on the plantar calcaneus, the spur, and its ligamentous attachment. Heel pads may, in acute cases, be placed temporarily on the foot. They may be placed directly into the shoe, onto cushioned innersoles, or incorporated into the construction of orthoses.

Cuboid pad

The cuboid pad (Fig. 17-16) affords a great deal of relief and comfort by supporting the cuboid bone along with its associated joints, ligaments, and tendons. This area of the foot is subject to fracture, subluxation, sprain, tearing of the ligamentous tissue, bursitis, synovitis, and peroneal tendonitis. In some instances of cuboid subluxation, manipulation

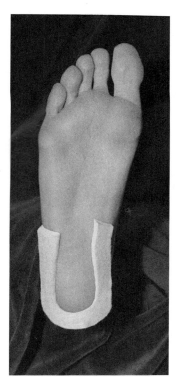

Fig. 17-14. Horseshoe heel pad.

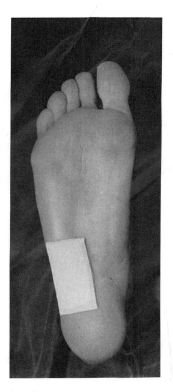

Fig. 17-16. Cuboid pad.

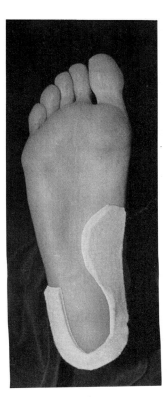

Fig. 17-15. Heel cobra or J pad.

of the cuboid is indicated and attempted by those with the ability to do so.[1]

The cuboid pad may, at times, spontaneously adjust a mildly subluxed cuboid by its upward thrust. The pad is usually made of 1/4-in. felt. It is approximately 1-1/2 in. wide and 2 to 3 in. long. The cuboid pad is skived at its edges. The actual length of the pad is determined by the distance from the calcaneocuboid articulation to the cuboid–fifth metatarsal articulation. The cuboid pad is placed directly under the cuboid bone and should not extend distally under the styloid process of the fifth metatarsal.

In acute cases the cuboid pad may be placed directly onto the foot in conjunction with a Low Dye strap. Follow-up treatment may consist of a cuboid pad in the shoe, attached to a removable innersole or incorporated into an orthosis.

Removable Elastoplast pad

The Elastoplast (Beiersdorf, Inc.) pad is primarily a forefoot pad, that is, the metatarsal pad and its accommodative modifications. It may, however, be used for bunions, tailor's bunions, and dorsal, medial, and lateral exostoses and lesions.

The pad is prepared for the foot, and a 3- to 4-in.-wide strip of Elastoplast is placed snugly around the forefoot to cover the first and fifth metatarsal heads. The nonadhesive surface of the

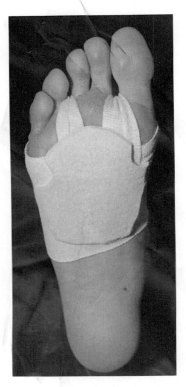

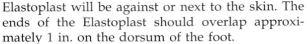

Fig. 17-17. Construction of removable Elastoplast pad.

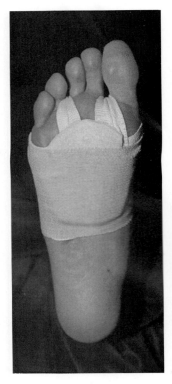

Fig. 17-18. Completed removable Elastoplast pad.

Elastoplast will be against or next to the skin. The ends of the Elastoplast should overlap approximately 1 in. on the dorsum of the foot.

Two strips of 5/8-in. tube gauze 6 to 8 in. long are stretched from end to end to remove any slack and then threaded through the first and third interspaces and placed firmly into the dorsal and plantar adhesive surfaces of the Elastoplast. Stretching the slack from the Tubegauze (Scholl Manufacturing, Chicago, IL) will, to some extent, keep the pad from migrating proximally toward the heel when the pad is worn. In order to prevent discomfort or a fissure at the plantar-medial crease at the base of the fifth toe, the Tubegauze should not be placed in the fourth interspace. To prevent the Tubegauze from being pulled loose, it should be placed to within an inch of the proximal edges of the Elastoplast (Fig. 17-17).

The pad is placed into position over the plantar tube gauze strips and pressed firmly into the adhesive. The entire dorsal and plantar surfaces are covered with a continuous strip of equal-width Elastoplast wrapped around the foot, with the nonadhesive surface exposed (Fig. 17-18). Care should be taken not to place the seam along the medial or lateral side of the foot but rather on the dorsum. If the first and fifth metatarsal heads are constricted, a curved portion of the Elastoplast may

be cut away exposing the heads. Any exposed adhesive edges should be trimmed.

The patient should be instructed to apply powder before wearing the pad and to remove the pad at night. The patient should also understand which surface is plantar and which interspaces are to be used for the Tubegauze.

Digital pads or shields

Digital lesions requiring padding are the following:

1. Painful hyperkeratotic lesions, that is, corns and calluses
2. Hyperkeratotic lesions with sequelae, that is, inflammation and tissue necrosis
3. Abscesses, ulcers, trauma, infection, and iatrogenic lesions
4. Congenital or acquired malformations and exostoses subject to pathologic conditions
5. Diabetic and peripheral vascular sequelae

Lesions, *regardless of cause, should not only be* medicated but shielded from weightbearing and from footwear. Padding, medications, and dressings are essential to facilitate healing by eliminating pressure and irritation, both of which reduce blood flow and retard healing.

Many prefabricated pads are available and are

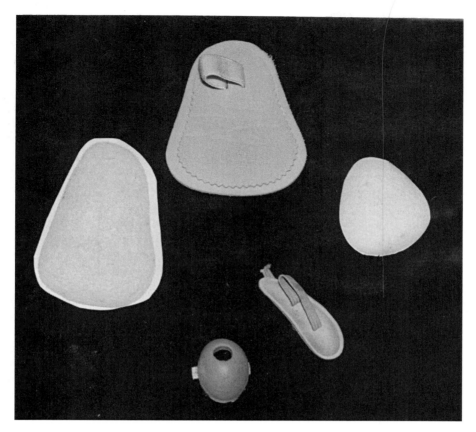

Fig. 17-19. *Bottom:* Prefabricated digital aperture pad and crest pad. *Top:* Left to right, Prefabricated metatarsal pad, sling pad for plantarflexing a digit or plantar cushion and metatarsal button.

time-saving. Prefabricated pads lend themselves to modifications and may be combined with other pads and materials. Bulk materials are available and at times preferable when fabricating a particular pad. Materials commonly employed for digital padding are felt, foam rubber, foam plastic, Rolofoam (tube foam) (Chicago Medical), Tubegauze (Scholls) Pedi-foam, Elastoplast, moleskin, and Dental Roll (Henry Schein, Chicago, IL).

Digital pads include aperture pads, crest pads, buttress pads, crescent pads, and interdigital pads.

Aperture pads

The digital aperture pad is usually fabricated from felt, foam rubber, foam plastic, or moleskin. Felt and foam tend to pack to a lesser thickness. A single thickness of moleskin gives little or no effective shielding as an aperture pad. A moleskin cover does afford some relief by absorbing friction and protecting the skin. Aperture pads are available in thicknesses of 1/16, 1/8 and 1/4 in. (Fig. 17-19).

In order to take advantage of the linear shape of the digit and phalanges, the aperture pad should be oblong or elongated with the aperture in the center or off-center. The aperture ensures that pressure is transferred from a lesion to adjacent bone, that is, the shafts of the phalanges.

Digital lesions such as those involving phalangeal heads, condyles, interdigital lesions, and various exostoses require an aperture larger than the affected lesion or area. It is also important that the thickness of the pad be at least a fraction higher than the lesion and underlying bone. Additional thickness is obtained by adding adhesive felt or foam to either end or both ends of the pad.

To prevent irritation to an adjacent toe, the dorsal aperture pad should be slightly narrower than the digit. The pad should be skived and should not be over the articulation of an interphalangeal or metatarsophalangeal joint.

Digital pads may be fastened to the toes with various adhesive strips, Gauztex (General Bandages, Morton Grove, IL), and lamb's wool. Lamb's wool should be applied loosely to allow for shrinkage due to hot water bathing. The apron-shaped

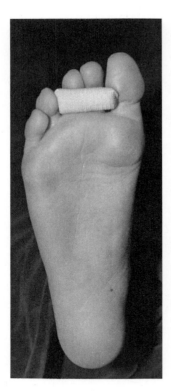

Fig. 17-20. Crest pad.

"Toe Shield" (Beiersdorf, Inc.) is excellent for adhering a pad to a digit.

The aperture in a pad makes an excellent receptacle for medications and gauze dressings.

Crest pad

The crest pad acquires its name from the crescent-shaped crest or sulcus at the plantar base of the toes at the metatarsophalangeal articulations (Fig. 17-20). The purpose of the crest pad is to mechanically dorsiflex and extend the digits by creating an upward thrust and placing weightbearing onto the padded plantar aspect of the toes. In doing so, the pad may alleviate painful lesions on a previously weightbearing distal end of a toe. The crest pad is also effective in dorsiflexing and elongating clawed or hammer toes as well as reducing the dorsiflexed head of a proximal phalanx. The crest pad is not always effective if the digit does not dorsiflex.

Prefabricated pads are available. Because the sulcus varies in depth with the length and amount of plantarflexion of the toes, prefabricated pads are limited in diameter and effectiveness. Crest pad rolls may be fabricated from dental rolls, felt, and foam rubber.

Dental Roll. Dental Roll may be effective in a very shallow sulcus or crest. Dental Roll is available in limited diameters and after some use it compresses with a loss of diameter and becomes hard. Consequently, the effect of the pad is not achieved.

Felt. Felt creates a firm-to-hard crest pad that is not always well tolerated by the patient.

Foam rubber. Foam rubber is soft and may be easily rolled into any effective diameter. Adhesive foam rubber makes a slightly more firm roll than the nonadhesive type. Foam rubber crest pad rolls retain their softness and diameter for a reasonable length of time and are more acceptable and better tolerated by the patient.

Fabrication. The amount of dorsiflexion of the toes should be determined. The foam rubber should then be rolled and fitted sufficiently to fill the crest and create a gentle comfortable lift to the digits. The crest roll should not be bulky and protrude beyond the distal end of the toes. The roll is then placed in the center of a piece of Elastoplast, 3 in. wide and approximately 6 in. long. The roll is then enclosed in the Elastoplast, which is folded from end to end. The Elastoplast is trimmed close to, but not exposing the ends of the roll.

An aperture is cut in the Elastoplast approximately 1/2 in. from the roll. The aperture cut should be straight across rather than a concave cut. A concave cut will create too large an aperture. This in turn will allow the crest roll to slide in a plantar direction out of the crest or dorsally away from the base of the toes. The excess Elastoplast is trimmed, leaving a tongue, if desired, over the dorsum of the metatarsophalangeal joints.

The crest pad roll may also be enclosed in a 5/8 in. Tubegauze, with the Tubegauze overlapping at the dorsal base of the toes and held together with a short strip of 1-in. fabric adhesive tape. Micropore adhesive is not strong enough for this purpose.

To place a crest pad under one toe may, in some instances, result in the pad working its way between the toes with resulting discomfort and rejection by the patient. It is therefore advisable to have the roll long enough to accommodate at least two toes. The crest pad should be snug and comfortable, but loose enough to slip over the toes without difficulty. The patient should be advised to remove the crest pad at night and not to wear it if interdigital discomfort occurs. Some patients object to the texture of the Elastoplast and prefer the Tubegauze.

Buttress pad

The purpose of the buttress pad is to shield or buttress the dorsum of the heads of the proximal phalanges and alleviate or prevent lesions on the dorsum of the toes.

The buttress pad is fabricated in the same manner as the crest pad. The buttress pad is the reverse of the

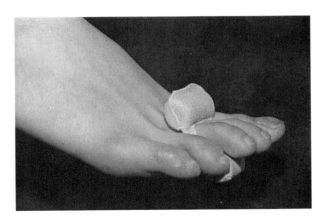

Fig. 17-21. Combination crest and buttress pad.

crest pad in that it is placed on the dorsum of the foot at the base of the toes.

The diameter of the buttress roll is determined by the depth of the sulcus between the base of the toes and the heads of the proximal phalanges. The roll, to be effective, must be as high or a fraction higher than the phalangeal heads.

If the metatarsophalangeal and interphalangeal joints are flexible there will be a tendency for the buttress pad to extend the digits and reduce the amount of dorsiflexion of the heads of the proximal phalanges. Unlike the crest pad, which is more effective with the reducible digit, the buttress pad is useful with both the reducible and the nonreducible digit.

Patients may be apprehensive or sceptical at first, but are then usually pleased to learn that their shoe will accommodate the crest or buttress pad.

Combination crest and buttress pad. The combination crest and buttress pad is used when there are symptomatic lesions at the dorsal and distal aspect of the toes (Fig. 17-21).

Fabrication. The combination crest and buttress pad is more conveniently made with Elastoplast. The diameter and length of the rolls is determined and they are then placed on a single strip of Elastoplast approximately 1 in. apart and approximately 1 in. from one end of the Elastoplast. The long end of the Elastoplast must be such that it can be folded over and between the rolls and onto the remaining Elastoplast. An aperture is cut between the rolls. A straight cut rather than a curved or concave cut will ensure that the aperture is not too large. If the aperture is too large the dorsal or plantar roll will not be in an effective position, that is, it will be too proximal on the dorsum or plantar aspect. The Elastoplast is trimmed proximally, leaving a small dorsal tongue over the metatarsophalangeal joints.

The crest, buttress, and combination pads are trimmed close to the ends of the rolls. Excessive Elastoplast between the toes is irritating. If the aperture in the Elastoplast is too small, one should attempt to stretch the Elastoplast before cutting nicks in either end of the aperture.

Crescent pads
Crescent pads derive their name from the crescent-shaped cut of the pad. Crescent pads may be fabricated from felt, foam rubber, and various other materials as well as moldable compounds. In addition to being applied to the foot, the crescent pad may also be placed in a shoe or incorporated into an orthotic or latex shield.

To accomplish an acceptable crescent cut, one should cut from one corner of the material to the opposite corner. Cutting well back in the scissors with the scissors angled, the crescent cut will be skived. If the skived crescent is placed next to the skin, the dorsal or outer surface of the crescent will be flush with the skin. The remaining outer edges are skived and will also be flush with the skin.

The depth of the crescent cut and the thickness of the pad are determined by the size of the area to be shielded, that is, the bunion or hammer toe. The pad should be fashioned and fitted to the area to be shielded and then transferred onto a Rolofoam sleeve, innersole, orthosis, latex shield, etc. The crescent shield, like all shields, must be as high as or a fraction higher than the symptomatic area if it is to be effective.

In most instances, the crescent pad is placed on the shaft of a metatarsal or phalanx shielding a lesion or exostosis. A small crescent pad applied to the distal aspect of a digit to shield a painful keratosis or open lesion, along with medication and dressing, is effective.

Crescent pads must conform to bone contours and the lesions to be shielded. Prefabricated pads of various sizes and thicknesses may be cut in half and the extending arms of the resulting U cut away, thus giving a crescent shape and eliminating side-to-side compression of the lesion.

Bunion shield. Prefabricated bunion shields are available but are limited in size and effectiveness. A particular 1/4-in. felt bunion shield with the aperture off-center may be too bulky but makes an excellent shield for lesions plantar to the first metatarsal head when employed with a butterfly sling over the hallux and held in place by the stocking and shoe (Fig. 17-22). Tubegauze may also be used for a sling.

The padding of a bunion shield should be crescent-shaped and adapt to the contour of the metatarsal head. There may be double pads, that is,

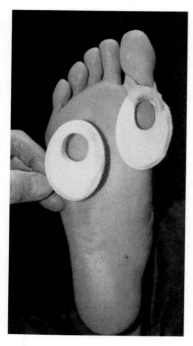

Fig. 17-22. Prefabricated felt bunion shield with butterfly sling for intractable plantar keratoma of the first metatarsal head.

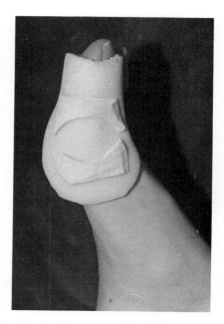

Fig. 17-24. Bunion shield demonstrating felt shield too narrow.

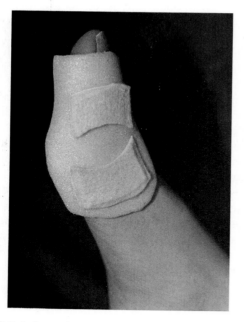

Fig. 17-23. Rolofoam sleeve with bunion shields.

proximal and distal to the head, or single, that is, proximal or distal to the first metatarsal head. In the case of a low-cut pump, the distal pad resting on the shaft of the proximal phalanx will be sufficient.

A strip of Rolofoam of sufficient diameter and long enough to extend from the interphalangeal joint to approximately 1 to 2 in. proximal to the metatarsal head is used. The Rolofoam is cut along its length, leaving a collar at least wide enough to encircle the shaft of the proximal phalanx. The crescent-shaped pads are cut and fitted to the individual foot. When the examiner is satisfied that the pads are adequate, they are then transferred to the Rolofoam (Fig. 17-23).

The actual buildups should be such that the proximal one rests along the shaft of the first metatarsal just proximal to the bunion, avoiding the first metatarsophalangeal joint. The distal buildup rests on the shaft of the proximal phalanx of the hallux, avoiding the joints proximal and distal to it. Care should be taken that the pads are wide enough from proximal to distal so as to disperse as much pressure as possible. A pad that is too narrow will be ineffective (Fig. 17-24).

The pads on the bunion shield may be of skived foam rubber or felt, usually 1/4 in. thick. The thickness, of course, is determined by the size of the exostosis. In some instances a thinner thickness may be sufficient. Stepped offset 1/8- or 1/16-in. thicknesses are used to obtain the desired thickness of the shield. It is important that the shields be as high as or a fraction higher than the exostosis to be shielded.

The excess Rolofoam is trimmed from the proximal portion along with any excess between the hallux and second toe. The finished shield may be covered with moleskin, Elastoplast, or the less bulky flesh-colored Micropore adhesive tape. A latex shield may be fabricated over a plaster cast of the bunion.

Patients with mildly symptomatic bunions may

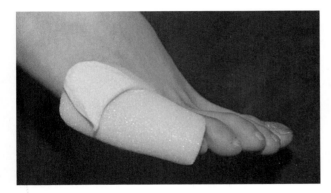

Fig. 17-25. Tailor's bunion shield on Rolofoam sleeve.

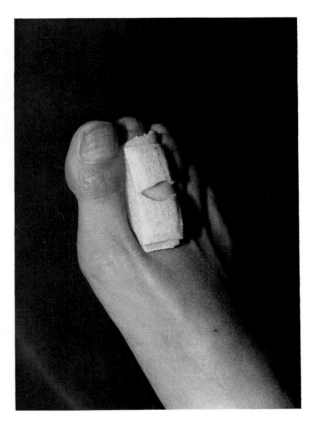

Fig. 17-27. Rolofoam sleeve with shields for dorsal lesions (may be proximal, distal, or both).

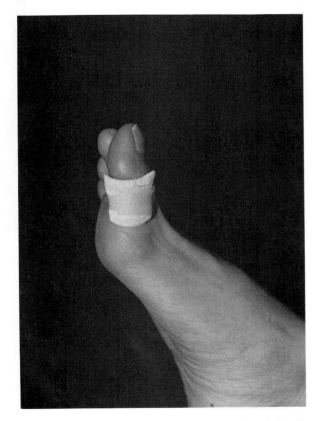

Fig. 17-26. Crescent felt pad with butterfly sling for pinch callus of the hallux.

prefer a shield of Rolofoam minus the padded buildup. The Rolofoam protects the skin from irritation by absorbing friction from the shoe.

Tailor's bunion pad. A Rolofoam sleeve is employed with a collar over the fifth toe extending proximally over the distal third of the fifth metatarsal. A crescent-shaped shield adequate to shield the tailor's bunion is fitted to the foot and then transferred to the Rolofoam. The crescent shield rests on

the shaft of the fifth metatarsal immediately proximal to the tailor's bunion (Fig. 17-25). In most cases a distal buildup is not required and may even prove uncomfortable if it rests on the metatarsophalangeal, or interphalangeal joints. A suitable covering for the shield is used.

Hallux pinch callus pad. Pinch callus lesions occur at the medial or medial-plantar aspect of the hallux and may involve an underlying necrosis or neurovascular inclusion. The pinch callus shield should be shaped, sized, and skived so that the pad rests on the shaft of the proximal phalanx proximal to the lesion, avoiding the joints distal and proximal to the pad. The pad may be transferred to a Rolofoam shield or fitted with a butterfly sling (Fig. 17-26). The butterfly sling should be snug but loose enough to be easily slipped on and off by the patient. With lesions that require medication and dressings, the shield can be applied to the skin and be a part of the dressing. In most cases 1/8- or 1/4-in. felt makes an adequate shield.

Digital pads. Smaller versions of the crescent pad are effective in protecting or buttressing lesions at the dorsal head of the proximal phalanges, the middle phalanges, and the distal end of the digits.

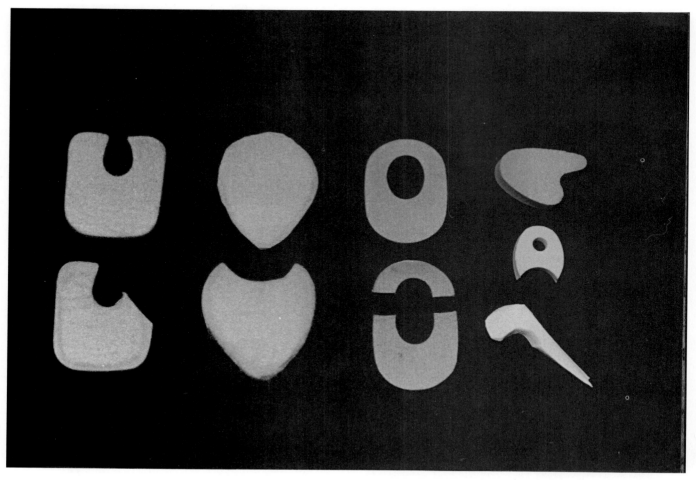

Fig. 17-28. Prefabricated pads for shielding and their modifications (*left*) and Interdigital pads (*right*).

Digital shields are designed and fitted to the individual problem and then transferred to a Rolo-foam sleeve (Fig. 17-27) or fitted with a butterfly sling. In acute cases with open lesions, an adhesive shield may be applied directly to the digit along with medication and gauze dressings.

Prefabricated aperture pads. Various digital prefabricated adhesive aperture pads are available (Fig. 17-28). The pads are usually oval with the aperture offset or in the center of the pad. The aperture should be larger than the lesion to be shielded. The aperture makes an excellent receptacle for medication when necessary. These aperture pads may be cut in half and used as crescent shields. Both prefabricated and fabricated digital aperture pads should rest on the shafts of the phalanges, not on the joints, and never on the eponychium. Larger prefabricated aperture pads are available from supply houses and can be used effectively elsewhere on the foot.

Interdigital pads

Interdigital pads (Fig. 17-28) serve the purpose of alleviating or preventing lesions along the medial, lateral, or webbed interdigital aspect of the toes. Interdigital lesions may be ischemic, diabetic, ulcerous, abscessed, or infectious, and may or may not be associated with a hyperkeratotic lesion. In most cases they are the result of the phalanx of one toe articulating with the phalanx of an adjacent toe. Interdigital lesions, for the most part, occur in one of the following three areas:

1. At the distal aspect of a toe. This lesion is usually due to the distal phalanx articulating with the opposite toe.
2. At the middle portion of a toe, often opposite the head of a proximal phalanx.
3. In the web of the fourth interspace and at times continuing up the medial aspect of the fifth toe. This lesion is the result of the head of the proximal phalanx of the fifth toe ar-

ticulating with the base of the proximal phalanx of the fourth toe. It is frequently accompanied by hyperkeratosis on the dorsum of the fifth toe.

Interdigital lesions are often associated with a companion lesion on the opposite toe.

Various prefabricated interdigital pads are available, or they may be fabricated from foam rubber or felt. Interdigital pads may be crescent- or comma-shaped, and when indicated have an aperture. The effective thickness of such pads is usually 1/8 to 1/4 in. Adhesive foam rubber or felt shield attached to Rolofoam sleeves is an excellent interdigital pad. Adhesive interdigital pads placed on interdigital skin for long periods of time should be avoided.

Distal interdigital lesions. The distal interdigital lesion requires a crescent-shaped pad immediately proximal to it resting on the shaft of the phalanx or a comma-shaped pad continuing down into the toe web. Both of these pads create a separation of the toes distally. Crescent-shaped pads attached to Rolofoam sleeves are effective. The crescent cut will face distally and next to the lesion.

Midtoe interdigital lesions. Midtoe lesions respond well to foam aperture pads and to crescent pads of foam or felt adhesive on Rolofoam sleeves.

Interdigital lesions of the toe web. Keratotic lesions of the toe web respond well to the comma-shaped pad when a notch is cut at the angle of the comma, thereby creating a gap in the pad at the area of the lesion and toe web. The toes rest on the pad distally with no pad at the web or base of the toes in the web.

When fabricated or prefabricated comma-shaped pads are used, the patient must be advised to wear the pad with the "tail" on top over the web. This prevents the pad from falling through the toes. If the lesion is distal or midtoe, the crescent faces distally. If the lesion is in the web, the crescent faces proximally.

The prefabricated 1/4-in. foam nonaperture interdigital pad is an excellent pad for modification into a notched or aperture pad. This pad is provided with a tail. It is also useful for separating toes when there is an abnormality in the nail grooves. More firm-to-hard prefabricated interdigital pads of a latex-type material and moldable compound materials are available for interdigital lesions. They are not always tolerated by the patient. A crescent-shaped, foam rubber Band-Aid type of prefabricated shield is available and effective for interdigital as well as other lesions of the foot.

Unless the interdigital shields are being used in conjunction with medication for open lesions, etc., the patient should be advised to remove the pads at night.

The butterfly sling

The butterfly sling is useful in the construction of a removable shield. With use, the center nonadhesive section between the two adhesive ends of the butterfly tends to roll or rope up. To prevent the roll from being too thick and uncomfortable it is wise to remove approximately one third of the longitudinal width from the desired length of 1-in. adhesive tape. This leaves a length of tape approximately 2/3 in. wide.

Holding the adhesive strip (adhesive side up) between the first and fourth and second and third fingers, a small nick is made with the scissors approximately 1/2 in. from each end of the adhesive. The resulting section is folded between the nicks toward the center. The strip is reversed and the nick is repeated on the opposite side. The section is folded toward the center to meet the opposite section so that no adhesive is exposed. This provides a nonadhesive center section with two adhesive ends. The end product is referred to as a "butterfly." To prevent the adhesive ends from tearing away from the center section of the butterfly, the nicks should not be cut too deeply.

The center portion of the sling or butterfly is placed between the toes resting on the web. The shield to be used is placed in its desired position and the adhesive ends of the butterfly are attached to the shield and reinforced with an additional piece of tape (Fig. 17-29).

If the sling is not resting on the toe web, the shield will slide from its effective position until the butterfly rests on the web, resulting in malposition of the pad and discomfort. The shield should be checked for effectiveness and easy removal, particularly for removal over the bulbous end of a digit. The patient should be advised to remove the shield at night and when bathing.

Removable shields using the butterfly sling

Hallux pinch callus shield. A crescent-shaped skived 1/4-in. felt shield is fitted to the shaft of the medial-plantar aspect of the proximal phalanx, proximal to the interphalangeal joint. The butterfly is attached to the shield, making sure the butterfly rests on the toe web. This shield transfers pressure or weightbearing from the interphalangeal joint to the shaft of the proximal phalanx.

Dorsal shield for the head of the proximal phalanx.

1. A 1/4-in. felt skived shield is fabricated to rest on the proximal phalanx proximal to the

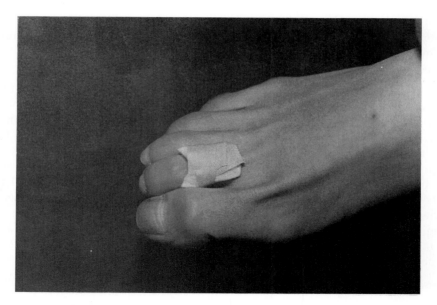

Fig. 17-29. One-quarter-inch felt crescent shield with butterfly sling.

phalangeal head. The butterfly is attached and the shield acts as a buttress pad.

2. An elongated skived 1/4-in. felt shield no wider than the digit with a hollow or aperture over the head of the proximal phalanx is fabricated for the toe. The distal portion rests on the middle phalanx, avoiding the distal interphalangeal joint. The proximal end rests on the shaft of the proximal phalanx, avoiding the metatarsolphalangeal joint. The butterfly is placed between the toes resting on the web. The pad is put in place and the butterfly is attached to the dorsum of the proximal end of the pad (Fig. 17-30).

Plantar first metatarsal head shield. A prefabricated or fabricated aperture bunion shield with the aperture off-center, or a sesamoid accommodative pad is used. The butterfly sling is placed over the hallux close to the web and attached to the pad which has been put into place on the plantar surface.

The butterfly sling pads stay in place with the stocking and will mold to the contours of the foot.

Summary

The word *doctor* originally meant expert, authority, teacher. Medical knowledge and techniques largely evolve within the framework of an apprenticeship system wherein seniors pass on knowledge and ideas to their juniors, who then strive to improve their inheritance and outshine their mentors.

The objectives of medicine are to promote health,

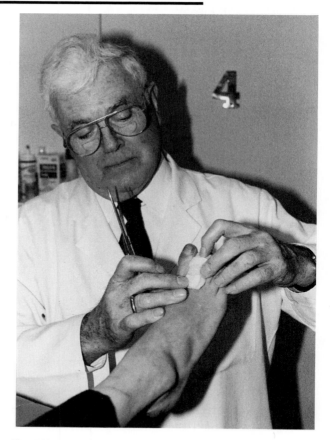

Fig. 17-30. Fitting the digital shield.

to restore health, to prevent disease, and to rehabilitate the patient. The doctor of podiatric medicine is steadfastly involved in each of these four objectives.

Adequate blood flow unhindered by pressure or

irritation is necessary for tissue granulation and complete healing. From its earliest days the profession of foot care has resorted to devising effective shields and devices to facilitate healing and to prevent chronic or acute weightbearing or pressure lesions. It is imperative, therefore, that the medical foot practitioner be well acquainted with the techniques, materials, and products (new and old) that are available for the protection or prevention of wounds, ulcers, abscesses, hyperkeratoses, malformations, etc. No amount of surgical or biomechanical procedures can entirely eliminate the need for palliative shielding. It is hoped, therefore, that the material, however briefly mentioned in this chapter, may be of assistance and guidance to the student and young practitioner, some of whom will most surely be innovators in their professional careers.

References

1. Blakeslee TJ: Morris JL: Cuboid syndrome and the significance of midtarsal joint stability, *J Am Podiatr Med Assoc* 77:12, 1987.
2. Dye R: *Natl Assoc Chiropod* 29:11, 1939.
3. Henley W: *Oxford dictionary of quotations*, 1979.
4. Johss MH: *Disorders of the foot and ankle*, ed 2, vol 3, Padding devices by Milgram, JE, Philadelphia, 1991, WB Saunders.
5. Kaplan C: *Padding and strapping*, Mt Kisco, NY, Futura. 1982.
6. Wu K: *Foot orthoses*, Baltimore, Williams & Wilkins. 1990.

ankle-foot orthoses

Notty Bumbo, Pedorthist

Neuromuscular and musculoskeletal conditions

Extrinsic vs. intrinsic AFOs
Extrinsic AFOs
Intrinsic AFOs

Footwear considerations for AFOs

Casting techniques and considerations for intrinsic AFOs
Casting method

Prescribing AFOs

Summary

While most foot and gait problems may be treated successfully with the standard methods of palliative care, foot orthoses, or surgical intervention, there are instances where another approach is necessary, either as a follow-up to the primary medical response, or as an initial treatment of choice. These instances include trauma, neuromuscular disorders, musculoskeletal disorders, or the need for extreme protection of the brittle diabetic foot. The circumstances for a more rigorous mechanical intervention are quite varied, but there are a few aspects they share in common: functional muscular weakness or loss in the lower extremity of one or more muscle groups; upper or lower motor neuron disease or trauma with accompanying spasticity or loss of tone; or loss of sensory functions within the lower extremity that may lead to tissue breakdown. These may present individually or separately.

When a patient presents with functional symptoms such as these, he or she is seldom an appropriate surgical candidate. Additionally, some pathomechanical conditions may be too advanced for the successful use of standard, functional foot orthoses. While palliative care, such as the debridement of lesions, is called for in some cases, it may not represent the full range of care available for the needs of the patient.

Ankle-foot orthoses, generally referred to as AFOs, include a range of devices that act to support, protect, or enhance the function of the foot and ankle during gait. AFOs can be divided into two categories: extrinsic, or conventional, with attachment to the outside of the shoe, and intrinsic, or plastic, which is worn inside the shoe. (*Extrinsic* and *intrinsic* are my designations for the two types of AFOs to aid with their differentiation over the course of this chapter.) AFOs are further categorized by what function the AFO must perform, for example, dorsiflexion assistance, ankle stabilization, or foot-ankle immobilization.

In general, all orthoses function with five goals in mind. Some of these goals may be concurrent, but in all instances, at least one of these following five goals is operable:[9]

1. Relief of pain by limiting motion or weight-bearing
2. Immobilization and protection of weak, painful, or healing musculoskeletal segments
3. Reduction of axial load
4. Prevention and correction of deformity
5. Improvement of function

This chapter presents an introduction to lower limb AFOs, describing the various types and their applications, and illustrates the casting technique employed as the initial stage of fabrication for intrinsic-style AFOs. This chapter also provides the practitioner with a description of AFOs and their applications, which will assist with the treatment of various neuromuscular and musculoskeletal disorders.

Neuromuscular and musculoskeletal conditions

There are numerous conditions that might call for the prescription of an AFO. Perhaps the most frequent application is for patients after a cerebrovascular accident (CVA), with a resultant loss in the dorsiflexors of the affected side. This situation usually results in footdrop, or toe drag gait, forcing extensor substitution, a circumducted gait, and the possibility of falling, particularly when the patient attempts to navigate any variation in the walking surface, such as stairs. An AFO for this type of patient would employ some type of dorsiflexion assistance, either a spring-loaded ankle joint in an extrinsic-style brace, or a leaf-spring-style intrinsic AFO. Lateral or medial ankle stability must be taken into account here, as the abductors are often affected as well. In nearly all post-CVA patients, there will be extensive physical therapy involved, and the application of the AFOs should be concurrent with the therapy.

There are numerous types of traumatic injuries that might call for the use of an AFO: crush injuries; relatively minor spinal cord injuries, resulting in tethered-cord syndrome; or any trauma that compromises the normal function of the foot and ankle, either temporarily, or permanently. The goal may be relief of pain, immobilization, improvement of function, or a reduction of axial loading. The type and scope of the trauma will determine the prescription, and the duration of use of the orthosis. It is important to determine the presence, type, and duration of edema before determining the type of device that will be most appropriate for the patient's needs. A related situation that may demand the use of AFOs is a surgical complication that results in nerve impairment or loss to the lower extremity. Patients in this group may require dorsiflexion assistance, ankle stabilization, or both.

Another condition that might call for the use of an AFO is a patient experiencing the post-poliomyelitis syndrome. While poliomyelitis is rare in the younger population of the United States, it is still found in many Third World countries, and among the population of this country born prior to 1955. There is an increasing number of poliomyelitis patients who are experiencing a secondary weakness in their affected limb many years

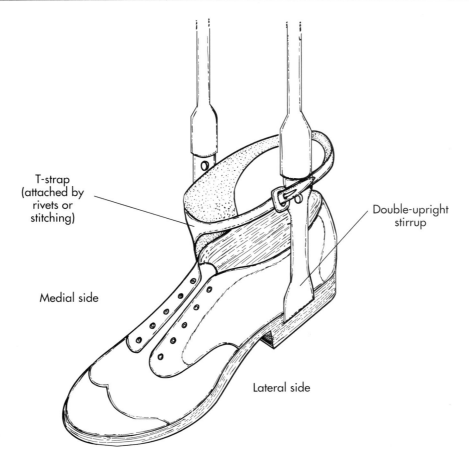

T-strap
(attached by
rivets or
stitching)

Medial side

Double-upright
stirrup

Lateral side

T-strap for intrinsic AFO
Lateral side attachment to control excess inversion/supination
Medial side attachment to control excess eversion/pronation

Fig. 18-1. Extrinsic AFO–Double-upright stirrup. Attached to plastazote-lined depth shoe, with hook-and-loop closure. Ankle joints use spring for dorsiflexion assistance.

later.[1,2,6,11] The original advice given to these patients when they recovered from the effects of the initial onset was to use the other limb more, and to exercise their other muscle groups for compensation. This was based on the belief that damage to the anterior horn cells had halted its progression, and that the overt physical effects were limited to the apparently affected areas only. It is now understood that the damage to the patient was more extensive than previously thought. The syndrome seems to appear later in the patient's life, in many instances creating weakness in the apparently unaffected side. The purpose of an AFO in these patients is to enhance the loss or increasing weakness of dorsiflexors, to stabilize laterally and medially, or to enhance both aspects at the same time. It should be noted that many of these patients have an accompanying limb shortening, which has often been untreated. Any such discrepancy in limb

length must be taken into account when considering an AFO (see Chapter 16).

Cerebral palsy is a condition that can vary in the degree of lower extremity involvement, ranging from a mild in-toeing, to a profound degree of scissoring, a nearly complete lack of dorsiflexion, and an inability to decelerate. While an AFO may be inadequate for the more extreme manifestations of cerebral palsy, the milder levels of involvement may be greatly aided with an AFO. It is essential that the degree of spasticity in such patients be carefully noted, as this will contribute to extreme pressure distribution against the shoe and the brace. These pressure areas should be duly padded, and in the application of an extrinsic type of AFO, a T strap should be used to counter ankle and subtalar inversion (Fig. 18-1).

In the diabetic Charcot's foot, there is a significant risk of ulceration and infection. While there are a number of methods that can be effective in healing subsequent tissue breakdown, customary shoe and orthotic therapies offer limited success for this foot condition. Because such patients are without sensation in varying levels of the lower leg, impact of the foot with the ground will be more extreme, as the patient requires some sensory feedback to enable ambulation. This increased shock contributes to the acceleration of the Charcot process. Such feet should be protected as much as possible to reduce the possibility of subsequent amputation. Any brace utilized for a diabetic patient must be very well padded, usually with Plastazote, to prevent tissue breakdown at pressure points. Diabetic patients must have their feet and orthoses examined by the practitioner or orthotist regularly for any signs of pressure. The padding material should be replaced whenever it becomes too compressed, soiled, or wrinkled, to prevent infection or ulceration.

AFOs are also employed in a corrective or assistive manner with children who are being treated for a wide array of congenital deformities, such as spina bifida, talipes equinovarus, and other congenital defects that affect the lower extremities. Often, the uses of an AFO in these situations are for a limited duration, with a certain amount of correction anticipated. In some cases, one type of bracing may be followed by another type in a serial approach to facilitate multiple corrections (e.g., in cases of mild talipes equinovarus or congenital gastocnemius equinus). A child's growth must be taken into account. The parents should be properly trained in putting on and removing the orthoses, examining the orthoses for wear or malfunction, and alerting the practitioner to the need for a new orthosis when the current one is outgrown. While night splints are appropriately considered AFOs, they are covered elsewhere in this book.

The prevention or correction of deformities encompasses a significant number of conditions that might require the use of an AFO. The more common conditions are:

1. Muscle imbalance around a joint, whether from upper or lower motor neuron paralysis or muscle disease

2. Muscle disease or other paralytic condition leading to unopposed gravitational forces

3. Progressive fibrous tissue diseases, such as Dupuytren's contracture

4. Lesions leading to reactive scarring, such as local trauma, burns, or inflammation involving joint structures or muscles

5. Arthritis, especially of the shoulders, elbows, and knees (and feet), leading to pain-induced inhibition of muscular action

6. A disrupted blood supply to a muscle or limb, such as Volkmann's ischemic contracture

7. Any painful state of bone, joint, or muscle where inhibition of muscle contraction occurs.[9]

An AFO used for the correction or prevention of a deformity might act to stretch, stabilize, assist (as with a spring or elastic strap), or resist. Again, the type and degree of the deformity defines the type of orthosis required. With children, it should be apparent that the younger the child is at the outset of treatment, the more effective the orthotic treatment will be.

Another important consideration is the stability of the knee joint whenever an AFO is to be prescribed. If there is limited motion, or a recurvatum at the knee joint, the practitioner should note this on the prescription. The resultant orthosis will be positioned in neutral, 5-degree dorsiflexion, or 5-degree plantarflexion, depending on the quality and range of motion available in the knee joint.

Extrinsic versus intrinsic AFOs

AFOs can be divided into two broad categories: extrinsic, which has been the type of AFO historically available, and intrinsic, which is a more recent development, brought about primarily by the advent of plastics and newer fabrication techniques. Extrinsic AFOs are attached to the outside of the patient's footwear, while intrinsic AFOs are worn inside the shoe. Extrinsic AFOs are usually constructed of combinations of metal, leather, and plastic, while intrinsic AFOs are constructed of plastic, and in some cases, of composite materials, such as carbon-fiber lay-ups.

The most important difference between extrinsic and intrinsic AFOs is that the intrinsic AFO is closer to the body and can perform its function more effectively. This is because the closer that the brace can be brought to the center of force, the greater the mechanical advantage. There are circumstances where an intrinsic AFO is not advisable, however, and the practitioner must note these conditions carefully before prescribing an orthosis. For example, if there is significant edema in the lower limb, whether fluctuating or chronic, an intrinsic AFO is not advisable. Even when the edema is post-traumatic, and expected to subside, the practitioner is advised to utilize an extrinsic AFO.

Another difference between extrinsic and intrinsic AFOs is that of cosmesis. An orthosis that may be hidden inside the shoe and under the pants leg provides a major psychological contribution to pa-

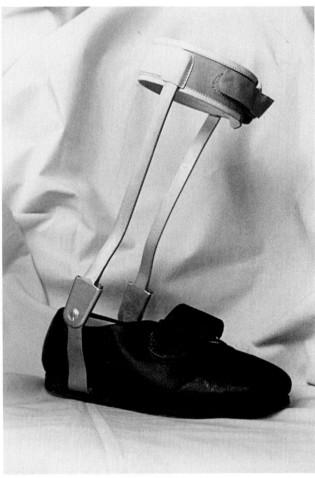

Fig. 18-2. Extrinsic AFO—Wire-spring Brace. Attached to athletic shoe. Note fleece-lined calf band with hook-and-loop closure. Provides moderate dorsiflexion assistance. (**A**). Extrinsic AFO attached to Plastazote-lined depth-style shoe (**B**).

tient compliance with the course of treatment. There are also a variety of colors of plastics available that can mimic skin tones quite closely, making the device less noticeable. It has also been demonstrated that in those instances where an intrinsic AFO can be used easily, it is more readily accepted by the patient.

AFOs are not an over-the-counter treatment modality. They are a prescribed device, and while there are a broad array of prefabricated orthoses available today, it should be noted that only about 20% of the patient population can be successfully fitted with a prefabricated orthosis.[5] Proper fit is crucial, as is the proper choice of orthosis. For example, a posterior leaf-spring AFO will not provide adequate ankle stabilization because the trim lines reduce the axial load-bearing abilities of the orthosis significantly. If the prescribing practitioner is not aware of the differences in the various AFOs, he or she should clearly state the pathologic

condition and symptoms to the orthotist, and allow the orthotist to make the proper selection.

Extrinsic AFOs

AFOs are put to fairly rigorous use, and any shoe that is considered for use with an AFO must be strong enough to perform the required task. Unfortunately, what makes a shoe adequate for this task will not always be acceptable to the patient on the basis of cosmesis. Blucher-type shoes are the traditional choice for extrinsic bracing because they are so well constructed, usually employing a steel shank, a leather sole, and a leather insole. These features allow the AFO to be attached to the shoe with little likelihood of separation during use. There has been, in recent years, some success in using athletic footwear with extrinsic AFOs, but there may be some compromise in longevity owing to the extraordinary stresses on the shoe relative to the durability of the components[5,7] (Fig. 18-2**A**).

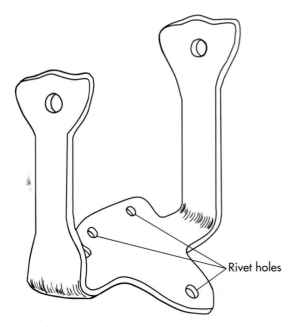

Fig. 18-3. Double-upright stirrup, extrinsic AFO-attachment to shoe.

Rivet holes

Another type of shoe that may be utilized is a depth-style shoe, some of which are constructed with a steel shank, and some with a wedge-type construction (Fig. 18-2**B**). As long as the insole and the outsole are strong enough to withstand the stresses of the AFO, and are capable of securing the rivets that are used to hold the brace to the shoe, then such shoes should be considered for this application. Regardless of the type of shoe chosen for use with an AFO, shoe wear should be carefully monitored, as excessive wear may contribute to a marked reduction in the efficacy of the orthosis.

Extrinsic AFOs are constructed from a combination of metal and leather components. There are two types of attachments for extrinsic AFOs: stirrup and caliper. Both of these attachments have variations, but the most common is the double-upright stirrup (Fig. 18-3). Caliper attachments employ either round fittings, or flat, box-type fittings (Fig. 18-4 **A** and **B**). The advantage of the caliper-style brace is that a number of the patient's shoes can be fitted with the box plate or round plate, with the need for only one upper brace section. The disadvantage of the caliper-type AFO is the sacrifice of a certain amount of strength when compared with the double-upright–stirrup-style AFO. There is also a lightweight dorsiflexion assist AFO called a wire-spring brace, which is effective for those patients demon-

strating weak dorsiflexors that do not require ankle stabilization (see Fig. 18-2**A**).

Most extrinsic-style AFOs use an ankle-joint component, which allows motion in plantar- and dorsiflexion. This motion may be spring-assisted, when there is a loss of function that must be replaced, or it can be restricted, when excessive motion would cause or accentuate existing pathomechanical conditions. It is important to communicate clearly to the orthotist the kind and amount of motion that is needed. This information will allow the orthotist to choose the proper ankle-joint configuration for the orthosis.[7]

All extrinsic AFOs require a method of attachment to the calf. The usual attachment is called the calf band, and uses either a strap-and-buckle closure or a D-ring and hook-and-loop closure system. This latter closure system is ideal for patients with limited strength or dexterity in their hands. Calf bands should be well-padded, and the inside surface, which contacts the limb, should have no seams that might cause tissue irritation. A soft leather, called orthopedic cow lining, is the usual material of choice, as it is quite durable while retaining its soft surface for a long time. Some calf bands utilize a steel posterior piece covered with padding and leather for extra durability.

The main body, comprised of the uprights, of an extrinsic AFO is usually fabricated with stainless steel, although some uprights are fabricated with aluminum stock to reduce weight, while the box or round-caliper shoe plates and stirrups are made from stainless steel because of the strength required at the shoe-orthosis interface.

Because extrinsic AFOs are made from a variety of materials, and because they usually contain a mechanical component (the ankle joint and closure system), the orthosis must be inspected regularly, at least every 6 months, unless malfunction of the brace requires more frequent attention by the orthotist. Maintenance of the orthosis includes lubrication of all joints, cleaning and replacing the calf band as needed, repairing or replacing the closure system as wear dictates, checking springs for wear, and checking attachment rivets, replacing them as needed.[4,5,7,8]

The fitting parameters for extrinsic AFOs, while not as rigorous as with intrinsic AFOs, still require proper fit for correct function and comfort. The width of the caliper attachment or the stirrup must be adequate to prevent the uprights of the orthosis from rubbing against the malleoli. The length of the uprights must be correct to allow the calf band to rest in the best location on the calf. The circumferential length of the calf band must not be too short or too long. Improper fit will result in an uncom-

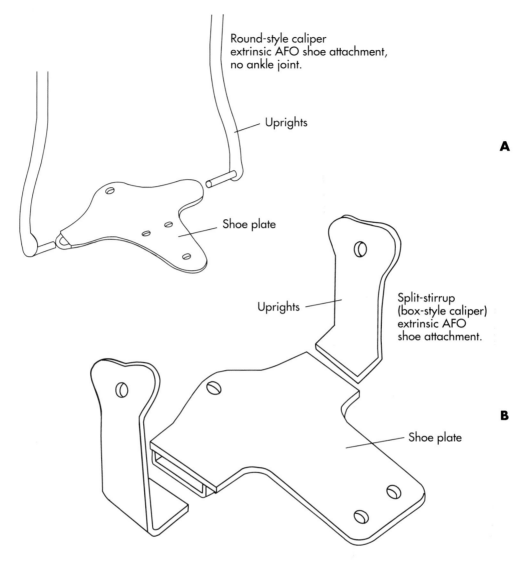

Fig. 18-4. (A) Round style caliper extrinsic AFO shoe attachment. (B) Split stirrup box-style caliper extrinsic AFO shoe attachment.

fortable, ineffective orthosis, and can contribute to the patient's rejection of the device. Good communication between all members of the team, the practitioner, the orthotist, the physical therapist, and the patient, is crucial to a successful outcome.

Intrinsic AFOs

Intrinsic AFOs refers to any type of AFO that is molded to fit closely to the foot and leg, and is worn inside the patient's footwear. Intrinsic AFOs are usually constructed from plastic, most often polypropylene, or in cases that require great strength, composite materials such as carbon-graphite or resin lay-ups. Some intrinsic AFOs have functional ankle joints designed to promote normal ankle flexion and extension. The manner in which the trim line of the orthosis is designed will determine the function of the orthosis, as well. The calf band of an intrinsic AFO is usually a continuation of the upright portion of the orthosis, while utilizing a hook-and-loop and D-ring closure system.

The most commonly utilized intrinsic AFO is called a posterior leaf-spring AFO. It is designed with a very narrow trim line, posterior to the malleoli, which acts as a dorsiflexion assistance brace. It is normally used whenever there is a loss or weakness of the dorsiflexors, but with associated adequate lateral and medial strength. The plantar portion of the orthosis usually extends to the sulcus of the toes, and the plantar aspect is dorsiflexed 5 degrees to the ankle, which serves to resist toe drag and assist toe-off (Fig. 18-5).

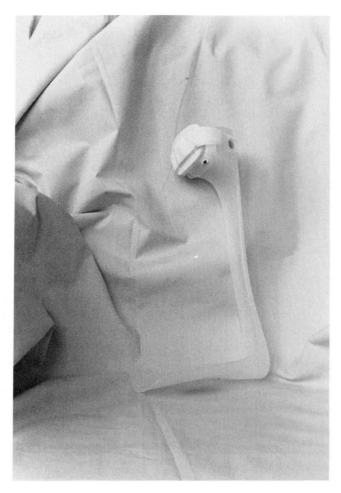

Fig. 18-5. Intrinsic AFO—Posterior Leaf-spring Brace. Very narrow posterior trim lines and long foot-bed provide excellent dorsiflexion assistance, no ankle stabilization.

In instances where greater lateral and medial ankle stabilization is required, the trim lines are carried more anteriorly, in some cases coming over the malleoli. When the malleoli are encompassed by the orthosis, the device must be appropriately padded over the prominences. The consequences of making the trim lines wider are a more rigid, as well as a bulkier appliance. This design also serves to restrict normal dorsi- and plantarflexion to a higher degree. This may be a necessary compromise to achieve the desired outcome (Fig. 18-6).

The alternative to the above style of orthosis is to insert an ankle joint mechanism into the orthosis, shown in Figure 18-7, p. 400. Note the posterior stop mechanism. This adjustable pin permits a specific amount of plantarflexion, with a fair degree of adjustability. This articulated orthosis allows functional ankle motion in the proper plane and restricts lateral and medial motion, while also providing dorsiflexion assistance in gait.[4,5,8]

In cases where there is a requirement for greater lateral or medial ankle stabilization, but there is adequate dorsi- and plantarflexory strength and function, an ankle-stabilizing orthosis provides good results. It is cosmetically acceptable, although it only provides minimal dorsiflexion assistance (Fig. 18-8, p. 401). Some ankle-stabilizing orthoses use ankle reinforcement to increase the strength and life of the device. The two most common techniques for such reinforcement are carbon-graphite struts at the level of the ankle, placed into a "sandwich" of polypropylene at the lateral and medial ankle, or a "rib," which is formed during the initial molding process (see Fig. 18-6). Because all plastics eventually fatigue, such reinforcing measures are beneficial, and are especially important when AFOs are used in heavier patients.

There are many variations on the intrinsic AFOs presented here. Each of the variations is based on specific patient needs, as pathomechanical influences and cosmesis, and general lifestyle considerations differ widely among a given patient population. Factors such as weight, edema, mobility, degree of severity of gross physical symptoms, age, and psychological resistance or readiness must be evaluated in decisions related to the prescription and final design of the orthosis.

The primary negative consideration for an intrinsic AFO is the sensitivity or insensitivity of the skin. While an intrinsic AFO is not precluded in the case of a diabetic patient, such patients should be monitored very closely for an increase in pressure at all bony prominences and an increased propensity for tissue maceration. Patients who display any signs of allergic response to rubbers, adhesives, or leather might require special consideration, and are better candidates for an extrinsic orthosis. Finally, because intrinsic AFOs are in nearly continuous contact with the skin, patients with a history of contact dermatitis should also be considered for an extrinsic brace.

Footwear considerations for AFOs

All types of AFOs are used in conjunction with a shoe or shoes. Extrinsic AFOs must be securely attached to a shoe, and intrinsic AFOs must be worn inside a shoe. The type of footwear chosen as part of the orthosis treatment is very important, therefore, and the choice of appropriate footwear should be thoroughly discussed with the patient. If the shoe style does not possess the necessary strength to allow for attachment of the orthosis, or adequate space inside to permit proper entry and fit of both brace and foot, then the orthosis will not be of use.

The most frequently used shoe style is the blucher. This is simply a shoe that has a lace closure system, a leather sole, a steel shank sandwiched between the sole and the insole, and a leather insole. The blucher is available in both women's and men's styles. Although this type of shoe is quite durable, it may not suit some patient's style consciousness, and the education process may prove difficult. It may also require some creative work on the part of the orthotist to reach an acceptable compromise.

Depth-style shoes are also excellent for both extrinsic and intrinsic AFOs. Because there is extra depth in the last design of these shoes, ranging from 1/8 to 3/16 in. in some brands, intrinsic AFOs usually fit inside them with little adjustment of the shoe or the brace. These shoes are also a style compromise for many people, but they are lightweight and durable, and are often available with other closure systems, such as the hook-and-loop. One type of depth shoe that is of particular interest is the open-to-toe shoe, so named because the shoe opens up to the toes to allow the foot to enter the shoe without flexing. Open-to-toe shoes are avail-

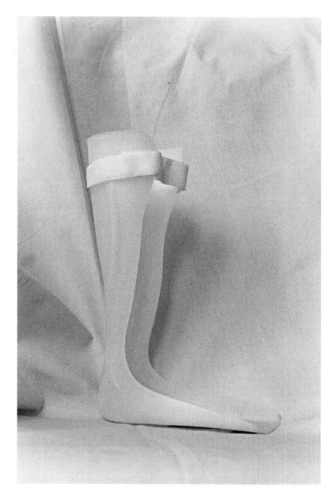

Fig. 18-6. Intrinsic AFO—Reinforced Ankle Stabilization Brace. Note generous anterior trim-lines, "rib" along lateral and medial sides extending just below malleoli, for increased rigidity. Minimal dorsi- and plantarflexion.

able in both a lace closure, and a hook-and-loop, D-ring closure system. This type of shoe is excellent for those patients with very flaccid, or very rigid feet, who have a difficult time getting their feet into more conventional footwear.

Athletic shoes are also quite effective with intrinsic AFOs, as most are made with a removable inlay that allows for additional room inside the shoe. Many athletic shoe styles are also appropriate vehicles for orthopedic modifications which might be necessary in addition to an AFO, such as lifts or rocker soles. Athletic shoes are not as appropriate for extrinsic AFOs, because their soles are not firm enough to hold rivets, and would allow the brace to pull away from the shoe. The structural integrity of the shoe-orthosis bond is crucial.

The shoe is just as important to the rehabilitation process as the orthosis. As such, it is important that shoe wear be examined at reasonable intervals,

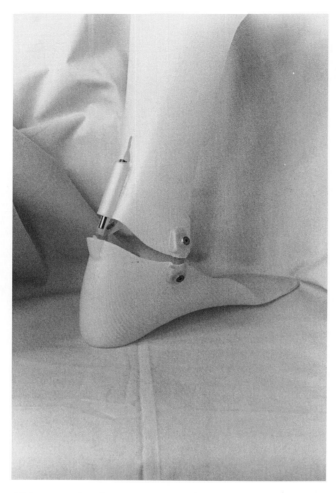

Fig. 18-7. Intrinsic AFO—Articulated-Posterior stop. Allows ankle dorsiflexion, limits plantarflexion, stabilizes ankle.

every 6 months, for example, as should the brace itself. Excessive wear on the heel or sole should be noted and repaired, so as not to compromise overall function of the orthosis. There may be a need to include some type of shoe modification, either for fit or for function, and these modifications should also be periodically reassessed for continuing effectiveness, as well as for structural integrity. Modifications such as SACH heels, rocker soles, heel and sole lifts, stretching, or closure system modifications will have to be performed on all shoes the patient will be wearing with the orthosis, in order to ensure continuity of the performance of the AFO.[10]

Casting techniques and considerations for intrinsic AFOs

Unlike an extrinsic-style AFO, an intrinsic AFO requires an impression cast of the patient's involved lower leg, usually distal to the knee. Except in those instances where a prefabricated orthosis can be used, the cast is necessary, and it should be taken by a person trained in the procedure. The position of the patient during the casting process is very important, both for the outcome of the cast, and for the patient's comfort. In the procedure listed below, it is evident that the process requires an adequate work area, good seating for the patient, and certain tools and materials to enable both the application of the plaster and its removal.

Casting method

1. Position the patient in the chair with ankle and foot at 90 degrees (Fig. 18-9**A**). Apply the stockinet from the knee to approximately 3 in. distal to the toes. In patients with generous hair growth on the leg and foot, it is wise to apply Vaseline (petroleum jelly) or another lubricant to the leg to prevent adhesion.

2. Apply rubber tubing to the anterior lower leg, centered over the tibia. Secure with

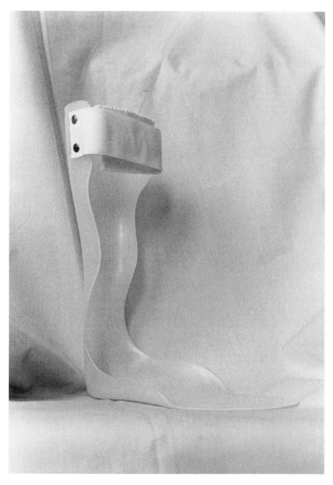

Fig. 18-8. Intrinsic AFO—Stabilizing Brace. With moderate dorsiflexion assistance. Note trim lines more anterior, especially distal to the ankle.

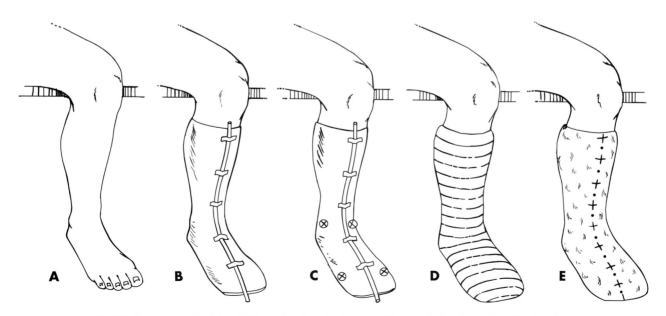

Fig. 18-9. Casting method for AFO production. Redrawn with permission from Jennifer Sanders, DPM (Pro Lab, USA: Brisbane, CA).

skin tape along the length of the tubing (Fig. 18-9**B**).

3. Using a cast pencil, mark the medial and lateral malleoli, styloid process, and medial eminence of the first metatarsal. Also mark bony prominences or any area that requires intrinsic accommodation (Fig. 18-9**C**).

4. Moisten all rolls of plaster (4-in. rolls) simultaneously. This ensures uniform drying and facilitates ease of removal from the leg. Apply the first roll to the distal foot using the entire roll. Allow the plaster to extend distally 2 in. beyond the toes. Apply the second roll beginning at the level of the ankle, continuous with the first roll, proximally to the level of the fibular head. Final cast thickness should be approximately three layers. Massage the plaster thoroughly while it is still wet, taking care to maintain the leg in its proper position throughout the procedure (Fig. 18-9**D**).

5. Use the cast pencil to mark the cast anteriorly for proper realignment after the cast is removed (Fig. 18-9**E**).

6. Using a blade or a cast cutter, cut the cast along the tubing anteriorly. Gently pry the cast apart and away from the leg and foot, and bring the marked edges back together again promptly. Minor adjustments to correct the forefoot-to-rearfoot relationship may be done while the cast is still pliable.

7. Remove the stockinet liner from the inside of the cast and allow the cast to dry thoroughly before sending it to the laboratory for fabrication.[11]

Prescribing AFOs

When the practitioner considers an AFO as part of the treatment and rehabilitation plan for a patient, there are a number of points to consider. The most crucial is clear communication with the patient, regarding the reasons for the recommendation of an orthosis; what the orthosis will do, and what it will not do; the expected duration of use; footwear considerations; cost; and finally, ease of use. The practitioner must remember that there will inevitably be a psychological reaction to the need for an orthosis, no matter how cosmetically acceptable the brace may be. Though the patient has a true need for the brace, and may even seem ready to do anything to alleviate his or her pain, discomfort, or poor function, this does not preclude rejection, for what may seem to the practitioner irrational reasons. Clear, considerate communication, and the influence of friends and family members, are often the key to patient acceptance of an orthosis.

This aspect of clear communication also extends to the orthotist. It is essential that the orthotist obtain the practitioner's guidance regarding the needs of the patient if the resulting orthosis is to properly meet the needs of that patient. The practitioner must clearly communicate all the biomechanical needs of the patient to the orthotist. Specific information should be solicited. Is the brace for dorsiflexion assistance? Does the ankle require stabilization? Does the knee joint exhibit any pathomechanical condition that might influence or be influenced by the orthosis, (e.g., genu recurvatum)? Does the patient have a limb length inequality? These questions should be clearly addressed in the prescription.

What other problems exist? Are there ischemic or neurologic conditions that may contraindicate the use of an intrinsic orthosis? Is there chronic or temporary edema? Is the edema fluctuating? Are there acute behavioral or psychological conditions that might affect the use of an orthosis? Are there other pathologic conditions, such as acute inner-ear imbalances, that might contribute to postural instability? Any condition that might affect the use of an orthosis should be duly considered and noted when appropriate in the prescription.[3]

The prescription for the actual orthosis is not the only part of the process that the practitioner must consider, however. The patient will require education on the application and use of the orthosis. This is particularly true in post-CVA patients, or in any patient who has clear impairment or loss of function, and needs gait retraining or training for putting on the brace itself. Physical and occupational therapists must rightly be considered a part of the rehabilitative team. In those instances where the brace is being prescribed for short-term rehabilitation only, the psychological impact on the patient will be less than on that patient who may require an AFO for a longer duration. In some instances, it may become desirable to have a trained psychotherapist available to assist with the process.

Cost is another factor that must be taken into consideration, as not all insurance carriers offer coverage for orthoses. Some carriers only offer coverage for extrinsic AFOs, and some only allow for prefabricated braces. Any one of these limitations may make the treatment plan difficult to carry out as planned. Since prefabricated AFOs do offer a savings when they can be successfully used, this may offer the patient some assistance with his or her medical needs.

Summary

There are many conditions which can benefit from the prescribed use of an AFO. As an adjunct to surgery, an alternative to surgery, or as a treatment of the first consideration, AFOs are an important addition to the practitioner's armamentarium. With a team approach, the practitioner can achieve the best possible results for the patient, and can contribute directly to an improvement in the lifestyle of the patient. By working in close concert with the patient, the orthotist, the physical and occupational therapist, and the pedorthist, the biomechanical needs of the patient can be successfully addressed by the practitioner. Practitioners should familiarize themselves with the entire range of AFOs available, and should be encouraged to develop a professional relationship with a competent, licensed orthotist.

References

1. Agre JC, et al: Late effects of polio: critical review of the literature on neuromuscular function, *Arch Phy Med Rehabil*, 72:923–931, 1991.
2. Birk TJ: Poliomyelitis and the post-polio syndrome: exercise capacities and adaption—current research, future directions, and widespread applicability, *Med Sci Sports Exerc* 25:466–472, 1993.
3. Bowker P, Bowler P, Condie D, Meadows CB, editors: *Ankle foot orthoses, Biomechanical basis of orthotic management*, Oxford, England, 1993, Butterworth-Heineman, pp 99–123.
4. Fishman S, et al: *Atlas of orthotics*, ed 2, St Louis, 1985; Mosby–Year Book, pp 199–210.
5. Koniuk W: Personal communication, May, 1994.
6. Kovindha A, Dean E: Clinical decision making in the management of the late sequelae of poliomyelitis, *Phys Ther* 71:752–761, 1991.
7. Lehmann J: *Lower limb orthotics*. In Redford J (editor) *Orthotics etcetera*, Baltimore, 1986, Williams & Wilkins, pp 278–300.
8. Meyer P: Lower limb orthotics, *Clin Orthop* 58–71, 1974.
9. Redford J, et al (editors): *Orthotics etcetera*, Baltimore, 1986, Williams & Wilkins, pp 1–20.
10. Rubin G, et al: The shoe as a component of the orthosis, *Orthot Prosthet* 30:13–25, 1976.
11. Trojan DA, et al: Electrophysiology and electrodiagnosis of the post-polio motor unit, *Orthopedics* 14:1353–1361, 1991.

serial plaster immobilization of congenital foot deformities

Richard Berenter, DPM
Daniel Kosai, DPM

Metatarsus adductus
    Serial plaster immobilization of metatarsus
      adductus
Tibial torsion vs. tibial position
    Serial plaster immobilization for tibial position
Talipes calcaneovalgus
    Serial plaster immobilization for talipes
      calcaneovalgus
Talipes equinoadductovarus
    Serial plaster immobilization procedure for
      talipes equinoadductovarus
Talipes equinus
    Serial plaster immobilization procedure for
      talipes equinus
Summary

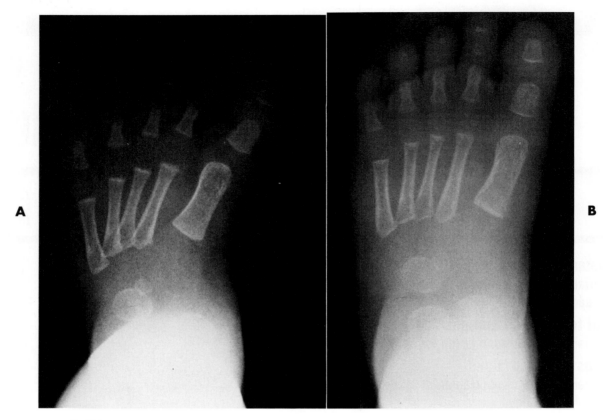

Fig. 19-1. Serial radiographs are useful to indicate if proper reduction of the deformity has occurred during serial cast immobilization. **A,** In this 1-year-old child, note a mildly increased metatarsus adductus angle, and an increase in the overlap of the metatarsal bases as well as the adducted appearance of the metatarsals from lateral to medial. **B,** After successfully applying four casts at weekly intervals, all of the above have been reduced without any sign of midtarsal joint disruption.

Podiatrists see and treat a variety of congenital abnormalities affecting foot position and function. Treatment options include both conservative and surgical care. Although different approaches to conservative care are available, optimal results are best achieved if treatment is initiated at an early age when the joint structures of the lower extremity usually exhibit a significant amount of mobility. As the child ages, the joint structures and surrounding soft tissues become more fixed. Therefore, efforts to change joint position in the older child not only take longer to accomplish but also increase the risk of joint dysfunction. External forces applied to the joints of the lower extremity via corrective casts may allow the limbs to redirect growth in a straighter configuration, thus preventing future deformities. Manipulation should always precede cast application in order to loosen any soft tissue contractures, thus maximizing the effectiveness of cast correction. Five to 10 minutes of carefully applied force directed at the abnormal segment is usually adequate to prepare the limb.[11] Once the casting is completed, a

proper course of maintainence therapy should be undertaken to prevent recurrence of the deformity.[12,13,44] Maintainence therapy includes the use of special shoes, a variety of splints, braces and bars, padding, and buttressing and generally lasts approximately twice as long as the casting time. Serial radiographs may be obtained during the course of treatment to ensure that proper correction is taking place at the appropriate joint level[29,53] (Fig. 19-1**A** and **B**). The purpose of this chapter is to provide the practitioner with a guide on how to apply a corrective cast for varying deformities, modifications of the process, and how to avoid potential problems.

Metatarsus adductus

Metatarsus adductus is a congenital deformity that causes in-toeing of the foot. *Metatarsus adductus* may be defined as a transverse plane abnormality in which the metatarsals are adducted relative to the lesser tarsus at Lisfranc's joint.[10,44,50] The literature

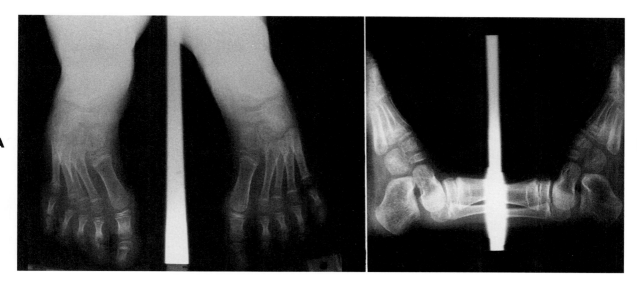

Fig. 19-2. **A** and **B**, These radiographs demonstrate an uncompensated metatarsus adductus deformity which developed as a result of chemical toxicity in a child treated for leukemia. Note an absence of pronatory changes such as the navicular articulating with a high percentage of the talar head on the dorsoplantar projection, the small talocalcaneal angles on both views, and the relatively high calcaneal inclination angle without faulting on the lateral film.

refers to this deformity by many different names including pes adductus, pes or metatarsus varus, pes or metatarsus adductovarus, metatarsus supinatus, hooked forefoot, C-shaped foot, pes internus, and others.[3–5,23,28,34,35] The compensated metatarsus adductus foot has also been given many names, including skewfoot, Z foot, and serpentine foot.[5,17,28,29,30,36] The incidence of this deformity has been reported to be approximately 1 per 1,000 births, but this may reflect only the severe cases, thus underreporting the true incidence.[9,53,54] The relative risk increases to 5% when one sibling has demonstrated the deformity.[54] It may be either unilateral or bilateral, but appears more often on the left side when only one foot is affected.[4,49] The etiologic theories proposed for metatarsus adductus include foot molding resulting from intrauterine pressure; genetic and hereditary factors; a shortened medial column (i.e., hypoplastic medial cuneiform); overpowering or contracted muscles, including the abductor hallucis, the tibial head of the flexor hallucis brevis, and the posterior or anterior tibial muscle; maternal hormonal influences; associated medical conditions; and environmental factors.*

Metatarsus adductus may appear as an isolated problem or in association with other deformities, neuromuscular disorders, or connective tissue syndromes. Therefore, the infant who exhibits metatarsus adductus should be inspected for other abnor-

malities such as talipes calcaneovalgus, vertical talus, clubfoot, dislocation of the hips, other torsional abnormalities of the leg and hip, arthrogryposis multiplex congenita, spina bifida, myelomeningocoele, and Friedreich's ataxia, as well as connective tissue disorders that may be associated with growth disturbances.[20,42,54] Clinically, a metatarsus adductus foot has a concave medial border, convex lateral border with a prominent styloid process, a wide first interspace, and an inability of the forefoot to abduct past the midline of the leg when the foot is stroked laterally.[50] Radiographs may be included in the clinical workup to assess the deformity, and to serve as a baseline for determining the effectiveness of treatment. Radiographic evaluation demonstrates the following typical changes: on the anteroposterior (AP) view an increase is seen in both the metatarsus adductus angle and the amount of overlap of the metatarsal bases, and a decrease in the amount of metatarsal adduction from medial to lateral.[50] In the absence of pronatory changes, the talocalcaneal angle is small. The lateral view also demonstrates an increase in overlap of the metatarsal bases. In addition, the calcaneal inclination angle is large and the talocalcaneal angle small in feet without severe pronatory changes (Fig. 19-2**A** and **B**). However, metatarsus adductus feet often do develop abnormal pronatory changes within the rearfoot and midfoot complex.[36,39] These changes may be explained as a consequence of improper treatment or shoe gear, the effect caused by ambulation, or weak ligaments or muscle imbalance as in

---

* References 9, 12, 17, 23, 26, 28, 35, 39, 40, 42, 50, 51, 53, 54.

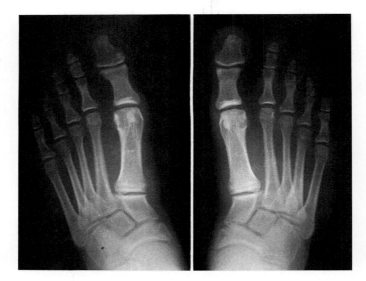

Fig. 19-3. This radiograph demonstrates a skewfoot in an adult patient with spondyloepiphyseal dysplasia tarda, X-linked recessive form. Unusual findings include a small bone size for the patient's stated age and a squaring-off of the ends of the tubular bones of the foot.

connective tissue syndromes. The net effect of abnormal pronation at the level of the midtarsal joint is the development of a skewfoot (also referred to as a serpentine or Z foot), which may be demonstrated radiographically by the following: an increase in the talocalcaneal angle on both the AP and lateral views, a decrease in the calcaneal inclination angle on the lateral view, an increase in the talar declination angle on the lateral view, the bisection of the talus falling plantar to the bisection of the first metatarsal on the lateral view, the presence of a medial column fault between the talonavicular, naviculocuneiform, or cuneiform–first metatarsal as demonstrated by angulation of the trabecular bone patterns on the lateral view, an abducted position of the cuboid on the calcaneus on the AP view, and an increase in the lesser tarsus abductus angle on the AP view with the navicular laterally displaced on the talar head. In addition to structural alterations that result from midtarsal joint compensation, a myriad of radiographic changes may be seen in patients with other associated abnormalities (Fig. 19-3). Consequently, a thorough neuromuscular examination should be performed along with an arthrometric evaluation to assist in ruling out associated conditions. Treatment for metatarsus adductus varies from nonintervention to a host of options including manipulation, casting, braces and night splints, and special shoes. If left untreated, children's feet often develop compensatory changes within the midtarsal joint and subsequent symptoms later in life.[4] A variety of theories have been proposed to help explain the involvement of the midtarsal joint. Children who toe in are

reminded to walk straight. Thus, the child consciously tries to turn the feet out by utilizing the peroneal muscle group, specifically the peroneus brevis, which is a strong pronator of the midtarsal joint. Secondly, the ligaments and tendons that surround and stabilize the midtarsal joint may be weak as a result of a connective tissue disorder. Another clue may be the ultimate effect that wearing shoes has on foot structure and function. When a metatarsus adductus foot is forced into a shoe which has less curvature built into the shoe's last, the midfoot experiences torque as a result of the laterally directed force on the medial aspect of the first metatarsal head and the stabilizing force on the lateral region of the heel. The amount of torque generated on the midfoot is proportional to the force and distance of the lever arm. Since the force originates through the first metatarsal head, the midfoot joint farthest away from the forefoot will have the longest lever arm, and thus experience the greatest amount of torque (Fig. 19-4**A** and **B**). This explains why abnormal midtarsal joint pronation or subluxation may ensue secondary to an untreated or improperly treated metatarsus adductus. The feet may give the appearance of being self-corrected or straight to the untrained eye, and it is because of this illusion that investigators in the past have erred in their assessment that the deformity had reduced spontaneously. When the cuboid is stabilized during treatment, the torque produced is directed at Lisfranc's joint, maintaining an intact and properly functioning midtarsal joint. Unfortunately, published follow-up investigations of nontreated feet have been inadequate in not addressing the effects

A

Pressure spots

B

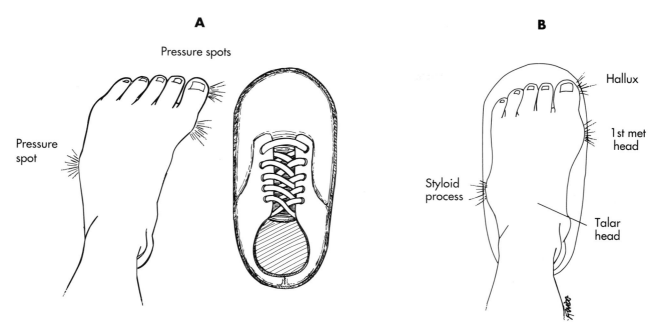

Pressure spot

Hallux

1st met head

Styloid process

Talar head

Fig. 19-4. A and **B**, A metatarsus adductus foot placed into a shoe constructed from a last with less curvature than the foot. Torque is generated through the foot as a result of the force couple produced from the pressure against the medial aspect of the shoe against the first metatarsal head, and the lateral aspect of the shoe against the lateral aspect of the heel or styloid process.

the deformity has later in life. Evaluation of adults with compensated metatarsus adductus demonstrates that a large proportion of patients present with symptoms attributable to midtarsal joint compensation such as plantar fasciitis, bunion deformities, hammer toes, neuromas, tendinitis, sinus tarsi syndrome, and osteoarthritis.[9,30,36,44,50] For this reason early intervention is recommended when the growth rate of the child allows reshaping of the foot at the level of Lisfranc's joint, thus preventing midtarsal joint compensation. Successful reduction of the deformity may be possible with proper use of corrective casts.[9,13,17,36,47,50] Routinely, the foot is then maintained in a corrected position through the use of straight-last shoes with a triplane heel wedge and buttressing added inside to prevent recurrence.

Serial plaster immobilization for metatarsus adductus

When the decision is made to apply a cast, the parents should be well informed regarding the procedure in order to alleviate any fears or unrealistic expectations they may have. Ideally, the appointment should be scheduled after the child has taken a nap and the parents should be reminded to bring a bottle of formula and a pacifier with them. Supplies necessary for casting should be sequestered and ready to use prior to starting the procedure, and may include (but are not limited to) a container of water, draping materials, tincture of benzoin compound (TBC), stockinet, Webril (Ken-

dall Company, Mansfield, MA) paper tape, and 3- to 4-in. rolls of extra-fast-setting plaster of Paris. To begin the process the infant's foot is manipulated or "warmed up" for approximately 10 minutes to loosen any soft tissue contractures. This step is vital in order to achieve the maximum correction possible during the casting process. In the technique of manipulation the involved foot is held such that the external force applied does not sublux or dislocate the midtarsal joint. The person manipulating the foot should stabilize the midtarsal joint by placing the thenar eminence of one hand onto the lateral aspect of the cuboid.[9,37,50] When manipulating the left foot the right hand should be used as the stabilizing force, and vice versa when performing the procedure on the right foot. The stabilizing hand is "cupped" about the back of the foot and the arm is gently supinated to rotate the heel into a slight varus attitude.[9,37,50] This maneuver places the cuboid more plantar and in closer proximity to the navicular, thus positioning the midtarsal joint in a more compact and stable configuration.

The opposite hand is used to apply a corrective force within the transverse plane. This is achieved by pinching the heads of the metatarsals between the thumb and index finger. The first web space of the hand should abut the medial aspect of the first metatarsal head, and the interphalangeal joints of the thumb and index finger should be hyperextended to ensure even pressure across the forefoot

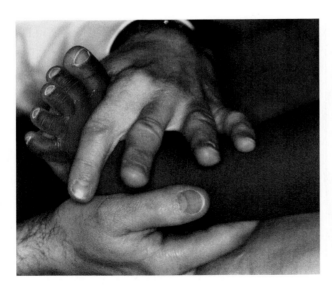

Fig. 19-5. Demonstration of the correct hand position for manipulating a metatarsus adductus foot prior to serial cast immobilization.

(Fig. 19-5). When applying the force, care is taken to direct the pressure parallel with the plantar aspect of the heel to maintain a perpendicular forefoot-to-rearfoot relationship. When external pressure is applied to the foot in this fashion the amount of torque generated is greater on the midtarsal joint than on Lisfranc's joint since there is a longer lever arm acting on the midtarsal joint. The navicular and cuboid will attempt to move laterally, but the stabilizing hand should be firmly in place to prevent any possibility of lateral or dorsal subluxation or dislocation of the midtarsal joint.[5,9] When performing the manipulation the ankle joint is maintained at a 90-degree angle. Accommodative contracture of the Achilles tendon may ensue if the ankle joint is plantarflexed when applying the cast, thus leading to potential symptoms as a result of the equinus produced. Therefore, it is important to be consistent and create sound habits when performing manipulation, since this technique is reproduced in an identical fashion when applying the cast. Manipulation should be performed for approximately 5 to 10 minutes to loosen any soft tissue contractures.[50] The importance of this step in the overall process cannot be overstated. Inadequate manipulation does not allow the soft tissues to stretch out, and the amount of change in the joint position that the cast captures will be minimal at best. Additionally, failure to stabilize the midtarsal joint can lead to the development of a rocker-bottom flatfoot and significant symptoms in the future.

At this point, TBC (tincture of Benzoin compound) may be applied to the foot and leg (Fig. 19-6). The advantage of using TBC is that it leaves a sticky residue which enables the cast padding to adhere to the underlying skin, thus preventing foot movement and possible irritation under a completed cast. It is essential to allow the TBC to dry thoroughly prior to initiating the next step. Small stockinet pieces may be used to enclose the proximal and distal ends of the cast, preventing frayed plaster edges from causing skin irritation (Fig. 19-7). Paper tape may be used to help attach the stockinet to the skin. Care should be taken to avoid having the distal piece of stockinet extend too far proximal. The possibility of the foot sliding under the stockinet should be taken into consideration, because it is particularly important to ensure that the region of Lisfranc's joint is secure under the cast in order that cast correction is maintained. Cotton Webril cast padding is then applied from distal to proximal (Fig. 19-8, p. 412). Likewise, it is imperative that a minimal amount of padding be applied over the midfoot to secure the foot in the corrected position beneath the cast. Areas of possible irritation, such as the posterior aspect of the heel, the malleoli, and the proximal edge of the cast, should be well protected with cast padding. Care should also be taken to avoid any wrinkling of the padding material, which could cause pressure points below the cast. One variation sometimes employed is to use lamb's wool over the skin creases at the anterior aspect of the ankle (Fig. 19-9, p. 412). This is helpful in preventing skin breakdown as a result of cast irritation.

After the padding is in place the cast is ready to be applied. The size of the child's foot dictates the width of the plaster rolls chosen. Typically, two 3-in.-wide rolls serve the purpose. To initiate the application process, the plaster roll is submerged in a basin of tepid water. If extra-fast-setting plaster is used, then the plaster should be left saturated after removal from the basin to allow adequate time to position the joints and properly manipulate the foot. The plaster is wrapped around the foot starting at the most distal aspect at the end of the toes. After two turns the stockinet hanging over the ends of the toes is folded back proximally and then covered with a few more layers of plaster (Fig. 19-10, p. 413). The plaster is then continued proximally up the foot to just above the ankle joint. A minimum of six layers along the entire course of the foot is mandatory to provide adequate strength to the cast. When proceeding up to the ankle joint it is essential to note that there are enough layers of plaster at the plantar and posterior heel region. When approaching the end of the roll, the last few inches of plaster may be folded onto itself and placed on the outside or lateral aspect of the ankle joint. The tag produced serves as a reference marker or starting point when the parents soak the cast off. This may be further

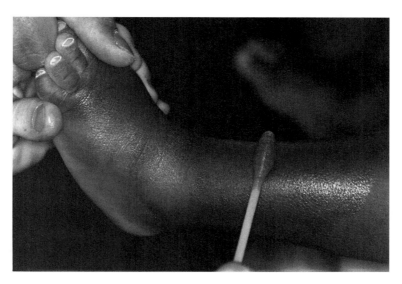

Fig. 19-6. Tincture of benzoin compound is applied to the infant's extremity to add a protective coating to the skin and minimize motion within the cast.

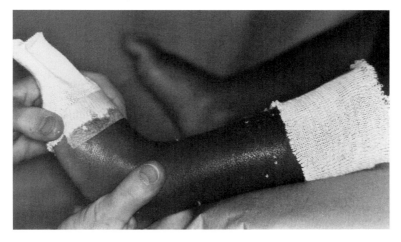

Fig. 19-7. Stockinet is applied under the most distal and most proximal aspects of the cast to reduce the likelihood of skin irritation.

identified by drawing an X over the tag area. After the first roll is applied, the foot should be stabilized and manipulated (as previously described) until the plaster hardens.

The first part of the casting procedure involves producing a slipper cast. Once the first roll has set, a second roll of plaster is applied starting at the point where the first roll ended proximally. The second roll is added to extend the cast up the leg (Fig. 19-11, p. 413). Once again, a minimum of six layers is necessary throughout the length of the cast to provide adequate strength. Similar to the distal end of the cast, the stockinet should be folded back over and sandwiched between a few layers of plaster to create a smooth proximal end to protect the skin. As with the first plaster roll, the last portion of the second roll may be folded and placed against the

lateral aspect of the cast to serve as a starting point when soaking the cast off (Fig. 19-12, p. 414).

Modifications of the casting process may include, but are not limited to, the following. One may decide not to incorporate a plaster tag at the end of the plaster roll if the cast is to be sawed off. The practitioner may decide to continue the cast up the thigh, creating a long-leg cast as a means of minimizing the effects of the posterior muscle groups, or realigning the knee joint position. Fiberglass casting material may be used to reinforce the cast, especially if the child is large or active, or if there is a possibility that the cast may get wet and weakened before the follow-up appointment. The amount and types of cast padding vary from none to copious amounts of various sorts. Absence of padding may leave the extremity susceptible to skin

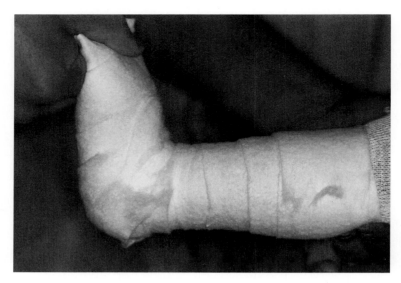

Fig. 19-8. Cotton Webril cast padding is applied to protect bony prominences. Care must be taken not to apply excessive amounts; this may lead to pistoning of the extremity within the cast and loss of correction.

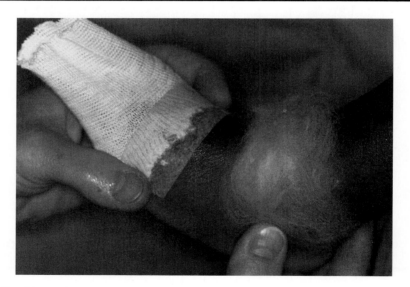

Fig. 19-9. Lamb's wool may be added to the anterior aspect of the ankle to further prevent skin irritation.

irritation. Too much material applied between the cast and skin may allow movement of the extremity below the cast, reducing the possibility of success.

Applying the first roll from the end of the toes and continuing up the leg is another modification employed. A second roll is then applied in a similar fashion to reinforce the cast. When the cast is constructed in this fashion the practitioner should be cognizant of the number of laminations and corresponding strength of the cast to avoid loss of correction secondary to foot movement below the plaster of Paris. One way to ensure that the cast is sufficiently thick and strong enough to maintain

correction is by using 4-in. rather than 3-in. rolls of plaster.

On average, most children receiving casts for metatarsus adductus require a total of four to eight casts. Cast changes are performed routinely on a weekly basis, but may be done more often or less often depending on the child's age, and the flexibility of the foot.[4,29] Parents should be instructed to soak the cast off a few hours prior to the next appointment, unless the practitioner anticipates using a cast cutter. It is important that parents be encouraged to remove the cast just prior to the next appointment to avoid any recurrence of soft tissue

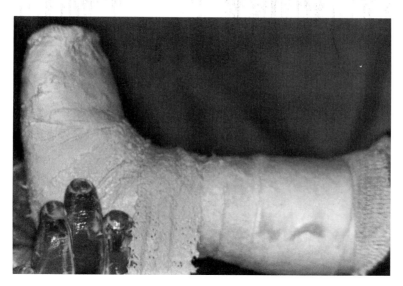

Fig. 19-10. The plaster is applied to the foot, producing a slipper cast that is then molded into the corrected position.

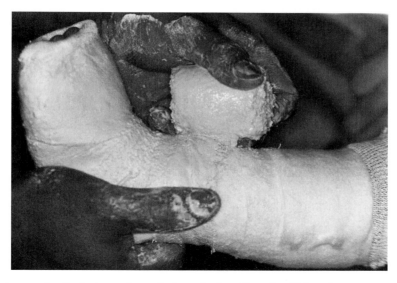

Fig. 19-11. A second roll of plaster is applied up the leg. Care should be taken to strengthen the junction of the two sections of the cast at the ankle joint.

contractures. Soaking the cast in a basin of warm water with vinegar may help loosen the plaster bonds, thus facilitating cast removal. Typically, the time necessary to remove a short-leg cast is approximately 30 minutes.

Tibial torsion versus tibial position

The ankle mortise is comprised of the medial and lateral malleoli, which are the distal extensions of the tibia and fibula, respectively. The talus is situated within the ankle mortise and functions primarily in the sagittal plane. The direction that the ankle mortise takes within the transverse plane

during ambulation is determined by the combination of both positional and torsional components of the lower leg.[41] Thus, the ability of the talus to dorsiflex and plantarflex toward the line of progression during gait is dependent on the resultant position of the ankle mortise within the transverse plane. Lack of talar function causes the foot to be lifted off the ground at the end of contact phase (an apropulsive gait) leading to the possible development of a soft tissue equinus deformity. In addition, the altered mechanics brought about by the abnormal gait pattern may lead to foot and knee disorders.[55] Although some external or lateral tibial torsion is expected until the growth plates are

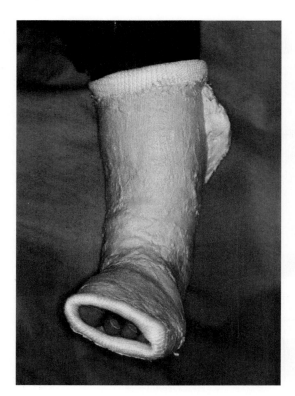

Fig. 19-12. The finished cast. Note the plaster tag at the lateral aspect of the cast. This tag serves to help identify the end of the roll to facilitate cast removal.

closed, benign neglect should be avoided since often children do not outgrow transverse plane abnormalities, but rather compensate at other segments of the axial skeleton, which may lead to joint dysfunction.

Transverse plane abnormalities of the leg may be divided into bony (torsional) vs. soft tissue (positional) causes.[41] Torsion is the amount of twisting that occurs in the longitudinal axis of the tibia and it affects the spatial relationship between the medial and lateral malleolus relative to the femoral condyles (malleolar position).[4,19,27,47,48] Another mechanism that may be responsible for altering malleolar position is the amount of gliding that occurs between the tibia and fibula during development.[1,41] It should be emphasized that the casting techniques typically employed for transverse plane leg deformities are done over a course of a few weeks and have little or no effect on the torsional component of the tibia. In addition, caution should be taken to avoid altering the spatial relationship between the tibia and fibula by generating a torque force at the level of the malleoli, since disruption of the syndesmosis and ankle joint subluxation may ensue.

Tibial position is another cause of transverse plane abnormalities of the leg. *Tibial position* may be defined as the transverse plane orientation of the proximal tibial joint surface relative to the femoral condyles (Fig. 19-13). As children grow and develop, the axial orientation of the leg on the thigh is dependent on the rotatory influences imposed by the capsule, muscles, and ligaments that cross the knee joint axis. On clinical presentation, the child will have no measurable abnormality of hip position, femoral torsion, malleolar position, or foot shape. In addition, the knees may be seen functioning in the sagittal plane. However, when the child walks, in the latter stages of swing phase the nonweightbearing foot will rapidly rotate medially or remain laterally rotated in the transverse plane producing an adducted or abducted foot position at heel-strike. The dynamic nature of this positional or soft tissue etiology is the result of imbalance between muscles crossing the knee joint, and helps distinguish tibial or joint position vs. torsion etiologies. In-toeing may be due to overpowering of the medial or internal rotators such as the medial hamstrings, medial head of the gastrocnemius, the popliteus, gracilis, or possibly the plantaris. The biceps femoris, tensor fascia lata, or lateral head of the gastrocnemius may be responsible for an out-toeing gait pattern. The primary goal in serial cast treatment of children with abnormal tibial position is to rotate the tibia on the femur in an attempt to place the ankle mortise toward the line of progression. One of the clinical examinations employed to evaluate tibial position is known as the tibial-fibular axial rotation test.[4,48] This examination enables the practitioner to establish a baseline reference of knee position as well as serving to document progression of the treatment regimen. With the child prone on the examination table, the knees are flexed to 90 degrees and the foot is placed in subtalar neutral position. The loading force placed on the foot is minimal since the foot is dorsiflexing with gravity, and as a result the foot is usually still in a plantigrade attitude with respect to the leg bisection. The first measurement performed serves as a reference and is known as the thigh-foot angle.[4,47] The angle between the thigh and foot is then measured after maximally rotating the leg medially or internally. Lastly, the leg is laterally or externally rotated to the end of its available range of motion and the thigh-foot relationship is determined.[13,19] Caution should be taken throughout this examination to ensure that the subtalar joint is maintained in its neutral position. An excessive amount of rotation in one direction over the other is indicative of a tibial position problem. Other tests that may be performed include placing the child supine and evaluating the amount of leg rotation at the knee joint. Clinical examination of a newborn's knee joint

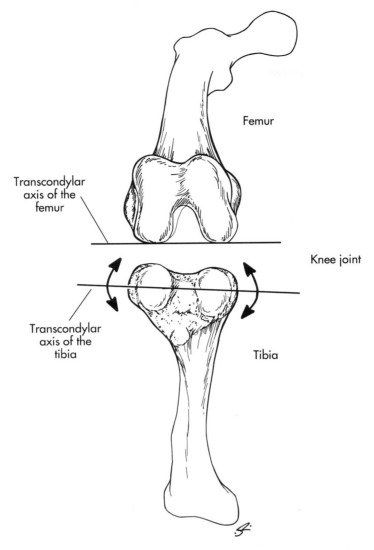

Fig. 19-13. Relationship between the femoral condyles and the proximal tibial plateau.

reveals approximately equal amounts of internal or medial vs. external or lateral motion. The average amount of transverse plane leg motion in infants is approximately 10 to 15 degrees while the knee is in the fully extended position. By the age of 4 years the fully extended knee will typically retain less than 5 degrees of leg motion within the transverse plane. A higher percentage of motion in one direction over the other is another indication of an abnormal tibial position.

Serial plaster immobilization procedure for tibial position

Serial plaster immobilization for tibial position begins similarly to the procedure described for metatarsus adductus. Manipulation should once again be performed for at least 5 to 10 minutes prior to the casting process in an attempt to loosen soft tissue structures. In order to accomplish proper manipulation, the clinician uses one hand to stabilize the distal aspect of the thigh, while the other hand rotates the leg in the appropriate direction with the knee joint maintained in a 30-degree flexed position. Although the materials used are the same as previously mentioned, the padding should continue past the knee joint and up the thigh. Once again, a rim of stockinet may be used on the proximal and distal ends of the cast to avoid skin irritation from the rough edges of the finished cast.

The first step involved with the plaster is the formation of a short-leg cast. If a foot deformity coexists with the genicular abnormality, then it should be addressed. Attention is then directed proximally to form a thigh cast, leaving the knee joint uncovered (Fig. 19-14). Next, the knee joint is flexed approximately 30 degrees and the leg is rotated into a corrected position. With the limb

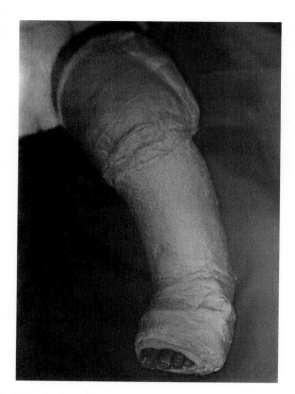

Fig. 19-14. A short-leg and thigh cast are applied separately, leaving the knee joint exposed.

maintained in this position, the proximal and distal ends of the cast are joined together with another roll of plaster[37] (Fig. 19-15). Similar guidelines described for the metatarsus adductus casting technique should be adhered to such as time intervals between cast changes, and the use of tags after applying each roll of plaster. This last guideline will make identifying the end of the plaster roll much easier for the parents when attempting to remove the cast. Once again, the parents should be encouraged to remove the cast the morning of the follow-up appointment rather than the night before to prevent loss of correction. Successful resolution of the condition is generally attained with two or three casts. The correction should be maintained with night splints for at least twice as long as the casting sequence.

Talipes calcaneovalgus

Talipes calcaneovalgus has been described as the most common congenital abnormality of the feet, occurring in approximately 1 in 1,000 live births.[54] It is often referred to as a congenital flexible flatfoot, congenital plantarflexed talus, or as the "up and out" deformity because of the foot being everted, abducted, and dorsiflexed against the leg[7,12,13] (Fig. 19-16). One must be careful to distinguish talipes calcaneovalgus from vertical talus

since they both demonstrate a similar appearance at birth.[16] However, vertical talus may be distinguished by the lack of motion at the subtalar and ankle joints within 6 months after birth, a negative calcaneal inclination angle, complete dislocation of the talonavicular joint, and a higher incidence of associated neuromuscular conditions. The anatomic deviation described in the literature for calcaneovalgus is the formation of a valgus inclination to the sustentaculum tali or middle facet with respect to the superior surface of the calcaneal body.[12]

A cause of intrauterine molding has been proposed since a higher incidence of children with calcaneovalgus are first-born from young mothers.[54] In addition, these children may be noted to have an increase in ligamentous laxity.[54] Talipes calcaneovalgus may occur unilaterally or bilaterally and is often seen in the presence of other congenital deformities of the feet and lower extremity. Examples reported in the literature include tibial bowing, congenitally dislocated peroneal tendons, and a 4% to 5% associated incidence of dislocated hip.[34,38,54] Although manipulation by itself has been advocated as a treatment option, treatment via serial plaster immobilization provides around-the-clock correction and thus a faster, more predictable outcome.[24] This avoids the potential pitfalls of inappropriate foot manipulation or compliance on the parents' part. The goal of treatment is to bring the foot plantigrade, and move the heel away from the valgus position.

Serial plaster immobilization procedure for talipes calcaneovalgus

The application of a short-leg cast to correct talipes calcaneovalgus is similar to the casting protocol for a metatarsus adductus with the exception of the manipulation technique employed prior to and during the casting process. The technique for manipulating a right-sided calcaneovalgus will be described. First, the practitioner cups the infant's heel in the palm of his or her right hand and applies an inversion-plantarflexion force. The thumb of the left hand is placed below the infant's right foot at the level of the plantar-distal aspect of the calcaneus. As the practitioner's right hand pulls down on the proximal posterior portion of the heel, the left thumb simultaneously applies a superiorly directed force in an attempt to rotate the rearfoot (talus and calcaneus) out of equinus.[14] The practitioner then places the lesser fingers of the left hand on the child's midfoot just anterior and distal to the ankle region and applies a plantigrade inversion force[14] (Fig. 19-17, p. 418). Care must be taken to apply the force at the level of the midtarsal joint. A force applied too distal at Lisfranc's joint may cause disrup-

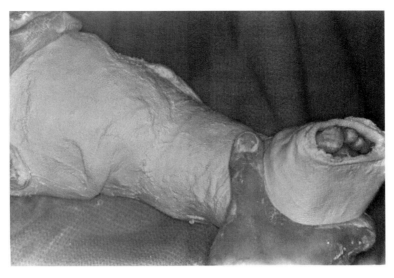

Fig. 19-15. The knee joint is flexed approximately 30 degrees, and the leg is rotated into a corrected position. The ends of the casts are then joined together with a roll of plaster.

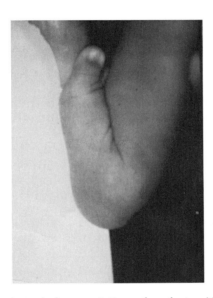

Fig. 19-16. A typical presentation of a foot with talipes calcaneovalgus.

tion or subluxation of the infant's forefoot. The protocol then repeats the same pattern previously described for preparing the first roll of plaster application. Following placement of TBC, Webril, and small pieces of stockinet, a 2- to 4-in. roll of plaster is applied from the end of the toes to above the ankle. The practitioner then positions the child's foot in the precise attitude described for manipulation, and maintains this "position of correction" until the first roll of plaster hardens (Fig. 19-18**A** and **B**). Once the foot has been brought plantigrade and in line with the leg, one or two additional casts are applied to

loosen the dorsolateral soft tissue structures and prevent recurrence of the deformity. Maintaining the correction is achieved via splints or shoe therapy.[12] An effective method utilized to create a splint is to bivalve the final cast and preserve the anterior half. The corrected foot is placed into the anterior splint and an elastic bandage is wrapped circumferentially about the child's foot and leg to maintain the desired position. Postcasting maintenance typically lasts approximately twice as long as the period of plaster immobilization.

Talipes equinoadductovarus

Talipes equinoadductovarus, or clubfoot, is a pedal abnormality recognized by ancient civilizations and first described in detail by Hippocrates in 300 B.C.[18] The incidence of clubfoot is approximately 1 per 1,000 births, and it occurs approximately twice as often in boys.[54] An increase in incidence has been reported in some Middle Eastern, North African, Mexican, and Polynesian populations.[52] Clubfoot presents bilaterally 50% of the time with a slight predilection for the right foot when unilateral.[49] The deformity may be classified as congenital or acquired, with the majority being of the idiopathic congenital variety.[8] Other congenital types include those secondary to spinal defects, arthrogryphosis multiplex congenita, and osteogenic and myogenic origins.[52] The majority of acquired clubfeet are neurogenic such as poliomyelitis and cerebral palsy.[25] The cause is unknown. Some theories include in utero mechanical factors, nerve lesions, heredity, arrested embryologic development, and environmental factors. Associated developmental deformities

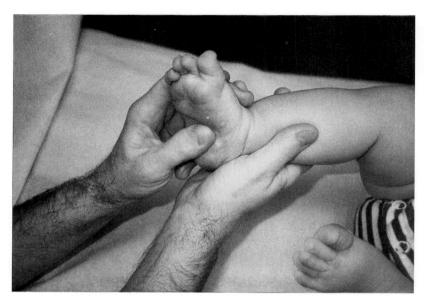

Fig. 19-17. Manipulation prior to cast correction of talipes calcaneovalgus.

include metatarsus adductus, congenital deformity of the hands, limb shortening, and a decrease in calf and foot size.[49]

Anatomically, clubfoot is classically described as being comprised of an adducted forefoot, a varus position of the heel, an ankle equinus, and an overall cavus appearance (Fig. 19-19). (This appearance resembles the embryonic foot position at the seventh to ninth week of development, lending some credence to the arrested embryologic development theory.) Several concepts regarding the evolution of the pathoanatomy of clubfoot have arisen through the years, the most popular being a primary deformity in the shape and position of the talus.[45,46] The body of the talus is inverted and internally rotated in the ankle mortise, with the head and neck deviated plantar-medially.[15] This condition leads to a medially displaced navicular and contractures of the posteromedial soft tissue structures, as well as an inverted and internally rotated calcaneus. Another model views the clubfoot as a spatial derangement of the lateral or medial column of the foot due to the inability of the talus and calcaneus to dorsiflex and rotate externally about the tibia.[6,43] The structures which prevent this rotatory motion are located between the fibula, talus, and calcaneus and consist of the calcaneofibular ligament, the posterior ankle capsule, the posterior talofibular ligament, and the peroneal retinaculum. A third theory focuses primarily on the subtalar joint.[32,33] The calcaneus is rotated internally in the transverse plane, resulting in medial displacement of the navicular and cuboid on the talus and calcaneus, respectively. The anterior aspect of the calcaneus moves beneath the head and

neck of the talus while the posterior aspect of the calcaneus moves toward the fibula. This also results in the previously mentioned soft tissue contractures. The final theory relates to the relative longitudinal development of the tibia and fibula.[45,46] Among the various medial structures that fail to develop properly is the posterior tibial, with its expansive insertion playing the largest role. The navicular subluxates medially off the head of the talus modifying the anterior talar axis, resulting in a medial deviation. The posterior tibial also contributes to the calcaneal equinus deformity.

Serial plaster immobilization procedure for talipes equinoadductovarus

A stepwise joint-by-joint correction of the clubfoot deformity is the most logical and leads to fewer complications (rocker-bottom foot or flattop talus).[1,9,47] As with any other congenital deformity manipulation prior to casting is essential to reduce the effects of soft tissue contracture. Attention is first directed to the midtarsal complex.[2] The technique will be described for casting a left-sided clubfoot. First, the practitioner places the left hand over the dorsal aspect of the infant's left midfoot corresponding to the navicular, and applies a downward force in the direction of plantarflexion and eversion in order to pronate the medial column of the infant's foot. Next, the infant's heel is grasped between the practitioner's right index finger and thumb, and everted and externally rotated (Fig. 19-20**A** and **B**, p. 421). In addition, the practitioner's right hand should attempt to pull the proximal posterior portion of the calcaneus plantigrade in an attempt to

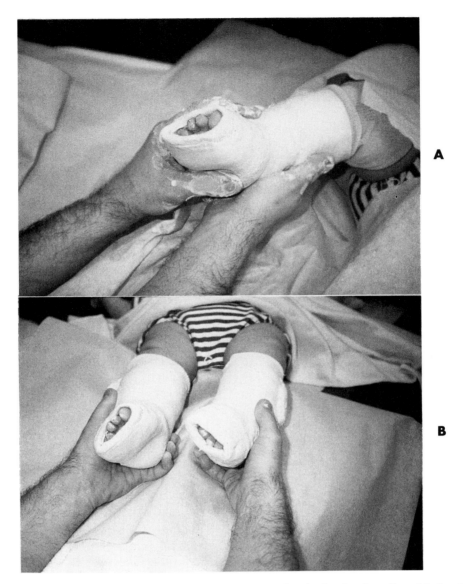

Fig. 19-18. A, Hand position during plaster application. Note that the forefoot is realigned in front of the rearfoot in a plantarflexed inverted position. **B,** Bilateral talipes calcaneovalgus deformity with completed short-leg casts.

reduce the equinus component. As a precaution, it is extremely important that the midtarsal complex be sufficiently relaxed and properly aligned prior to addressing the equinus in order to prevent the development of a rocker-bottom deformity. On completion of the below-knee portion of the cast, the application of plaster is continued above the leg to form a long-leg cast with the knee maintained in a flexed position of approximately 30 degrees (Fig. 19-21, p. 421). The purpose of continuing the cast above the knee is to reduce the effect of the gastrocnemius muscle as well as to address any associated genicular abnormality that may be present (Fig. 19-22, p. 422). An alternative method of plaster application is to first apply a slipper cast with the foot in an equinus attitude.[21,22] Once the midtarsal complex has been relaxed, the varus and adductus components addressed, and this portion of the cast has dried, the foot is placed in a dorsiflexed position as the remainder of the cast is applied. The primary concern with this method is possible soft tissue impingement at the level of the anterior ankle.

Talipes equinus

The amount of ankle joint dorsiflexion within a given lower extremity may be defined as the angle formed in the maximum dorsiflexed flexed position by the plantar plane of the foot and the longitudinal bisector of the leg. In the average newborn, this

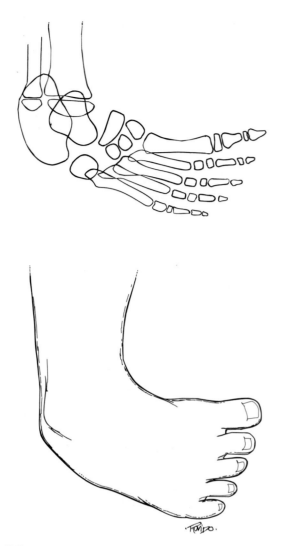

Fig. 19-19. Schematic representation of a talipes equinoadductovarus foot.

Distally, these two muscles join together and form a common tendinous insertion, the Achilles tendon, which attaches to the posterior aspect of the calcaneus. With the knee in the fully extended position, both the soleus and gastrocnemius muscles are at their resting length. As the knee is flexed, the distance between the origin and insertion of the gastrocnemius is decreased, thereby allowing an increase in ankle joint dorsiflexion when the equinus is solely due to a tight gastrocnemius.[31] However, if there is limitation in ankle joint dorsiflexion both with the knee flexed and extended, then a soleus or ankle bony equinus may mask the presence of an underlying contracted gastrocnemius. Use of stress films and interpreting the end of the range of dorsiflexion as solid or soft help distinguish between a tight soleus muscle vs. a bony ankle block (see Chapter 11).

Many congenital afflictions of the lower extremities have reduced ankle joint dorsiflexion angles as a result of spasticity or shortening of the achilles tendon complex, or secondary to bony alterations of the segments that constitute the ankle joint. These congenital conditions include abnormalities such as talipes equinoadductovarus, congenital convex pes valgus (vertical talus), connective tissue syndromes causing growth disturbances, cerebral palsy, muscular dystrophies, other syndromes of mesenchymal origin, and neuromuscular conditions.[49] In addition, there are a large number of children who are born with a congenitally shortened gastrocnemius-soleus complex in the absence of any other significant findings. When the patient's equinus component is unrecognized or left untreated, subsequent compensatory changes may ensue within the involved extremity causing significant symptoms or future disability. Compensatory changes for a talipes equinus include midfoot subluxation via midtarsal joint oblique axis pronation (development of a rocker-bottom flatfoot), knee joint hyperextension, and externally rotating the hips while decreasing stride length and rate. The backward displacement of the tibia that results in hyperextension of the knee joint is referred to as genu recurvatum and along with midtarsal joint subluxation is a mechanism to bring the heel down to the ground. Genu recurvatum may lead to internal knee derangement and osteoarthritis, and the development of a rocker-bottom flatfoot ultimately leads to a myriad of pronatory sequelae including degenerative arthritis and disability. As a result, children with equinus should have a course of treatment directed at lengthening the superficial posterior muscle group to prevent the damaging effects secondary to compensation.

angle typically approaches 70 to 75 degrees and reduces in the first few weeks of life to approximately 50 degrees.[14,31] The term talipes equinus refers to those feet which have a reduced amount of ankle joint dorsiflexion available at birth. When evaluating a patient with suspected limitation of dorsiflexion, the amount of ankle joint motion and quality of the endpoint of motion should be evaluated both with the knee in extension and in flexion. The two muscles that comprise the superficial posterior compartment are the soleus and gastrocnemius muscles.[31] The origin of the soleus arises from the lateral aspect of the leg from the fibular head, whereas the gastrocnemius has both a medial and lateral head originating at the medial and lateral epicondyles of the femur respectively.

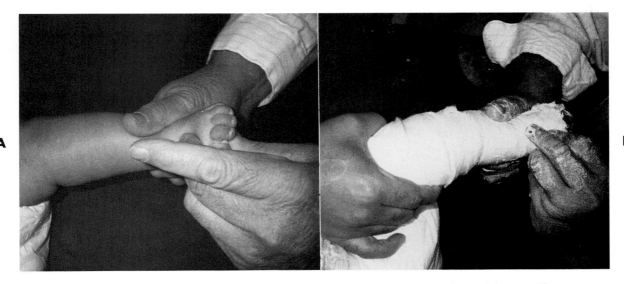

Fig. 19-20. A, Manipulation prior to plaster application in a child with a clubfoot deformity. The calcaneus is distracted, everted, and externally rotated, while the medial column is pronated at the level of the midtarsal joint. **B,** Application of the corrective forces after application of the short-leg cast.

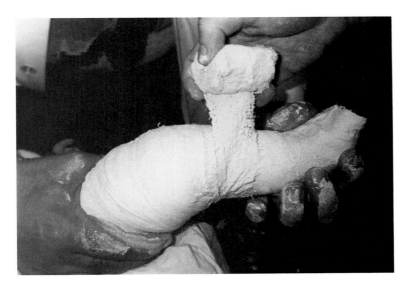

Fig. 19-21. The cast is extended above the knee, which is maintained in a flexed position of approximately 30 degrees.

Serial plaster immobilization procedure for talipes equinus

Serial plaster immobilization for talipes equinus should be restricted to children with limited ankle joint dorsiflexion secondary to soft tissue contracture of the superficial posterior muscle group. Proper evaluation of ankle joint motion should always be performed prior to casting. The practitioner should work on the assumption that there may be an underlying gastrocnemius equinus present when clinical examination demonstrates limitation of ankle joint dorsiflexion with the knee in the flexed position. As a result, a long-leg cast applied with the knee in the extended position is necessary to ensure that the gastrocnemius muscle is placed on stretch. The cast application process begins by applying a slipper cast to the foot and ankle with the foot dorsiflexed to resistance. After applying the first plaster roll, the examiner inverts the child's heel to place the cuboid below the

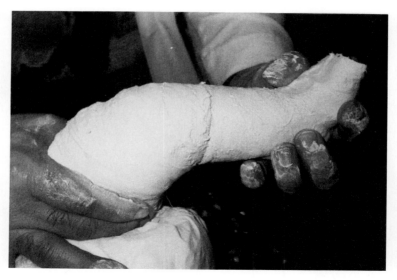

Fig. 19-22. Correction of talipes equinoadductovarus with the use of a long-leg cast.

navicular. In this position the midfoot is stabilized in a compact orientation. Consequently, when a dorsiflexory force is applied to the plantar plane of the foot, the cuboid is restricted by the navicular superiorly, and is therefore unable to dorsally subluxate at the oblique midtarsal joint (calcaneocuboid joint). The next step is to continue the cast up the leg and apply a thigh cast in a fashion similar to that described in the section on serial plaster immobilization for the tibial position. The final roll of plaster is used to bridge the thigh and leg segments. As the plaster sets, the knee should be held gently in an extended position. Care should be taken not to hyperextend the knee joint in the final position in order to prevent joint derangement. In instances where one is attempting to increase ankle joint range of motion in the ambulatory child, a below-the-knee cast may be employed. This is appropriate in that the child will normally maintain the knee in an extended attitude during ambulation, thereby adequately stretching the posterior musculature with each step.

Summary

Some of the common congenital foot deformities requiring treatment include metatarsus adductus, tibial position, talipes calcaneovalgus, clubfoot, and talipes equinus. Although treatment options include both conservative and surgical methods, an attempt at nonsurgical intervention should be considered in the child under 2 years of age, with the best results attained in the child under 1 year of age. This precludes unnecessary surgery, and allows for the reduction of associated soft tissue adaptation. Con-

sequently, it is imperative that the practitioner understand the principles and proper techniques when utilizing conservative modalities.

References

1. Badelon OB, Bensahel H, Folinais D, et al: Tibiofibular torsion from the fetal period until birth, *J Pediatr Orthop* 9:169–173, 1989.
2. Bensahel H, Huguenin P, Themar-Noel C: The functional anatomy of clubfoot, *J Pediatr Orthop* 3:191–195, 1983.
3. Berg E: A reappraisal of metatarsus adductus and skewfoot, *J Bone Joint Surg [Am]* 68:1185–1196, 1986.
4. Bleck E: Developmental orthopaedics. III: toddlers, *Dev Med Child Neurol* 24:533–555, 1982.
5. Bleck E: Metatarsus adductus: classification and relationship to outcomes of treatment, *J of Pediatr Orthop* 3:2–9, 1983.
6. Carroll N, McMurtry R, Leete S: The pathoanatomy of congenital clubfoot, *Orthop Clin North Am* 9:225, 1978.
7. Cohen L, Cohen M: Congenital calcaneovalgus, *J Am Podiatr Assoc* 66:10, 1976.
8. Coleman S: *Complex foot deformities in children*, Philadelphia, 1983, Lea & Febiger.
9. D'Amico JC: Congenital metatarsus adductus: an overview, *Arch Podiatr Med Foot Surg* 3:1–10, 1976.
10. Engel E, Erlick N, Krems I: A simplified metatarsus adductus angle, *J Am Podiatr Assoc* 73:620–628, 1983.
11. Galluzzo AJ, Hugar DW: Congenital metatarsus adductus: clinical evaluation and treatment, *J Foot Surg* 18:16–22, 1979.
12. Ganley JV: Calcaneovalgus deformity in infants, *J Am Podiatr Assoc* 65:405–421, 1975.
13. Ganley JV, McDonough MW: Clinical discourse . . . torsional problems in children, *Arch Podiatr Med Foot Surg* 3:55–67, 1976.
14. Giannestras NJ: Recognition and treatment of flatfeet in infancy, *Clin Orthop* 70:10–29, 1970.
15. Goldner JL: Congenital talipes equinovarus—fifteen years of surgical treatment, *Curr Pract Orthop Surg* 4:11–23, 1969.
16. Greenberg AJ: Congenital vertical talus and congenital calcaneovalgus deformity: a comparison, *J Foot Surg* 20:189–193, 1981.

17. Haber J: Surgical treatment of metatarsus adductus, *Arch of Podiatr Med Foot Surg* 3:17–23, 1976.

18. Irani RN, Sherman MS: The pathological anatomy of idiopathic clubfoot, *J Bone Joint Surg [Am]* 45:45, 1963.

19. Jakob RP, Haertel M, Stussi E: Tibial torsion calculated by computerised tomography and compared to other methods of measurement, *J Bone Joint Surg [Br]* 62:238–242, 1980.

20. Kite H: Congenital metatarsus varus, report of 300 cases, *J Bone Joint Surg [Am]* 32:500–506, 1950.

21. Kite H: Some suggestions on the treatment of clubfoot by casts, *J Bone Joint Surg [Am]* 45:406, 1963.

22. Kite JH: *The clubfoot*, New York, 1964, Grune & Stratton.

23. Kite JH: Congenital metatarsus varus, *J Bone Joint Surg [Am]* 49:388–397, 1967.

24. Larsen B, Reimann I, Becker-Andersen H: Congenital calcaneovalgus, *Acta Orthop Scand* 45:145–151, 1974.

25. LeNoir JL: *Congenital idiopathic talipes*, Springfield, Ill, 1966, Charles C Thomas.

26. Lichtblau S: Section of the abductor hallucis tendon for correction of metatarsus varus deformity, *Clin Orthop* 110: 227–232, 1975.

27. Malekafzali S, Wood MB: Tibial torsion—a simple clinical apparatus for its measurement and its application to a normal adult population, *Clin Orthop* 145:154–157, 1979.

28. Marcinko DE, Iannuzzi PJ, Thurber NB: Resistant metatarsus adductus deformity (illustrated surgical reconstructive techniques), *J Foot Surg* 25:86–94, 1986.

29. McCauley J, Lusskin R, Bromley J: Recurrence in congenital metatarsus varus, *J Bone Joint Surg [Am]* 46:525–532, 1964.

30. McCormick DW, Blount WP: Metatarsus adductovarus, *JAMA* 141:449–453, 1949.

31. McCrea J: *Pediatric orthopedics of the lower extremity: an instructional handbook* Mt Kisco, NY, 1985, Futura.

32. McKay D: New concept of and approach to clubfoot treatment I. Principles and morbid anatomy, *J Pediatr Orthop* 2:347, 1982.

33. McKay D: New concept of and approach to clubfoot treatment II. Correction of the clubfoot, *J Pediatr Orthop* 3:10, 1983.

34. Pappas AM: Congenital posteromedial bowing of the tibia and fibula, *J Pediatr Orthop* 4:525–531, 1984.

35. Peabody CW, Muro F: Congenital metatarsus varus, Presented at the Annual Meeting of the American Orthopaedic Association, Toronto, June 27, 1932, pp 171–189.

36. Peterson H: Skewfoot (forefoot adduction with heel valgus), *J Pediatr Orthop* 6:24–30, 1986.

37. Ponseti IV, Becker JR: Congenital metatarsus adductus: the results of treatment, *J Bone Joint Surg [Am]* 48:702–711, 1966.

38. Purnell ML, Drummond DS, Engber WD, et al: Congenital dislocation of the peroneal tendons in the calcaneovalgus foot, *J Bone Joint Surg [Br]* 65:316–319, 1983.

39. Reimann I: Pathology of congenital metatarsus varus and its relationship to other congenital deformities of the foot, *Orthop Clin North Am* 9:219–224, 1978.

40. Reimann I, Werner H: Congenital metatarsus varus, a suggestion for a possible mechanism and relation to other foot deformities, *Clin Orthop* 110:223–226, 1975.

41. Rosen H, Sandick H: The measurement of tibiofibular torsion, *J Bone Joint Surg [Am]* 37:847–855, 1955.

42. Rushforth G: The natural history of hooked forefoot, *J Bone Joint Surg [Br]* 60:530–532, 1978.

43. Scott WA, Hoskings SW, Catterall A: Clubfoot: observations on the surgical anatomy of dorsiflexion, *J Bone Joint Surg [Br]* 66:71–76, 1984.

44. Sgarlato TE: A discussion of metatarsus adductus, *Arch Podiatr Med Foot Surg* 1:35–40, 1973.

45. Simons G: Symposium: current practices in the treatment of idiopathic clubfoot in the child between birth and five years of age I, *Contemp Orthop* 17:63, 1988.

46. Simons G: Symposium: current practices in the treatment of idiopathic clubfoot in the child between birth and five years of age II, *Contemp Orthop* 17:161, 1988.

47. Staheli LT: Torsion—treatment indications, *Clin Orthop* 247: 61–66, 1989.

48. Staheli LT, Engel GM: Tibial torsion: a method of assessment and a survey of normal children, *Clin Orthop* 86:183–186, 1972.

49. Tachdjian M: Pediatric orthopedics, Philadelphia, 1990, WB Saunders.

50. Tax HR, Albright T: Metatarsus adducto varus, a simplified approach to treatment, *J Am Podiatr Assoc* 68:331–338, 1978.

51. Thomson S: Hallux varus and metatarsus varus, a five-year study (1954–1958), *Clin Orthop* 16:109, 1960.

52. Turco VJ: Clubfoot. In *Current problems in orthopedics*, New York, 1981, Churchill Livingstone.

53. Votta JJ, Weber RB: A nonsurgical treatment regimen for metatarsus adductus utilizing orthoses, *J Am Podiatr Assoc* 7:69–72, 1981.

54. Wynne-Davies R: Family studies and the cause of congenital club foot—talipes equinovarus, talipes calcaneo-valgus and metatarsus varus, *J Bone Joint Surg [Br]* 46:445–463, 1964.

55. Yagi TY, Sasaki T: Tibial torsion in patients with medial-type osteoarthritic knee, *Clin Orthop* 213:177–182, 1986.

lower extremity treatment modalities for the pediatric patient

Ronald L. Valmassy, DPM

Introduction
Pediatric lower extremity splinting and
    bracing techniques
    Type and level of deformity
    Type of splint
    Age of the child
    Length of treatment
    Determining the extent of correction
    Modifications to impede subluxatory changes
        and maintain normal anatomical relationships
    Appropriate shoes for splints
Splinting and bracing devices
    Denis Browne splint
    Fillauer splint
    Uni-bar
    Ganley splint
    Friedman Counter splint or Flexosplint
    Brachman skate
    Langer pediatric counter rotational system splint
    Twister cables
    Wheaton brace
    Wheaton bracing system
    Tibial Torsion Transformer
    Plaster or fiberglass splint
    Circular Torqheel

Pediatric shoe therapy
    Tarso-medius shoe
    Conventional last shoe
    Inflare last shoe
    Outflare last shoe
    Bebax shoe
Pediatric orthoses
    History
    Shoe inserts
Summary

Introduction

Although children suffer from a vast array of potential problems which may affect their lower extremities, angle-of-gait disturbances as well as flatfooted conditions are present in a significant number of children requiring treatment. In order to implement appropriate therapy, the practitioner must be aware of which pediatric musculoskeletal problems may be outgrown and which problems require treatment. A complete knowledge and sound understanding of all normal developmental landmarks must be appreciated by the practitioner prior to deciding if a presenting complaint is abnormal. Coupled with this basic understanding, the practitioner must then utilize his or her clinical skills, which include appropriate history taking, gait evaluation, biomechanical evaluation, muscle testing, and radiographic examination, to arrive at a final treatment recommendation. At this point, the practitioner may then explain the findings to the child's parents, noting the severity of the condition, the likelihood of the condition resolving spontaneously, and, if not, what appropriate treatment measures may be anticipated. It is at this point that the practitioner and parents agree on what course of treatment is best suited for the child's problem. The purpose of this chapter is to present the indications for the appropriate use of pediatric splinting, bracing, and orthotic therapy for the pediatric patient. Appropriate guidelines for the use of each device are presented as well as possible complications arising from their use. Night splints, braces, shoes, commercially available shoe inserts,

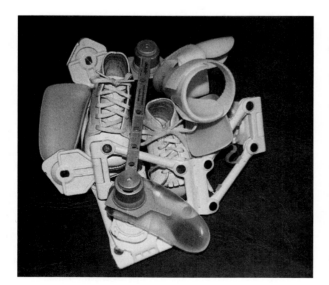

Fig. 20-1. A variety of night splints, braces, shoes, and orthoses are available for use in treating podiatric lower extremity deformities.

and functional foot orthoses are addressed (Fig. 20-1).

Pediatric lower extremity splinting and bracing techniques

A host of lower extremity splints, braces, and bars have been available for numerous years to assist in the treatment of lower extremity pediatric deformities. The various devices have been designed to be utilized following periods of serial plaster immobilization or, in many cases, in lieu of that form of therapy. Additionally, the various devices may be utilized following corrective surgery of the lower extremity to maintain or enhance the results achieved at the time of surgery. In all cases, care must be taken to not only prescribe the appropriate device for the specific musculoskeletal condition but also to understand the variables for successful implementation of the device. Prior to prescribing any specific night splint or bracing system, the practitioner should be aware of all the variables inherent to this form of therapy. The variables listed in Table 20-1 should be considered when prescribing one of the devices.

Type and level of deformity

Night splints and braces may be appropriately utilized for a host of lower extremity soft tissue and osseous malalignment problems. Although the splints are considered to be more effective in correcting deformities attributable to soft tissue contractural involvement, they may also be utilized for some osseous pathologic conditions. Prior to undertaking the use of any of these devices, the practitioner should be aware of any significant family history for a similar type of problem. This may result in a somewhat less-than-successful conclusion to the treatment regimen. Generally speaking, internal and external femoral torsions do not respond well to splinting techniques.[26,36,37] Because the majority of the devices are fixed to the feet or in some cases at the knee, it is difficult for

Table 20-1
Variables involved in prescribing splints and braces

- Type and level of deformity
- Type of splint
- Age of child
- Length of treatment
- Determining the extent of correction
- Modifications to impede subluxatory changes and maintain normal anatomic relationship
- Appropriate shoes for splints

appropriate pressure to be placed proximal enough to precipitate any measurable osseous changes. It should be noted, however, that the vast majority of children with an internal or external femoral torsion generally assume a position of comfort while sleeping. Since this represents approximately one half to two thirds of the child's early life, specific soft tissue adaptation may occur. Generally speaking, infants and children with an internal femoral torsion or internal femoral position sleep on their stomachs with their legs and feet rotated in an internal position. Conversely, those infants and children with an external femoral torsion or external femoral position generally assume a position in which their feet and legs are rotated externally. Owing to this positioning, soft tissue contracture affecting the capsular, ligamentous, and musculature structures occur, thereby reinforcing the abnormal position. Ultimately, this is significant in that all children who have either a marked internal or external femoral torsion will additionally have some degree of soft tissue contracture.

Additionally, those youngsters with a primary internal femoral position or external femoral position will also have increased soft tissue adaptation due to the same type of sleeping positions. Therefore, congenital soft tissue contracture may occur primarily in some children or may occur secondary to an osseous deformity, as described above. Arguably then, night splints may be utilized effectively in either condition to primarily alter the sleeping position and thereby secondarily stretch associated contracted soft tissue structures.[9,15] Internal or external tibial position and torsion problems may be addressed via splinting and bracing. It should be noted that the techniques may be the primary method of treatment in some cases or as an adjunctive procedure in more severe cases. In cases where serial plaster immobilization is utilized initially, splints and braces may then be utilized to maintain the correction. Because tibial position problems are attributable to soft tissue contractures about either the medial or lateral aspect of the knee, improvement may be attained via these treatment modalities. True internal tibial torsion may be affected by a variety of the splints because constant traction on the distal tibial epiphysis is capable of introducing an increased amount of external tibial torsion.[32,42,44] As external tibial torsion generally represents an overdevelopment or overtwisting of the segment, bracing techniques may be unsuccessful. However, since it is difficult to determine to what extent the torsion may ultimately develop, splints may be utilized to inhibit additional outward deflection of the segment. It is important for the practitioner to realize that although splints that are attached to shoes may appear to correct tibial torsion problems, the level of correction is often attained at the child's knee. This is due to the large range of transverse plane rotation that is present in the developing child's knee. This range of motion is easily influenced by constant internal or external rotation forces caused by a distal force, as from a night splint.

Specific foot conditions such as metatarsus adductus, talipes equinovarus, and talipes calcaneovalgus may all be addressed via specific splinting techniques.[2,5,17,20,39] However, it is essential that the practitioner determine the extent and severity of the deformity to ensure that more aggressive treatment may not be initially required. Although mild cases of any of the above may improve via regular stretching, shoe therapy, and splinting techniques, moderate-to-severe cases unquestionably require more aggressive treatment. In cases where the severity requires surgical intervention or treatment with serial plaster immobilization techniques, splinting and bracing become a secondary line of treatment. In those cases, the splints and braces are utilized to maintain the corrections achieved by the more aggressive treatments as opposed to being solely responsible for the complete resolution of the deformity.

Type of splint

Over the years, a host of splints and braces have been developed to assist in the development of a normal lower extremity. When selecting a splint, a series of variables must be considered. Certain devices are designed to address specific foot and leg deformities. Later in this chapter, each of the devices is explained in greater detail. At this point, one must determine if the device is to correct one deformity or a combination of deformities. It should be noted that it is common for multiple deformities to be present. For example, a metatarsus adductus foot type may be exacerbated by the presence of an internal femoral torsion or position or possibly an internal tibial torsion or position. Conversely, a talipes calcaneovalgus foot type may be exacerbated by the presence of an external femoral torsion or external femoral position or possibly an external tibial torsion or position. For completeness' sake, one must also be aware of the "windswept" foot deformity, wherein the structures of one extremity are internally rotated while the same structure of the other limb is externally rotated.[36,38] In cases of multiple deformities, one should employ splints and braces that are capable of affecting each of the involved areas. Therefore, initial selection of the splint or brace should be made in relationship to the type of deformity that is being treated. In cases where one has chosen to utilize a device that is affixed to the patient's shoe, selection may be based on the materials used and the fabrication of the device, its overall flexibility or rigidity, ease of application, and, finally, the actual cost of the device.

Age of the child

The age of the child being treated with a splint or brace must also be considered when electing to utilize this form of therapy. As a rule, any device that may force a child to sleep in a supine position should be avoided until after the age of 3 months. It has been reported that the incidence of a child younger than 3 months aspirating fluids is greater when the child is forced to sleep in the supine position.[36,42] Because the "golden age" for treatment of pediatric rotational and torsional abnormalities is generally under 1 year of age, the most successful treatment results are generally obtained between the ages of 3 and 12 months.[20] Unfortunately, as many of the more common rotational deformities are only evidenced after a child has initiated ambulation, most treatment plans are not initiated until this time. Most of the various splinting techniques are well tolerated by the pediatric patient up to the age of 2 or 3 years, at which time the child may become uncomfortable or agitated by the restrictive nature of the splint or brace. Interestingly enough, after the age of 4 most children understand that the modality being used is for their benefit and may therefore adapt to the splinting. In regard to specific deformities, the effectiveness of splints and braces on femoral torsion and position problems may only exist for a few years. Although developmental changes in this segment may occur up to the age of 13 or 14, successful alterations of femoral rotation problems are best achieved under the age of 5 years.[15,25,26] Position problems affecting the tibia are generally problematic up to the age of 3 or 4. At that age, the conditions generally resolve owing to the normal tightening effect of the developing knee joint. However, because an internal tibial position is responsible for precipitating a significant amount of instability with concomitant tripping and falling in the 1- to 3-year-old child, treatment is generally recommended. In terms of true tibial torsion problems, one must note that most external transverse plane rotation of the tibia is completed by the age of 7 or 8. Therefore, the conclusion of normal development of this segment would preclude any attempt at treatment beyond that age. Although significant external tibial torsion problems do not occur as frequently, the same developmental and treatment considerations exist for that condition as well.[38,44]

In regard to specific foot problems, the pathologic conditions best suited to treatment via splinting and bracing techniques are best treated at an early age. In cases where a talipes equinovarus deformity is unchallenged before age 1, splinting techniques are generally ineffective. In cases of a metatarsus adductus or talipes calcaneovalgus, splints and braces may be effective up to the age of 2 or 3, but only in their milder forms. In more severe cases, the most successful use of splints generally follows implementation of surgical intervention or serial plaster immobilization.

Length of treatment

Prior to the initiation of treatment via splints and braces, the practitioner should recommend a general approximation in regard to the actual length of the treatment interval. It is imperative that the parents of the child not only be presented with the rationale regarding this form of therapy, but also with an idea regarding the appropriate time involved. In the broadest sense, the deformity being evaluated must be treated for a time adequate enough to clinically alter positional torsional changes and then be maintained in that corrected position for an additional period of time. In cases specifically involving femoral torsion or femoral position problems, one can generally anticipate a treatment period extending from approximately 12 to 18 months.[44] During this time, the practitioner should be able to clinically appreciate a measurable change in the deformity. If there is no appreciable change elicited over a period of 6 to 10 months, then it is likely that the child's problem may not respond even with continued treatment. Regardless of treatment, approximately 10% of these deformities persist into adult life.[31,32] Therefore, it is sometimes appropriate to terminate treatment when no changes become evident.

In cases involving an internal or external tibial position, the period of treatment depends on whether serial plaster immobilization was utilized. In cases where this was employed as an initial measure, the casting sequence would generally encompass a period of time extending from 4 to 6 weeks. Following this, a splint or brace is utilized for approximately twice as long as a plaster immobilization, that is, 8 to 12 weeks. In cases where serial plaster immobilization was not employed, then the overall treatment would encompass 3 to 6 months. Tibial torsion problems, if treated successfully via serial plaster immobilization, may not require additional splinting after correction has been achieved. In cases where the splint or braces represent the primary form of therapy, the treatment regimen extends for approximately the same length of time as femoral rotation problems, that is, 12 to 18 months.[40,42]

In regard to foot deformities, talipes equinovarus, metatarsus adductus, or talipes calcaneovalgus require varying degrees of splinting or bracing, depending on severity. If the initial treatment involves serial plaster immobilization, then the splinting or bracing period generally lasts for at least twice as long as the casting sequence. In more severe cases, where surgery preceded the period of serial plaster immobilization, the bracing and splinting period might extend to three times the length of the casting sequence. Overall, the splinting or bracing system should be utilized as much as possible throughout the day. A younger child should wear the brace or splint while sleeping at night as well as during naps. If the brace or splint is flexible or is worn on only one limb, then the device may be utilized for longer periods of time throughout the day.[39,42]

Determining the extent of correction

The child's ability to tolerate a splint often depends on a number of variables. The most significant involves the angle of correction of the splint or brace. Over the years, a common prescription provided for any internal leg, knee, or foot deformity was for a Denis Browne bar set at 45 degrees abducted bilaterally with reverse-last shoes. In some instances, the bar was initially set at 60 degrees abducted bilaterally.[44] Although this type of bar and shoe modification is tolerated by some children, many will not wear the bar, often because they cannot tolerate the degree of correction. If a child is initially unable to wear a splint or brace because of excessive correction and subsequent discomfort, further efforts, even with the reduction of correction, are generally unsuccessful. Because of this, it is imperative that the practitioner calculate the total degree of external leg rotation available when attempting to utilize a splint or brace for any internally deviated limb segment. For example, available external femoral rotation should be added to available external knee rotation, and this number then added to the degree of external tibial torsion. This number would then represent the total available external motion present in this child. If the total range of motion was 30 degrees (hip) plus 15 degrees (knee) plus –10 degrees (tibial torsion), then the maximum available external rotation for this limb would be 35 degrees. If this child were placed in a bar initially set at 45 degrees externally rotated, it would be unlikely that the child would tolerate the correction. This measurement should be calculated for both limbs and utilized appropriately.

One method of dealing with the correction is to initially set the splint or bar at a minimum degree of external rotation. This allows the child to become accustomed to the alteration of the environment as well as to the introduction of a new force or pressure on the limb. The child is then seen in 2 weeks and monthly thereafter to increase the external correction to a tolerable position. If at any point the child is unable to adapt to the corrected position, some reduction of that position is required. Care must be taken not to be overly aggressive while implementing this form of therapy, as cases of avascular necrosis of the femoral head have been reported.[9,36,37] In children with unilateral tibial rotation problems, the practitioner should be aware that unilateral bracing systems are available and that these eliminate any concern regarding the preceding discussion.[13] Where a splint or brace is being used to alter an external femoral or tibial rotation problem, the device is most appropriate in altering the child's sleeping position. In these cases, care must be taken to avoid aggressive rotation of the limb into an adducted position. It is essential that the practitioner be aware of the possibility of a night splint or brace causing an unstable or dislocatable hip to actually dislocate. Because a dislocatable hip cannot be accurately diagnosed, either clinically or radiographically, beyond 4 months of age, a child with an externally deviated limb may have this problem. Because the motion of hip adduction and internal rotation is responsible for dislocating a dislocatable hip, caution must be exercised not to excessively adduct the child's limbs. Since the goal of this treatment is to alter the sleeping position of the child, a corrected position of approximately 25 to 45 degrees abducted may be sufficient to effect such a change. It is inappropriate to set the correction to a negative or internal value, as this has the greatest potential for subluxing the child's hip.[5,15,19,37]

Modifications to impede subluxatory changes and maintain normal anatomic relationships

One of the long-standing concerns regarding splinting and bracing techniques involves the potential for the device to precipitate subluxatory changes in the developing child's foot. Normal structural and functional alterations of the lower extremity should not be achieved at the expense of midtarsal and subtalar joint stability. It is essential to note that the majority of splints and braces act initially at the point of least resistance, which is the foot. Therefore, prior to the initiation of any force being directed into the tibia, knee, femur, or hip, the midtarsal and subtalar joints of the foot will necessarily be affected first.[30,34,36,44] In order to eliminate the possibility of this occurring, several modifications may be introduced into the more static or stationary devices to minimize this possibility. Placing a 15 to 20 degree varus bend in the bar portion of specific splints (e.g.,

Ganley, Denis Browne, Fillauer) and placing a triplane or varus wedge in the heel seat of each shoe is advisable.[34,44] The combination of these two antipronation measures maintains the subtalar joint in an inverted position, which results in locking of the midtarsal joint. Thus, when an external force is directed against the internally rotated limb, the foot moves as a unit, thereby maintaining its structural stability and integrity. In some cases where the splint or brace is available in a variety of widths, the practitioner should measure the distance across the child's shoulders or the distance from one anterior superior iliac spine to the other and add an inch. Either measurement may be utilized to then select the appropriately sized bar.[42,44]

Appropriate shoes for splints

As a rule, a stiff-countered leather-soled shoe is advisable for mounting to any of the splinting or bracing systems necessitating a shoe. Although some of the splints and braces may be utilized in conjunction with an existing shoe, the practitioner should evaluate the shoe for any evidence that it may have adapted to the deformity. For example, a child with a metatarsus adductus deformity may have broken down the existing shoes to the point where the deformity could be exacerbated. If this is the case, the shoe should not be utilized. When possible, open-toed shoes should be utilized for adequate ventilation and to provide room for growth. If a closed-toe shoe is selected, then the toe box of the shoe should be cut away for the same purpose. This can easily be accomplished with a skiving knife or surgical blade. In cases where the shoes are to be worn for a prolonged period of time, they can be cut along the vamp and into the tongue to allow for expansion of the foot width.

Table 20-2
Splinting and bracing devices utilized in the treatment of pediatric lower extremity musculoskeletal deformities

- Denis Browne splint
- Fillauer splint
- Uni-bar
- Brachman skate
- Ganley splint
- Langer Counter Rotation System splint
- Friedman counter splint or Flexosplint
- Twister cables
- Wheaton brace
- Wheaton bracing system
- Tibial Torsion Transformer
- Plaster or fiberglass splint
- Circular Torqheel

Splinting and bracing devices

The various types of splints and braces that are utilized in the correction of angle-of-gait deformities are listed in Table 20-2 and described below.

Denis Browne splint

This splint was initially described and utilized by its developer in Great Britain in 1934. Although this splint has been utilized for the treatment of congenital convex pes planovalgus, internal and external femoral and tibial pathologic conditions, as well as talipes calcaneovalgus and metatarsus adductus, the splint was originally described for the treatment of talipes equinovarus.[5,10,11,39] The splint was developed in an attempt to avoid the inevitable complications and resultant immobility that were created by the prolonged serial plaster immobilization, tenotomies, and open reduction techniques employed at the time.[22] Sir Denis Browne believed that a more rapid correction could be achieved with his splint because the foot could be kept active while the shape was being corrected. Additionally, he believed that the position of one foot would be capable of controlling the other foot during treatment. Presently, the Denis Browne splint continues to be utilized with a wide variety of applications. It is available with bar widths ranging from 4 to 14 in. (Fig. 20-2**A** and **B**). The splint must be attached to an appropriate leather-soled shoe. It is typically affixed by a series of rivets or set screws which are affixed into pre-existing holes in some prescription pediatric shoes.

Fillauer splint

The Fillauer splint (Markell Corp., Yonkers, NY) is a variation of the Denis Browne splint. The primary modification of this device is that its basic construction is altered by replacing the screw plate with a clamping system (Fig. 20-3**A** and **B**). This modification simplifies application of the shoe to the bar and allows the patient to reuse the shoe once treatment has been terminated or during periods of ambulation when the bar is not being utilized. Although this allows the use of a variety of shoes, a stiff leather-soled shoe is preferable, because the clamping system often distorts a more flexible shoe.

Uni-bar

The Uni-bar (Spectra Industries, Richard Manufacturing Co., Memphis, TN) is yet another type of Denis Browne bar. This bar is equipped with a ball-and-socket type of friction joint at each footplate (Fig. 20-4, p. 432). This allows for limitless adjustment of the footplate within all three body

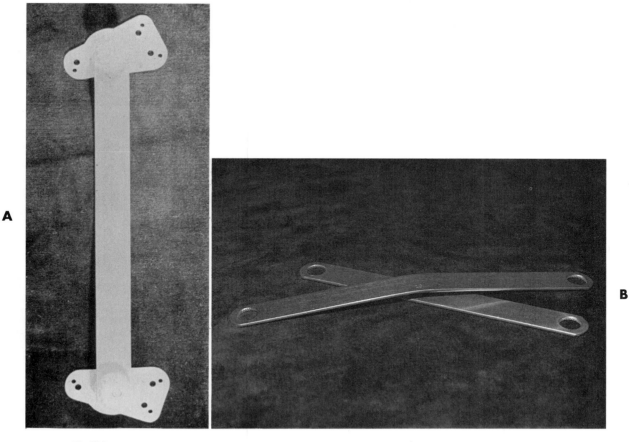

Fig. 20-2. A, Denis Browne splint. B, Denis Browne splint demonstrating a 15-degree bend in the frontal plane. This decreases the likelihood of subtalar and midtarsal joint subluxation occurring as the forefoot is abducted during treatment.

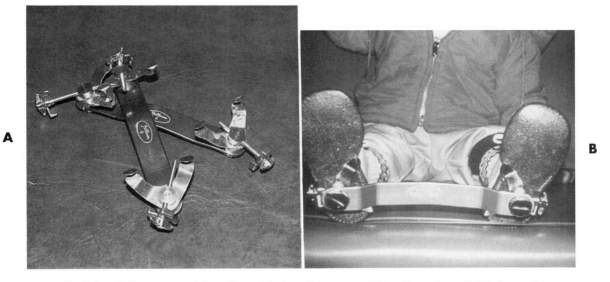

Fig. 20-3. A, Fillauer-type night splint with clamping system. This allows the splint to be easily dispensed. Additionally, the clamping system is appropriate for use with a variety of shoes. B, Fillauer splint attached to a child's shoes. (Courtesy of Markell Corp., Yonkers, NY.)

planes. It allows the practitioner to set each footplate at an angle that not only corrects the foot in the transverse plane but stabilizes the subtalar and midtarsal joints in the frontal plane as well. This eliminates the necessity of bending the bar. This bar is available in one length only. After determining the appropriate width for the bar, the practitioner snaps off the excess material on the bar and moves the footplate to the proper position (Fig. 20-5).

The molded plastic construction allows for straightforward in-office application and adjustments. Again, a stiff-soled high-top shoe is preferable. Overall, this device generally functions more effectively in infants and smaller children, as its plastic components tend to fatigue and crack with use in the older child.[44]

Ganley splint

The Ganley splint (Chicago Medical Supply, Chicago) is indicated for the treatment of the following: internal or external femoral torsion or position, internal or external tibial torsion or position, metatarsus adductus, talipes calcaneovalgus, talipes equinovarus, or any combination of these.[20] The device was developed by James Ganley, D.P.M. who noted that none of the available splints were effective in appropriately treating combination foot and leg disorders. He subsequently developed this splint to deal with those problems. The splint is constructed of a variety of metal pieces, which include four footplates and three bars (Fig. 20-6). Two shank bars and one torque bar are included in the kit. The splint is available in only one size, with the torque bar ultimately being cut to the desired width. The footplates are affixed to the soles of the shoes and are secured with clinching nails.[25,26]

These nails do not pull out easily, and they turn onto themselves during application to the splint. The shoes are split to allow correct placement of the forefoot relative to the rearfoot. The ability to effectively alter forefoot and rearfoot positions in both the transverse and frontal planes makes the Ganley device a unique splinting system.

In regard to treating specific deformities with the Ganley splint, the following modifications should be noted. Treatment of a metatarsus adductus deformity requires that the shoe be split at the level of Lisfranc's joint and that a 7- to 10-degree abducted position of the forefoot to rearfoot be attained with the shank bar (Fig. 20-7). Additionally, the forefoot should be slightly everted to the rearfoot to plantarflex the anteromedial column, as this is what maintains the metatarsals in an ab-

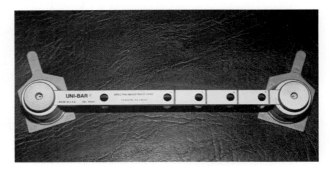

Fig. 20-5. Uni-bar. Note that the bar may be snapped along any of the inscribed indentations to allow for a custom fit. This bar has been adjusted to an 8-in. length.

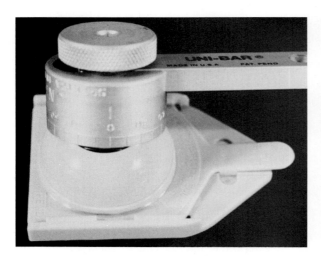

Fig. 20-4. Completely adjustable footplate component of the Uni-bar allows for correction in all body planes.

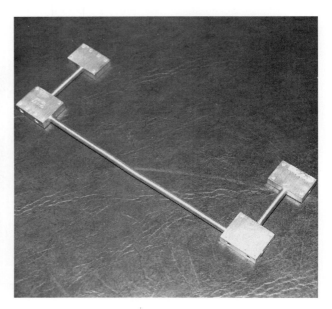

Fig. 20-6. The Ganley splint consists of four foot plates, two shank bars, and one torque bar.

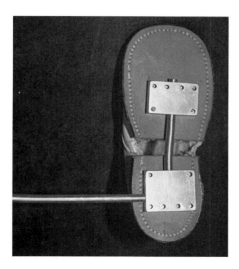

Fig. 20-7. Desired forefoot-to-rearfoot correction may be established following articulation of the shoe and bending of the shank bar.

ducted position. If a talipes calcaneovalgus is being treated, the shoes are split at the same level as for metatarsus adductus. The shank bar is utilized and the forefoot is placed in an adducted and plantar-flexed position. In treating internal rotation problems, the torque bar is placed between the two rearfoot plates. In treating an external rotation problem, the torque bar is placed between the two forefoot plates. If a metatarsus adductus or talipes calcaneovalgus deformity is being treated as an isolated deformity, the torque bar need not be utilized. Conversely, if a more proximal deformity is being treated without any foot involvement, then the shank bar need not be utilized. The Ganley splint is worn by the child only when sleeping. Ambulating with the device in place is discouraged.[25,26]

Friedman Counter Splint or Flexosplint

The Friedman counter splint (Friedman Counter Splints, Inc. Westtown, PA.) is utilized to specifically treat internal femoral rotation problems. The device works by altering the child's sleeping position by restricting internal rotation of the limb during sleeping or napping. The splint consists of a flexible 6-in. piece of leather which is riveted to the heel counter of the child's shoes. The device is available in several lengths and is sized according to the child's shoes. The approximate angle of correction can be set according to the numbers marked on the device itself. The splint pulls the child's heels together and externally rotates the lower extremities, thereby allowing unlimited motion of the lower extremities in any direction except internally. The device is simple to utilize, is easily adapted to by the child, and generally meets with parental approval.

The Friedman counter splint is not as specific as other devices and this limits its use. There is some concern regarding the likelihood of this device subluxing a dislocatable hip because it maintains the limbs in an adducted position. The Friedman Flexosplint is similar to the counter splint. It is supplied in only one adjustable size, however.

Brachman skate

This device was developed by Brachman in the early 1940s as a primary treatment modality for talipes equinovarus.[8] It was initially referred to as a reciprocal ambulatory skid plate or skate (Fig. 20-8). Following its introduction for talipes equinovarus, Brachman suggested that it could also be used to treat metatarsus adductus, internal and external positional hip problems, talipes calcaneovalgus, and balancing and gait problems associated with spastic disorders.[27] Brachman believed that his skate could correct these deformities by providing a broad base of support with subsequent improvement of balance. It was developed to allow for normal movement and designed to be worn 24 hours/day. The device is yet another modification of the original Denis Browne bar. The primary difference is that one or two parallel crossbars are affixed to the child's shoe between two aluminum plates. This arrangement allows the device to be freely movable in the direction of correction, but restricts motion in the abnormal position. The angle of correction is then established with a set pin that is placed between the two aluminum heelplates. Therefore, a bar set at an angle of 35 degrees abducted would not allow internal rotation beyond that point. However, it would be capable of allowing unrestricted external rotation beyond that angulation. It has been suggested that the device be utilized for children between the ages of 6 months and 8 years, being utilized initially as a night splint only.[44] Recommendations for appropriate use suggest increasing the wearing time until the device could be worn 24 hours/day. Although the device was designed to be utilized in a dynamic fashion for a wide range and variety of conditions, it is more appropriate to use it solely as a night splint. Marked dynamic external rotation precipitated by this device during gait could result in subluxatory problems at the level of the midtarsal and subtalar joints. Additionally, excessive stress directed at the developing child's knees within the transverse plane is an additional concern. Furthermore the device is restrictive in that it can only be utilized effectively on smooth, flat surfaces.[44]

Langer Pediatric Counter Rotation System Splint

The Langer Pediatric Counter Rotation System splint (Langer Corp., Deer Park, NY) introduced in

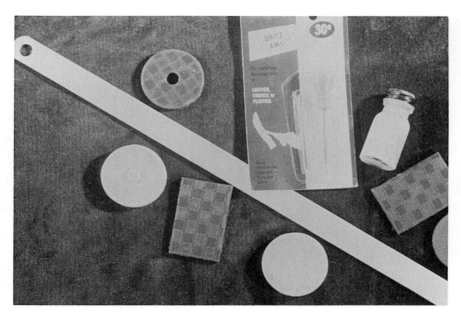

Fig. 20-8. Components of Brachman skate.

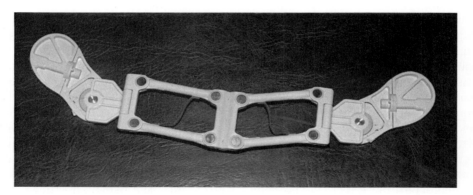

Fig. 20-9. Langer Pediatric Counter Rotation System splint.

1982, is the most flexible and best tolerated of all the available splinting or bracing systems. Its ease of application, success in resolving lower extremity rotational problems, and degree of parental acceptance mark it as an excellent modality. The system is best used to treat internal and external rotational problems of the hip, femur, knee, and tibia, or any combination of those deformities.[16,44] Additionally, the splint may be utilized as an adjunct to the management of mild forms of cerebral palsy. Although the splint allows for adjustment of the forefoot to the rearfoot on the frontal plane, there is no available mechanism to correct transverse plane deformity. The splint is comprised of two fully movable, hinged, rectangular crossbars and two footplates (Fig. 20-9). The splint is available in only one size and is intended to be utilized for the prewalker up to a 7- or 8-year-old child. It may be used for up to 24 hours/day by the prewalker, because its hinged mechanism allows for normal, unencumbered crawling. Since the shoe is attached with a super cement and accelerator, any type of shoe may be worn. Although shoes with rubber or vinyl soles are easily affixed to this splint, the uppers of these types of shoe are generally inadequate to maintain appropriate foot position on the splint. In cases where treatment for metatarsus adductus is also needed, then an appropriately padded straight-last or tarsal outflare shoe may be utilized (Fig. 20-10).

Twister Cables

Twister cables were initially developed to assist in the treatment of spastic gait disorders present primarily in children with cerebral palsy. Since that time, they have been utilized to treat all internal and external rotational problems of the lower extremity.

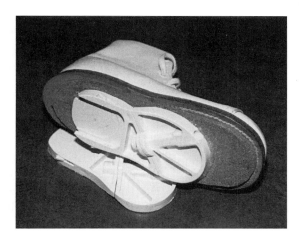

Fig. 20-10. Straight-last shoe affixed to footplate.

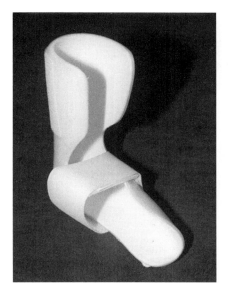

Fig. 20-11. Wheaton Brace.

The cable system develops a twisting movement around the longitudinal axis of the limb which precipitates either an internal or external force. The arm of activity extends over the entire length of the limb and ultimately transmits its force to the foot. This derotational movement is countered by a balance force on the opposite side of the body. If this does not occur, compensatory realignment of the pelvis and contralateral limb makes corrective attempts ineffectual. The device consists of a leather waistband with a flexible joint attachment which allows unrestricted movement of flexion and extension. These joints are, in turn, attached to a 7.5-mm five-layer flexible spring, or shafting wire, which extends from the greater trochanter to an outside calf band and finally to the shoe. The shafting wire is coiled into a helix and enclosed in a rubber sheath. The cables are spring-loaded so that when the child places the foot on the ground, the tension from the cables forces the legs to abduct in response to the degree of tension placed on the shafting wire. The device may be utilized for 24 hours or only during waking hours in the older child. The cable system has been utilized for the prewalker up through 8 to 10 years of age. Although used quite extensively in the past, twister cables have not been prescribed as frequently in recent years owing to the significant degree of torque applied to a developing child's lower extremity. Even when the shoes are appropriately wedged or a foot orthosis is utilized, marked significant forces can be directed by the cable system. Overcorrection and excessive forces applied by the cables are capable of adversely affecting the joints of the leg as well as alignment of the limbs.[44]

Wheaton Brace

The lightweight, thermoplastic Wheaton brace (Wheaton Brace Co., Carol Stream, IL.) is designed for the primary treatment of metatarsus adductus in infants and children aged up to 4 years. It is a new application of the three-point treatment principle for metatarsus adductus. It is effective because the three points of fixation work in a balanced fashion to initiate a corrective force against the deformity (Fig. 20-11). The first point of fixation is distal, which places an abduction force beyond the hallux. This effectively treats any associated hallux varus secondary to a tight abductor hallucis brevis tendon. The second point of fixation maintains the calcaneus securely in place and minimizes subtalar joint pronation. The third point of fixation is maintained by a Velcro strap, which is tightened against the apex of the deformity. The brace is useful in the treatment of metatarsus adductus in three ways: (1) It acts as a primary treatment that is capable of replacing serial plaster immobilization; (2) it acts as an adjunctive treatment, thereby shortening the period of plaster application, and (3) it acts as a retentive device to be utilized after appropriate correction has been achieved.[13] The brace is available in two series representing a variety of sizes. The metatarsus adductus series, which is utilized for infants up to 8 months of age, demonstrates a 15 degrees plantar-flexed ankle position designed to prevent iatrogenic foot subluxation during correction. In the TEV-CRB series, the ankle is maintained at a 90-degree angle in order that the older, ambulatory child may be more mobile. Generally, the same brace may be used for the duration of the treatment, which is approximately 3 months. The brace is not effective in the treatment of totally inflexible, rigid deformities.[13] Generally speaking, this type of deformity is more amenable to surgical intervention.

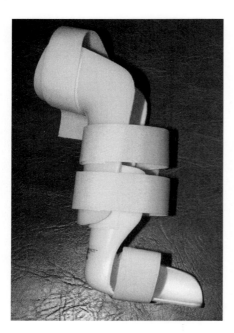

Fig. 20-12. Wheaton bracing system.

Wheaton bracing system

The Wheaton bracing system incorporates the lower leg portion described above for the Wheaton brace with an additional thermoplastic upper leg component for the treatment of metatarsus adductus, talipes equinovarus, and internal or external tibial torsion or position. This upper component is designed to maintain the knee in a 90 degrees flexed position and, when combined with the lower portion, allows for torque correction of the tibial component (Fig. 20-12). By overlapping the two components, the practitioner can choose an infinite number of corrected positions. Additionally, by adjusting the position of the two portions, compensation may be achieved for growth of the leg during correction. The benefits of this system are as follows: (1) The device treats the tibial component directly without simultaneously twisting the femur or hip; (2) the knee is maintained in an appropriately flexed position; (3) in cases of unilateral deformity, only the involved side is treated; (4) the system is easily adjustable for growth, thereby eliminating the necessity for multiple replacements; and (5) associated foot disorders may be treated in conjunction with tibial rotation abnormalities. The upper component is available in four sizes and may be utilized in children up to 4 years of age.

Tibial Torsion Transformer

Developed by Brewer Medical Companies, Jacksonville, FL, this device attempts to correct rotational deformities affecting the tibia. With this device, the tibia is maintained in a corrected position with the knee in a flexed position. The device is manufactured of metal with correction achieved by a series of nut and bolt adjustments. The device cannot be used to treat any associated foot problems. These must be treated with an additional device.

Plaster or fiberglass splint

Rather than utilizing one of the commercially available splints or braces, the practitioner may elect to fabricate a custom splint in cases where serial plaster immobilization has been utilized in the treatment of a lower extremity problem. The practitioner may bivalve the last cast in the series (Fig. 20-13) or may fabricate a new splint at the conclusion of the casting sequence (Fig. 20-14**A–D**, p. 438). A variety of materials may be utilized, including plaster, rigid fiberglass, or flexible 3M Scotchcast Soft cast (3M Healthcare. St. Paul, MN). In all instances, the inner surface should be well padded and the parent fully instructed in the appropriate application of the splint.

Circular Torqheel

The Circular Torqheel (Markell Corp.) is a dynamic device used in the treatment of internal or external rotation problems. The Circular Torqheel is a rubber lift that attaches to the heel of the child's shoe. The cleats, which are arranged in a radial pattern, bend under weightbearing, thereby exerting a torque or twist on both feet and legs. When utilized as marked (right and left), they introduce an external torque at heel contact. They may be utilized in reverse fashion to produce an internal rotation. If the deformity is unilateral, then only one cleat is utilized. Care must be taken to prevent excessive subtalar joint and midtarsal joint pronation and excessive torquing of the knee. Excessive motion at these joints may be minimized through the use of functional foot orthoses or varus shoe wedging utilized in combination with the Torqheel.[8,26,32]

Pediatric shoe therapy

Shoes serve a protective function and should be utilized when the child initiates ambulation. If the developing child's foot does not demonstrate any significant degree of deformity, then flexible-soled, nonsupportive types of shoes are generally recommended. In cases where some degree of deformity is noted, as with metatarsus adductus, talipes equinovarus, talipes calcaneovalgus, or flexible flatfoot deformity, a more supportive deformity-specific shoe should be utilized. In cases of a normal foot, a good shoe must be properly fitted and have the same

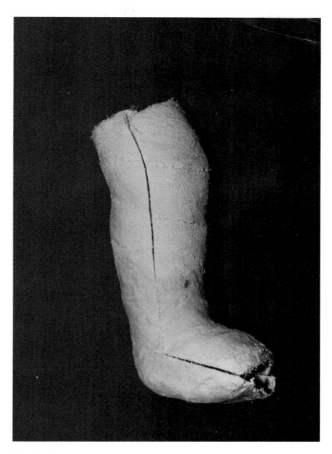

Fig. 20-13. Bivalved cast. Following the application of appropriate padding, this may be utilized as a night splint.

general shape as the child's foot. As the child grows older, the shoe should become somewhat stiffer, with the shank capable of promoting both support and enough rigidity to act as a rigid lever when the child starts to ambulate in a propulsive fashion. A well-constructed shoe is fashioned of leather for durability and has an average heel height of 3/32 in. for infants and 3/8 in. for children.[44] More recent innovations include both low-top and high-top athletic-style shoes[28] with firm heel counters and supportive midsoles (Fig. 20-15, p. 439). Since a child's foot may grow quite quickly, it is not uncommon for the shoe size to change three or four times in 1 year. Because of this, the child's shoes may be purchased with approximately 1/2 in. of additional length in the toe box to allow for rapid growth.

When utilizing a shoe to assist in the correction of foot abnormalities, one should be aware of the uses and indications for the various shoes. There are three basic styles of pediatric orthopedic shoes. The prewalker style is an open-toed shoe which laces to the exposed digital area for easy application. This type of shoe allows additional room for growth and owing to its open style minimizes maceration to the

digits. The prewalker shoe is generally constructed over a straight last and is available only in infant sizes. The clubfoot prewalker appears similar in the toe box area, but is constructed over an outflared last (Fig. 20-16, p. 439). The addition of a strap over the instep assists in maintaining the foot in a secure position (Fig. 20-17, p. 439).[6] The Oxford style is a low quarter-shoe that laces below the ankle to the level of the midfoot and resembles a normal shoe. Since a child under 24 to 30 months old has a rounded calcaneus without definition, this shoe should be avoided in that age group, as it will easily slip off. The high-top boot generally laces from above the ankle to the level of the forefoot. This is a standard high-top pediatric shoe available in multiple styles and degrees of correction. When utilizing a prescription shoe for a pediatric patient, the practitioner should prescribe the style and last of the shoe according to the deformity. There are four basic lasts utilized in the construction of pediatric shoes: (1) the straight last, (2) the conventional last, (3) the inflared last, and (4) the outflared last. The shoes utilized in the treatment of pediatric deformities are listed in Table 20-3, p. 439.

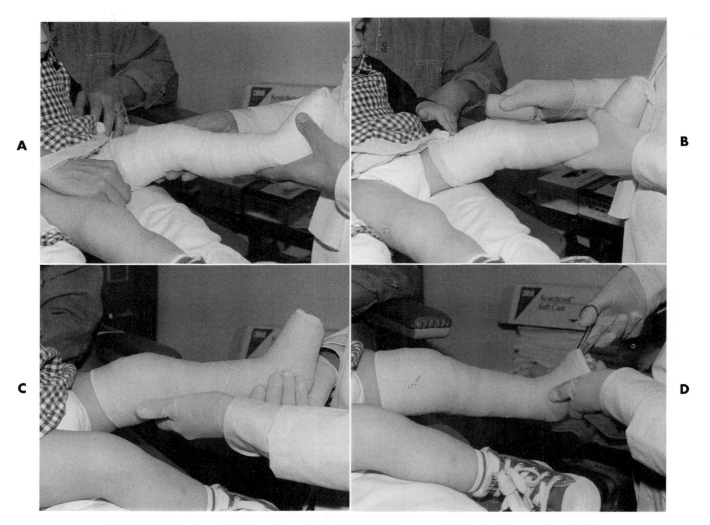

Fig. 20-14. Fabrication of night splint with flexible Soft Cast material. **A,** Stockinet and webril applied. **B,** Application of splinting material. **C,** Maintaining the foot and leg in the appropriate corrected position. **D,** Removal of flexible splint with scissors.

Tarso-medius shoe

This is an example of a shoe constructed over a straight last. There are two types of straight-last shoes—the symmetric and the nonsymmetric. The symmetric type has no corrections or wedges built into the shoe and does not appear to have a specific right or left side (Fig. 20-18, p. 440). Closer inspection demonstrates that the tongue of the shoe is stitched into the medial portion of the shoe's upper, thereby delineating a right or left shoe. The nonsymmetric straight-last shoe has a longer extended heel counter and may have either a Thomas heel to prevent pronation or a valgus heel to promote forefoot abduction. As a rule, this shoe is the most versatile in the treatment of the majority of pediatric foot problems. This shoe can easily accommodate triplane or varus heel wedges to decrease pronation in the child with a flexible flatfoot. This shoe is also

effectively utilized in children with a flexible metatarsus adductus or in children who have undergone serial plaster immobilization for metatarsus adductus and who require postcasting retention of the correction. In cases where metatarsus adductus has been successfully treated and a metatarsus primus varus remains, this shoe is capable of stretching the contracted abductor hallucis brevis muscle. In these cases, a triplane heel wedge is utilized to maintain subtalar and midtarsal joint integrity with an additional 1/4-in. adhesive felt pad placed along the medial aspect of the toe box.[44] This buttressing effect places an abduction force on the forefoot while the rearfoot is stabilized by the wedge. An additional portion of adhesive felt may be added to the area of the cuboid on the lateral aspect of the shoe to act as a fulcrum in the overall correction of the forefoot. Use of this type of correction for 6 to 12 months may

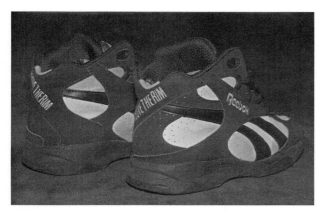

Fig. 20-15. High-topped athletic shoes with firm heel counters and supportive midsoles.

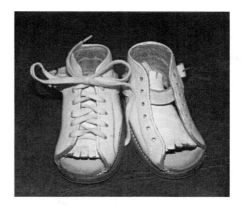

Fig. 20-17. The strap overlying the instep of the prewalker shoe assists in maintaining the foot in a secure position.

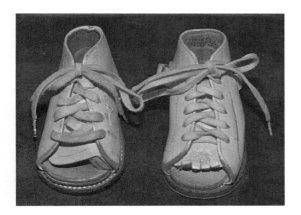

Fig. 20-16. *Left:* Standard prewalker style. *Right:* Clubfoot prewalker with outflare last construction.

Table 20-3
Shoes utilized in the treatment of pediatric lower extremity musculoskeletal disorders

- Tarso-medius shoe
- Conventional last shoe
- Inflare last shoe (tarsal supinator)
- Outflare last shoe (tarsal pronator or tarsal outflare)
- Bebax shoe
- Ipos shoe

be appropriate, depending on the response of the child to treatment.

Conventional last shoe

The conventional last shoe is constructed with a reinforced heel counter and inner longitudinal arch in a Goodyear welt design. The shape of the shoe is designed to fit comfortably and firmly from the heel to the ball of the foot. This type of shoe, with its rounded toe box, allows the foot and toes to spread to their fullest and does not restrict normal foot motion. Although this shoe is typically worn by children without lower extremity deformity, its style easily accommodates wedges and other modifications for minor lower extremity problems.

Inflare last shoe

The inflare or C-shaped last is designed to apply firm pressure to the lateral aspect of the forefoot and at the level of the calcaneocuboid joint. This com-

bination of forces creates a degree of adduction designed to position the child's foot in a more supinated attitude. Although this inflared last does not correct or resist excessive pronation, it is useful in cases of flexible flatfoot deformities, external femoral or tibial rotation problems, and tibia angulation problems. The shoes are also useful in treating mild cases of talipes calcaneovalgus or following correction of that deformity with serial plaster immobilization (Fig. 20-19).

Outflare last shoe

The outflare last shoe tends to pronate both the subtalar and midtarsal joints. Additionally, this shoe places pressure on the medial aspect of the first metatarsal head, which causes abduction of the forefoot; the medial aspect of the calcaneus, which leads to abduction of the rearfoot; and the lateral aspect of the calcaneocuboid joint, which serves as a fulcrum for the two aforementioned forces.[44] There are two basic types of shoes constructed over this last—the tarsal pronator and the tarsal outflare shoe. The tarsal pronator shoe utilizes a stiff heel counter, a valgus heel, and a 1/8-in. lateral outer sole wedge. This shoe has classically been prescribed for angle and gait disturbances secondary to femoral and tibial rotation problems, as well as

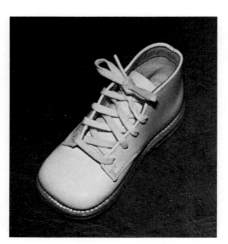

Fig. 20-18. Tarso-medius shoe.

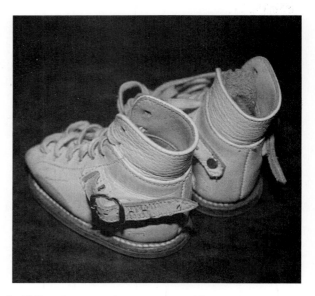

Fig. 20-19. Inflare last shoes. Note modification of additional leather stitched above each heel counter. This was added to assist in maintaining the child's foot securely within the shoe.

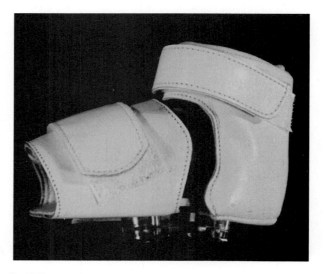

Fig. 20-20. Bebax shoe.

metatarsus adductus. This combination of shoe modifications is capable of abducting the angle of gait by limiting internal rotation of the tibia. Additionally, the marked outflared construction of the shoe places an abduction force on the metatarsus adductus deformity. Although the appearance of a metatarsus adductus may improve cosmetically with the use of this shoe, it may occur at the expense of subluxing the developing child's foot. As the shoe "breaks" at the level of the midtarsal joint rather than at Lisfranc's joint, correction may occur at the inappropriate level. Because of this, care must be utilized when prescribing this shoe. In cases where a tarsosupinator shoe is not available for treatment of a talipes calcaneovalgus, this shoe may be effectively reversed for therapy of that deformity.

The tarsal outflare shoe is also constructed over an outflare last, but has a less rigid shank and a flexible spring heel. It does not incorporate a valgus heel or sole and is less aggressive in introducing a significant subluxation force against the child's foot. Because of this, the shoe is more appropriately utilized in the treatment of metatarsus adductus deformities.

Bebax shoe

The Bebax (Broadwest Corp., New York, NY) is a leather shoe split through the sole with separate soleplates attached to each portion. The shoe has a freely movable forefoot and rearfoot portion similar to the arrangement previously described for the Ganley splint. This shoe is available only in paired sizes. Owing to the universal joint located on each footplate, the forefoot-to-rearfoot relationship may be adjusted without limitation (Fig. 20-20). Thus, this device may be utilized in the treatment of various congenital abnormalities, including metatarsus adductus and talipes calcaneovalgus. Al-

though the device has been recommended as an alternative form of treatment for deformities requiring serial plaster immobilization, it appears to work best in milder, more flexible deformities. Overall, this shoe is not able to direct sufficient force to the specific levels of involvement to adequately correct the less flexible deformities.[44]

Ipos shoe

The Ipos shoe (Chicago Medical Corp.) is another articulated shoe. Available in various sizes, it provides even tension across the forefoot to correct metatarsus adductus conditions. As with similar devices, this shoe is best suited to address the more flexible forms of deformity or as maintenance bracing following serial plaster immobilization. There is some question as to whether this shoe is capable of producing adequate pressure at the specific points necessary to effect a change.

Pediatric orthoses
History

Prior to reviewing the various devices available for pediatric flexible flatfoot conditions, it is appropriate to briefly review the history of this form of therapy. In 1845 an English chiropodist, Durlacher, described the use of a built-up shoe insert fashioned of leather.[1] This was the earliest report of attempting to build up a flatfoot by effectively altering the position of the foot within the shoe. In 1874 the English orthopedic surgeon Hugh Owen Thomas attempted to decrease flatfooted conditions by addressing treatment to the outer sole of the patient's shoe. He added a medial extension to the heel of the shoe to extend shank support distally to the talonavicular joint. This modification continues to be utilized in a variety of pediatric prescription shoes to this day.[23,26] In 1907 Royal Whitman, an American orthopedic surgeon, addressed the various mechanical components associated with the flexible flatfoot condition. He was instrumental in influencing other healthcare practitioners to consider flatfooted conditions as being severe enough to warrant attention and eventual treatment. He was one of the first physicians to recognize the correlation between marked flatfooted problems and painful postural problems. In the early 1890s he developed a metal foot brace which was utilized extensively in the treatment of flatfoot conditions.[26,27] In 1912 Percy Roberts, developed a metal foot brace which functioned similarly to the Whitman brace.[1] Essentially, the Roberts plate attempted to control the foot by maintaining the calcaneus in a vertical position. In the 1920s a chiropodist, Otto Schuster, combined the two aforementioned devices into the Whitman-Roberts brace.[1,29] This device was more efficient and better tolerated. In 1958, Merton Root, a podiatrist, developed an orthotic device made of thermoplastic and fashioned over a nonweightbearing plaster model of the foot.[33,34] This device has proved to be the model for all functional foot orthoses to this date.

In 1967 the UCBL (University of California Biomechanics Laboratory) device was developed by J.W. Campbell and W.H. Henderson.[21] This polypropylene device functioned like a heel stabilizer and was capable of effectively maintaining the

calcaneus in a perpendicular attitude. In 1981 Richard Blake, a podiatrist, developed the inverted orthotic device, which was a modification of the Root functional foot orthosis.[4] The modified positive cast construction of the inverted device produced a heel cup which could be inverted from 25 to 75 degrees. Essentially, the device was developed to function as a true functional foot orthosis with the incorporation of an aggressive varus heel position. Although the above-mentioned are not the only types of devices that have been successfully utilized over the years, they have been used with the greatest degree of success by a wide variety of practitioners. Over the years a host of other devices and modifications of the above devices have been utilized to alter the abnormal forces and resultant problems precipitated by a flexible flatfoot condition. The devices listed in Table 20-4 represent the more commonly utilized shoe inserts for the treatment of this condition.

Shoe inserts

During the normal development of the child's foot, the calcaneus functions in an everted position. During the first years of life this everted position reduces so that the calcaneus eventually assumes a perpendicular attitude relative to the weightbearing surface. This developmental process should be completed by the age of 7 years and corresponds to the development of the longitudinal arch as well as a reduction in overall subtalar joint motion. Based on clinical evaluation, the average position of the calcaneus upon the initiation of ambulation may be as much as 7 degrees everted.[30,31] A position of 10 to 12 degrees of calcaneal eversion may be noted in a small percentage of children, particularly those with severe pes planus. This is often associated with a marked internal or external femoral or tibial torsion

Table 20-4
Wedges and orthoses utilized in the treatment of pediatric lower extremity musculoskeletal disorders

- Triplane wedge
- Over-the-counter supports
- Whitman plate
- Roberts brace
- Shaffer plate
- Whitman-Roberts plate
- Heel stabilizer
- Root functional foot orthosis
- UCBL (University of California Biomechanics Laboratory)
- Blake inverted orthosis
- Gait plate

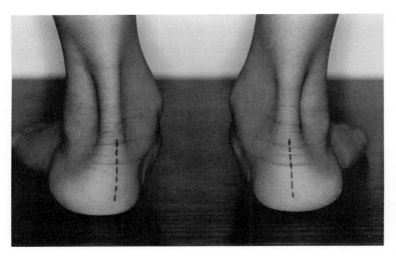

Fig. 20-21. A 12-year-old boy with abnormal foot position secondary to a compensated transverse plane deformity. Note excessive calcaneal eversion, prominent talar head, and marked midtarsal joint subluxation.

or position, or in compensated gastrocnemius equinus or talipes calcaneovalgus. As the normal reduction of calcaneal eversion is approximately 1 degree per year, the following formula may be utilized to determine the approximate degree of normally acceptable calcaneal eversion: 7 degrees minus the child's age equals normal calcaneal eversion.[41] Any significant eversion beyond this is indicative of excessive pronation. Another case of abnormal pronation occurs in instances where the "degree of eversion" falls within normal limits for a child, yet there is an overriding deforming force which could possibly maintain the foot in that position throughout development. A child who demonstrates an abnormally everted calcaneus during development is a candidate for treatment. The philosophy regarding the initiation of treatment in these cases is to protect the child's foot against any abnormal pronation force which may be originating from the foot, leg, or hip (Fig. 20-21). Because the child's foot completes the majority of its functional development by the age of 7 years, it is essential that normal forces be transmitted throughout the dorsal and plantar aspects of the medial longitudinal arch with preservation of the talonavicular articulation. To accomplish this, treatment often includes a combination of in-shoe wedges along with the use of the previously described splints or braces. When attempting to alter the position of a developing child's foot, a host of factors must be considered. These include the type and level of the deformity, the extent of compensation, the child's age, the child's weight, and the degree of activity.[30]

Triplane wedge
One of the simplest and most effective methods

of controlling subtalar joint pronation and associated calcaneal eversion is through the use of a triplane wedge. The triplane wedge is so named because it is capable of affecting foot function within the three cardinal body planes. Specifically, it promotes frontal plane inversion of the calcaneus, transverse plane abduction of the talus, as well as sagittal plane dorsiflexion of both the talus and calcaneus. The wedge is a pad constructed from 1/4-in. material such as cork or black piano felt so that the calcaneus is supported in a more supinated position. This wedge is constructed to fill the heel seat portion of a shoe in its entirety. The wedge is fashioned from the appropriate material, with the distal-medial quadrant being traced on the superior surface of the wedge. The material is then tapered away from this high point with a grinding sander. The distal margin of the quadrant is tapered slightly to minimize plantar skin irritation (Fig. 20-22). The wedge may be placed in any of the previously mentioned pediatric shoes and is secured with an adhesive. Owing to its ease of fabrication, several pairs may be made for use in various shoes. The triplane wedge is effective for treatment of abnormal pronation in the early walker. It may be utilized effectively in the pediatric patient between 1 and 2 years of age regardless of the cause of the abnormal pronation forces. Additionally, it is effective in conjunction with various other treatment modalities in an attempt to maintain the foot in a more stable position. An example of this is the use of a triplane wedge in a shoe affixed to one of the previously described splints or braces. The effect of the wedge maintains the subtalar joint in a supinated position which subsequently locks the midtarsal joint. Therefore, when an abduction force is introduced into the

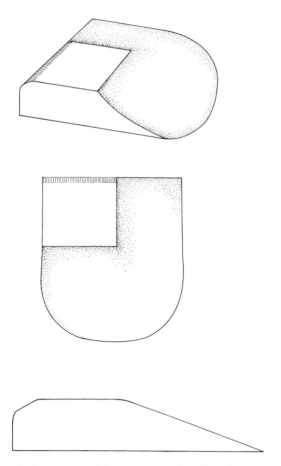

Fig. 20-22. Three views of the triplane wedge. Note that the high point is represented by the distal-medial quadrant of the wedge.

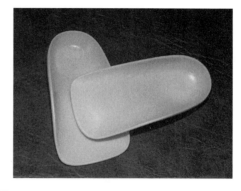

Fig. 20-23. Prefabricated pediatric orthoses. These are available in a wide range of sizes and widths and may be fabricated from numerous materials.

foot and leg by the splint, the midfoot is maintained in a stable position, decreasing the likelihood of forefoot subluxation. The triplane wedge is less effective in ambulatory children who demonstrate marked abnormal subtalar joint pronation with excessive calcaneal eversion and in children weighing more than 30 lb.[45]

Prefabricated orthoses

In cases where the ambulatory patient demonstrates marked eversion that cannot be adequately controlled with the triplane wedge or with prescription shoes, one may consider utilizing one of the various over-the-counter devices that are available for children. Although the responses with this type of device are not always favorable, the over-the-counter device may function well enough that casting for prescription devices may be postponed. Various orthopedic supply houses, as well as a host of orthotic laboratories, provide a variety of prefabricated devices. These are generally fabricated over "average" foot models and are available in a variety of sizes and widths (Fig. 20-23). The materials vary

from plastic to rubber to cork and are all amenable to having additional posting added by the practitioner. In most instances, the practitioner finds that these devices are much more effective when an extrinsic forefoot or rearfoot post, or both, are added. This may be accomplished in the office utilizing a variety of readily available materials such as cork or rubber.

The following four devices represent some of the earliest attempts at correcting the pediatric flatfoot. Although they are not used as extensively as they previously were, they are still available and remain the treatment of choice for some practitioners. Of note is the fact that some of the principles employed in their development exist as standard modifications on today's functional foot orthoses.

Whitman plate. This was developed by Royal Whitman in 1907 and was considered a "corrective device for abnormal foot pronation." The device was originally fashioned of metal with a high medial flange extending to the first metatarsophalangeal joint and a short lateral flange (Fig. 20-24). When a child with an everted calcaneus stepped on the device, the lateral flange tilted the device upward so that the medial flange was driven into the talar head. This forced the wearer to contract the posterior tibial, flexor hallucis longus, and flexor digitorum longus muscles in an attempt to relieve the pain. It was believed that this would function to increase muscle tone and strength. This theory was based on the commonly held physiologic belief at that time, which stated that the muscles were the primary weightbearing supports of the arch. If the physiologically weak muscles could be strengthened, then the device could ultimately be discontinued. The Whitman plate as originally designed was never widely utilized due to the discomfort it caused.[1,23] However, the concept of elevated medial and lateral flanges was

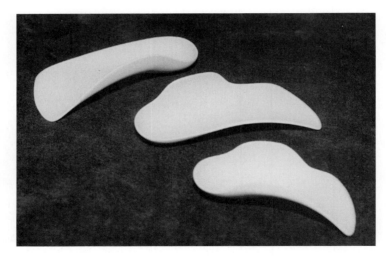

Fig. 20-24. *Left:* Whitman plate. *Center:* Roberts brace. *Right:* Whitman-Roberts plate.

instrumental in leading to the higher heel cups used in subsequent devices.

Roberts brace. This was developed by Percy Willard Roberts who followed the conceptual design initiated by Royal Whitman. Roberts recognized the difficulty of utilizing the uncomfortable Whitman brace and attempted to improve supination of the foot by cupping the calcaneus and forcing it to invert (Fig. 20-24). Although better-tolerated and more effective than other devices, the Roberts brace does not address or support either the arch or forefoot area of the foot. This device most likely represents the first attempt at developing a true heel stabilizer.

Shaffer plate. This type of device represents one of the original methods of attempting to utilize an insert that more closely contoured the foot's plantar surface. Based on the Whitman plate, the device originally encompassed a medial arch flange, but only to the midnavicular area. This device is not commonly utilized, as it functions primarily as an arch support. It should be utilized only in those cases where minimal control is required.

Whitman-Roberts plate. This type of device evolved from the previously described devices. It originally incorporated the higher medial arch flange of the original Whitman plate and the higher lateral flange of the Roberts plate (see Fig. 20-24). It generally functions by restricting abnormal motion through the rigidity of its flanges, as opposed to improving abnormal foot function as in treatment with functional foot orthoses.[26,35]

Heel stabilizers

Over the years, a variety of devices aimed at specifically restricting subtalar joint pronation by reducing frontal plane motion of the calcaneus have

been developed. The classic form of therapy for restricting marked degrees of calcaneal eversion has evolved around the use of heel stabilizers. There are five different types of heel stabilizers available: types A, B, C, D, and E. They are generally fabricated of fiberglass or polypropylene. Each device incorporates high medial and lateral flanges which extend to points just inferior to the malleoli. Their aggressive flanges makes them particularly useful in the younger patient with a significant degree of subtalar joint pronation associated with marked calcaneal eversion. The devices are generally better tolerated by the early walker and young child as opposed to the adolescent or adult. In cases of extreme eversion, as seen in ligamentous laxity or residual talipes calcaneovalgus deformities, the device may prove more beneficial than a standard type of functional foot orthosis. In cases of unrestricted eversion, there is a tendency for the calcaneus to slide off a standard functional foot orthosis even if a deeper heel cup is utilized. The heel stabilizer generally functions best in conjunction with a stiff-countered shoe. It is my opinion that when a heel stabilizer is poorly tolerated, ineffective in restricting significant degrees of abnormal pronation, or unsuccessful in alleviating symptoms, then the child may be considered a candidate for surgical intervention.[24,41,42]

Type A stabilizer. This device is utilized primarily to decrease abnormal subtalar joint pronation with associated excessive calcaneal eversion. It functions by firmly grasping the medial and lateral borders of the calcaneus, thereby limiting frontal plane motion of the rearfoot. This does not address any specific forefoot deformity and is therefore limited in its overall application.

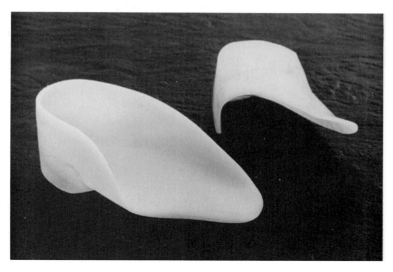

Fig. 20-25. Type C heel stabilizer.

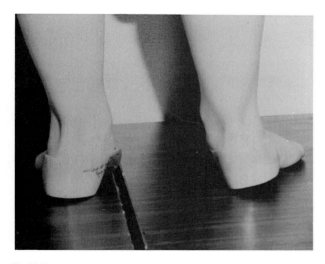

Fig. 20-26. Four-year-old child with marked calcaneal eversion secondary to congenital gastrocnemius equinus. Inability to alter foot function or symptoms using conservative measures resulted in surgical lengthening of the tendon.

Type B stabilizer. This device combines the principles of the type A stabilizer along with an attempt to control both the midfoot and forefoot. The device extends distally to the metatarsal heads and is similar to a functional foot orthosis in size and dimensions. An extended medial flange extends beyond the talonavicular joint. This type of device is useful for mild to moderately pronated foot types and is constructed over a neutral-position suspension cast. It is my belief that other devices described in this section, specifically the Root functional foot orthosis and the Blake inverted orthosis, are superior to this device in controlling moderate degrees of flexible pes planus deformities.

Type C stabilizer. In cases where moderate-to-severe flexible flatfoot conditions exist, this type of stabilizer may be beneficial. The type C stabilizer has a medial flange that extends distally along the entire medial aspect of the foot to the level of the first metatarsophalangeal joint. The extended lateral flange extends to just proximal to the fifth metatarsophalangeal joint (Fig. 20-25). This device is useful in restricting frontal plane motion of the calcaneus as well as excessive transverse plane movement of the forefoot relative to the rearfoot. This device is also fabricated over a neutral-position suspension cast. If severe pronation forces are not capable of being addressed with this device, then the practitioner should carefully note the extent and level of any complicating factors. Typically, the child who does not improve with this type of heel stabilizer may be best served by surgical intervention (Fig. 20-26).

Type D stabilizer. See Gait Plate, below.

Type E stabilizer. See Gait Plate, below.

Root functional foot orthosis

This device was developed by Merton Root in an attempt to improve foot function by addressing specific musculoskeletal and joint deformities. The goal of the Root functional foot orthosis is to maintain both subtalar and midtarsal joint stability by addressing leg, rearfoot, and forefoot deformities. The device is designed to function in a dynamic fashion during the heel contact, midstance, and propulsive phases of gait. This device represents the first truly functional type of foot orthosis to be utilized for the correction of a host of lower extremity disorders (Fig. 20-27). The device is

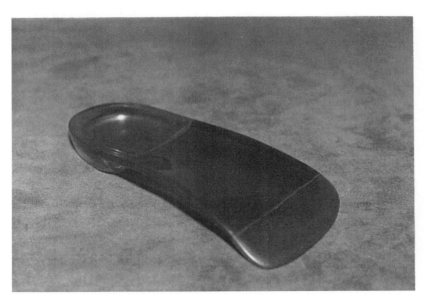

Fig. 20-27. Root functional foot orthosis.

fashioned over a properly obtained neutral-position off-weightbearing cast of the foot. The cast should correspond with whatever forefoot varus or valgus deformities were noted in the musculoskeletal examination and should be appropriately corrected with intrinsic or extrinsic posting. Rearfoot posting, either flat or inverted by 4 or 6 degrees with appropriate motion added, is generally prescribed to assist in controlling heel contact pronation. Although the device was originally fabricated of rohadur, it is now made from a host of materials including polypropylene, graphite, and graphite composites. When utilizing this device in the pediatric patient with a flexible flatfoot condition, several considerations must be addressed. Because the device functions at specific points in the gait cycle, it is generally advised that treatment be initiated when the child develops a propulsive or heel-to-toe type of gait pattern. This typically occurs at the age of 3 or 4 years, and corresponds to the child's ability to climb upstairs or downstairs without having to keep both feet on each step.[41,42] However, one should be sensitive to the fact that excessive calcaneal eversion may often be identified in the beginning walker. In these cases, whatever device is successful in maintaining the foot in a more normal position should be utilized as soon as possible. Since the previously described wedges and over-the-counter devices are inadequate in treating severe deformities, heel stabilizers or functional foot orthoses may be utilized even prior to the age of 3 or 4 years.

When treating the pediatric patient with the Root type of functional foot orthosis, the parent should be advised that the device will lose its effectiveness as the child's foot grows and develops. As a rule, this type of device is generally replaced when the child has grown the equivalent of two full shoe sizes. This generally corresponds to the distal margin of the orthosis reaching the midshaft portion of the metatarsals. Additionally, the heel cup will also be narrower at this point as well. Because of this, most root type devices will last approximately 2 years.

Functional foot orthoses should be changed whenever any of the following occur:

1. The device reaches the midshaft portion of the metatarsals.
2. The soft tissue surrounding the calcaneus is no longer properly seated in the heel cup.
3. The child complains of pain caused by the device.
4. The parents note an alteration in the gait pattern.
5. The practitioner notes an alteration in the gait pattern.
6. There is a return of the original symptoms if these in fact were the presenting concern.

Careful monitoring of the pediatric patient utilizing functional foot orthoses includes follow-up visits every 6 months. This results in an appropriate and timely change of the device when necessary. If the device is used specifically to treat a severe flexible flatfoot deformity, care should be taken to eliminate any excessive degree of structural forefoot varus or soft tissue supinatus angulation affecting

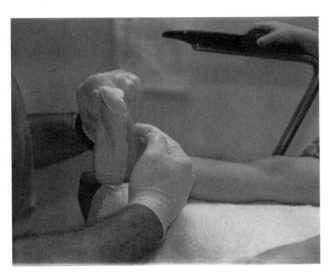

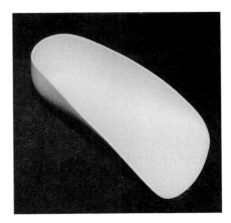

Fig. 20-29. UCBL device.

Fig. 20-28. Appropriate hand position used in obtaining a negative cast in a pediatric patient. Note that the right hand is placing a mild plantarflexing force on the medial column of the child's foot.

the longitudinal axis of the midtarsal joint. If the full complement of the inverted deformity is captured and then "corrected" by intrinsic or extrinsic forefoot posting, the deformity will be forcibly maintained by the orthosis. It is believed that if this occurs, the device will in fact be capable of inhibiting normal frontal plane rotation and development of the forefoot. To avoid this, the practitioner should place a mild plantarflexion force on the medial column of the child's foot. This force should be placed dorsal to the first and second metatarsal cuneiform articulations (Fig. 20-28), and should result in a marked decrease in the measurable inverted forefoot position. Additionally, this assists in artificially increasing the medial arch of both the negative and positive casts, thereby leading to a greater degree of medial column plantarflexion.[23]

Additional modifications for the Root type of orthosis for this deformity include having the device poured in an inverted fashion, thereby increasing the varus cant of the rearfoot. This procedure should be noted on the orthotic prescription sheet and should be carried out by the orthotic laboratory. Typically, the degree of inversion may range from 5 to 10 degrees. Additionally, higher medial and lateral heel cups up to 25 mm deep may be requested. A long rearfoot post with a medial flange or outflare may also be requested in an attempt to decrease excessive frontal plane motion of the foot. The combination of these modifications proves effective in maintaining the child's foot in a more normal and stable position. In cases where there is insufficient correction achieved with these modifications, the practitioner should consider the use of

an inverted orthosis (see Blake Inverted Orthosis, below).

In cases where a child is being treated for an angle-of-gait deformity associated with a flexible pes planus, the practitioner should caution the parents regarding the eventual cosmetic effect of the device.[14] Owing to the axis of motion of the subtalar joint, any limitation of frontal plane eversion of the calcaneus will result in a similar increase in adduction of the forefoot. Therefore, if the abnormal subtalar joint pronation and calcaneal eversion are properly controlled, the result will be that of a vertical calcaneus with increased adduction of the forefoot. Conversely, one should note that a similar situation occurs in cases of an inverted calcaneus with an adducted gait. This situation is generally caused by a high degree of forefoot valgus which is inadequately compensated through the longitudinal axis of the midtarsal joint. In these cases, the rearfoot becomes markedly inverted to allow the lateral column of the foot to contact the ground. As rearfoot supination and calcaneal inversion occur, an accompanying marked adduction of the forefoot may be noted. In this instance, the functional foot orthosis not only allows the calcaneus to function more closely to the perpendicular by elevating the lateral column of the foot, but it will also improve the cosmetic appearance of the foot by increasing the abducted position of the forefoot.

UCBL (University of California Biomechanics Laboratory)

In 1967 this device was developed at the University of California Biomechanics Laboratory in San Francisco for the treatment of flexible flatfoot conditions.[1,21] The device is fashioned over a weight-bearing impression of the foot and is typically fabricated from thin, lightweight, semirigid polypropylene. In its present form, the device has been

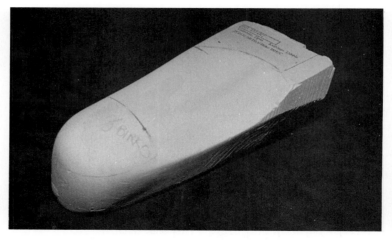

Fig. 20-30. Plaster correction for 25 degrees inverted orthoses.

utilized for all types and forms of flexible flatfoot conditions. It is essentially a combination of the Whitman-Roberts plate and the type C heel stabilizer. The device has high medial and lateral flanges which are joined in the heel area to form a deep heel cup (Fig. 20-29). The flanges extend distally to an area just proximal to the metatarsophalangeal joints. The device is used extensively in the treatment of flexible flatfoot deformities. Its deep flanges and heel cup have also made it the treatment of choice for the more significant forms of pes planus, as seen in various neuromuscular diseases. Because of this, the device has attained widespread use for the treatment of apropulsive and pronated feet in children with cerebral palsy. Overall, its success depends on its ability to restrict abnormal motion rather than by initiating normal movement and function, as is provided by the Root type of device. Unfortunately, its design and bulk make it difficult to utilize comfortably in most shoes.

Blake inverted orthosis

This device was initially developed to counteract the marked degrees of abnormal subtalar joint pronation in runners and other recreational athletes. The unique mechanics of running coupled with its predilection toward greater degrees of foot pronation has made treatment of many running-related injuries extremely challenging.[3,4] Although practitioners were able to effectively alter the abnormal forces encountered in those patients with the Root type of functional foot orthosis, the overall results were often less than satisfactory.

The Blake device represents an aggressive correction of the standard off-weightbearing neutral-position cast. The key to the success of this device lies in its ability to effectively invert the rearfoot using a marked plaster modification to the heel,

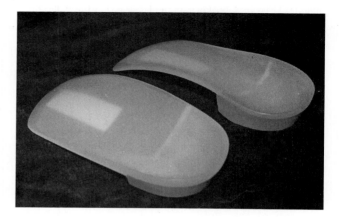

Fig. 20-31. Blake inverted orthoses. Note deep heel cups and flat rearfoot posts.

arch, and forefoot area of the positive cast (Fig. 20-30). The completed cast may be inverted to any desired degree, with 25 degrees being the standard. Corrections of as little as 15 degrees to as great as 75 degrees may be utilized. When fabricated properly, the device contours to the medial longitudinal arch. Because of this, there is seldom a tendency to develop any degree of lateral ankle instability. As a rule, this device is capable of correcting an everted calcaneus at an approximate ratio of a 5:1 correction up to 5 degrees of eversion. Therefore, when attempting to correct a 5 degrees everted calcaneus, a 25 degrees inverted orthosis should be utilized. If calcaneal eversion is above 5 degrees, then a 7:1 ratio appears more appropriate. For example, a 7 degrees everted calcaneus should be corrected via a 50 degrees inverted orthosis. As a rule, pediatric patients generally require greater correction for the same degree of calcaneal eversion as seen in an adult patient. This is due to the marked degree of inherent

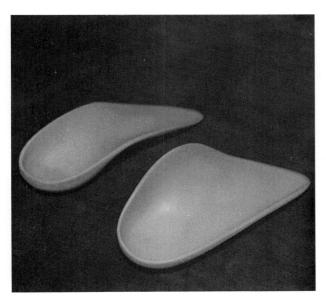

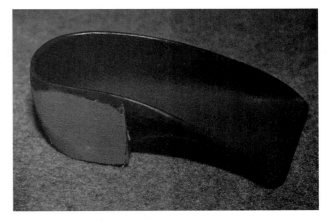

Fig. 20-33. Type D heel stabilizer, to promote foot abduction during gait.

Fig. 20-32. *Left:* In-toe gait plate, to promote foot adduction during gait. *Right:* Out-toe gait plate, to promote foot abduction during gait.

flexibility and increased subtalar joint range of motion.

In addition to the plaster modifications previously described, the device also benefits from some additional standard features. These include an accommodative plantar fascial groove, an increased heel cup height of approximately 25 mm, and a flat rearfoot post, all of which increase the overall antipronation effects of the device (Fig. 20-31). Since the Blake device controls abnormal foot function through its inverted heel cup rather than by maintaining an inverted or everted forefoot correction, it generally may be utilized for a longer period of time than the standard Root functional foot orthosis. Additionally, the depth and shape of the heel cup will generally accommodate the developing child's foot for a longer period of time. For these reasons, it is not unusual for a Blake type of functional foot orthosis to function effectively for a minimum of 3 years in a developing child. For a complete discussion of the applications of this device, see Chapter 22.

Gait plates

This is a rigid type of orthotic device which has been employed for years in an attempt to physically alter the appearance of an adducted or abducted gait pattern. Although gait plates have been utilized primarily to effect a cosmetic alteration of an abnormal gait pattern, they are also capable of effectively placing a stretching motion on tight capsular ligamentous and tendinous structures. Gait plates may be fashioned to promote either in-toeing or out-toeing (Fig. 20-32).

The most commonly utilized device is the outtoeing type of gait plate, which may be utilized in cases where abnormal foot adduction is caused by an internal femoral torsion or position, or an internal tibial torsion or position. The effect of the device is related to its ability to angulate the fashion in which the ball of the foot bends within the shoe. The gait plates should be rigid and the shoe flexible in order to achieve the desired result.[26,43] The device is fabricated with a lateral flange that extends beyond the fourth and fifth metatarsophalangeal joints to approximately the level of the distal interphalangeal joints of the fourth and fifth digits. No portion of the device extends plantar to the other metatarsophalangeal joints. In its original form, the device was fashioned from a flat piece of metal or plastic and conformed to an outline of the patient's shoe. No attempt was made to support or control the rearfoot with a heel cup or extrinsic posting.

The device effects angular changes in gait by altering propulsion of the foot. In gait, weight stresses pass along the lateral aspect of the foot across the metatarsals and then move distally out through the hallux. When the patient utilizing an out-toed gait plate attempts to push off over the lateral aspect of the foot during propulsion, the distal-lateral flange inhibits that motion. The foot therefore falls medially to allow dorsiflexion at the first, second, and third metatarsophalangeal joints. As this occurs, the net effect is that the forefoot is forced to abduct. As greater pronation occurs, a greater amount of abduction is generated. Therefore, the child's shoe cannot break at a right angle to the direction of walking unless the foot toes out. Toeing off the lateral aspect of the foot is not possible and ultimately requires external pivoting of the limb in propulsion.

Although the gait plate will improve the appear-

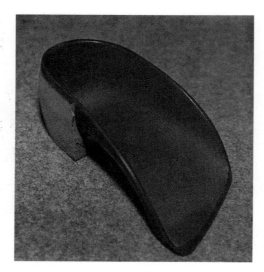

Fig. 20-34. Type E heel stabilizer, to promote foot adduction during gait.

ing the overall cosmetic appearance of the foot in gait. A recent modification which I have prescribed with success is a Blake type of inverted orthosis incorporating a standard type of lateral out-toe flange. Overall, this type of device is superior to the type D gait plate in its ability to control abnormal subtalar and midtarsal joint compensatory pronation.[43] Additionally, the lateral out-toe flange is most effective in promoting some degree of cosmetic change in the appearance of the gait pattern. Generally speaking, this type of device is better tolerated than the type D heel stabilizer and the control point affecting the calcaneus is less obtrusive than the antipronation effect created by the stabilizer's higher heel cup.

Although adducted gait patterns are cosmetically and functionally undesirable, the practitioner should also be concerned about significant out-toe or abducted gait patterns. This type of problem may be associated with an external femoral torsion or position, an external tibial torsion or position or, in some cases, with an occult unilateral or bilateral dysplasia of the hip. In those instances where a marked unilateral external foot and leg position is noted, care must be taken to rule out a congenitally dislocated hip. Externally rotated limbs generally cause a child to initiate ambulation at a later stage of development and most typically promote a significant apropulsive, pronated type of gait. In these instances, the force of gravity falls medial to the subtalar joint axis of motion and leads to marked subtalar joint and midtarsal joint pronation with associated forefoot abduction. In cases such as this, the out-toe type of gait plate improves both the angle of gait and limits the degree of subtalar and midtarsal joint pronation. The device is fashioned so that the angulation of the anterior aspect of the gait plate tapers immediately from the hallux interphalangeal joint to a point proximal and lateral to the fifth metatarsal head (Fig. 20-34). This functions like the out-toe type of gait plate in that it alters the flexing point of the foot by limiting motion of the metatarsophalangeal joints. With limitation of joint motion at the medial three metatarsophalangeal joints, the child's foot is forced to roll laterally in the propulsive phase of gait. The result is that the foot adducts and supinates as well. A standard in-toe type of gait plate may be constructed similarly to the out-toe type of gait plate previously described, with the exception of the flange placement. One type of out-toe gait plate is the type E heel stabilizer. This device incorporates a long medial flange that extends distal to the first, second, and third metatarsophalangeal joints. As in the standard type of out-toe gait plate, this device forces the foot to roll out early during the gait cycle. In turn, this initiates

ance of the child's gait and may minimally stretch some soft tissue structures about the hip, care must be exercised because the device will increase pronation. More recently, the device has been fabricated over a neutral-position cast of the child's foot. In this fashion, some contouring in control of the rearfoot may be accomplished. The device may be prescribed in cases where there is minimal eversion present and one wants to primarily alter the angle of gait. This type of device is generally referred to as a reverse Roberts plate. An additional modification of the device was accomplished with the development of the type D heel stabilizer.[26,43] This device not only enlarged the lateral flange but also incorporated an aggressive medial and lateral rearfoot flange. This further confined the heel and supported the talonavicular joint (Fig. 20-33). One must note that as this device attempts to both abduct the foot and control excessive pronation, significant cosmetic improvement of the foot in gait may not be evidenced. As previously noted, alterations in frontal plane positioning of the calcaneus result in transverse plane alteration of the forefoot as well. As a general rule, every degree of calcaneal eversion that is controlled by an orthosis results in an increased adduction of the foot to that same degree (e.g., 6 degrees of calcaneal eversion that is controlled by a functional foot orthosis to a perpendicular position adducts the foot by approximately 6 degrees). Whereas a standard orthosis would further adduct the foot when placing the calcaneus in a perpendicular position, a type D heel stabilizer maintains the child's foot to the same degree of adduction, but with a perpendicular calcaneus. Overall, this stabilizes the function of the child's foot without negatively influenc-

supination of the foot. This type of device is generally most effective when treating the previously noted external deformities. In cases where marked abduction and calcaneal eversion is present, a Blake type of inverted orthosis incorporating the distal medial flange is more appropriate.

Summary

It is essential that today's healthcare practitioner be capable of carefully diagnosing pediatric lower extremity developmental disorders. Because the child's foot remains adaptable and plastic during the first 7 or 8 years of development, every effort should be made to allow the osseous and soft tissue structures to develop normally. When utilizing any of the splints, braces, and shoe or orthotic devices described in this chapter, the goal should be directed toward that end. In some instances, early initiation of a treatment plan will result in an improvement of gait and the development of a normally functioning lower extremity. In other cases, the deformity may persist because of the extent of its severity or because treatment was delayed until an older age. In those cases, functional foot orthoses are the treatment of choice and generally represent a lifelong treatment plan. In those instances, parents should be assured that the devices will be capable of decreasing the likelihood of such common lower extremity deformities as patellofemoral dysfunction, heel spur syndrome, plantar fasciitis, hallux abductovalgus, and hammer toe deformities.[42]

It is hoped that the appropriate use of the devices presented in this chapter will allow the practitioner to provide effective and efficient care for his or her pediatric patients.

References

1. American Academy of Orthopedic Surgeons: *Atlas of orthotics: biomechanical principles and application,* St Louis, 1975, Mosby–Year Book, p 232.
2. Bell JF, Grice DS: Treatment of congenital talipes equinovarus with the modified Denis Browne splint, *J Bone Joint Surg* 26:803, 1944.
3. Blake RB, Ferguson H: Foot orthosis for the severe flatfoot in sports, *J Am Podiatr Med Assoc* 81:10, 1991.
4. Blake RL: Inverted orthotic technique, *J Am Podiatr Med Assoc* 76:275, 1986.
5. Bluhm M: Modification of the Denis Browne splint, *J Bone Joint Surg* 29:767, 1946.
6. Blumenfield I, Kaplan N, Hicks EO: The conservative treatment of congenital talipes equinovarus, *J Bone Joint Surg* 28:248, 1946.
7. Bordelon RL: Correction of hypermobile flatfoot in children by molded insert, *Foot Ankle* 1:143, 1980.
8. Brachman P: *Foot therapy for children,* Chicago, 1966, Podiatry Books, p 106.
9. Brachman P: In-toeing and out-toeing in infants and children, *J Am Podiatr Assoc* 49:111, 1959.
10. Browne D: Talipes equinovarus, *Lancet* 2:969, 1934.
11. Browne D: Splinting for controlled movement, *Clin Orthop* 8:94, 1956.
12. Bunch WH, Reagy ND: *Principles of orthotic treatment,* St Louis, 1976, Mosby–Year Book, p 41.
13. Chong A: *Is your child walking right?,* Wheaton, Ill, Wheaton Resource Corp.
14. Connolly J, Regen E, Hillman JW: Pigeon toes and flatfeet, *Pediatr Clin North Am* 17:301, 1978.
15. Crane L: Femoral torsion of the lower extremity. *Am J Phys Anthropal* 3:255, 1945.
16. CRS, *Pediatric Counter Rotational System, clinical prospectus,* Deer Park, NY, 1982, Langer Biomechanics Group.
17. DeValentine S: *Foot and ankle disorders in children,* New York, 1992, Churchill Livingstone.
18. Elftman H: Torsion of the lower extremity, *Am J Phys Anthropol* 3:255, 1945.
19. Fabry G, MacEwen GD, Shandshards AR, Jr: Torsion of the femur: a follow-up study in the normal and abnormal conditions. *J Bone Joint Surg [Am]* 55:726, 1973.
20. Ganley JV: Calcaneovalgus deformity in infants, *J Am Podiatr Med Assoc* 65:407, 1975.
21. Henderson WH, Campbell JW: *UCBL—Shoe insert casting and fabrication,* Technical Report 53, Biomechanics Laboratory, University of California at San Francisco and Berkeley, 1967.
22. Kennedy JM: *Orthopedic splints and appliances,* London, 1974, Bailliere Tindall, pp 106,128.
23. Kirby KA, Green DR: Evaluation and non-operative management of pes valgus foot. In De Valentine (ed): *Ankle disorders in children,* New York, 1992, Churchill Livingstone, pp 295–327.
24. Levitz ST, Whiteside LS, Fitzgerald T: Biomechanical foot therapy. In Scurran B: *Clinics in podiatry—applied biomechanics,* Philadelphia, 1984, WB Saunders, pp 721–735.
25. Lynch ER: The Ganley splint, *Clin Podiatr* 1:517, 1984.
26. McCrea JD: *Pediatric orthopedics of the lower extremity,* Mt Kisco, NY, 1985, Futura.
27. Moore JW, editor: *Clinical orthopedic handbook,* ed 2, Chicago, 1978, William School College of Podiatric Medicine, p 61.
28. Nigg BM, editor: *Biomechanics of running shoes,* Champaign, Ill, 1986, Human Kinetics.
29. Redford J: *Orthotics etcetera,* ed 2, Baltimore, 1980, Williams & Wilkins, p 346.
30. Root ML: A discussion of biomechanical considerations for treatment of the infant foot, *Arch Podiatr Med Foot Surg* 1:41, 1973.
31. Root ML, Orien UP, Weed JH: *Normal and abnormal function of the foot,* Los Angeles, 1971, Clinical Biomechanics.
32. Schuster RD: In-toe and out-toe and its implications, *Arch Podiatr Med Foot Surg* 3:28, 1976.
33. Schuster RO: A history of orthopedics in podiatry, *J Am Podiatr Med Assoc* 64:332, 1974.
34. Sgarlato TE: *A compendium of podiatric biomechanics,* San Francisco, 1971, California College of Podiatric Medicine.
35. Spencer AM, Person VA: Casting and orthotics for children. In *Clinics in podiatry: symposium on podopediatrics,* Philadelphia, 1984, WB Saunders.
36. Tachdjian MO, editor: *Pediatric Orthopedics,* Philadelphia, 1972, WB Saunders, pp 1277, 1323, 1331.
37. Tax HR: Dangers posed to the hips of infants by counter splints used to treat internal rotation of the legs, *J Am Podiatr Assoc* 65:54, 1975.
38. Tax HR: *Podopediatrics,* ed 2, Baltimore, 1985, Williams & Wilkins, pp 314, 373.
39. Thomson SA: Treatment of congenital talipes equinovarus

with a modification of the Denis Browne method and splint, *J Bone Joint Surg* 24:291, 1942.

40. Tracy HW: Treatment of congenital metatarsus varus with Denis Browne splints, *South Med J* 61:939, 1968.
41. Valmassy RL: Biomechanical evaluation of the child, *Clin Podiatr Med Surg* 1:563, 1984.
42. Valmassy RL: Torsional and frontal plane conditions of the lower extremities. In Thompson, P: *Introduction to podopediatrics,* London, 1993, WB Saunders, pp 27–46.
43. Valmassy RL: The use of gait plates for in-toed and out-toed deformities, *Clin Podiatr Med Surg* 11:211-217, 1994.
44. Valmassy RL, Lipe L, Falconer R: Pediatric treatment mo-
dalities of the lower extremity, *J Am Podiatr Med Assoc* 78:69–80, 1988.
45. Valmassy RL, Terrafranca N: The triplane wedge, *J Am Podiatr Med Assoc* 76:12, 1986.
46. Wenger DO, Mauldin D, Speck G, et al: Corrective shoes and inserts as treatment for flexible flatfoot in infants and children, *J Bone Joint Surg [Am]* 71:800, 1989.
47. Whitman R: The importance of positive support in the curative treatment of weak feet and a comparison of the means employed to assure it, *Am J Orthop Surg* 11:215, 1913.
48. Whitman R: Observations of forty-five cases of flatfoot with particular reference to etiology and treatment, *Boston Med Surg J* 118:598, 1898.

athletic shoes

Jane A. Denton, DPM

Running
Cycling
Downhill skiing
Soccer
Football
Baseball
Tennis
Basketball
Dance
Summary

The design and construction of athletic shoes depends on the particular kinetic and physical demands of the sport for which they are worn. Over the years, shoes have evolved, as have technology, playing surfaces, habits of the population, and knowledge of the biomechanics of a sport. Footwear for running, skiing, cycling, soccer, football, baseball, tennis, basketball, skating, and several forms of dance are examined in this chapter. The movements of a sport, recurrent injuries that might be sustained, the terrain on which the sport is played, and the equipment used are all factors in the design and construction of athletic shoes.

Running

Relative to other sports, much research has been done on the biomechanics of running and on running shoes. The mechanics of sprinting differ from those of distance running. There is also much individual variation in running style and biomechanical efficiency. Classically, the long-distance heel-striker lands on the lateral heel with the foot supinated. Very quickly, the foot pronates, absorbing shock in response to ground reaction force. Weight is transferred from laterally toward medially as the midfoot and forefoot load. In the propulsive phase of running, the heel lifts off the ground as the foot resupinates, becoming a rigid lever. During moderate speed running on flat terrain, ground reaction force reaches two to three times body weight. Running downhill or changing running style or shoes may also affect the magnitude of the ground reaction force.[5]

The long-distance running shoe should help control excessive motion and attenuate shock in running. For the person who pronates abnormally, certain features are recommended. The heel counter, usually made of plastic, should be firm when squeezed. If it extends medially or there is an additional external heel counter, it reinforces pronation control. Higher-density material in the medial midsole resists the pressure and motion of pronation. An insole board adds torsional rigidity to the shoe. If the insole board is full-length, it is also known as full board–lasted. If there is no insole board it may be called slip-lasted. If the insole board extends only proximal to the forefoot, it is known as combination-lasted.

Shoes should be tried on at the end of the day when the foot may be somewhat swollen. Any pads, socks, or inserts used while running should be worn when selecting the shoe. Often there is inconsistency among the shoe companies as to what is considered a standard size. Even within the same company, the sizing may not be consistent from year to year or from model to model. In fact, the athlete's foot itself changes over time, widening and lengthening as soft tissue structures stretch with use. Thus, trying on the shoe for fit is essential before purchase. On standing, there should be a thumb's-width distance between the end of the longest toe and the end of the shoe. When one foot is slightly bigger than the other, fit the bigger foot.

A stable well-fitted shoe enhances motion control leading to fewer overuse injuries such as tendinitis. Wearing orthoses in running shoes may help with motion control problems, but occasionally orthoses can create fit problems in the shoe. The presence of the orthosis adds volume to the shoe and places the heel slightly higher in the shoe. Minor adjustments to the orthosis, removing the insole of the shoe, and purchasing a shoe with a deeper heel counter help alleviate the problem. If possible, purchase the shoe after getting orthoses, not before, in order to ensure a good fit.

The fit of the shoe is critical. An ill-fitting shoe can produce injuries such as blisters, black toenails, corns, ingrown toenails, and pressure irritation. Because most running shoes are made for men, women have a more limited selection, especially if they have small or narrow feet. Some companies offer shoes in several widths. Variable width lacing, with widely spaced eyelets that cinch a shoe around a narrow foot, may help. Adding more fill inside a shoe, such as a flat insole, may also help. Many women with a wide forefoot, but narrow heel, opt for the wider shoe to avoid pressure irritation, but consequently have heel slippage problems. A partial solution might be a tongue pad, padding the heel collar, changing the lacing pattern (thus tightening the heel collar) or the use of a forefoot insole. If the foot is still too wide for the shoe in the forefoot, the stitching on the foxing over the upper in the area of pressure can be released without compromising the longevity of the shoe. In cases where no modification works, running shoes can also be custom-made.

Shoe construction is important in dealing with certain running injuries. In Achilles tendinitis, there needs to be sufficient lift in the rearfoot compared to the forefoot (at least 5/8 in. higher in the rearfoot). Shoes with thin midsoles and a low heel raise should be avoided or heel lifts should be inserted. Those prone to ankle sprains should avoid a high lift or a shoe worn excessively laterally. The athlete with recurrent stress fractures should not wear a shoe with an old compressed midsole and the shoe should help control abnormal pronation. For athletes with pain in the ball of the foot, sufficient padding in the insole with a supportive firm midsole works well.

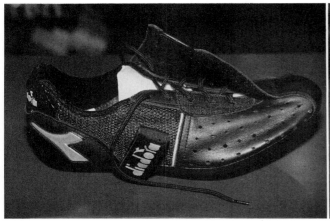 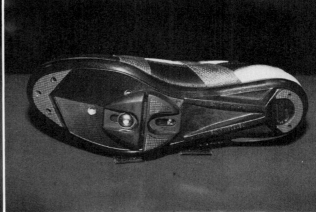

Fig. 21-1. A, Cleated cycling shoe. **B,** Cleat on cycling shoe.

Different training habits may require different shoes and insoles. A trail runner might prefer running in a trail shoe with a heavier tread for better traction and less slippage. A faster, competitive runner may want to train in racing flats on hard workout days. These flats are running shoes with far less cushion and support than the average training shoe. The midsoles in the racing flats are thinner, the cut of the shoe is narrower, and the height of the heel counter is lower. If orthoses are used in racing flats or cleats, a full-length orthosis might be recommended for motion control in the forefoot as the runner lands on and pushes off the ball of the foot. In this situation, orthoses of softer materials are often better-tolerated because of the flexibility of the device and its ability to contour to the foot. However, the orthosis needs to be sufficiently narrow to fit the thin, shallow racing shoe.

Cycling

Cycling shoes are currently categorized into cleated, clipless, mountain bike, and touring shoes, although several of these categories may overlap. Cleated shoes are generally used with road or racing bicycles (Fig. 21-1A). The uppers are a combination of vented leather and mesh with laces or Velcro over a tongue cinching the shoe on the foot. Occasionally a dual closure (Velcro straps over laces) system is used. The toe box is quite rigid to protect the toes against the toe clip attached to the pedal. The outsole is lightweight and very rigid so as to minimize wasted motion in the foot and maximize the power from the hip and thigh directed into the bike pedal.[3] The cleat is attached to the outsole under the ball of the foot (Fig. 21-1B). There is about 10 to 15 degrees of play in the cleat position to accommodate variation in individual anatomy in the transverse plane. A small

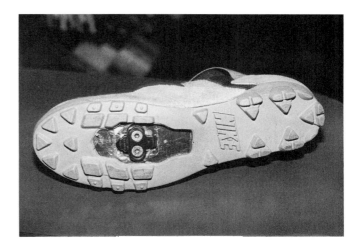

Fig. 21-2. Recessed clipless shoe.

metal rise on a standard pedal engages the horizontal linear recess in the cleat. The toe clip has a leather band which when tightened across the cleated shoe and foot secures it on the pedal, increasing the efficiency of the stroke, especially the upstroke.[3] For some cyclists the cleat and toe clip system feels harder to disengage than the clipless system. The prominence of the cleat on the plantar aspect of the shoe is awkward for walking and walking on it eventually wears down the cleat. The rigid sole does not bend, as does a walking shoe.

A number of clipless bike shoe models are available. One early model by Look (Salt Lake City, UT) uses a mechanism similar to ski bindings for disengaging the foot and shoe from the bike pedal. The bike shoe is fitted with specific hardware on the outersole and clicks into a compatible pedal. By twisting the heel away from the bike, the shoe disengages from the pedal. The mechanism also has

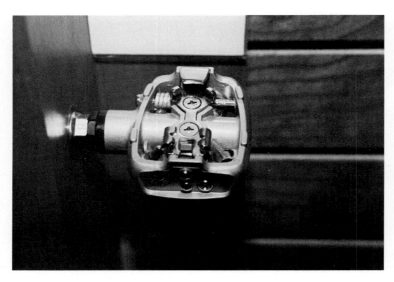

Fig. 21-3. Compatible clipless pedal.

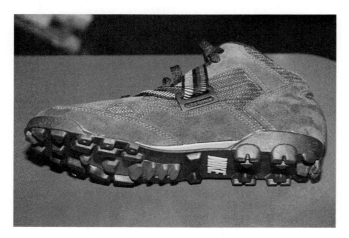

Fig. 21-4. Mountain bike shoe with clipless system and tread.

a screw which when tightened or loosened can change how tightly the shoe is held onto the pedal. Ten to 15 degrees of play is also available in this clipless system to allow for individual anatomic variation in the transverse plane. Because of the many clipless shoes on the market, some models are often compatible with other brands. The specific hardware to be applied to the sole of the shoe is purchased as part of the pedal system. Shimano (Irvine, Calif.) (Figs. 21-2 and 21-3) has a system in which the affixed hardware is recessed into the depth of the shoe so that there is no bulky prominence on the plantar aspect when walking.

In sports where the shoe is rigid, such as road cycling, skiing, and skating, a full-length rigid orthosis can be used. Because of the very snug fit of these shoes, in-shoe casting or tracings of the insole and pitch of the shank may be necessary for exact contour match between the orthosis and the shoe.

Mountain bike shoes are generally not cleated because of the necessity of getting on and off the bike quickly in uneven or steep terrain. Instead they are usually clipless with a specially designed outsole. (Fig. 21-4). Other mountain shoes have transverse ridges which grip but do not engage the pedal, as do the shoes of the clipless system. The design of the outsole usually has a moderate amount of tread to negotiate walking on trails. The outsole tends to be less stiff than racing or road bike shoes and easier to walk on. The upper may be a combination synthetic mesh with suede or leather foxing which often comes in a midcut height. The upper may have Velcro straps or ties or a combination of the two for cinching the foot into the shoe.

Touring shoes are often used on road bikes. They have neither cleats nor the clipless mechanisms. The upper is usually low-cut, vented leather or suede combined with mesh. The outsole is semirigid enabling the touring cyclist who might also tour occasionally on foot to walk more comfortably. They are generally comfortable but less efficient cycling shoes.

Downhill skiing

Downhill skiing is one of the most popular winter sports. A rigid plastic ski boot holds the foot and ankle tightly dorsiflexed. With knees bent and body weight shifted forward, the skier maintains balance and control by exerting ever-changing pressure through the boot bound onto skis, which cut and glide through the snow. Ski boots are molded rigid polyurethane shells which encase the foot and come up to the lower shin. There is a selection of front-entry, rear-entry, and midentry (hybrid) boots (Figs. 21-5, 21-6, and 21-7). The front entry boot shell

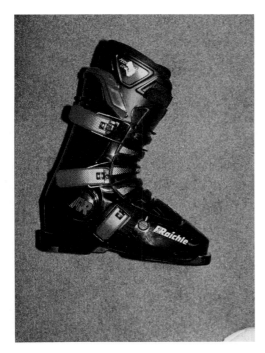

Fig. 21-5. Front-entry ski boot.

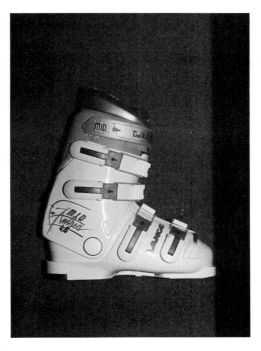

Fig. 21-7. Midentry ski boot.

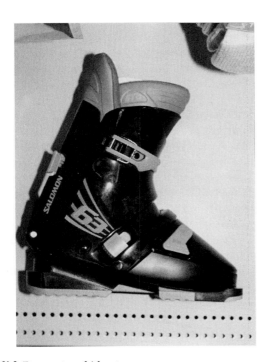

Fig. 21-6. Rear-entry ski boot.

overlaps anteriorly and has four buckles which fasten in front. They generally fit tightly and offer good support, though they are more difficult to put on than the rear-entry boots. The rear-entry boot has a separate plastic shell posteriorly which fastens to the main body of the boot with only one buckle. Some feel the rear-entry boot is comfortable and

easy to put on, but that the separate rear shell provides insufficient support and allows too much rearward movement. The midentry boot has a hinged rear panel which allows for ease of putting on and taking off the boot.[4]

Attachments on a ski boot can be adjusted for better control, positioning, and fit of the foot. Flex adjustors allow more or less resistance to forward flexion in the boot. A forward lean adjustor allows more or less forward lean at the top of the boot, thereby changing weight distribution anteriorly or posteriorly. A forefoot adjustor tightens the boot across the front of the foot, allowing better fit and control in the forefoot. Similarly, in the rearfoot there may be an instep cable which tightens across the heel and top of the rearfoot to allow for better fit and control. A cant adjustor changes the varus tilt of the shaft of the boot to better align the boot with the angle of the lower leg. The inner boot is a soft liner which insulates the hard plastic shell and cushions the lower leg, ankle, and foot. Wedges or orthoses can be put inside the inner boot to achieve better edging and more efficient biomechanical control.

Soccer

Soccer is an increasingly popular sport in the United States and is thought to be the most popular sport worldwide. Although it is usually played on a grass field, soccer is also played indoors and on turf fields. A soccer team has 11 players: five forwards (offensive players), five backs (defensive players), and one

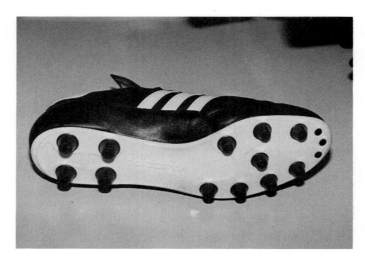

Fig. 21-8. Soccer shoe.

goalie. However, the strategic conformation of the players may vary. Soccer is primarily a forward-running sport where the ball is dribbled, passed, kicked, or trapped with the lower extremities. Other movements such as juggling and volleying require adept foot and leg skills as well. The player's upper extremities may not handle the ball (exception: the goalie), but the player may thrust the ball with the head, shoulders, and trunk.

The soccer shoe must allow the player to "feel the ball." It fits the foot snugly in the upper which is usually made of leather or imitation leather. It must fit with the player's socks and shin guards on. At the back of the shoe there is an Achilles tab, designed to protect the tendon. Inside there is usually a nylon lining and a very narrow insole. The last is narrow allowing maximal contact between the leather upper and most of the foot surface for ball control. The plantar aspect of the soccer shoe has 10 or more cleats which act as traction devices as well as shock absorbers (Fig. 21-8). The cleats are often made as a molded unit with a rubber or synthetic semiflexible outsole. More experienced players might use replaceable screw-in cleats. The more cleats placed in the heel, the greater the traction or strain on the Achilles tendon. In a susceptible adolescent player, this could lead to Sever's disease. The harder the surface, the shorter the cleat. Indoor soccer shoes have no cleats but rather a wedge design like a running shoe for shock absorption.

Football

In football, the predominant motion depends on the position played. Receivers and running backs primarily move forward with quick lateral cuts, turns, and high steps to avoid defenders. The defensive backs often mirror these motions. Linemen gener-

ally run less but require strength and traction to block, sprint, and tackle at the snap of the ball. Football is a contact sport in which the injury rate is among the highest of all sports. Improvement in football shoe design as well as other football equipment has contributed to fewer injuries. However, synthetic turf, which is harder and fixes the foot more firmly than natural turf, may contribute to more severe injuries in cases of turf toe, ankle, and knee injuries, abrasions, and contusions. Wet or dry conditions of the turf also affect foot fixation and the injury rate.[2]

Today's football shoes differ from those in the past by number, design, conformation, and composition of cleats (Fig. 21-9). An older conventional shoe had only seven cleats each 3/4 to 1 in. long with narrow tips. These fewer, longer, conically shaped, narrow-tipped cleats on the older shoe fixed the foot firmly to the ground. Medical recommendations were to shorten the length, widen the diameter, and increase the number of cleats on the sole of the football shoe, making it more like a soccer-style shoe.[6] A 1985 ruling for nonprofessionals required a minimum of 12 cleats, no longer than 1/2 in. long and 7/16 in. wide at the tip.[1] Some models have detachable cleats for replacement. Turf models generally have more cleats, which are shorter in length. The upper of football shoes is usually made of a combination of mesh, nylon, and leather. The linemen's shoes tend to be heavier with a three-quarter top or higher cut, whereas receivers may prefer a lower-cut, lighter shoe.[1] There is usually a midsole of ethyl vinyl acetate (EVA) material, higher in the rearfoot, lower in the forefoot. There is often a steel shank for protection against turf toe. The outsole is generally a synthetic polyurethane-like material, although some are rubber. The sizing of the shoe may range up to men's size 16 or 17 because of the larger

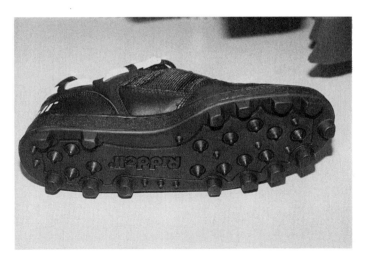

Fig. 21-9. Football shoe.

profile of the football player compared with athletes in other sports.

Baseball

Baseball is a popular sport in the United States, Central America, Canada, and Japan. Motion in baseball involves straight-ahead sprinting, rounding bases, sliding, batting, throwing, and pitching. It may be played on natural or, less commonly, on artificial turf. Baseball shoes are cleated shoes with fewer cleats than football shoes (Fig. 21-10). Generally the cleats are squared and made either of molded rubber, polyurethane-like material, or metal. (Metal cleats are usually not allowed in Little League or softball.) Some models come with detachable replacement cleats. Turf cleats are shorter and more numerous. The uppers on a baseball shoe are generally low-topped leather combined with mesh or nylon, although higher cuts are available. Traditionally the tongue folds over the proximal laces. Usually there is an EVA-wedged midsole for cushioning.

With the preceding field sports, orthoses can be used. For best motion control they can be rigid and of standard length. In baseball and soccer shoes, the orthoses should be narrow, have relatively low heel cups, and little or no post in order to fit the profile of the shoes. Soft forefoot extensions are used if space permits. Football shoe orthoses may be rigid and of standard length. Because of the higher three-quarter cut, wider, posted devices are often well tolerated.

Tennis

Movements in tennis are sprints, quick stops and starts, side-to-side movements, and the serve.

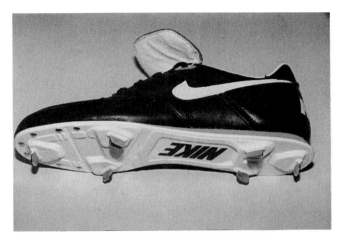

Fig. 21-10. Baseball shoe.

Whereas 20 years ago most tennis shoes consisted of a low-cut canvas upper, little or no midsole, and a plain outsole, today's shoes offer more support, better cushioning and traction, and improved durability. The upper of tennis shoes usually comes in leather for firm support with ventilation holes for breathability. There should be ample length and width in the toe box to prevent "tennis toe," which is a reflection of repeated bruising of the toenail by chronic shoe pressure. The midcut or three-quarter top shoes provide some protection against ankle sprains (Fig. 21-11). The midsole is wedge-shaped and higher in the heel, taking the strain or pull off the Achilles tendon. The shoe is lower in the forefoot but thick enough to provide cushioning. The outsole should be wide enough to provide a stable base against ankle sprains. There are often customized areas on the underside of the outsole. Toe pivot markings facilitate spinning on the big toe joint (Fig. 21-12). Flex grooves under the ball of the foot aid

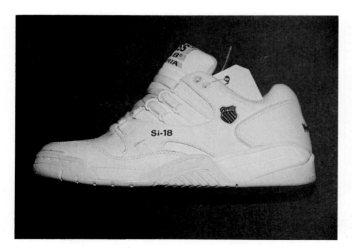

Fig. 21-11. Tennis shoe.

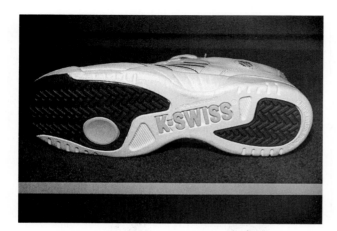

Fig. 21-12. Outsole of tennis shoe.

forefoot flexion. The medial outsole may extend onto the upper in the area of the great toe, preventing wear from toe drag.

Basketball

Movements in basketball include forward running, lateral cuts, jumps, and backward or side-running to avoid or guard an opponent. Like tennis shoes, basketball shoes have evolved from an uncushioned canvas high-topped shoe to one that provides better support and shock absorption (Fig. 21-13). The uppers are typically vented, leather high-tops providing some ankle protection. The heel counters should be firm for rearfoot motion control. The midsole, usually of an EVA or polyurethane material, is wedged higher in back than in the front. In general, the basketball shoe has a thicker midsole than most other court shoes, providing more shock absorption on landing from jumps. The rubber or

synthetic outsole usually has a specific pattern such as creases in the forefoot easing jumping or a pivot circle under the big toe joint.

Orthoses for court sports such as tennis and basketball can be rigid, standard-length, wider-posted devices depending on the particular shoe gear. Forefoot extensions are helpful because of the time spent jumping, pivoting, and landing on the forefoot.

Dance

Dance shoes vary in design and construction depending on the type of dance performed. Modern dance, diverse and free-form, is usually performed barefoot or, rarely, with a modern-dance shoe. That shoe is really a half-shoe with a thin leather sole in the forefoot, nothing in the heel, and a strap securing it around the ankle (Fig. 21-14). In theatre dance, such as musicals and opera, shoe gear may be heels or oxfords, pointe shoes, or bare feet, depending on the particular costume or effect desired. Theater, jazz, and tap dance all use character shoes on occasion (Fig. 21-15). This is a black leather shoe with a semiflexible leather sole, a somewhat rounded toe, a strap across the instep, and a fairly broad based 1 1/2- to 2-in. heel. In tap dance, the metal taps are nailed into the tips of the forefoot and onto the heel of character shoes (Fig. 21-16). Ballroom dance shoes for women usually have a 2- to 3-in. narrow heel and tapered toe box. Men's ballroom shoes resemble men's character shoes and are a black leather tie-up shoe with a thin semiflexible leather sole and small 1/2-in. heel (Fig. 21-17). Jazz shoes are similar in appearance to ballroom shoes but are much more flexible in the sole. The thin narrow leather sole may be full or split for more flexibility. More recent innovations in jazz shoes include a boot style as well as rubber on the outsole of the forefoot to prevent slippage.

Ballet is a unique dance form which utilizes ballet slippers, pointe shoes and, less often, character shoes. In ballet, "turn-out," primarily from external hip rotation, is essential. There are five formally defined positions and very specific movements which are incorporated into ballet choreography. Ballet slippers, also called technique shoes, are used by younger female dancers as well as male dancers (Fig. 21-18). Experienced female dancers use pointe shoes as well as technique shoes. Technique shoes are usually soft black, pink, or white leather or canvas shoes, with a flexible, narrow, and very short leather sole. There is usually a thin elastic strap across the instep and a drawstring encircling the top of the shoe to better hold the shoe on the foot. The top of the ballet slipper, unlike tie-up jazz shoes, is open on the dorsum of the foot, much like a pump.

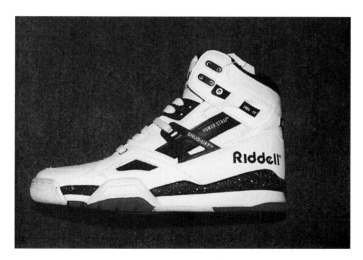

Fig. 21-13. Basketball shoe.

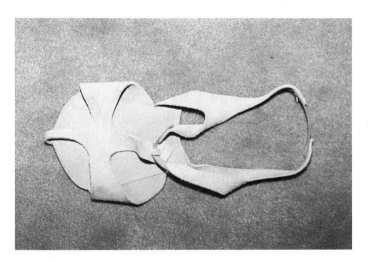

Fig. 21-14. Modern dance shoe.

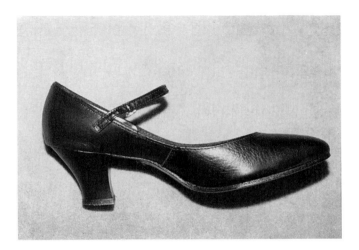

Fig. 21-15. Woman's character shoe with heel.

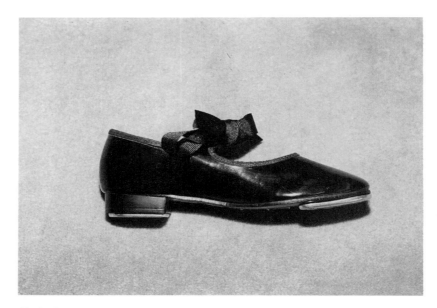

Fig. 21-16. Child's tap shoe.

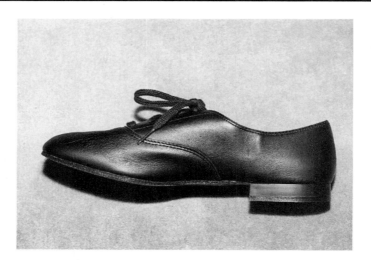

Fig. 21-17. Man's character shoe.

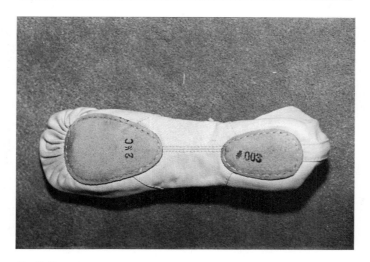

Fig. 21-18. Ballet slipper, split sole.

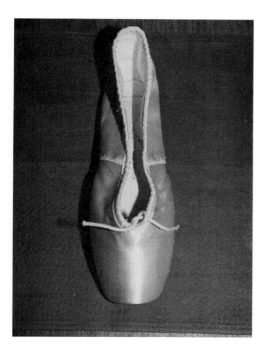

Fig. 21-19. Pointe shoe.

After the young female dancer develops strength, demonstrates good alignment of the lower extremities, and has competent technique, she may go "en pointe" or "on toe," usually between the age of 9 and 12 years old. In the pointe shoe, the body's weight is supported primarily by the tips of the first and second rays.

The pointe shoe or toe shoe is usually a pinkish satin fashioned over a fabric made very stiff in the toe box (Fig. 21-19). This helps to hold the dancer's foot en pointe. The midfoot fabric is not stiff, but a drawstring helps the shoe fit snugly around the dancer's foot. The general shape of the shoe should match the individual dancer's foot. Different brands and models of pointe shoes vary in stiffness, shank, and vamp length, and toe box shape. A stiffer, longer shank and vamp provide more support for the en pointe foot although more advanced dancers prefer a more flexible shoe for aesthetic reasons. These stronger dancers often break, soften, or remove part of the shank in order to have a more arched appearance to the foot. In the rearfoot of the pointe shoe, 1-in.-wide satin ribbons are sewn into the shoe and then wrapped around the ankle for support. Elastic sewn under the ribbons and coursing around the front of the ankle provides some support as well. The pointe shoes themselves are not durable, soften quickly, and as they do so, contribute to high injury rates among ballet dancers. Ill-fitting toe shoes can also create problems of blisters, corns, ingrown toenails, and subungual hematomas.

Summary

Different sports require different shoes. The predominant motions in a sport determine the design and construction of the shoe. The shoe for one sport may be sturdy and well-cushioned, whereas another sport requires a flexible lightweight shoe. Owing to anatomic and biomechanical variation, aesthetic preference, level of competence, varied playing surfaces, position of play, economic factors, and changing technology, the choice of shoe may vary as well, even within one sport. Shoes for sport have changed over the years, but the sport-specific shoe is here to stay.

References

1. Cheskin M, Sherkin K, Bates B: *Complete handbook of athletic shoewear,* New York, 1987, Fairchild.
2. Culpepper M, Nieman K: An investigation of shoe-turf interface using different types of shoes on Poly-Turf and Astro-Turf: torque and release coefficients, *Ala J Med Sci* 20:387–390, 1983.
3. Faria I: Energy expenditure, aerodynamics and medical problems in cycling, *Sports Med,* Winter 1:43–63, 1992.
4. Hogen J: 30 unbeatable boots, *Snow Country* 1993, p 127.
5. Miller D: Ground reaction forces in biomechanics of distance running. In Cavanagh P, editor: *Biomechanics of distance running,* 1990, Human Kinetics, Champaign, IL.
6. Torg J: Athletic footwear and orthotic appliances, *Clin Sports Med* 1:157–175, 1982.

the inverted orthotic technique: its role in clinical biomechanics

Richard L. Blake, DPM
Heather Ferguson, MS, B App Sci (POD)

Initial patient presentation
Establishing a diagnosis
Correlation between diagnosis and gait
Initiation of biomechanical treatment
Follow-up correlation between gait changes and symptom response
Manufacturing the inverted orthotic technique
    Negative casting
    Pouring process
    Positive cast corrections
    Prescription writing for the inverted orthotic technique
    Common modifications to inverted orthotic therapy
    Overcorrection modifications
    Undercorrection modifications
5-to-1 rule
Concept of serial orthoses
Summary

The treatment of abnormal gait patterns is a vital part of the practice of podiatry. Abnormal motion, whether excessive, limited, or out of normal sequence, can create problems. Recognizing abnormal patterns, and then changing those patterns, can successfully help a myriad of maladies. The degree of correction needed in each situation is unknown, although the clinician will gradually develop a sense of the change needed. The clinician analyzing patients within the realm of podiatric biomechanics requires a variety of treatment options. This great variety of modalities, which does help many patients, has given this area an element of mystery. For any given injury, many treatments do help. Yet the clinician must analyze the success or failure of any modality in two vital areas: (1) percentage of abnormal gait changed, and (2) percentage of symptom response.

Since subtleties of gait producing injury can be difficult to detect, and since symptom response can be varied with even ideal changes, this area will remain more an art than a science for many years to come. However, this area is challenging, rewarding, and marked by success. Improved biomechanical therapy will lower the number of surgical procedures. Many surgeries presently done will be avoided by perfecting clinical biomechanical treatment. Patients are seen daily where one physician had recommended surgery, or just living with the chronic pain, only to have complete resolution of the

symptoms with biomechanical application. This chapter focuses on one approach to clinical podiatric biomechanics which has proved very successful in caring for injured athletes and nonathletes alike. We highlight the orthotic technique routinely utilized in this approach—the inverted orthotic technique.[1–6]

Initial patient presentation

Most patients present to a practitioner's office because of pain. It may be purely podiatric, limited to foot or ankle soreness or, in most sports medicine offices, the pain may be above the ankle, in the low back, hip, thigh, knee, or lower leg. Any of these painful areas may be caused or aggravated by abnormal function. It is also common for patients to present with a myriad of concomitant injuries requiring attention. Although the cause may be systemic, this is rare. Normally, the cause is overuse, with a strong biomechanical predisposition. For example, if all the pain is on one side of the body, consider limb length discrepancy, correction of which is but one part of the process in biomechanical therapy (Fig. 22-1).

When a patient presents with pain, there are four basic steps that must be addressed. These are:

1. Establishment of a diagnosis
2. Correlation between diagnosis and gait (Fig. 22-2)
3. Initiation of biomechanical treatment
4. Follow-up correlation between gait changes and symptom response

As these four areas are reviewed, many common biomechanical principles will be discussed. It is

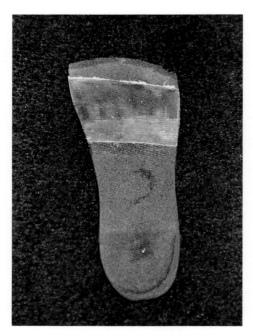

Fig. 22-1. Full-length lift to sulcus for short side with a 1/16-in. polypropylene cap preventing breakdown at the distal edge of the orthotic device.

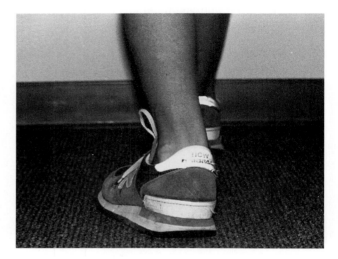

Fig. 22-2. Midstance and propulsive phase pronation of the left side observed in gait causing or aggravating Achilles tendinitis. Observe heel eversion past vertical.

essential to evaluate the biomechanics of each injury from the initial visit. The study of biomechanics requires that you constantly test theories, and modify those theories as necessary. Are tight calf muscles causing the Achilles tendon strain (Fig. 22-3) and will a simple heel-lift help? Is the runner's knee injury related to overpronation, and will varus heel wedges (Figs. 22-4 and 22-5) and new anti-

pronation shoes (Fig. 22-6) remedy the situation? The well-trained practitioner can diagnose and treat these problems, and many others, with authority.

Establishing a diagnosis

On completion of the initial visit, it is important to establish a working diagnosis. It is normally not

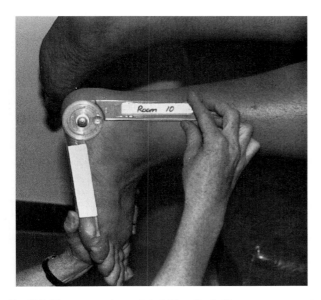

Fig. 22-3. Demonstration of Achilles flexibility measurement with a goniometer.

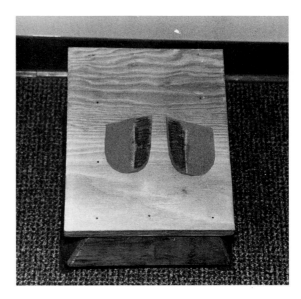

Fig. 22-4. Varus heel wedges of 6 degrees (3/8 in.) to assist in controlling excessive subtalar joint pronation.

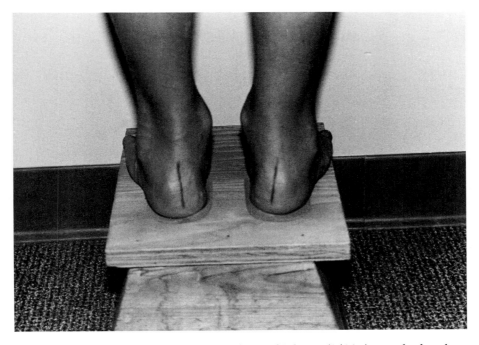

Fig. 22-5. Slightly inverted heel positioning with use of 4 degree (1/4-in.) varus heel wedges.

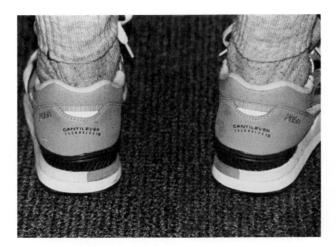

Fig. 22-6. Antipronation running shoes designed to prevent excessive rearfoot or calcaneal eversion.

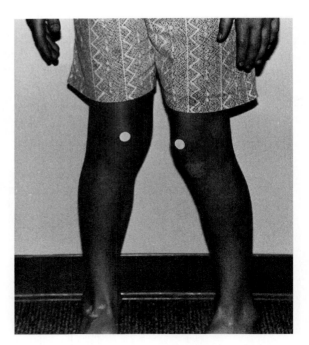

Fig. 22-7. Internal patellar position in a patient with chondromalacia patellae symptoms and excessive subtalar joint pronation.

Table 22-1
Common injuries and their classic causes

Injury	Cause
Morton's neuroma	Excessive midtarsal pronation
Fourth metatarsal stress fracture	Excessive subtalar supination with unstable fifth metatarsal
Tibial sesamoiditis	Plantarflexed first ray
Plantar fasciitis	High arched foot with midtarsal joint collapse
Cuboid syndrome, peroneal tendinitis	Excessive subtalar joint supination
Posterior tibial tendinitis	Excessive subtalar joint pronation
Achilles tendinitis	Tight Achilles tendon; excessive subtalar joint pronation; compensation for short leg
Tibial stress fractures	Poor shock absorption; excessive subtalar joint pronation with pull of posterior tibial tendon
Chondromalacia patellae	Excessive subtalar joint pronation with internal femoral rotation (Figure 22-7)
Medial meniscus contusion	Excessive subtalar joint supination
Hamstring strain	Tight hamstrings; excessive subtalar joint pronation
Piriformis syndrome, sciatica	Excessive subtalar joint pronation
Sacroiliac sprain	Excessive subtalar joint supination

essential to establish an accurate diagnosis at this time to initiate treatment. A complete biomechanically oriented historical review cannot only help make the diagnosis, but will begin to lay the foundation for the important steps of treatment. Review the common causes of injury by formulating questions touching on these areas. The general categories regarding the cause of an injury are weak muscles, tight muscles, training errors, structural problems, improper equipment, nutritional deficiencies, and improper technique. Therefore, ask questions pertaining to the biomechanics of the injury along with the common specific injury-related questions. Is there swelling? Is there ecchymosis? Did the patient feel a tear, pop, or snap? For example, the following seven questions typify the seven areas of injury cause of an Achilles tendinitis:

1. Have you ever had a bad ankle injury and did not have restrengthening therapy?
2. Do you routinely stretch your Achilles tendon or calf before and after exercise?
3. What was your training like during the 2 weeks prior to your injury? Were there any changes?
4. Have you ever been told you have a short leg, flat feet, or high arches?
5. What type of shoe gear were you wearing when you were injured? Were your shoes worn-out?
6. What has your diet been lately? Do you get enough calcium? Are you a vegetarian?
7. Have you ever been told that your technique is different or "funny?" Have you recently made any technique changes?

It is a simple task to ask similar questions for any area of pain. All these questions, along with the examination findings, will help develop a tentative working diagnosis based on the area of injury and the possible cause. Every injury also has common causes that are considered "classic." Table 22-1 lists some common injuries and their classic causes. Always rule these in or out in your workup when presented with these injuries. Although Table 22-1 is only a partial list, it focuses on common causes which should not be overlooked. For example, chronic chondromalacia patellae should always be treated with quadriceps strengthening, and biomechanical treatment for excessive pronation control (Fig. 22-7).

Correlation between diagnosis and gait

Gait analysis is crucial in understanding the biomechanics of any injury. It is important to first look for patterns of motion. Watch the patient walk barefoot, then with shoes, then with shoes and any inserts (even over-the-counter [OTC] inserts) they may be wearing. If the patient was injured participating in a sport that requires running, watch the running gait style. Is it the same pattern as with walking, or is it different? If the patient participates in another sport (e.g., aerobic dance, race walking, tennis, bowling), have the patient demonstrate his or her technique as best as possible. This may require that the spouse or a friend videotape the workout for your review. In most sports, there are repetitive motions, for example, the footwork in bowling, golfing, tennis

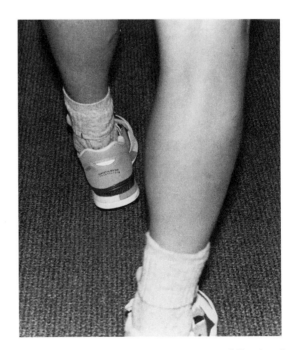

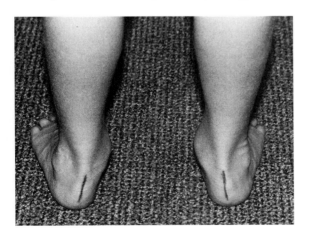

Fig. 22-8. Severely everted heel position secondary to excessive subtalar joint pronation.

Fig. 22-9. Excessive subtalar joint supination following heel contact of left foot.

serves, and step aerobics. Observe this pattern and correlate where the stress is placed with the injury site. There are many classic injuries that occur as a result of this repetitive asymmetric motion. For example, left-sided Morton's neuroma in a right-handed golfer may be a result of the foot roll from medial to lateral on the forward power swing of a drive.

There are four common patterns to look for as you begin to correlate the diagnosis with the gait. These four patterns will help design inserts to remedy the situation. They are (1) excessive subtalar joint pronation (Fig. 22-8), (2) excessive subtalar joint supination (Fig. 22-9), (3) inadequate shock absorption, and (4) changes related to limb length discrepancy (Fig. 22-10). Recognition of these four common patterns and combinations of these patterns (e.g., poor shock absorption with excessive subtalar pronation) is a key starting point in the treatment of biomechanically related symptoms. As this information is grouped with the understanding of differences between feet, asymmetric functioning (i.e., excessive pronation of the right foot and poor shock absorption of the left foot), and estimations of the degree of force of these abnormal motions (i.e., mild, moderate, or severe pronation forces), appropriate biomechanical support can be initiated. Table 22-2 briefly outlines the common gait changes seen in each of these four categories.

After recognition of the abnormal motion the checklist in Figure 22-11 **A** is used to further categorize the changes by asymmetry and degree of force. This enables an accurate clinical model to be framed in which treatment may be addressed. The specifics of each walking or running evaluation should be filled in (e.g., walking with Avia aerobics shoes and orthoses). Figure 22-11 **B** and **C** shows specific examples of gait findings and treatment recommendations.

Initiation of biomechanical treatment

When biomechanical treatment is employed, it is important to thoroughly understand the various options available in all four categories as well as the amount or percentage of correction required to improve any given condition. Some injuries require a slight correction of the abnormal motion to completely resolve the symptoms. Other injuries need marked correction, or even overcorrection, for

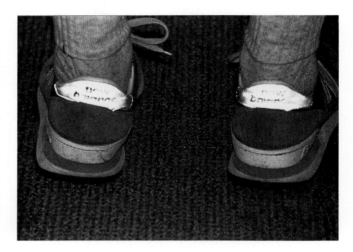

Fig. 22-10. Greater heel eversion of the longer left side in a patient with 3/8-in. shorter right leg.

Table 22-2
Gait categories and their common gait findings

Gait categories	Common gait findings
Excessive subtalar joint pronation	Arch collapse; heel eversion; abduction twist of heel at heel-lift; internal patellar rotation at heel contact
Excessive subtalar joint supination	Lateral heel instability at contact phase; varus thrust at ankle and knee; no internal patellar rotation at heel contact
Inadequate shock absorption	Excessive heel jarring; no arch movement; shock wave up to low back
Changes due to limb length discrepancy	Shoulder drop; excessive side-to-side motion of trunk; dominance to one side; asymmetric foot motion; asymmetric arm swing

Name: Patient _____

Tentative Diagnosis: _____

☐ Walking   Category _____

☐ Running   Category _____

CLINICAL OBSERVATIONS

EXCESSIVE PRONATION

Right *Left*

☐ ☐ Heel eversion

☐ ☐ Arch collapse

☐ ☐ Abductory twist

☐ ☐ Internal patellar rotation

EXCESSIVE SUPINATION

☐ ☐ Lateral heel instability

☐ ☐ Varus thrust ankle/knee

☐ ☐ No internal patellar rotation

INADEQUATE SHOCK ABSORPT.

☐ ☐ Heel jarring

☐ ☐ No arch movement

☐ ☐ Shock waves legs

LIMB LENGTH DISCREP. (LLD)

☐ ☐ Shoulder drop

☐ ☐ Side-to-side motion

☐ ☐ One side dominance

☐ ☐ Asymmetric foot motion

☐ ☐ Asymmetric arm swing

STRUCTURAL FINDINGS

1. _____
2. _____
3. _____
4. _____
5. _____
6. _____
7. _____

GAIT CATEGORIES

Right

☐ Excessive pronation

☐ Excessive supination

☐ Inadequate shock absorption

☐ LLD

Left

☐ Excessive pronation

☐ Excessive supination

☐ Inadequate shock absorption

☐ LLD

DEGREE OF FORCE

(Circle when applicable)

Mild, moderate, severe

Mild, moderate, severe

Mild, moderate, severe

Mild, moderate, severe

Mild, moderate, severe

Mild, moderate, severe

Mild, moderate, severe

Mild, moderate, severe

TREATMENT RECOMMENDATION CATEGORIES

Right

☐ Control pronation

☐ Control supination

☐ Increase shock absorption

☐ Correct LLD

Left

☐ Control pronation

☐ Control supination

☐ Increase shock absorption

☐ Correct LLD

Initial treatment recommendations (specific)

_____

_____

_____

_____

Fig. 22-11. Correlation of gait abnormalities and treatment recommendations. **A,** Blank form.

Name: Patient, John

Tentative Diagnosis: Left Posterior Tibial Strain

☒ Walking   Category AVIA 2050

☐ Running   Category _____

CLINICAL OBSERVATIONS

EXCESSIVE PRONATION

	Right	Left
Heel eversion	☐	☒
Arch collapse	☐	☒
Abductory twist	☐	☒
Internal patellar rotation	☐	☒

EXCESSIVE SUPINATION

	Right	Left
Lateral heel instability	☐	☐
Varus thrust ankle/knee	☐	☐
No internal patellar rotation	☐	☐

INADEQUATE SHOCK ABSORPT.

	Right	Left
Heel jarring	☒	☐
No arch movement	☐	☐
Shock waves legs	☐	☐

LIMB LENGTH DISCREP. (LLD)

	Right	Left
Shoulder drop	☒	☐
Side-to-side motion	☐	☐
One side dominance	☒	☐
Asymmetric foot motion	☒	☐
Asymmetric arm swing	☒	☐

STRUCTURAL FINDINGS

1. 10° Forefoot varus right/2° left
2. 1/4" long left leg
3. _____
4. _____
5. _____
6. _____
7. _____

GAIT CATEGORIES

Right
- ☐ Excessive pronation
- ☐ Excessive supination
- ☒ Inadequate shock absorption
- ☐ LLD

Left
- ☒ Excessive pronation
- ☐ Excessive supination
- ☐ Inadequate shock absorption
- ☒ LLD

DEGREE OF FORCE

(Circle when applicable)

Mild, moderate, severe
Mild, moderate, severe
(Mild,) moderate, severe
Mild, moderate, severe

Left
Mild, (moderate,) severe
Mild, moderate, severe
Mild, moderate, severe
Mild, (moderate,) severe

TREATMENT RECOMMENDATION CATEGORIES

Right
- ☐ Control pronation
- ☐ Control supination
- ☒ Increase shock absorption
- ☐ Correct LLD

Left
- ☒ Control pronation
- ☐ Control supination
- ☐ Increase shock absorption
- ☒ Correct LLD

Initial treatment recommendations (specific)

- Moderate pronation control (L) with 25° inverted
- Arch support (R) Root balancing with 5/32" poly for mainly shock absorption
- Begin lift therapy with 1/8" full-length lift (R) foot

Fig. 22-11, cont'd. Correlation of gait abnormalities and treatment recommendations. **B,** For a male patient with left posterior tibial strain.

Name: Patient, Jane
Tentative Diagnosis: Right Chondromalacia Patellae

☐ Walking   Category
☒ Running   Category Etonic stable air with worn-
                              out orthoses

CLINICAL OBSERVATIONS
EXCESSIVE PRONATION
                        Left
Right
☒ ☐ Heel eversion
☒ ☐ Arch collapse
☒ ☐ Abductory twist
☒ ☐ Internal patellar rotation

EXCESSIVE SUPINATION
☐ ☒ Lateral heel instability
☐ ☒ Varus thrust ankle/knee
☐ ☒ No internal patellar rotation

INADEQUATE SHOCK ABSORPT.
☐ ☐ Heel jarring
☐ ☐ No arch movement
☐ ☐ Shock waves legs

LIMB LENGTH DISCREP. (LLD)
☒ ☐ Shoulder drop
☐ ☐ Side-to-side motion
☒ ☐ One side dominance
☒ ☐ Asymmetric foot motion
☐ ☐ Asymmetric arm swing

STRUCTURAL FINDINGS
1. 1/8" short right side
2. severe posterior tibial dysfunction (R)
3. 5–6 forefoot valgus deformity bilateral
4.
5.
6.
7.

GAIT CATEGORIES

Right
☒ Excessive pronation
☐ Excessive supination
☐ Inadequate shock absorption
☐ LLD

Left
☐ Excessive pronation
☒ Excessive supination
☐ Inadequate shock absorption
☒ LLD

DEGREE OF FORCE

(Circle when applicable)
Mild, moderate, (severe)
Mild, moderate, severe
Mild, moderate, severe
Mild, moderate, severe

Mild, moderate, severe
Mild, (moderate,) severe
Mild, moderate, severe
Mild, (moderate,) severe

Initial treatment recommendations (specific)
• (R) severe pronation control with 35° inverted
  orthosis and 1/8" varus shoe midsole wedge
  and possible Kirby modification
• 1/8" full length lift for short right side
• (L) orthotic device with high lateral heel cup,
  and lateral extension extrinsic rearfoot post
  (Root Device)

TREATMENT RECOMMENDATION CATEGORIES

Right
☒ Control pronation
☐ Control supination
☐ Increase shock absorption
☐ Correct LLD

Left
☐ Control pronation
☒ Control supination
☐ Increase shock absorption
☒ Correct LLD

Fig. 22-11, cont'd. C, for a female patient, with right Chondromalacia Patellae.

a period of time to reduce the inflammatory response. There are levels of sophistication of the different modalities designed to help correct abnormal motions or positions. Yet, greater sophistication is not necessarily correlated with better function. One should thoroughly examine the function produced by modality, comparing function with and without the modality, to understand the change produced. The worse-looking inserts in a bag of inserts may actually produce the best function. Analysis of function should guide treatment planning. However, it is important to remember that full correction, or even overcorrection (Fig. 22-12) may be necessary to completely resolve the symptoms.

Do not settle for less correction when the symptoms remain or recur. Figure 22-13 demonstrates the range of corrections seen with treatment modalities.

It is important to evaluate the degree of correction of any treatment modality, as well as to evaluate the two sides separately. The correction response to similar inserts, shoes, or exercises tends to be asymmetric. A key goal in clinical biomechanics is to achieve symmetry of function between the two sides. The common errors in this area are (1) accepting less than complete or overcorrection when symptoms are slow to respond, (2) accepting less than the desired correction on the noninjured side, and (3) not recognizing when the treatment actually

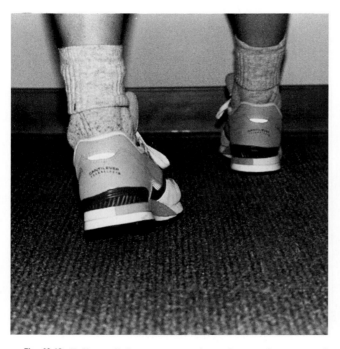

Fig. 22-12. Full to slight overcorrection of severely pronated right foot with 35 degrees inverted orthotic devices and stable antipronation shoes. Note that during contact phase the right foot stays slightly inverted. Relaxed calcaneal stance position was a 5-degree everted right foot. Note that the left foot remains inverted in propulsive phase.

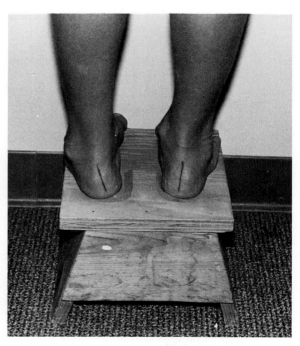

Fig. 22-14. Overcorrection with resultant lateral instability noted with 6 degrees varus heel wedge on the left side with complete correction on the right side (right heel actually standing slightly inverted).

Modality Evaluated: _____ (check appropriate box)

Right	Left
☐ overcorrection	☐ overcorrection
☐ complete correction	☐ complete correction
☐ significant correction	☐ significant correction
☐ good correction	☐ good correction
☐ slight correction	☐ slight correction
☐ negligible correction	☐ negligible correction
☐ negative correction	☐ negative correction

Fig. 22-13. Degree of correction noted per modality.

causes a negative result, providing a "negative" correction (i.e., actually increasing pronation in the attempt to design an antipronation device).

It is useful for many practitioners to correlate the following seven categories with estimations of correction. When dictating charts, or discussing the change produced with patients, it is helpful to use percentages. The percentage correlations with category are as follows:

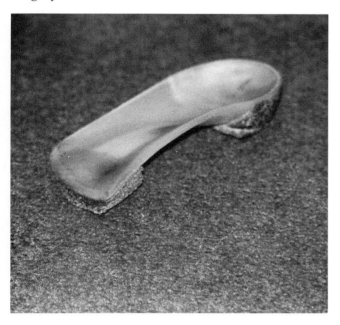

Fig. 22-15. Top medial view of 4-degree varus wedging applied to anterior edge and rearfoot posting of a functional foot orthotic device.

Category	Correlation (%)
Overcorrection (Fig. 22-14)	>100
Complete correction	90–100
Significant correction	70–90
Good correction	50–70
Slight correction	20–50
Negligible correction	0–20
Negative correction	–

Any insert, and any shoe, can produce any correction. A simple heel-lift may produce a significant correction of abnormal motion, whereas a custom-made functional foot orthosis may result in a negative correction. The degree of force potentially generated by various inserts may be somewhat predictable (i.e., more force with a plastic custom-made insert vs. a heel wedge); however, individual feet are treated, not generalizations.

Focusing on shoe inserts, and their realm in clinical podiatric biomechanics, all of the common functions affected by the prescription must be fully evaluated. The nine common functions of the foot affected by any shoe or shoe insert are:

1. Arch support (medial column support)
2. Heel eversion/control
3. Heel inversion control
4. Lateral column support
5. Metatarsal support
6. Shock absorption
7. Propulsive phase stability
8. Slight forward transference of weight

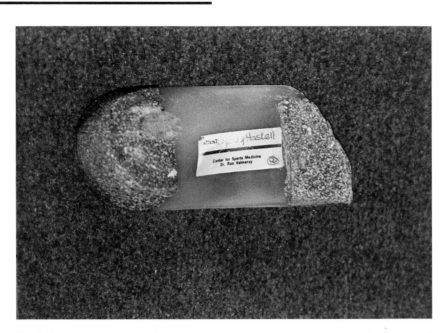

Fig. 22-16. Bottom view of 4-degree varus wedging applied to the anterior edge and rearfoot posting of a functional foot orthotic device.

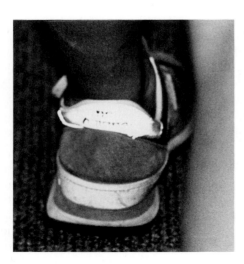

Fig. 22-17. Valgus heel canting with a functional foot orthotic device for the left foot poured 3 degrees everted and capturing a 15-degree forefoot valgus deformity. This prevents chronic lateral ankle sprains and produces rearfoot pronation.

9. Smooth transfer of weight following heel contact

Every insert should produce a positive or negligible effect on all nine areas, even though the degree of change will vary for any function. There should never be a negative effect in any area that could produce an injury while trying to address another injury. Based on these nine areas, a proper working shoe or insert should support the medial (1) and lateral (4) columns of the foot, control heel inversion (2) and eversion (3), absorb shock (6), support the metatarsals (5), allow for propulsive phase stability (7), produce a slight forward transfer of weight (8), and smoothly transfer weight following heel contact (9). Specific inserts can be designed to affect one of these functions more than another without producing other problems. Therefore, an arch support that stabilizes the medial column should never make the lateral column unstable, producing lateral instability or poor shock absorption.

There are three other specific functions that may be incorporated into an insert. These are (1) various area accommodations (i.e., sub-second metatarsal, plantar fascial); (2) varus heel canting (Figs. 22-15 and 22-16); and (3) valgus heel canting (Fig. 22-17). The inserts with these specific functions, however, should never violate the other functions. The goal of shoe insert therapy is normal, smooth functioning of both feet.

Follow-up correlation between gait changes and symptom response

As gait is changed with shoes or inserts, or both, symptom response should be carefully monitored.

The initial working diagnosis is first correlated with the four common gait patterns. Treatment is then initiated to alter the gait. These treatments have many options, with the initial treatment typically based on three factors: (1) severity of the injury, (2) chronicity of the injury, and (3) severity of the abnormal force. These factors help the clinician understand the need for correction of the situation—simple correction, moderate correction, or advanced correction.

Figure 22-18 is designed to function as a guide to assist the clinician in the initial management. Following the initial treatment, changes can be made with careful review of function and symptom response. There are many instances where multiple corrections, occurring over months, are required. It is also important to remember that two or three or all four of the abnormal gait categories may exist in the same patient and in different degrees between the two feet. This was presented in Figure 22-11. Table 22-3 shows how the clinician may use these "implied need" categories to increase or decrease the correction in each gait category. This is based on the effects on function and response of the symptoms to treatment. Also included in Table 22-3 is the typical increase in pronation control if a 35 degrees inverted orthotic device provides inadequate pronation control. Since several abnormal functions may exist in the same foot or leg, an understanding of the use of the inverted orthotic device must be coupled with correction of the other three gait categories. Failure of the inverted orthotic technique may occur as a result of improper correction of a limb length discrepancy, poor shock absorption, or excessive supination (normally due to a high inverted landing heel position with excessive pronation following). In some severe cases, full correction of all four categories must be obtained. For example, the four gait patterns are treated in the same foot as follows:

Gait category	Treatment degrees
Excessive pronation:	35 degrees inverted technique with Kirby modification
Excessive supination or antisupination	High lateral heel cup (23–30 mm); lateral extension, extrinsic rearfoot post; Denton modification; forefoot valgus extensions; lateral midsole wedges (heel to full foot) (Fig. 22-19)
Inadequate shock absorption	Motion ground into rearfoot post; shock-absorbing material as full-length or sulcus length topcover (Fig. 22-20); shock-absorbing shoes

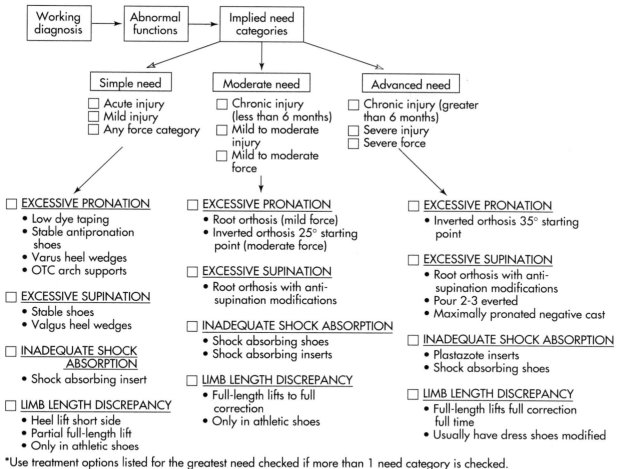

Working diagnosis → Abnormal functions → Implied need categories

Simple need
- ☐ Acute injury
- ☐ Mild injury
- ☐ Any force category

Moderate need
- ☐ Chronic injury (less than 6 months)
- ☐ Mild to moderate injury
- ☐ Mild to moderate force

Advanced need
- ☐ Chronic injury (greater than 6 months)
- ☐ Severe injury
- ☐ Severe force

☐ EXCESSIVE PRONATION
- Low dye taping
- Stable antipronation shoes
- Varus heel wedges
- OTC arch supports

☐ EXCESSIVE SUPINATION
- Stable shoes
- Valgus heel wedges

☐ INADEQUATE SHOCK ABSORPTION
- Shock absorbing insert

☐ LIMB LENGTH DISCREPANCY
- Heel lift short side
- Partial full-length lift
- Only in athletic shoes

☐ EXCESSIVE PRONATION
- Root orthosis (mild force)
- Inverted orthosis 25° starting point (moderate force)

☐ EXCESSIVE SUPINATION
- Root orthosis with anti-supination modifications

☐ INADEQUATE SHOCK ABSORPTION
- Shock absorbing shoes
- Shock absorbing inserts

☐ LIMB LENGTH DISCREPANCY
- Full-length lifts to full correction
- Only in athletic shoes

☐ EXCESSIVE PRONATION
- Inverted orthosis 35° starting point

☐ EXCESSIVE SUPINATION
- Root orthosis with anti-supination modifications
- Pour 2-3 everted
- Maximally pronated negative cast

☐ INADEQUATE SHOCK ABSORPTION
- Plastazote inserts
- Shock absorbing shoes

☐ LIMB LENGTH DISCREPANCY
- Full-length lifts full correction full time
- Usually have dress shoes modified

*Use treatment options listed for the greatest need checked if more than 1 need category is checked.

Fig. 22-18. Flowchart for initial biomechanical treatment based on implied need.

Table 22-3
Increasing/decreasing correction of the gait patterns

Abnormal gait pattern	Implied need			
	Simple	Moderate	Advanced	Severe
1. Excessive pronation	• Low dye taping • Stable antipronation shoes • Varus heel wedges • OTC arch supports	• Root orthosis (mild force) • Inverted orthosis 25° starting point (moderate force)	• Inverted orthosis 35° starting point	• Inverted orthosis 35° starting point • Varus wedge midsole shoes • Kirby correction • Fettig correction
2. Excessive supination	• Stable shoes • Valgus heel wedges	• Root orthosis with antisupination modifications	• Root orthosis with antisupination modifications • Pour 2 to 3 everted • Maximally pronated negative cast • Lateral midsole/outersole wedges	
3. Inadequate shock absorption	• Shock absorbing insert	• Shock absorbing insert • Shock absorbing shoes	• Plastazote inserts • Shock absorbing shoes	
4. Limb length discrepancy	• Heel lift (1/8″ to 1/4″) short side • Partial full length lift • Only in athletic shoes	• Full length lift up to full correction • Only in athletic shoes	• Full-length lifts full correction full time • Usually have to have dress shoes modified	

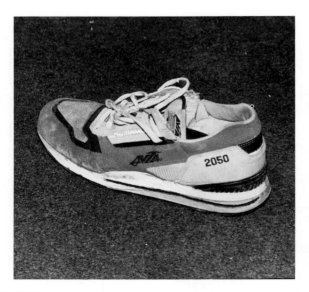

Fig. 22-19. Korex valgus midsole wedge of 1/8 in. seen along the lateral aspect of the shoe from the heel to the level of the metatarsal head.

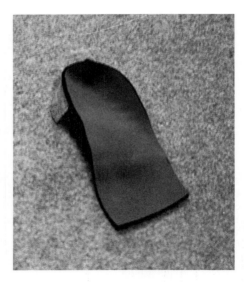

Fig. 22-20. One-eighth-inch spenco sulcus length for shock absorption as topcover for a functional foot orthosis.

Limb length discrepancy	Full length, full-time use of full correction (applied to outersole of dress shoes or under orthotic devices in athletic shoes) (Fig. 22-21)

Manufacturing the inverted orthotic technique

Negative casting technique

The inverted orthotic technique is a positive cast modification. The standard Root device is normally made with the bisection of the heel on the negative cast poured perpendicular to the supporting surface. This is also termed 0 degrees or vertical. The inverted orthotic technique uses the same neutral suspension cast as the Root device. With this cast, the subtalar joint is held in its neutral position, and both axes of the midtarsal joint are maximally pronated. Care is taken not to deform the plantar surface and to fully pronate the midtarsal joints. The fourth and fifth toes are used to stabilize the foot and must be held in their neutral position to the metatarsals, neither dorsiflexed nor plantarflexed.

Once the negative cast is removed from the foot, it is placed on a supporting surface. The heel is bisected by using a tangent through the lateral curve of the heel as a parallel line. It is essential to place the plaster on the foot smoothly and evenly to allow accurate reading of the heel curve between the lateral malleolus and the lateral plantar fat pad (Fig. 22-22). A parallel line tangent to this curve is drawn

on the posterior aspect of the negative cast. For better visualization, the negative cast is held in position where the tangential line is perpendicular to the supporting surface, and then the bisection line is drawn. This line in its relationship to the supporting surface represents the amount of forefoot-to-rearfoot angulation present. There are three possible general positions of this posterior heel bisection line to the supporting surface. These are (1) the vertical position with no forefoot-to-rearfoot angulation or deformity (Fig. 22-23); (2) the everted position with an inverted forefoot-to-rearfoot deformity (i.e., forefoot varus or forefoot supinatus) (Fig. 22-24); and (3) the inverted position with an everted forefoot-to-rearfoot deformity (i.e., forefoot valgus or plantar-flexed first ray).

Pouring process

It is standard practice to pour the negative cast with the heel vertical to the supporting surface. If there is a forefoot-to-rearfoot angulation or deformity, a wedge of material must be placed under one side of the forefoot (metatarsal head) area to maintain the heel in a vertical position while the plaster of Paris is being poured into the cast. It is important to use a separating medium in the negative cast (e.g., green soap) to allow for easy removal of the positive cast from the negative cast. Plaster splints may be necessary to achieve depth in this pouring process since the inverted technique normally requires high heel cups. Pouring the cast too shallow and then inverting it 25 degrees or more will leave a lateral heel area that is too small to make a 21- or 25-mm heel cup (fairly standard for the inverted technique). Blue dye is used in making the positive cast, so there

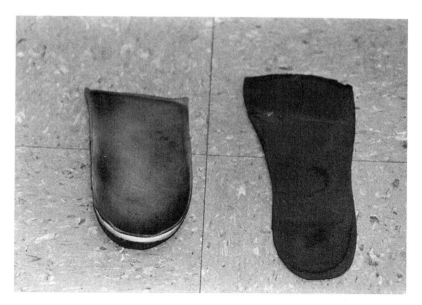

Fig. 22-21. Sulcus length lift of 1/8 in. for short right side seen next to the orthotic device (normally under the orthotic device in the shoe).

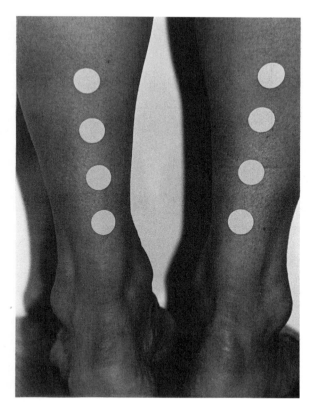

Fig. 22-22. The area demonstrated here between the inferior aspect of the lateral malleolus and the superior aspect of the plantar lateral fat pad will form a line parallel to the heel bisection line on a negative cast.

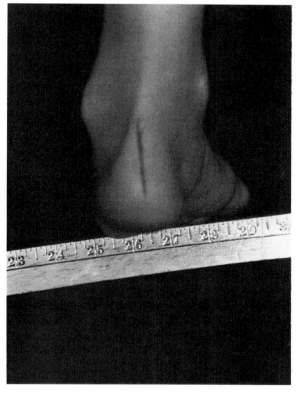

Fig. 22-23. No forefoot-to-rearfoot deformity is noted. In the negative cast the heel bisection rests in a vertical position.

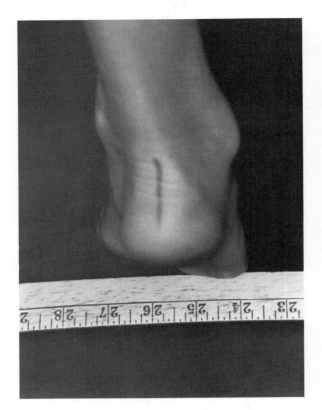

Fig. 22-24. Forefoot varus or supinatus is noted. In the negative cast the heel bisection rests in an everted position.

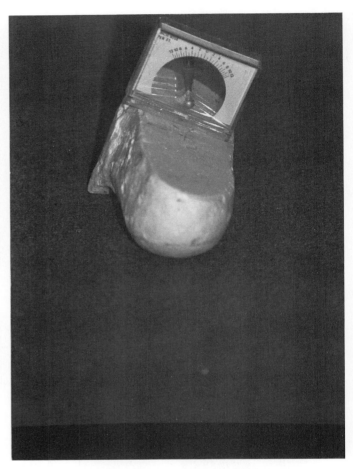

Fig. 22-25. After pouring the positive cast vertical, the anterior platform is applied—in this instance, 15 degrees inverted.

is an easily observed distinction between the positive cast and the original foot. Because the pressing process may break the positive cast, a tongue depressor is placed down the middle of the positive cast when the plaster is still wet. This makes it much easier to repair the cast if it breaks.

Positive cast corrections

When the negative cast is poured in a vertical position, the top surface of the positive cast should be parallel with the supporting surface when the heel bisection is vertical. When adding the anterior platform with the inverted orthotic technique, the nail under the first metatarsal head places the top surface inverted a minimum of 15 degrees (Fig. 22-25). This places the weight onto the fifth metatarsal head. In the presence of a prominent fifth metatarsal styloid process, the weight may be shifted to this area. In this instance, a second nail is needed under the fifth metatarsal head to lift the styloid process off the supporting surface. Normally then, the first or medial nail must be reset to retain the correct overall degrees of inversion. Then the anterior platform is applied with plaster. The technique requires a large bowl of plaster. After the platform has dried, and the excess plaster has been removed, the top angle on the positive cast is

rechecked. Normally, a devil's level is utilized for this measurement.

In many circumstances, the full everted forefoot deformity (i.e., forefoot valgus or plantarflexed first ray) is placed into the anterior platform. This is the Fettig modification, named after podiatrist Dr. Mathias Fettig (Fig. 22-26). Fettig introduced this technique for those patients in whom the inverted correction would potentially sacrifice both lateral column (antisupination) support and metatarsal support. The sequencing of nail application is crucial: Place the medial nail first, angulating the top surface X degrees more inverted than the pouring correction ordered. The X degrees is the amount of the everted deformity present. For example, if the original pouring request was 35 degrees inverted, and there was 8 degrees of forefoot valgus, the original nail is placed 43 degrees inverted. A lateral nail is then placed under the fifth metatarsal head, rotating the top surface to bring the overall correction to the degrees ordered. In the example above, the medial nail placed the top surface 43 degrees

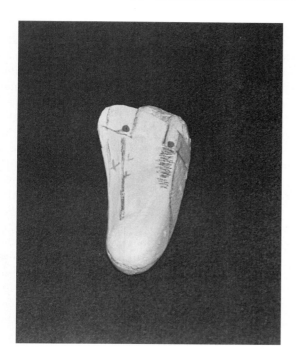

Fig. 22-26. The positive cast for a patient with a 25-degree inverted pour, and 7 degrees of forefoot valgus balanced (known as the Fettig modification). Two nails are needed with an abrupt forefoot valgus support indicated by the marked area. The plantar fascial accommodation is also marked.

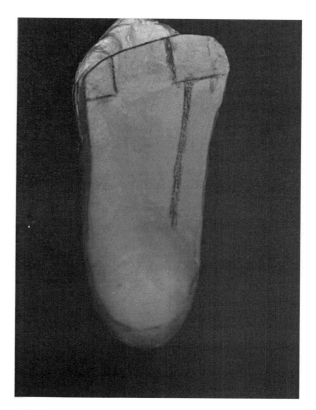

Fig. 22-28. Four vital aspects of the positive cast: (1) flat fifth metatarsal area parallel to the anterior platform, (2) rounded lateral heel expansion, (3) no medial heel expansion, and (4) marked area for plantar fascial accommodation (from the first metatarsal bisection to the medial calcaneal tubercle).

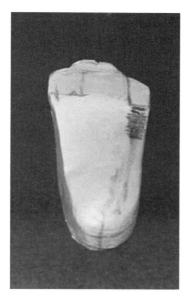

Fig. 22-27. Demonstration of the area with the abrupt forefoot valgus support.

inverted, and the lateral nail derotates the cast back to 35 degrees inverted.

It is important to remember that the medial nail is placed first and that the lateral nail is placed second. With both the styloid process modification and the Fettig modifications, an abrupt transition is made from the lateral anterior platform onto the

fifth metatarsal shaft in the classic Root style (Fig. 22-27). This is key to maximizing lateral column support. When placing plaster on the lateral foot expansion, it is kept parallel to the anterior platform as it is applied. It is normally 3 mm in thickness. It is easy to err and apply this plaster at an oblique angle to the fifth metatarsal platform. This creates a lateral edge in the orthotic device that either cuts up into the patient's foot or is skived away from the foot allowing the patient to slip laterally off the orthotic device. The lateral expansion at the heel area should be rounded and allow the orthotic device to gradually separate from the foot as the heel cup gets higher (Fig. 22-28). A common mistake is to not accommodate for the high lateral heel cup of (commonly) 21 to 25 mm. The rounding of the lateral heel should be as high as the plastic heel cup to be made. The transition from the lateral heel cup expansion medially around the posterior aspect of the heel should stop just onto the medial one half of the heel near the posterior heel bisection. There should be minimal to no medial heel expansion.

The medial arch expansion uses one bowl of plaster on a foot of average size. The technician should make a smooth transition from the medial

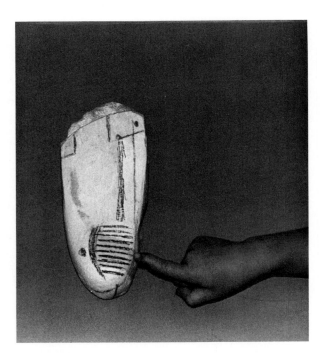

Fig. 22-29. Area skived for the Kirby modification medial to the plantar contact point. The plantar fascial accommodation, 2 mm high by 5 mm wide, is also clearly marked.

aspect of the anterior platform proximally to the medial calcaneal tubercle area. The arch height as finally designed should be slightly higher than the arch height in the classic Root technique. The arch should be smooth, with the height of the arch at the navicular-cuneiform joint (peak). There should be no "peaking" in any other area. Two common incorrect areas of peaking are the first metatarsal shaft, and the first metatarsal-cuneiform joint. Both of these areas become painful when the height of the arch culminates there. The transitions from distal to proximal and from lateral to medial should be smooth and gradual. The fourth metatarsal shaft should not be covered with any plaster unless a small "divot" exists. Once the arch expansion has been applied, a 2-mm-high by 5-mm-wide plantar-fascial accommodation (ridge) is applied from the first metatarsal bisection to the medial calcaneal tubercle. This minimizes the irritation on the plantar fascial medial slip against the medial arch as the first ray plantarflexes in propulsion. The groove or dimpling effect this produces in the medial arch dramatically stiffens the arch area, adding greatly to the antipronation effect of the orthotic device.

Other modifications

Kirby modification. The Kirby modification affects the medial heel area of the positive cast (Fig. 22-29). When inverting the heel, the more rounded the plantar surface of the heel, the less the inversion force produced by the orthotic device. The flatter the plantar surface of the heel, the more inversion force produced by the orthotic device. The Kirby modification, first described by Dr. Kevin Kirby, makes a rounded heel into a flat heel medial to the plantar heel contact point.[7,8] Normally, 3 to 4 mm of plaster from this medial one half to two thirds of the heel area is removed (inskived), taking care to keep the contact point untouched. The technician finds the contact point by rubbing the plantar surface on a "marked" supporting surface in order to identify the contact area or point area. The rounded area medial to this point is then flattened from the posterior heel to the medial calcaneal tubercle area. When ordering an extended Kirby, this flattening is continued distal to the talonavicular joint. The Kirby or extended Kirby is used for moderate to severe pronators to increase the force on the medial side of the subtalar joint axis overall. Removing plaster from this area of the cast produces the opposite effect on the orthotic device, thereby increasing the pressure of the material controlling pronation.

Lateral heel modification. The lateral heel modification increases the expansion from 1/8 to 1/4 in. in selected cases. This should be ordered under the following conditions:

1. Lateral heel irritation from previous orthoses is a complaint.
2. The external angle of gait is greater than 15 degrees, producing excessive lateral heel contact.
3. A high forefoot varus deformity is present (>5 degrees).
4. A high rearfoot varus is present (>8 degrees), producing excessive lateral heel contact.
5. There are soft, delicate heel fat pads.
6. The feet are severely pronated, with lateral displacement of the plantar heel fat pad.
7. The inverted orthotic devices require over 30 degrees of correction.

Medial column modification. The medial column modification increases the support under the midfoot (navicular, first cuneiform, first metatarsal base). Whereas the inverted orthotic technique and the Kirby modification place the major medial column correction in the heel area, selected cases need much greater midfoot correction. In these instances, the peaking of the arch is normally under the first cuneiform, tapered distally and proximally from that area. It is analogous to adding a Schaeffer correction to a standard Root orthotic mold. Owing to the greater sensitivity of the soft tissue in this area vs. the medial heel area, and the foot's need to plantarflex the first metatarsal in propulsion, mul-

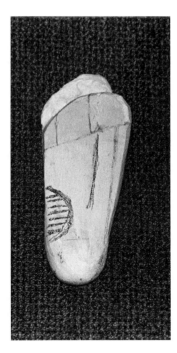

Fig. 22-30. Feehery modification for greater lateral column support.

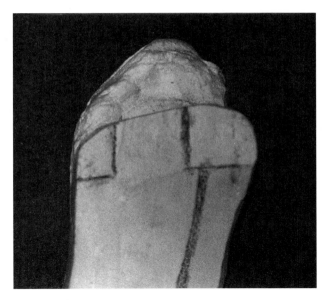

Fig. 22-31. Metatarsal arch modification. The area between the first and fifth metatarsal platform is skived out approximately 1/8 in. for greater metatarsal support.

tiple adjustments are common when using this modification. The common orthotic cases in which this technique is used are:

1. Midfoot collapse into a previously made orthotic device
2. Posterior tibial dysfunction foot type
3. External angle of gait 20 degrees or greater in which arch collapse is prevalent
4. Equinus foot type with severe midfoot collapse
5. Flexible pes cavus feet in which medial column collapse is prevalent

Feehery modification. The Feehery modification increases the support under the lateral column, specifically under the cuboid (Fig. 22-30). Normally, an inskive 3 mm deep is centered over the cuboid along the lateral column, tapering distally to the fifth metatarsal base and proximally to the anterior one third of the calcaneus. First described by Dr. Ray Feehery, this technique has become a useful modification for generalized lateral column support for patients with excessive supination and cuboid pain, and instances where greater stability of the peroneus longus is desired, that is, in cases of first ray symptomatology and lateral ankle soreness.

Metatarsal arch modification. Finally, another common modification is the metatarsal arch modification (Fig. 22-31). Normally, when applying the anterior platform, the area between the first and fifth

metatarsal heads is skived approximately 1/16 in. This places the second through fourth metatarsal heads slightly higher than the first and fifth metatarsal heads. This produces the best forefoot stability, with the medial and lateral sides of the forefoot bearing the most weight during gait. This is very important in propulsion. A goal of orthotic therapy is to have the midtarsal joint maximally pronated and the medial and lateral columns stable as the heel lifts off the ground. If one of the central three metatarsals is lower than the outer two, teetering can occur. For example, if the second metatarsal is lower than the first (as in a metatarsus primus elevatus iatrogenically produced in bunion surgery), the medial column will be unstable in propulsion and the forefoot will pronate onto the first metatarsal. This propulsive phase pronation allows the first metatarsal to gain further weightbearing; however foot alignment is now abnormal and pronation problems can arise.

It is desirable to have the forefoot stable as the weightbearing load is applied during heel-lift to allow push-off to be centered through the foot. In gait, push-off should occur centrally through the second and third metatarsals. The metatarsal arch modification is an attempt to achieve this metatarsal or forefoot stability. The inskiving on the positive cast (which translates to second- through fourth-metatarsal uplifting) may be increased to 1/8 in. or greater. The common problems for which this is ordered include most forefoot problems, when extra stability is needed, and gait findings where propulsive phase pronation is prominent.

Table 22-4
Common variations of inverted prescription

Type of correction	Type of prescription			
Higher correction (A–F)	Type A 35 degrees inverted 25-mm medial heel cup	Type B 35 degrees inverted 25-mm medial heel cup Kirby if rounded heel	Type C 35 degrees inverted 25-mm medial heel cup Kirby 3/16-in. polypropylene Medial extension post	
	Type D 45 degrees inverted 25-mm medial heel cup 3/16-in. polypropylene Medial extension post	Type E 45 degrees inverted 25-mm medial heel cup Kirby 3/16-in. polypropylene Medial extension post	Type F 45 degrees inverted 25-mm medial heel cup Extended Kirby Medial arch correction 3/16-in. polypropylene Medial extension post	
Standard inverted orthotic device* Pronation/ supination corrections (G–J)	Type G 25 degrees inverted Fettig modification 1/8-in. Korex sub- 4th–5th metatarsals as forefoot extension	Type H 35 degrees inverted Fettig modification 25-mm lateral heel cup 1/8-in. Korex sub- 4th–5th metatarsals as forefoot extension	Type I 35 degrees inverted Fettig modification Feehery modification 25-mm lateral heel cup Denton modification 3/16-in. Korex sub- 4th–5th metatarsals as forefoot extension Lateral post extension	Type J 45 degrees inverted Fettig and Feehery modifications 25-mm lateral heel cup 3/16-in. Korex sub- 4th–5th metatarsals as forefoot extension Lateral post extension Denton modification
Shock absorp-tion corrections (K–M)	Type K 25 degrees inverted Spenco topcover sulcus length Birkocork/crepe posting 4–6 degrees pronation motion into post	Type L 35 degrees inverted Spenco topcover sulcus length Birkocork/crepe posting 4–6 degrees pronation motion into post 1/8-in. Spenco horse-shoe heel padding	Type M 45 degrees inverted Rest same as type L	

* Moderate pronation

Prescription writing for the inverted orthotic technique

Once the positive cast is made, any type of material, from foams to rigid plastics can be used to fabricate the inverted orthotic device. The standard prescription for an inverted orthotic device is:

1. Polypropylene, 5/32 in.
2. Polypropylene extrinsic rearfoot post flat-posted with 0 degrees of motion
3. Inverted pouring position of 25 degrees
4. Width to the bisection of the first metatarsal shaft
5. Plantar fascial accommodation, 2 to 3 mm
6. Medial and lateral heel cups, 21 mm
7. Distal edge straight, not rounded, from me-dial to lateral to maximize propulsive phase stability.

Table 22-4 provides an overview of the common variations of the standard prescription. Listed are six common variations, starting from the standard

prescription and moving toward increasing higher medial column pronation correction. Also listed are four common variations for patients with pronation and supination problems, better described as medial and lateral column needs. Three variations of the standard prescription are listed, providing for greater shock absorption. Because of the infinite possibilities each patient presents with, these three variations of the standard prescription are only a beginning. As Figure 22-18 suggests, greater or lesser support of the initial orthotic device is dictated by the patient's response. Figure 22-18 shows that the inverted technique is appropriate for excessive pronators in the "advanced" and "more advanced" categories. Table 22-4 lists 14 common prescriptions for this technique that we prescribe routinely. The three pouring positions commonly used are 25, 35, and 45 degrees inverted.

Figure 22-32 lists these 14 common prescriptions as they relate to clinical measurements (relaxed calcaneal stance position [RCSP] and neutral calca-

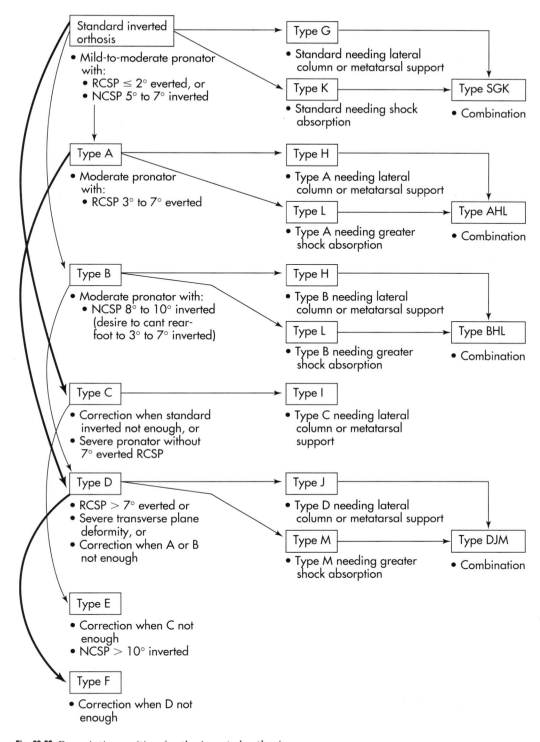

Fig. 22-32. Prescription writing for the inverted orthosis.

neal stance position [NCSP]), gait findings (mild pronator, moderate pronator, severe pronator, tendencies for supination, poor shock absorption), and biomechanically related symptoms (excessive pronation, excessive supination, inadequate metatarsal support, poor shock absorption). Figure 22-32 also demonstrates how these 14 prescription variables are integrated into a larger schematic and how they may be combined. For example, a moderate pronator secondary to 7 degrees of tibial varum angulation with an NCSP of 7 degrees inverted and an RCSP of 0 degrees (vertical) would normally get the

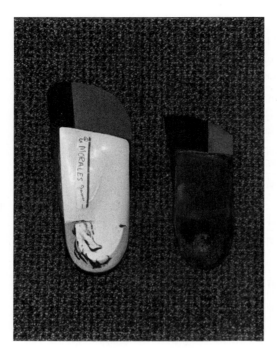

Fig. 22-33. Sulcus length Spenco topcovers with right-sided 1/8-in. Korex sub-fourth and fifth metatarsal heads and left-sided 1/8-in. Korex sub-second to fifth metatarsal heads. Both are used to support the lateral column and metatarsals.

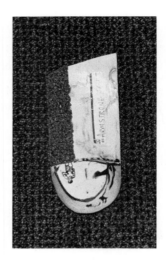

Fig. 22-34. Denton modification shown utilizing Birkocork material as fill for lateral column support distal to the rearfoot post smoothed at the distal edge of the orthosis.

standard inverted orthotic device. However, if gait evaluation showed poor shock absorption bilaterally, and by history multiple inversion sprains had occurred on the right side, then type SGK would be prescribed for the right and type K for the left. It is important to remember that an asymmetric prescription, based on asymmetric needs, is common. Table 22-4 lists the pouring position and common prescription variables. Therefore, type K includes all the prescription variables of the standard inverted orthotic device plus a Spenco topcover (sulcus length), Birkocork or crepe posting, and 4 to 6 degrees pronation motion in the rearfoot post.

With reference to the standard inverted orthotic device prescription (see above), type SGK is therefore a combination of this device and types G and K. The prescription would read

1. All standard device variables, except rearfoot post prescription (changed in type K)
2. Birkocork or crepe posting with 4 to 6 degrees of pronation motion ground into the post (from type K)
3. Spenco topcover sulcus length (from type K)
4. Fettig modification (from type G)
5. Korex 1/8 in. sub-fourth to fifth metatarsals as forefoot extension (Fig. 22-33) (from Type G)

Type K would be (1), (2), and (3), above.

Another example (see Fig. 22-32, Table 22-5) is a 42-year-old runner with chondromalacia patellae (right-sided); severe left side internal femoral torsion (transverse plane deformity); severe pronation in gait with ligamentous laxity; 10 degrees forefoot valgus angulation with Morton's neuroma symptoms bilaterally; and RCSP 5° everted bilaterally. From Figure 22-32 the correction for the right side would be type I (type C needing metatarsal support), and the correction for the left side would be type J (type D needing metatarsal support). From Table 22-4, the prescription for the right (type I) would be:

1. Polypropylene, 3/16 in. (changed from standard 5/32 in. in type C)
2. Polypropylene extrinsic rearfoot post flat-posted with 0 degrees of motion (same as standard) with medial (type C) and lateral (type I) post extensions
3. Inverted pouring position, 35 degrees
4. Width to the bisection of the first metatarsal shaft (same as standard)
5. Plantar fascial accommodation (same as standard), 2 to 3 mm
6. Medial (type C) and lateral (type I) heel cups, both 25 mm
7. Straight distal edge (same as standard)
8. Kirby medial heel modification (type C)
9. Fettig and Feehery modifications (type I)
10. Denton modification (type I) (Fig. 22-34)
11. Leather or vinyl topcover with 3/16-in. Korex sub-fourth to fifth metatarsals as forefoot extension (Type I).

From Table 22-4 the prescription for the left (type

Table 22-5
Summary of initial inverted prescription

RCSP*	Severity of pronation	
	Moderate	Severe
<2 degrees everted	25 degrees inverted	35 degrees inverted *or* 25 degrees inverted with Kirby
3–7 degrees everted	35 degrees inverted	45 degrees inverted *or* 35 degrees inverted with Kirby
>7 degrees everted	45 degrees inverted	45 degrees inverted with Kirby

* *RCSP*, relaxed calcaneal stance position.

Dr: _____ Date: _____ Due Date: _____
Patient Name: _____

Pouring instructions: Inverted R _____ L _____ Vertical R _____ L _____
Kirby R _____ L _____ Extended Kirby R _____ L _____
Fettig R _____ L _____ Denton R _____ L _____
Feehery R _____ L _____
Metatarsal arch modification R _____ L _____
Medial column correction R _____ L _____
Lateral heel modification R _____ L _____

Rearfoot posting:
    6° Motion R _____ L _____
    4° Motion R _____ L _____
    0° Motion R _____ L _____
    Post extension: Medial R _____ L _____ Lateral R _____ L _____

Width: Normal R _____ L _____ Bisection R _____ L _____ Maximum R _____ L _____
Heel cup heights:
    Medial R _____ L _____ Lateral R _____ L _____

Polypropylene thickness:
    1/8" _____ 5/32" _____ 3/16" _____ 1/4" _____

Posting material:
    Polypro _____ Birkocork _____ Crepe _____

Topcovers:
    1/8" Spenco _____ 1/16" Neolon _____ Vinyl _____ Leather _____
    Full length R _____ L _____ Sulcus length R _____ L _____
                          Orthotic length R _____ L _____

Forefoot extensions:
    Material: _____
    Metatarsals supported: _____
Special comments: _____
                  _____
                  _____
                  _____

Fig. 22-35. Sample prescription sheet (inverted technique).

Dr: _____ Date: _____ Due Date: _____
Patient Name: _____

Pouring instructions: Inverted R __35__ L _____ Vertical R _____ L _____
Kirby R __X__ L _____   Extended Kirby R _____ L _____
Fettig R __X__ L _____   Denton R __X__ L _____
Feehery R __X__ L _____
Metatarsal heel modification R _____ L _____
Medial column correction R _____ L _____
Lateral heel modification R _____ L _____

Rearfoot posting:
  6° Motion R _____ L _____
  4° Motion R _____ L _____
  0° Motion R __X__ L _____
  Post extension: Medial R _____ L _____ Lateral R __X__ L _____

Width: Normal R _____ L _____ Bisection R __X__ L _____ Maximum R _____ L _____
Heel cup heights:
  Medial R __25__ L _____ Lateral R __25__ L _____

Polypropylene thickness:
  1/8" _____ 5/32" _____ 3/16" __X__ 1/4" _____

Posting material:
  Polypro __X__ Birkocork _____ Crepe _____

Topcovers:
  1/8" Spenco _____ 1/16" Neolon _____ Vinyl __X__ Leather _____
  Full length R _____ L _____ Sulcus length R __X__ L _____
                    Orthotic length R _____ L _____

Forefoot extensions:
  Material: __3/16" Korex____
  Metatarsals supported: _____4/5_____
  Special comments: _____
       _____
       _____
       _____

Fig. 22-36. Sample prescription sheet (inverted technique): type I—right foot.

J) would be the same as type I, except for a 45 degrees inverted pouring position, and no Kirby modification. Table 22-5 also may help the practitioner focus on the prescription pouring position based on only the RCSP and degree of observed pronation (moderate or severe), which is correlated with Figure 22-32. Figure 22-35 is a sample prescription sheet for ordering these variables. All prescription variables described in this chapter are included on this form. Right and left sides are separated, since this technique emphasizes the asymmetry between right and left. Figure 22-36 is the same prescription sheet with type I ordered for the right foot described above.

Common modifications to inverted orthotic therapy

Overcorrection modifications

Once the orthotic device prescribed has been received back from the laboratory, some adjust-ments may be necessary to achieve optimal results. It is essential to correlate gait changes (with and without orthoses) and symptom response. As Figure 22-13 outlines, it is important to observe the foot and leg function in reference to "ideal" function. Utilizing percentages of correction is an excellent way of managing this clinical task. If you observe walking and running in the moderate-to-severe pronator for whom you have prescribed new inverted orthotic devices, estimate the correction of that pronation individually for the right and left sides. The seven common observations made are the following:

1. *Overcorrection* (>100%). The pronator has now become a supinator, with contact phase lateral instability. The lower extremity cannot tolerate this motion, since pronation must occur just following heel contact to absorb shock, allow for knee flexion, and move in the same direction as the pelvis, hip, knee, and lower leg.

When overcorrection is observed, eight common

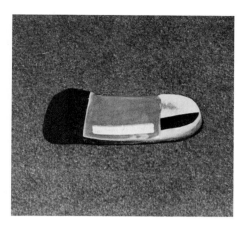

Fig. 22-37. Darkened area showing part of the medial aspect of the rearfoot post removed because of overcorrection.

adjustments to the orthotic device are attempted, one at a time, to preserve optimal control. These are:

a. Inskiving or removing the medial one half of the extrinsic rearfoot post (Fig. 22-37).

b. Narrowing the width to the normal lateral aspect of the first metatarsal head.

c. Lowering the medial aspect of the heel cup, down to 17 or 15 mm from the normal 21 to 25 mm.

d. Thinning the arch and medial heel areas on the top of the orthotic device to decrease the pressure, and increase flexibility.

e. Adding a 1/8-in. felt pad to the lateral one third of the heel cup area next to the heel itself (reverse temporary Kirby).

f. Adding a 1/8- to 3/16-in. Korex support under the fourth and fifth metatarsal heads just distal to the orthotic device.

g. Adding a 1/8-in. Korex valgus wedge under the lateral one fourth of the plantar surface of the rearfoot post, and the plantar surface of the distal lateral corner of the orthotic device (temporary Fettig). This support under the distal lateral corner is normally 1 in. long by 1 in. wide to provide adequate surface area for support and increased contact area.

h. Adding a Denton modification.

It is important that the laboratory provide the practitioner with the positive casts. We give these casts to our patients for storage and possible future use. If the above adjustments do not reverse the overcorrection, or if the patient wants the temporary adjustments listed above to become permanent, it is common to have the laboratory lower the correction, normally 15 degrees, and re-press another orthosis from the lower correction. Sometimes this is accomplished by re-rounding the heel and removing the Kirby modification. The Kirby modification pro-

vides such a significant varus force, that it is fairly easy to overcorrect an abnormal foot position and produce lateral instability. Table 22-6 summarizes these adjustments based on categories of overcorrection.

2. *Complete correction* (90%–100%). The alignment is now considered perfect. The abnormal pronation motion has been completely eliminated. Following heel contact, no pronation motion is present when gait is observed from behind. Additionally no midfoot collapse in midstance or propulsion is observed as the patient walks towards you.

In order to treat most lower extremity injuries appropriately, complete or full correction of abnormal pronation should be attained. We have found that many injuries only improve once complete correction has been attained. However, it should be noted that in some instances injury response may be slow, even when complete correction is achieved. The purpose of this chapter is to show that complete correction, when needed, may be achieved for any given patient. If the clinician is not routinely utilizing the inverted technique with a Kirby, Fettig, Feehery, or Denton modification, or utilizing full leg length difference treatment, then complete correction of most patients' problems is probably not being achieved on a routine basis. Clinicians who routinely underprescribe the correction of their orthoses often perform more surgeries for intractable pain or are simply allowing the patient to live with more pain. Later in this chapter the concept of serial correction is presented in greater detail. To summarize the above discussion, several important points must be emphasized: (a) Undercorrection of abnormal motion may delay or prevent complete injury healing. (b) The expectations of orthotic therapy should be (i) the prescribed orthotic device should produce a 100% change in abnormal foot and leg function; (ii) orthotic therapy should produce a 100% symptom response by changing foot function. (c) Orthotic therapy, like most therapies, is a process with the initially ordered orthosis representing the starting point—it is a means to the end, not the end itself.

When complete correction is attained for one function, the patient may still develop problems with other areas. Remember, the four common areas of biomechanical involvement are excessive pronation, excessive supination, inadequate shock absorption, and limb length discrepancy. Primary treatment of one of these four areas may negatively affect the other three areas. Follow-up evaluation is crucial. Listen to the patient's complaints. Complete correction of the abnormal pronation may cause a functional leg length difference—and symptoms, if more antipronation inversion is required on one

Table 22-6
Treatment modifications for overcorrection

Mild overcorrection (eliminate)

1. Inskive medial one half of rearfoot post
2. Decrease the orthotic width medially
3. Lower medial one half of heel cup
4. Decrease thickness of medial arch and medial heel cup

Moderate overcorrection (add)

1. Above four items (as needed)
2. Add reverse temporary Kirby
3. Add 1/8 to 3/16-in. support under fourth and fifth metatarsal heads
4. Add 1/8-in. valgus wedge to heel and distal lateral edge or orthotic device
5. Add 1/8 to 1/4-in. valgus midsole to outersole wedge heel or full foot to shoes (Fig. 22-38)
6. Denton modification

Major overcorrection (change orthosis)

1. Consider 15 degrees less inverted (i.e., 40 degrees down to 25 degrees) with Fettig applied
2. Remove Kirby (if applied) with repress
3. Consider Root technique
4. Variation on above 10 items in the mild-to-moderate overcorrection categories, if overcorrection still occurs with new orthotic devices

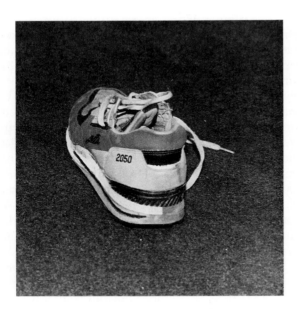

Fig. 22-38. Valgus midsole wedge of 1/8 in. applied for moderate orthotic overcorrection.

side. If the higher-corrected side was the long side originally, the device will function as if a lift was placed under the wrong side (the long side). The practitioner should check the standard pelvic and hip landmarks with the patient standing with his or her orthoses. If one side is higher, lifts are placed under the shorter side to balance the discrepancy. Complete correction may make the patient slightly unstable in side-to-side sports. Three-quarters or high-top shoes for these sports are mandatory when any orthotic device is utilized, particularly when full correction is noted. The excessive pronator, fully corrected, may also have problems related to inadequate shock absorption. The patient may complain that the orthotic device is "too hard," or that the shins, knees, or back is bothering him or her. At times, a simple Spenco topcover is helpful; however, 4 to 6 degrees of pronation motion ground into the rearfoot post, or removal of the post, is sometimes needed. Sometimes, changing to a more flexible or thinner plastic is necessary. It should be noted that there does not appear to be a loss of pronation control with Spenco topcovers or increasing post motion; however, removing the post or changing to a more flexible material can dramatically decrease the control of abnormal motion.

3. *Significant correction* (70%–90%). Most initial orthotic devices fall into this category. Complete correction has not been attained, yet significant change in abnormal motion has been achieved. The change is dramatic enough that a gradual break-in period is required. The box on p. 491 is a copy of a patient "break-in" educational sheet. If symptom

Sample patient instruction sheet

Instructions for wearing orthotics

It takes approximately 1 to 6 weeks to become accustomed to wearing orthoses. During this adjustment period, there may be some awareness in the form of foot or leg discomfort or direct irritation to the skin. Usually, this is part of normal body adjustment and resolves within a short period of time. To minimize discomfort, the following instructions may be helpful:

1. Wear the orthoses for 1 hour the first day and 2 hours the second day, increasing the time by 1 hour each day so that by the end of the first week, you are wearing the orthoses 7 hours a day. Children usually adapt more rapidly than adults. This schedule need not be strictly adhered to, as it may be necessary for you to divide the wearing time during the day. Do not be discouraged if your adjustment period is slower.
2. To minimize skin irritation, the orthoses should be worn with socks or stockings during the break-in period.
3. Discuss with your doctor the different types of shoes that you may wear with the orthoses.
4. The removable insole present in most athletic shoes should be removed and replaced by the orthoses. If the insole is flat and has no arch or heel reinforcement, it may be placed on top of the orthoses. A flat surface provides the best results.
5. If the orthoses squeak in your shoes, apply talcum powder to the inside of the shoes. Paraffin wax may also be applied to the front of the orthoses if needed.
6. The orthoses may be cleaned with soap and lukewarm water, but hot water will damage them.
7. If the orthoses or stabilizing device on the bottom are broken or damaged, notify the office at your earliest convenience.
8. Growing children should be re-evaluated every two shoe sizes.
9. Call the office if you have any difficulties or questions about the use or care of orthoses.
10. Remember, orthoses are designed to work with—not in place of—the physical therapy and rehabilitation program designed for your specific injury.
11. There are many instances where greater or lesser correction of your orthotic devices may be necessary to achieve maximal symptom relief. This may require simply modifying your present orthoses or redesigning a new orthotic device. Please keep the molds given to you for possible future use.
12. Many patients need a specific pair of orthoses for athletics, a different, less bulky, pair for dress shoes, and a third pair for another special function (e.g., high-heeled shoes, ski boots, dance shoes). Communicate with your doctor if you sense this need.

response is slow, Figure 22-32 will help the clinician design a better functioning orthotic device. Even though complete correction is not attained, shock absorption complaints may be heard, with similar remedies as previously listed utilized to improve shock absorption. A variety of inserts may produce a significant change in function. Sometimes, the simplest insert may produce the required change in function and symptom response, whereas a more sophisticated insert may cause abnormal motion and aggravate symptoms. A common mistake is to judge function by appearance rather than gait evaluation. It is common to evaluate four or five pairs of shoes at an office visit in order to choose the most stable pair. When a patient presents with several inserts, it is easy to assume the most sophisticated must be the best. It is important when trying to maximize stability to observe each insert, and judge it on its own merits.

Normally, when significant correction is obtained, it is safe to allow the patient to break in the insert, and not expect to make any modifications for at least 3 to 6 months. This degree of correction is usually void of shock absorption complaints, but they may occur. This correction does make a shift in weightbearing. The weightbearing for a pronator is shifted into a more lateral position. Symptoms of peroneal and iliotibial band strain may be similar to those seen in complete or overcorrected inserts. The practitioner should not attempt to lower the correction or help with these break-in complaints, although this may be necessary ultimately. Initially, the patient is placed on a more gradual breaking-in regimen and stretching exercises are started for the strained muscle groups. Several easy iliotibial band stretches also stretch the peroneals. However, the weight shift may affect any muscle group that is now being utilized or stressed more. Ice massage, anti-inflammatory or muscle relaxant medication, and activity modification may be required to help with these adjustments. It is crucial to advise the patient that there should be no pain in this process, and that adjustments are more the rule than the exception. This will help the patient to gradually accommodate to the device and ease his or her expectations regarding the number of office visits and the expense.

It is at the significant or good correction stages where complacency with the orthotic device prescribed is common, and potentially in error. Many injuries need complete or overcorrection from the prescribed insert in order to be completely resolved. It is acceptable to allow a 2- or 3-month period of utilization of the "good" to "significant" corrected insert, while observing symptom response. However, if the symptomatic response is slow, orthotic

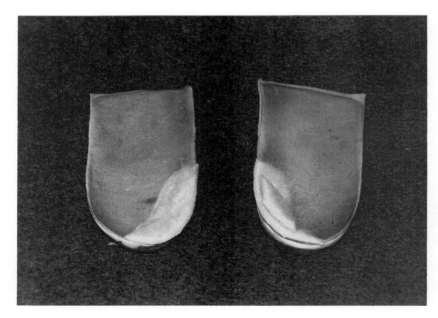

Fig. 22-39. "Temporary Kirby" effect of 1/4-in. felt placed into the medial heel area of the orthotic device for varus cant of the rearfoot. One of us (R.L.B.) uses this temporary padding daily to gain an extra 10% to 20% of rearfoot pronation control.

Table 22-7
Treatment modifications for undercorrection

Mild undercorrection (for inserts producing significant or complete correction)
　1. Medial heel cup made of felt or rubber padding (temporary Kirby)
　2. 3 degrees varus anterior Korex posting and additional rearfoot posting
　3. 1/8-in. varus forefoot extension
　4. 1/8-in. varus outersole or midsole wedging
Moderate undercorrection (for inserts producing good correction)
　1. *(1)* and *(2)* above
　2. 1/4-in. varus forefoot extension
　3. 1/4-in. varus outersole and midsole wedging
　4. Medial arch filler (polypropylene, Birkocork, Korex)
　5. Felt arch support under or over present topcover distal to temporary Kirby
*Major undercorrection (for inserts producing slight correction)
　1. Minimal 15 degrees inverted pour (with Kirby)
　2. Wider and thicker plastic on new orthotic device
　3. Higher medial heel cup with medial extension rearfoot post
　4. 1/4-in. varus outersole or midsole wedging
*Monumental undercorrection (for inserts producing negligible or negative correction)
　1. Minimal 25 degrees inverted pour (with Kirby)
　2. Wider and thicker plastic on new orthotic device
　3. Higher medial heel cup with medial extension rearfoot post
　4. 1/4-in. varus outersole or midsole wedge

* Compare these prescriptions with the new insert prescription utilizing the flow sheet in Figure 22-32 (i.e., if type B is undercorrected, order type D). Normally, it is best to utilize the modifications from Figure 22-32 and above that produce the greatest change in each prescription variable (i.e., if 10 degrees pouring change, and a 15-degree pouring change is given above, use the greater change).

modification must be performed as outlined in Figure 22-32. In some instances, temporary changes such as varus posting with Korex, applying a "temporary Kirby" to the medial heel cup area (Fig. 22-39), adding a Morton's extension or forefoot varus extension, or a combination of these three can

change the present orthotic device to a slightly overcorrected insert, thereby avoiding fabrication of a new insert. These modifications are summarized in Table 22-7.

　4. *Good correction* (50%–70%). This stage of correction can produce significant and complete relief

of symptoms, as can slight and negligible correction. Subtle mechanical changes for injuries produced by repetitive overuse may make major contributions to the patient's rehabilitation. The patient will be aware of improved stability at this stage. As with complete and significant corrections, the clinician may feel that a 2- or 3-month period to follow symptom response is necessary before considering a new insert or making adjustments (see Table 22-7). At this degree of correction, the practitioner must be more demanding in regard to recommending the type of shoes the patient wears. Even though the foot gear is crucial for all inserts, the foot gear must be stability-focused with good correction (i.e., anti-pronation athletic shoes). Foot gear becomes more important when the correction is significantly less than complete.

Patients normally present with an injury on one side—the "bad" side; the noninjured side is the "good" side. Patients normally function in a biomechanically unstable fashion on one side—the "bad" side. It is important to note how the two sides match up: injury vs. noinjury ("bad" vs. "good") and more unstable vs. more stable ("bad" vs. "good"). Table 22-8 summarizes the possible combinations, and defines them as "bad," if injured or less stable. Therefore, there are many instances when patients present to the office with two "bad" sides. Their injured side is their "bad" side because of the pain, and they attempt to favor the other side. The noninjured side, also typically known as their "good" side, may be their less stable side, sometimes by a significant degree. Mechanically, this is considered a "bad" side. The "good side syndrome" occurs when the noninjured "good" side is not good in regard to stability. The patient really does not have a "good" leg to stand on, and there are many reasons why this will interfere with rehabilitation. These include the following:

a. Normal treatment of the injury can tend to strengthen the injured side more than the noninjured side owing to the pain-reduction focus. The more stable side thus gets even more stable, and a greater imbalance can exist. This imbalance can lead to other injuries on the noninjured (weaker) side as activity resumes.

b. When inserts are prescribed, greater focus is placed on the injured side. Greater correction may be ordered for the injured side, even though it may initially be more stable. This increases the imbalance, making the "good" side even less sound. Even if greater correction is not prescribed, it may be achieved anyway. The clinician normally will accept less correction than desired on the side that is noninjured vs. a more critical judgment of the function of the insert on the injured side. Again, the weaker, more unstable side becomes even more unstable.

c. As the legs function in gait, a dominant side usually exists. It is the side that is used more—the side you step off a curb with, the side you depend on more, the usually stronger side—and this may be related to many factors, including whether you are right- or left-handed. If the dominant side is injured, the patient will continue to use it more if the nondominant side is unstable—if the "good" leg is "bad." This slows rehabilitation. The more stable the clinician can make the unstable, noninjured side, the more efficient the rehabilitation process. If the nondominant side is injured, it is easier to shift weight (unweighting the injured side) if the dominant side is stable. However, the dominant side is often unstable and the patient does not have a good leg to rely on.

Thus, recognition of the "good side syndrome" focuses the clinician less on which side is injured, and more on how each side is functioning. The authors recommend a greater focus on the noninjured side, when this side is the less stable. There are many instances when adjustments or remakes of the devices are an attempt to achieve greater correction on the noninjured side only.

Undercorrection modifications

5. *Slight correction* (20%–50%). The pronator is now less pronated, but the change is minimal. Subtle changes can produce excellent symptomatic response, however. This pronation control can occur in three areas: pronation range of motion, pronated positioning, and pronation velocity. Computerized gait analysis has demonstrated that slight range of motion or positional changes may coincide with marked changes in pronation velocity. To the naked eye, the changes may appear minimal, but the patient feels more stable, and pain may be diminished. It is very difficult to become efficient in observing velocity changes since the motion occurs in 1/60th or 1/20th of a second (one to three video frames). Changes in pronation range or position are easier to observe. Therefore, observations should be compared with patient response, both functionally and symptomatically.

Figure 22-32 offers assistance with understanding how to change prescriptions to a higher correction when slight, negligible, or negative correction has been accomplished. A review of this figure demonstrates the typical patterns of correction to higher support generally required if the first orthotic device was not adequate in controlling abnormal pronation. The two general patterns shown in Figure 22-32 for increasing pronation control are:

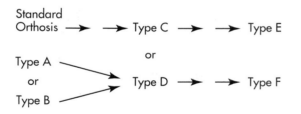

These changes are only necessary when the treatment modifications for undercorrection (listed in Table 22-7) were unsuccessful, or a more permanent version of this higher correction is desired. For example, when the correction variables listed in Table 22-7 for moderate undercorrection are successful in controlling the motion and symptoms, yet a more permanent version is sought to avoid long-term use of varus midsole wedging (Fig. 22-40) and add-on padding, a new orthotic device should be prescribed. This may only be necessary for one foot. We routinely send only one orthosis back to the laboratory for higher correction.

Figure 22-11 began the discussion on "degree of force" of each of the four gait categories. It is in the *subjective* nature of the estimation of amount of "pronation force" that leads to incomplete initial prescription writing where slight, negligible, or negative correction is attained. It is the biomechanical examination and gait analysis that gives us information as to the severity of the abnormal force which must be controlled. Table 22-5 assisted with the focusing of force and resting calcaneal stance position of the overpronator.

The common prescription writing problem normally occurs with undercorrection of the initial insert, following inadequate recognition of severe pronation forces. Figure 22-41 *refines* Table 22-5 with the initial inverted orthotic prescription based on RCSP and a clearer identification of those patients who fit into the "severe" category.

6. *Neglible correction* (0%–20%). There is no noticeable change with this correction. The severe pronator is still pronating severely. Figure 22-32 will help to design a new insert. Normally, this represents only one side that the clinician underestimated. Hopefully, Figure 22-41 will help the clinician to recognize those patients to be categorized as "severe" pronators. Recall also the "good side syndrome." The side most commonly undercorrected is the noninjured or "good" side. This side, however, may be the more unstable of the two sides, thereby requiring more correction.

7. *Negative correction* (–%). This is the worst possible outcome with foot inserts. The new inserts actually increase, not decrease, abnormal motion. Like overcorrection, this new insert may cause more harm than good. This occurs quite often with severe pronators. When the insert does not control the pronation, the insert only lifts the patient higher in the shoe, thereby making the foot more unstable and ultimately accelerating the abnormal pronation. It is common for this type of insert to irritate the patient's arch as the patient pronates through the insert. The inexperienced clinician may then lower the arch, making the orthotic device more comfortable, never recognizing that more medial column antipronation control is necessary. When symptoms persist, surgery may be performed in an attempt to alleviate the chronic pain symptoms. Therefore, it is crucial that the clinician recognize and treat these inadequate orthotic responses.

5-to-1 rule

One method of estimation of correction for the severe pronator is the "5-to-1 rule." Five degrees of plaster correction produces 1 degree of calcaneal inversion (rearfoot change). Measurement of the RCSP is therefore crucial in this determination. For example, a patient presents with left-sided posterior tibial dysfunction, and possible tear. The RCSP is 2 degrees everted on the right side and 10 degrees everted on the involved left side. Utilizing the 5-to-1 rule in an attempt to bring the rearfoot back to a vertical position, a 50-degree inverted orthotic correction should be ordered. If we utilize Figure 22-41, a type F insert (see Table 22-4) should be ordered. Type F would probably give slightly better correction than a 50-degree inverted orthotic device without the extended Kirby, medial arch correction, and medial extension of the rearfoot post. Therefore,

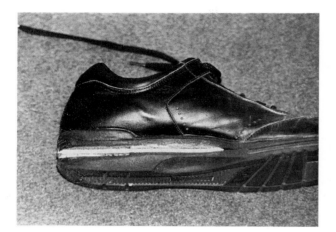

Fig. 22-40. A 1/4-in. heel and 1/8-in. midfoot varus midsole wedging for pronation control.

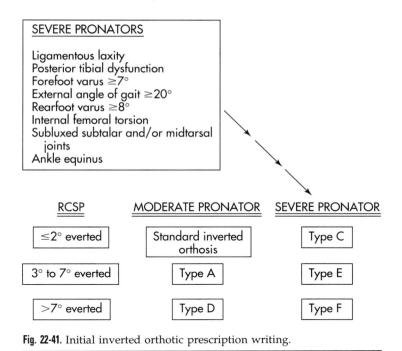

Fig. 22-41. Initial inverted orthotic prescription writing.

Table 22-8
Injury sides vs. stability sides

	Stability sides	
Injury side	Less stable	More stable
Injured side	Injured side less stable ("bad" side)	Injured side more stable ("bad" side)
Noninjured side	Noninjured side less stable ("bad" side)	Noninjured side more stable ("good" side)

these two formulas are fairly similar for most patients. The 5-to-1 rule is a good check on the data presented in Table 22-4 and Figures 22-32 and 22-41.

However, the patient response may be different from 5-to-1, which exists only as an average; "10-to-1" or "12-to-1" responses are not uncommon in achieving full correction. Therefore, a severe pronator with an RCSP of 10 degrees everted and an unknown 10-to-1 response rate will require a 100 degrees inverted orthotic technique for full correction. The technique reaches its highest correction at 70 degrees inversion with Kirby or extended Kirby modifications. There are so many technical difficulties in the manufacturing process above 70 degrees correction that the benefits are outweighed by the difficulties. Imagine trying to press an inverted orthotic device on a 70-degree inverted heel. Fortunately, medial shoe wedging, either midsole or outersole, may address the extra degrees when full correction is necessary for full symptomatic response. Medial shoe wedging produces an average

Table 22-9
Common shoe wedge corrections

Amount of wedge	Amount of heel correction
1/8"	1.5°
1/4"	3°
3/8"	4.5°
1/2"	6°

2-mm to 1-degree change in heel position. Table 22-9 lists the common changes. Therefore, for full correction, a 10-degree everted left foot secondary to a damaged posterior tibial tendon, with a 10-to-1 response rate from the inverted orthotic device, will require a 70-degree inverted device and 1/4-in. medial shoe wedge. A 15-degree everted heel secondary to ligamentous laxity and severe genu valgum deformity would require a 70-degree inverted orthotic device and a 1/2-in. medial shoe

Table 22-10
Prescription variables for different orthoses off same cast

Prescription variable	Running	Walking	Dress
Heel cups	21 mm medial and lateral	18 mm medial and lateral	12–15 mm medial and lateral
Width	Maximum width	Width to first metatarsal bisection	Width just medial to 1st interspace
Thickness	3/16-in. polypropylene	5/32-in. polypropylene	1/8-in. polypropylene
Post	0 degrees motion	4 degrees/4 degrees motion	No post or short post 4 degrees/4 degrees motion
Topcover	1/8-in. Spenco to sulcus	1/16-in. Neolon to sulcus	Vinyl to sulcus with 1/16-in. Neolon forefoot extension

wedge to bring the foot 13 degrees toward vertical. This combination often functions more efficiently than an ankle-foot orthosis and should be attempted prior to performing a rearfoot fusion.

Concept of serial orthoses

Orthotic therapy is a process. The goal of biomechanical treatment is to improve one problem without creating another. The goal of this chapter is to give the practicing clinician valuable treatment options. The practitioner must have high expectations for his or her orthotic therapy, namely, 100% symptom response and 100% biomechanical control.

It is important to emphasize to the patient that full correction may require many modifications. Gait analysis is the only viable way to evaluate these patients. Most initially-prescribed orthotic devices provide only partial correction. For the athlete, the initial orthotic device may be excellent for walking, but may only provide partial control for running. Or, the device may be excellent for running, and overcorrected for walking. One of us (R.L.B.) estimates that 30% of his running orthotic devices are overcorrected for walking, and should not be used for walking. However, 70% may be used for both activities. Yet, if complete correction is necessary for symptom relief, two orthotic devices (two different prescriptions) are normally necessary. Therefore, a great many patients require different pairs for walking and running. New prescriptions are dictated by the initial symptom response, the initial correction observed in gait, the left vs. right foot (treat separately), the prescription options available, type and level of activity, and type of shoe.

Poor shoes can destroy the gains achieved by excellent orthotic devices. As shoes wear out, good shoes may also become sources of poor symptom response. When treating an injury biomechanically, the focus must be toward achieving complete stability as a solid foundation for successful rehabilitation. With a solid foundation, other factors necessary for complete rehabilitation may be more successfully managed. These include strength, flexibility, inflammation, nutrition, training, and scar tissue.

To achieve full biomechanical control, it is not uncommon that three pairs of orthotic devices are initially necessary. A pair is made for the dress shoes, a pair is made for walking or hiking shoes, and a pair is made for athletic or running shoes. More correction is prescribed for the athletic shoes, since running activities produce a greater force throughout gait. The dress shoe orthotic device is narrower, thinner, and in general, less supportive than the walking or hiking orthotic device. Generally, the most important device is first prescribed (i.e., running), with further devices being made as symptom response and activity mandate. Table 22-10 lists the common prescription changes for these three common types of orthotic devices.

For example, a moderate pronator with complaints of a right posterior tibial tendinitis for 6 months presented for treatment. Because of the chronic nature of the complaint, orthotic devices were prescribed for all shoes. RCSP was 2 degrees everted bilaterally with excessive pronation noted throughout midstance into propulsion. Utilizing Figure 22-32, a standard inverted orthotic device was prescribed for running, walking, and dress shoes. Table 22-10 lists the common changes prescribed for these three orthotic devices from the same 25-degree inverted positive cast.

Summary

The inverted orthotic technique is an effective tool for changing abnormal function. Whereas the Root technique was initially described as an end in orthotic therapy, the inverted technique is a means of achieving better foot and leg function. The inverted technique is part of a process. There are 14 commonly prescribed inverted orthotic devices, with many variations. Each patient demands individualization of the process based on many variables. These include biomechanics, shoes, activities, injuries, expense, and other health issues (e.g., age).

Greater or lesser degrees of correction may be needed to help a patient with shin pain this year, and runner's knee pain in 3 years. The biomechanics clinicians most skilled at understanding this process will accomplish the most for their patients. The patients most informed about the process will seek fine-tuning as changes in shoes, activity, and symptoms come about. It is crucial that the orthotic laboratories be aware of this process so that new techniques can be incorporated into orthotic therapy. It is the responsibility of the prescribing practitioner to place this demand upon the laboratory, and to be actively involved in seeing that the laboratory accurately follows these techniques.

References

1. Baitch SP, Blake R; Finnegan P.: Biomechanical analysis of running with 25 inverted orthotic devices, *J Am Podiatr Med Assoc* 81:647–652, 1991.

2. Blake RL: Inverted functional orthosis, *J Am Podiatr Med Assoc* 76:275–276, 1986.

3. Blake RL, Ferguson H: Foot orthosis for the severe flatfoot in sports, *J Am Podiatr Med Assoc* 81:549–555, 1991.

4. Blake RL, Ferguson H: The inverted orthotic technique: a practical discussion of an orthotic therapy, *JBPM* 48:25–29, 1993.

5. Blake RL, Denton I; Ferguson H: TL-61 versus Rohadur orthoses in heel spur syndrome, *J Am Podiatr Med Assoc* 81:439–442, 1991.

6. Blake RL, Ferguson H: Update and rationale for the inverted functional foot orthosis, *Clin Podiatr Med Surg* 11:311–337, 1994.

7. Kirby KA: Rotational equilibrium across the subtalar joint axis, *J Am Podiatr Med Assoc* 79:1, 1989.

8. Kirby KA: The medial heel skive technique, *Precision Labs Newsletter*, July–August 1992.

index

A

Abduction, in congenital hip dislocation, 233(f), 234
Abductor hallucis brevis
    anatomy, 26
    tendinitis, 80
Accelerometer, for measurement of motion, in computerized
        gait evaluation, 198–199
Achilles tendinitis, 80
    gait and, 464(f)
Adhesive tape, for palliative padding and strapping, 368–369
AFOs (ankle-foot orthoses), 391–403. See also Ankle-foot
        orthoses (AFOs)
Age, and splinting in children, 426
Ankle-foot orthoses (AFOs), 391–403
    casting techniques for, 400, 401(f), 402
    extrinsic, 395(f)–397(f), 395–397
    extrinsic versus intrinsic, 394–399
    footwear for, 399–400
    intrinsic, 397–400, 398(f)–401(f), 402
        posterior leaf-spring brace for, 397, 398(f)
        reinforced ankle stabilization brace for, 398, 399(f)
    musculoskeletal conditions for, 392–394
    neuromuscular conditions for, 392–394
    prescription for, 402
Ankle mortise, in biomechanical examination of children, 264
Ankle rocker, in contact phase of gait cycle, 34, 34(f)
Ankles
    in active propulsion phase of gait cycle, 47, 47(t)
    anatomy, 2(f)–4(f), 2–3
    axis of, 3, 4(f)–7(f)
    biomechanical examination, in children, 260–265
    biomechanical examination of, 136(f)–137(f), 137
    in contact phase of gait cycle, 39, 39(t), 41, 41(t)
    dorsiflexion, 3–5, 4(f), 6(f)–7(f)
    equinus of, in children, 260–264
    lateral, instability, 75
    in midstance phase of gait cycle, 43, 43(t)
    motion, 3, 5, 7(f)
        kinetic chains in, 5, 7, 8(f)–9(f)
    in passive lift-off phase of gait cycle, 51, 51(t)
    physiology, 3, 4(f)–9(f), 5–8
    plantarflexion, 3(f), 3–4, 6(f)–7(f)
    in swing phase of gait cycle, 54, 54(t)
Antalgic gait, in children, 228
Anteroposterior shear
    during contact phase of gait cycle, 37, 39(f)
    during midstance phase of gait cycle, 42, 42(f)
    in passive lift-off during gait cycle, 50, 50(f)
Antipronation running shoes, 466(f)
Antiversion syndrome, femoral, 250
Aperture pads, 378, 378(f), 381(f), 381–382
Apley's compression test, 127(f)
Aponeurosis, plantar, physiology, 23(f)
Apophysis, calcaneal, 67
Arch pads, longitudinal, for shoes, 357, 358(f)
Arthritis, and gait abnormalities, in children, 240–241
Ataxic gait, 176(f), 176–177, 230
Athletic shoes, 451–461
    for baseball, 457, 457(f)
    for basketball, 458, 459(f)
    for cycling, 453(f)–454(f), 453–454
    for dance, 458–461, 459(f)–461(f)
    for downhill skiing, 454–455, 455(f)

    for football, 456–457, 457(f)
    for running, 452–453
        antipronation, 466(f)
    for soccer, 455–456, 456(f)
    for tennis, 457–458, 458(f)
Avascular necrosis, 67
    orthotics for, 67
Axis
    ankles, 3, 4(f)–7(f)
    definition, 2
    fifth ray joint, 31–32, 32(f)
    first ray, 24, 24(f)
    metatarsophalangeal joints, 28–29, 29(f), 32
    midtarsal joint, 15–16, 16(f)
    and midtarsal joint stability, 17, 18(f)
    variations in, 6(f)–7(f)

B

Back injuries, low, from running, 114, 116(t), 116–118,
        117(f)–119(f)
Back pain, foot orthotics for, 106–107
Barlow's maneuver, in hip dislocation, in children, 234(f), 235
Baseball, shoes for, 457, 457(f)
Basketball, shoes for, 458, 459(f)
Basket weave strap, 371, 371(f), 372, 372(f)
Bebax shoe, for children, 438, 438(f)
Biomechanical examination, 131–147
    of ankles, 136(f)–137(f), 137
    of calcaneus, 143(f)–144(f), 145
    of children, 243–277
        angle of gait in, 248
        ankle mortise assessment in, 264
        calcaneal position in, 248–249, 249(f)
        clinical evaluation, 247–276
        congenital convex pes valgus in, 267–268, 268(f)
        coxa vara in, 254–255
        evaluation of shoe wear in, 246, 247(f)
        family history in, 245
        femoral component, 249–251
        foot and ankle joint in, 260–265
        genu recurvatum in, 258
        genu varum and genu valgum in, 258–260
        growing pains in, 246
        hallux valgus in, 274–276, 275(f)–276(f)
        head tilt in, 247
        hip evaluation in, 249–254, 251(f)–254(f)
        during initial visit, 244–247
        knees in, 255–260
        level of activity and, 246–247
        metatarsus adductus in, 269–274, 270(f)–273(f)
        midtarsal joint in, 269
        neuromuscular developmental milestones in, 244–245
        participation in sports and, 247
        patellar position in, 247–248, 248(f)
        perinatal history for, 244
        shoulder and pelvis level in, 247
        sleeping and sitting positions and, 245, 245(f)–246(f)
        talipes calcaneovalgus in, 265–267, 266(f)–267(f)
        tarsal coalitions in, 268–269
        tibia in, 255–260, 256(f)–257(f)
        tibial position and, 256–258, 257(f)
        tibial torsion and, 255–256, 256(f)

Biomechanical examination—cont'd
  of children—cont'd
    tibial valgum in, 260
    tibial varum in, 260
    transverse plane in, 249–251, 251(f)
  evaluation form for, 146–147
  of first metatarsophalangeal joint, 138, 139(f), 141
  of first ray position, 137–138, 138(f)
  of forefoot position, 143(f), 143–144
  of hip abduction and adduction, 133, 134(f)
  of hip extension, 133, 134(f)
  of hip flexion, 133, 133(f)
  hip joint measurement in, 132, 132(f)
  hip range of motion in, 132(f)–133(f), 132–133
  instruments for, 132
  of knee position, 133, 134(f)–135(f), 136
  layout for, 132, 132(f)
  of limb length, 145, 145(f)
  of malleolar position, 135(f)–136(f), 136–137
  of neutral calcaneal stance position, 144(f), 145
  physical setting for, 132, 132(f)
  posture and, 144(f), 145
  of resting calcaneal stance position, 143(f), 145
  stance measurements in, 144–145
  of subtalar joint, 139(f)–142(f), 141–143
  of tibial position, 143(f), 144
Biomechanical treatment
  degree of correction in, 472(f), 472–474, 475(t)
  initiation, 468, 472–474
  response to, 474–476, 475(f), 475(t)
Blake inverted orthosis, 446, 446(f)
  in talipes calcaneovalgus, in children, 267(f)
Bleck's classification, of metatarsus adductus, 270, 271(f)
Blount's disease, in children, 259
Body planes, 2
Bones, growth of, and gait abnormalities in children, 231
Braces
  for ankle-foot orthoses
    reinforced ankle stabilization, 398, 399(f)
    wire-spring, 395, 395(f)
  for children
    Roberts, 442
    Wheaton, 433(f)–434(f), 433–434
  posterior leaf-spring, for ankle-foot orthoses, 397, 398(f)
Brachman skate, 431, 432(f)
Budding splint, for fracture or sprain, 372(f), 372–373
Buddy splint, as palliative strapping, 372(f), 372–373
Bunion pads, 383–385, 384(f)
Bunions, tailor's, 80
Butterfly sling, as palliative padding, 387–388, 388(f)
Buttress pads, 282–283

C

Cadence
  definition, 157
  in gait cycle, 35
Calcaneal stance position
  neutral, 144(f), 145
  resting, 143(f), 145
Calcaneus
  anatomy, 8, 9(f)
  apophysitis of, 67
  biomechanical examination of, 143(f)–144(f), 145
  everted, 62(f), 65
  inverted, 62, 62(F)
    with everted forefoot, pathologic changes with, 89
    with inverted forefoot, pathologic changes with, 90
    with perpendicular rearfoot to forefoot, pathologic
      changes with, 89
  position of, in biomechanical examination of children,
    248–249, 249(f)
  spurs in, 67–68
  vertical, 62(f)

Calcaneus gait, 174
  in children, 229, 230(f)
Calf muscles
  in active propulsion phase of gait cycle, 48, 48(t)
  in contact phase of gait cycle, 40(t), 40–41
  in midstance phase of gait cycle, 43–44, 44(t)
  in passive lift-off phase of gait cycle, 52, 52(t)
  in swing phase of gait cycle, 55
Calibration, of electronic output, in computerized gait evalua-
    tion, 185–186
Callus pads, 385(f), 385–386
Cameras, for measurement of motion, in computerized gait
    evaluation, 197–198
Capsulitis, 68
Casting
  for ankle-foot orthosis, 400, 401(f), 402
  corrective. See Serial plaster immobilization
  impression, 279–294. See also Impression casting
  negative, in inverted orthotic technique, 476, 477(f)–478(f)
  positive, in inverted orthotic technique, 478(f)–481(f),
    478–481
Caterall's classification, of Legg-Calve-Perthes disease (coxa
    plana), 238
Cerebellar gait, 176(f)
Cerebellum, evaluation of, in neuromuscular examination, 211,
    211(t)
Cerebral palsy, ankle-foot orthoses for, 393
Cerebrovascular accident, ankle-foot orthoses for, 392–393
Charcot's foot, ankle-foot orthoses for, 393–394
Children
  biomechanical examination of, 243–277. See also Biomechani-
    cal examination, of children
  braces for
    Roberts, 442
    Wheaton, 433(f)–434(f), 433–434
  gait abnormalities in, 228–233. See also Gait abnormalities, in
    children
  orthotics for, 439(t), 439–449, 440(f)–448(f). See also Orthotics,
    for children
  shoes for, 434–439, 437(f), 437(t), 438(f)
  splints for, 425–428, 428(t), 428–434, 429(f)–434(f)
  tibial torsion transformer for, 434
  twister cables for, 432–433
Chondromalacia patellae, subtalar joint pronation and, 466(f)
Circular Torqheel, for children, 434
Clawtoe deformity, 68–69
Closed kinetic chain
  in ankle motion, 5, 7, 8(f)–9(f)
  in first metatarsophalangeal motion, 28–29, 29(f)
  in first ray motion, 24–25, 25(f)
  in gait evaluation, 153–154, 154(f)–155(f), 156
  in midtarsal joint motion, 19–21, 20(f)–21(f), 23(t)
  and orthotics fitting, 336(f)
  in subtalar joint motion, 11–12, 13(f)–14(f)
Clubfoot, serial plaster immobilization for, 417–419,
    420(f)–422(f)
Cobb's angle, in childhood scoliosis, 239(f)
Cobra palliative heel pad, 378, 379(f)
Compartmental syndrome, 124–125, 128(f)
Computerized gait evaluation. See Gait evaluation, com-
    puterized
Contact phase. See Gait cycle, contact phase of
Convex pes valgus, congenital, 267–268, 268(f)
Cork
  for orthotics, 317
  as palliative padding, 374
Corrective casts, for congenital foot deformities, 405–422. See
    also Serial plaster immobilization
Counter pad, for shoes, 357(f), 358
Counter splint, Friedman, 431
Coxa plana, 237(f), 237–238
Coxa vara, in children, 254–255
Cranial nerves, evaluation of, in neuromuscular examination,
    209(t), 209–211, 210(f)

Creep, and orthotics materials, 313, 314(f)
Crescent pads, palliative, 383–386, 384(f)
  digital pads as, 383–386, 384(f)–385(f)
  hallux pinch callus pads as, 385(f), 385–386
  prefabricated aperture, 386, 386(f)
  Tailor's bunion pads as, 385, 385(f)
Crest pad, 357(f), 358, 382, 382(f)
Cuboid pad, 358–359, 378–379, 379(f)
Cuneiform bones. See Rays
Cycling, shoes for, 453(f)–454(f), 453–454

D

Dance, shoes for, 458–461, 459(f)–461(f)
Dancer's pad, for shoes, 357, 357(f)
Data, in computerized gait evaluation
  collection and storage, 183–184
  presentation, 186, 187(f)
Data sampling, in computerized gait evaluation, 184–185
Data smoothing, in computerized gait evaluation, 184, 184(f)
Decay phase, of walking, 33
Denis Browne splint, 428, 429(f)
Denton modification, in inverted orthotic technique, 484(f)
Developmental milestones, neuromuscular, in biomechanical examination of children, 244–245
Development phase, of walking, 33
Devil's tractor, in pediatric hip evaluation, 252, 252(f)
Diagnosis, gait and, 467(f), 467–468
Diaphragm, anatomy, 99–100
Digital pads, palliative, 380–388
  buttress pads as, 382–383
  crescent pads as, 383–386, 384(f)–385(f)
  crest pad as, 382, 382(f)
Digital strap, for fracture or sprain, 372
Dorsiflexion, 3–5, 4(f), 6(f)–7(f)
Downhill skiing, shoes for, 454–455, 455(f)
Drift, in computerized gait evaluation, 185
Dynamic acetabulum, 27, 27(f)
Dynamic load, response to, in orthotic materials, 321(t), 321–322
Dysdiadochokinesia, exam for, 211
Dysmetria, examination for, 211
Dystrophic gait, 174(f)

E

Elastoplast pad, palliative, 379–380, 380(f)
Electromyography, in computerized gait evaluation, 199
Electronic output, in computerized gait evaluation, 185–186
Equinus
  of ankle, in children, 260–264
  spastic, in children, 261
Euler angles, in computerized gait evaluation, 196, 197
Eversion. See specific structures
Exostosis
  first ray, 69
  retrocalcaneal, 77
    orthotics for, 77
Extensor hallucis longus, tendinitis, 80
Extraocular movements, in neuromuscular examination, 210(f), 210–211
Extremities
  lower, range of motion study of, for orthotics, 296–297
  shortened, in children, 230–232
Extrinsic ankle-foot orthosis, 395(f)–397(f), 395–397
  vs. intrinsic ankle-foot orthosis, 394–399
Extrinsic muscles
  in active propulsion phase of gait cycle, 49, 49(t)
  in contact phase of gait cycle, 41, 41(t)
  in midstance phase of gait cycle, 44–45, 45(t)
  in passive lift-off phase of gait cycle, 53, 53(t)
  in swing phase of gait cycle, 55
Eyes, in gait evaluation, 162, 164(f)

F

Facet joints, spinal, biomechanics, 107–108, 108(f)
Fasciitis, plantar, 76
Feehery modification, in inverted orthotic technique, 481, 481(f)
Felt, as palliative padding, 374
Femoral antiversion syndrome, 250
Femoral epiphysis, slipped, in children, 238(f), 238–239
Femur, evaluation of, in biomechanical examination of children, 249–251
Festinating gait, 176(f)
Fiberglass splints, for children, 434, 435(f)–436(f)
Fibula, stress fractures of, 79
Filauer splint, 428, 429(f)
First metatarsal-first cuneiform exostosis, 69
First metatarsophalangeal joint. See Metatarsophalangeal joint, first
Flexor digitorum longus, tendinitis, 81
Flexor hallucis brevis, anatomy, 26
Flexor hallucis longus, tendinitis, 81
Flexosplint, 431
Foam, for orthotics, 317
Foam rubber, as palliative padding, 374
Foot
  in biomechanical examination of children, 260–265
  congenital deformities of, serial plaster immobilization for, 405–422. See also Serial plaster immobilization
  development of, 439–440
  pronation, 105–106
  running injuries of, 125–130, 129(f)
Football, shoes for, 456–457, 457(f)
Footdrop gait, in children, 230, 230(f)
Foot types, 60–62
  classification, 85–93, 87(f)–88(f), 89(t)
    methodology, 86–88, 87(f)–88(f)
    studies on, 86
  pathologic changes with, 88–92
Footwear. See Shoes
Force
  measurement, by computerized gait evaluation, 191(f), 193–196, 195(f)–196(f), 200(f)
  and orthotic materials, 312
Force time integrals, in computerized gait evaluation, 195(f)–196(f)
Forefoot
  adductus of, in children, 272(f)
  biomechanical examination of, 143(f), 143–144
  everted
    with everted rearfoot, pathologic changes with, 91
    with inverted calcaneus, pathologic changes with, 89
    with perpendicular rearfoot, pathologic changes with, 90
  inverted
    with everted rearfoot, pathologic changes with, 92
    with inverted calcaneus, pathologic changes with, 90
    with perpendicular rearfoot, pathologic changes with, 91
  perpendicular
    with everted rearfoot, pathologic changes with, 91–92
    with perpendicular rearfoot, pathologic changes with, 90–91
  perpendicular to rearfoot, with inverted calcaneus, pathologic changes with, 89
  position, in gait evaluation, 168–169, 171, 171(f)
  running injuries of, 128–130
  supinatus, in frontal plane, 64–65
  types, pathologic changes with, 89(f), 89–92
  valgus, 170(f)–171(f)
    positive casting in, 479(f)
  valgus in frontal plane, 63(f), 65
  varus, 170(f)–171(f)
    in frontal plane, 62(f)–63(f), 62–64
    negative casting in, 478(f)
Forefoot rocker, in contact phase of gait cycle, 34, 34(f)
Forward flexion test, 109, 111(f)
Fourth metatarsal bone, 31

Fractures
    strapping and padding for. *See* Pads; *Strapping*
    stress. *See* Stress fractures
Freiberg's disease, 67
Friedman counter splint, 431
Frontal plane
    forefoot supinatus in, 64–65
    functional disorders in, 62–65
    valgus in, 62(f)–63(f), 65
        forefoot, 63(f), 65
    varus in, 62(f)–63(f), 62–64
        forefoot, 63–64
        rearfoot, 62–63
Functional disorders
    in frontal plane, 62–65
    in sagittal plane, 65
    in transverse plane, 66
Functional foot orthotics, diagnosing problems with, 327–348.
        See also Orthotics
Functional symmetry, assessment, in running injuries, 116–118,
    120(f)

G

Gait
    and Achilles tendinitis, 464(f)
    angle of, in biomechanical examination of children, 248
    antalgic, in children, 228
    ataxic, in children, 176(f), 176–177, 230
    biomechanics, 109–110, 110(f)–111(f)
    calcaneus, 174
        in children, 229, 230(f)
    cerebellar, 176(f)
    childhood limp in, 224(f)–225(f), 224–228, 226(t)–228(t). *See
        also* Limp, in children
    and diagnosis, 467(f), 467–468
    festinating, 176(f)
    first metatarsophalangeal joint in, 28
    first ray in, 25–26, 26(f)
    footdrop, in children, 230, 230(f)
    in lower motor neuron dysfunction, 174, 175(f)–176(f), 176
    motions during, 23(t)
    in myopathies, 173, 174(f), 176(f)
    in myopathy, 173, 174(f), 176(f)
    in mysthenia gravis, 174(f)
    neurologic, in children, 228–230, 229(f)–231(f)
    paralytic, in children, 228–230, 229(f)–231(f)
    patterns, 468, 468(t)
    phasic
        double float, 161(f)
        double stance, 161(f)
    spastic, in children, 230, 231(f)
    Trendelenburg, 176(f)
        in children, 225, 225(f)
    upper motor neuron dysfunction in, 176(f), 176–177
Gait abnormalities
    in children, 228–233
        arthritis and, 240–241
        bone growth and, 231
        under five years, etiology, 227(t)
        from hip dislocation, 233(f)–237(f), 233–236
        knee problems and, 241
        limp and loss of supporting structures in, 232
        osteomyelitis and, 240
        paralysis and, 228–230, 229(f)–231(f)
        scoliosis and, 239(f)–240(f), 239–240
        and slipped capital femoral epiphysis, 238(f), 238–239
    treatment, response to, 474–476, 475(f), 475(t)
    and treatment recommendations, 469(f)–471(f)
Gait cycle, 32–55
    angle of gait in, 35, 35(f)
    base of, 35, 35(f)
    biomechanics, 36(f)–37(f), 36–37
    cadence in, 35

    initial double support in, 33(f), 34
    midstance phase, biomechanics, 109, 110(f)
    single limb support in, 33(f), 34–35
    stance phase, 33(f)–34(f), 33–34
        active propulsion during, 33(f), 34, 45(f), 46–50
            ankle joint in, 47, 47(t)
            anteroposterior shear in, 46, 46(f)
            calf muscles in, 48, 48(t)
            extrinsic muscles in, 49, 49(t)
            hip joint in, 46, 46(t)
            in horizontal plane, 46, 46(t)
            intrinsic muscles in, 48–49, 49(t)
            knee joint in, 46, 46(t)
            longitudinal axis in, 47(f), 48
            midtarsal joint in, 47(t), 47–48
            oblique axis in, 47(f), 48
            pretibial muscles in, 48
            subtalar joint in, 47, 47(t)
            vertical load in, 46, 46(f)
        contact phase of, 33, 33(f), 33–34, 34(f), 37–41, 39(f)
            ankle joint in, 39, 39(t), 41, 41(t)
            ankle rocker in, 34, 34(f)
            anteroposterior shear in, 37, 39(f)
            calf muscles in, 40(t), 41
            extrinsic muscles in, 40–41, 41(t)
            forefoot rocker in, 34, 34(f)
            ground reaction forces in, 37, 39(f)
            heel rocker in, 34, 34(f)
            hip joint during, 38, 39(t)
            horizontal plane in, 37–38, 39(t)
            intrinsic muscles in, 41, 41(t)
            knee joint in, 38, 39(t)
            longitudinal axis in, 40
            midtarsal joint in, 40(t)–41(t), 40–41
            oblique axis in, 40
            pretibial muscles in, 40(t), 40–41
            subtalar joint in, 39–41, 40(t)–41(t)
            vertical load in, 37, 37(f)
        midstance phase of, 33(f), 33–34, 42(f), 42–45
            ankle joint in, 43, 43(t)
            anteroposterior shear in, 42, 42(f)
            calf muscles in, 43–44, 44(t)
            extrinsic muscles in, 44–45, 45(t)
            hip joint in, 42, 43(t)
            horizontal plane in, 42, 42(t)
            intrinsic muscles in, 44, 44(t)
            knee joint in, 42–43, 43(t)
            longitudinal axis in, 43
            midtarsal joint in, 43, 43(t)
            oblique axis in, 43
            pretibial muscles in, 43
            subtalar joint in, 43, 43(t)
            vertical load in, 42, 42(f)
        passive lift-off during, 33(f), 34, 50(f), 50–53
            ankle joint in, 51, 51(t)
            anteroposterior shear in, 50, 50(f)
            calf muscles in, 52, 52(t)
            extrinsic muscles in, 53, 53(t)
            hip joint in, 50, 51(t)
            in horizontal plane, 50, 51(t)
            intrinsic muscles in, 52(t), 52–53
            knee joint in, 51, 51(t)
            in longitudional axis, 51, 51(t)
            midtarsal joint in, 51, 51(t)
            in oblique axis, 51–52
            pretibial muscles in, 51(t), 52
            subtalar joint in, 51, 51(t)
            vertical load in, 50, 50(f)
        of running, evaluation of heel during, 120(f)
    step in, 35, 35(f)
    stride length, 35, 35(f)
    swing phase, 33(f), 33–34, 36, 37, 37(f), 53–55, 54(f)
        ankle joint in, 54, 54(t)
        calf muscles in, 55
        extrinsic muscles in, 55

ground reaction forces in, 53
hip joint in, 54, 54(t)
horizontal plane in, 54, 54(t)
intrinsic muscles in, 55
knee joint in, 54, 54(t)
longitudinal axis in, 54–55
midtarsal joint in, 54, 55(t)
oblique axis in, 55
pretibial muscles in, 55, 55(t)
subtalar joint in, 54, 55(t)
terminal double support in, 33(f), 34
traditional, 160(f)
walking, 160(f)
Gait evaluation, 150–154, 151(f)–155(f), 156, 157(f)
computerized
calibration in, 185–186
comparison of waveforms in, 192
data collection and storage in, 183–184
data presentation in, 186, 187(f)
data sampling in, 184–185
data smoothing in, 184, 184(f)
in determining need for treatment, 180–181
for documentation of progress, 181
drift in, 185
durability of equipment for, 186
electromyography in, 199
empirical approach to, 182–183
errors in, 192
force time integrals in, 195(f)–196(f)
impulses in, 195, 195(f)
joint power in, 201–202, 202(f)
kinematics in, 200–201
kinetics in, 200–201
limits of confidence in, 190
measurement of force in, 193–196, 195(f)–196(f)
measurement of motion in, 196–199, 197(f)–198(f)
accelerometers for, 198–199
cameras for, 197–198
Euler angles for, 196, 197
goniometers for, 197
projection angles for, 196–197
screw displacement axes for, 196–197
stereometer for, 197–198
measurement of pressure in, 193
mechanical analysis in, 199, 200(f)
modeling approach to, 181–182
normal values in, 180
precision of, 189
for prediction of high-risk patients, 180
sagittal plane balance in, 199–200
sensor calibration in, 185–186
statistical aspects of, 190–192
subject-test interaction in, 186–188
technical aspects of, 183–188
uses of, 180–181
validity of, 189–190, 191(f)
variability among subjects, 192
variations in, 191–192
crosschecking and, 171, 173
dynamic, 153–159, 155(f), 159(f)–172(f), 161–173
eyes in, 162, 164(f)
forefoot position in, 168–169, 171, 171(f)
forms for, 151(f–152(f),)155(f)
hips in, 163, 167(f)
kinetic chains in, 153–154, 154(f)–155(f), 156
knee position in, 165, 168(f)
line of progression in, 171, 172(f)
phasic observations in, 171, 172(f)
plantar lesions and, 156, 157(f)–158(f)
Q angle in, 163, 165, 167(f)
rearfoot position in, 165–168, 169(f)–170(f)
sensors for, 153(f)
shoulders in, 162–163, 165(f)–166(f)
site location for, 161–163, 163(f)–171(f), 165–169, 171
static, 153–154, 154(f)–155(f), 156

subtalar joint position in, 165–168, 169(f)–170(f)
subtalar joint range of motion in, 154, 155(f), 156, 157(f)
systems for, 150–152, 151(f)–154(f)
TBFR sequence for, 161–163, 163(f)–171(f), 165–169, 171
tibial position in, 165, 168(f)
Gait homunculus observed relational tabular (GHORT),
156–157, 159(f), 164(f)
Gait plates, for children, 447(f)–448(f), 447–449
Galeazzi's sign, in hip dislocation, in children, 233(f), 234–235
Ganley splint, 430, 430(f)–431(f)
Gastrocnemius equinus, 65, 260
Gastrocnemius-soleus, congenital equinus of, 260–261
Genu recurvatum, in children, 258
Genu valgum, in children, 258–260
Genu varum, in children, 258–260
GHORT (gait homunculus observed relational tabular),
156–157, 159(f), 164(f)
Gibney strap, 371, 372(f)
Glass transition temperature, and orthotic materials, 314, 315(t)
Gluteus maximus, paralysis of, in children, 228, 229(f)
Goniometers
measurement of motion by, in computerized gait evaluation,
197
for measurement of tendon flexibility, 465(f)
in pediatric hip evaluation, 252, 252(f)
Ground reaction force
in contact phase of gait cycle, 37, 39(f)
orthotics and, 347(f)
in swing phase of gait cycle, 53
Growing pains, in children, 246

H

Hallux abducto valgus, in first metatarsophalangeal joint, 29
Hallux extensus, 69
Hallux limitus, 69–70, 70(f)
Hallux, palliative strapping for, 373
Hallux pinch callus pads, 385(f), 385–386
Hallux rigidus, in first metatarsophalangeal joint, 29
Hallux valgus, 70–73, 72(f)
in children, 274–276, 275(f)–276(f)
in first ray, 24–25, 25(f)
Hammer toe deformity, 73–74
Hammock effect, in first metatarsophalangeal joint, 27(f), 27–28
Hamstrings, weakness, and gait abnormalities in children, 229,
230(f)
Head tilt, in biomechanical examination of children, 247
Heel, evaluation, during stance phase of running, 120(f)
Heel cup irritation, from orthotics, correction of, 341–342,
342(f)–344(f)
Heel grip, for shoes, 357, 358(f)
Heel height differential, of shoes, and fit of orthotics,
334(f)–335(f), 334–336
Heel modification, lateral, in inverted orthotic technique, 480
Heel pads, palliative, 378(f)–379(f), 378–379
aperture pad as, 378, 378(f), 381(f), 381–382
cobra pad as, 378, 379(f)
cuboid pad as, 378–379, 379(f)
digital pads as, 380–388
horseshoe pad as, 378, 379(f)
removable elastoplast pad as, 379–380(f)
Heel rocker, in contact phase of gait cycle, 34, 34(f)
Heel spur pads, 358, 359(f)
Heel stabilizers, for children, 442–443, 443(f)
Heel strike, biomechanics, 109, 110(f)
Heel wedges, varus, 465(f)
Hemihypertrophy, in children, 232
Hip rotation test, 120, 122(f)
Hips
abduction and adduction, measurement, 133, 134(f)
in active propulsion phase of gait cycle, 46, 46(t)
biomechanical examination of, 132(f)–134(f), 132–133
in children, 249–254, 251(f)–254(f)
during contact phase of gait cycle, 38, 39(f)

Hips—cont'd
in contact phase of gait cycle, 38, 39(t)
dislocation of, in children, 233(f)–237(f), 233–236
assymetric inguinal and buttock skinfolds in, 233(f), 234
causes, 234
diagnosis, 234–236
with limited abduction, 233(f)
radiography in, 235(f), 235–236
treatment, 236, 236(f)–237(f)
ultrasonography in, 236
extension, measurement, 133, 134(f)
flexibility, evaluation, 121(f)
flexion, measurement, 133, 133(f)
in gait evaluation, 163, 167(f)
in midstance phase of gait cycle, 42, 43(t)
in passive lift-off phase of gait cycle, 50, 51(t)
range of motion measurement, 132(f)–133(f), 132–133
running injuries of, 116t, 118–122, 121(f)–122(f)
in swing phase of gait cycle, 54, 54(t)
Horseshoe pad, for heels, 378, 379(f)
Hypermobile first ray, 69
Hypotonia, exam for, 211

I

Ilfeld splint, for hip dislocation in children, 236, 237(f)
Iliac spine, assessment, in running injuries, 116, 117(f)
Iliotibial tract, irritation, from running injuries, 122
Impression casting, 279–294
for ankle-foot orthoses, 400, 401(f), 402
modified techniques, 292–294, 293(f)
negative, 280–281
errors in, 328–329, 329(f)
hand position for, 445(f)
materials for, 280–281
for orthotics, 297–298, 298(f)
techniques for, 280
neutral suspension technique, 282–290, 284(f)–287(f), 293(f)
accuracy of, evaluation of, 288, 289(f), 290
advantages and disadvantages of, 284, 288
plaster application in, 283–284, 285(f)–287(f)
positive, 293(f), 294
prone casting technique, 290, 290(f)
semiweightbearing technique, 291–292, 292(f), 305–306
of subtalar joint, neutral position for, 281(f)–283(f), 281–282
vacuum technique, 290–291, 291(f), 306
Impulses, in computerized gait evaluation, 195(f)
Inflare last shoe, for children, 437, 438(f)
Innominates, biomechanics, 109
In-shoe accommodation(s), 359, 360(f)
Inskiving, 487, 487(f)
Intention tremor, exam for, 211
Interdigital lesions, palliative padding for, 387
Interdigital neuroma, 74–75
Interdigital pads, palliative, 386(f), 386–387
Interosseous talocalcaneal ligament, anatomy, 8–9
Interosseus ligaments. See First ray joint
In-toe gait plate, 447(f)
Intrinsic ankle-foot orthoses, 397–400, 398(f)–401(f), 402
posterior leaf-spring brace for, 397, 398(f)
reinforced ankle stabilization brace for, 398, 399(f)
Intrinsic muscles
in active propulsion phase of gait cycle, 48–49, 49(t)
in contact phase of gait cycle, 41, 41(t)
in midstance phase of gait cycle, 44, 44(t)
in passive lift-off phase of gait cycle, 52(t), 52–53
in swing phase of gait cycle, 55
Inversion. See specific structures
Inverted orthotics, Blake, 446, 446(f)
in talipes calcaneovalgus, in children, 267(f)
Inverted orthotic technique, 463–495
Denton modification in, 484(f)
diagnosis in, 465, 466(f), 466(t), 467
Feehery modification in, 481, 481(f)

Kirby modification in, 480, 480(f)
lateral heel modification in, 480
manufacturing process in, 476–481, 477(f)–481(f)
medial column modification in, 480–481
metatarsal arch modification in, 481, 481(f)
negative casting in, 476, 477(f)–478(f)
overcorrection modifications in, 486–491, 487(f)–490(f), 488(t)
patient presentation for, 464(f)–466(f), 464–465
positive casting in, 478(f)–481(f), 478–481
pouring process in, 476, 478
prescription writing for, 482(t), 482–486, 483(f)–486(f), 485(t)
5-to-1 rule in, 492–494, 493(f), 493(t)
undercorrection modifications in, 490(t), 491–492, 492(f)
Ipos shoe, for children, 438–439

J

Joint power, in computerized gait evaluation, 201–202, 202(f)
J strap, 371–372

K

Kinematics, in computerized gait evaluation, 200–201
Kinetic chains
in ankle motion, 5, 7, 8(f)–9(f)
in first metatarsophalangeal motion, 28–29, 29(f)
in first ray motion, 24–25, 25(f)
in gait evaluation, 153–154, 154(f)–155(f), 156
in midtarsal joint motion, 19–21, 20(f)–21(f), 23(t)
in subtalar joint motion, 11–12, 12(f)–14(f)
Kinetics, in computerized gait evaluation, 200–201
Kirby modification, in inverted orthotic technique, 480, 480(f)
Kirby's method, for subtalar joint examination of children, 265, 266(f)
Knees
in active propulsion phase of gait cycle, 46, 46(t)
anatomy, 127(f)
biomechanical examination of, 133, 134(f)–135(f), 136
in children, 255–260
biomechanics of, 123(f)
in contact phase of gait cycle, 38, 39(t)
and gait abnormalities, in children, 241
in midstance phase of gait cycle, 42–43, 43(t)
in passive lift-off phase of gait cycle, 51, 51(t)
position, in gait evaluation, 165, 168(f)
running injuries of, 122–124, 124(f)–127(f)
in swing phase of gait cycle, 54, 54(t)
Kohler's disease, 67

L

Langer Pediatric Counter Rotation System splint, 431–432, 432(f)–433(f)
Lasègue's sign, 116, 119(f)
Lasts, for shoes, 351(f)
pediatric, 435
Legg-Calve-Perthes disease
Caterall's classification, 238
in children, 237(f), 237–238
Leg length discrepancy, 101–105, 105(f)–107(f)
compensation for, in children, 232
shoe lifts for, 104–105, 360–363, 363(f), 464(f), 477(f)
Legs, running injuries of, 124–125, 128(f)
Lifting, physiology, 101, 104(f)
Lift therapy, for leg length inequality, 104–105, 360–363.363(f).464(f), 477(f)
Limb length, biomechanical examination of, 145, 145(f)
Limbs, measurement, in running injuries, 118, 121(f)
Limp, in children, 224(f)–225(f), 224–248, 226(t)–228(t)
contractures and, 232
psychogenic, 232–233
Line of progression, in gait evaluation, 171, 172(f)

LMN (lower motor neuron), dysfunction, and gait abnormalities, 174, 175(f)–176(f), 176
Loading response, of subtalar joint, 14(f)
Longitudinal arch pads, for shoes, 357, 358(f)
Low back, running injuries, 114, 116(t), 116–118, 117(f)–119(f)
    curvature assessment in, 116, 118(f)
Low back pain, foot orthotics for, 106–107
Low Dye strap, 369–371, 370(f), 372(f)
Lower extremities. See also specific structures
    anatomy, 1–57
    physiology, 1–57
Lower motor neuron (LMN), dysfunction, and gait abnormalities, 174, 175(f)–176(f), 176
Lumbosacral angle, 96, 97(f)
Lumbosacral joint, biomechanics, 109

M

Malleolus
    anatomy, 2, 2(f)
    position, biomechanical examination of, 135(f)–136(f), 136–137
Manual muscle testing, in neuromuscular examination, 212, 212(t)–214(t), 214, 215(f)–219(f)
McMurray's test, 126(f)
Mechanical analysis, in computerized gait evaluation, 199, 200(f)
Medial column modification, in inverted orthotic technique, 480–481
Meniscus, tears of
    Apley's compression test for, 127(f)
    McMurray's test for, 126(f)
Mental status, in neuromuscular evaluation, 209
Metatarsal arch modification, in inverted orthotic technique, 481, 481(f)
Metatarsal head, pain in, from orthotics, correction of, 346–348, 347(f)
Metatarsal pads, 356–357, 357(f), 375, 375(f)–378(f), 375–378
Metatarsals. See Rays
Metatarsophalangeal joints
    biomechanical examination, 138, 139(f), 141
    dorsal pain in, from orthotics, correction of, 345–346, 347(f)
    fifth, 32
    first, 27–31, 29(f)–30(f)
        anatomy, 27(f), 27–28
        axis, 28–29, 29(f)
        in gait, 28
        hammock effect in, 27(f), 27–28
        kinetic chains, 28–29, 29(f)
        pathophysiology, 29
        and propulsion, 29–30, 30(f)
        range of motion in, 30–31
    fourth, 32
    lesser, 32
    second, 32
    third, 32
Metatarsus adductus
    Bleck's classification of, in children, 270, 271(f)
    in children, 269–274, 270(f)–273(f)
    in first ray, 25
    serial plaster immobilization for, 406(f)–414(f), 406–413
Midfoot, running injuries of, 128
Midsole wedge, valgus, 476(f), 488(f)
Midstance phase. See Gait cycle, midstance phase
Midtarsal joint
    in active propulsion phase of gait cycle, 47(t), 47–48
    anatomy, 14(f), 15
    axis, 15–16, 16(f)
    in biomechanical examination of children, 269
    in contact phase of gait cycle, 40(t)–41(t), 40–41
    interdependence with subtalar joint, 16(f), 17
    ligaments, 15
    locking position, 18–19, 20(f)
    in midstance phase of gait cycle, 43, 43(t)

    motion of
        kinetic chains in, 19–21, 20(f)–21(f), 23(t)
        windlass effect and, 21–22, 23(f)
    osseous locking mechanism in, 17–19, 18(f)–20(f)
    in passive lift-off phase of gait cycle, 51, 51(t)
    physiology, 15–23
    planal dominance in, 16(f), 16–17
    range of motion in, 22
    stability, axis and, 17, 18(f)
    supination of, 14(f), 15
    in swing phase of gait cycle, 54, 55(t)
Mitered hinge, and planal dominance, 10, 10(f)
Modeling approach, in computerized gait evaluation, 181–182
Morton's extension, for shoes, 358, 359(f)
Motion
    during gait cycle, physiology, 36(f)–37(f), 36–37
    measurement, in computerized gait evaluation, 199, 200(f)
Motion analysis, in running injuries, 116–118, 120(f)
Motor function, evaluation, in neuromuscular examination, 212, 212(t)–214(t), 214, 215(f)–219(f)
Muscle imbalance, spinal, 101
Muscles, primary disease of, and gait abnormalities in children, 230
Muscle stretch reflex (MSR), in neuromuscular examination, 214, 217–218, 220(t)
Muscle testing
    in hip injuries, 119
    manual, in neuromuscular examination, 212, 212(t)–214(t), 214, 215(f)–219(f)
Myasthenia gravis, gait in, 174(f)
Myopathies, gait in, 173, 174(f), 176(f)
Myotactic reflex, 214, 217–218, 220(t)

N

Navicular, stress fractures, 78, 128
Negative casting, in inverted orthotic technique, 476, 477(f)–478(f)
Negative impression casting, 280–281. See also Impression casting, negative
Neurologic examination, 209–220, 220(t)
Neurologic gait, in children, 228–230, 229(f)–231(f)
Neuroma, interdigital, 74–75
    orthotics for, 75
Neuromuscular examination
    cerebellar evaluation in, 211, 211(t)
    cranial nerve evaluation in, 209(t), 209–211, 210(f)
    extraocular movements in, 210(f), 210–211
    mental status evaluation in, 209
    motor evaluation in, 212, 212(t)–214(t), 214, 215(f)–219(f)
    muscle stretch reflexes in, 214, 217–218, 220(t)
    neurologic examination in, 208(t), 208–220, 220(t)
    Romberg test in, 220
    sensory evaluation in, 219–210, 220(t)
    superficial reflexes in, 218–219, 220(t)
Neuromuscular junction, and gait abnormalities, 173–174, 174(f)
Neuromuscular sequencing, in gait, 175(f)
Neutral calcaneal stance position, 144(f), 145
Neutral position, of subtalar joint, 12–13
Neutral spinal biomechanics, 108
Neutral suspension casting technique, 282–290, 284(f)–287(f), 293(f)
Non-neutral spinal biomechanics, 108
Nystagmus, exam for, 211

O

Open kinetic chain
    in ankle motion, 5
    in first metatarsophalangeal joint motion, 28–29, 29(f)
    in gait evaluation, 153–154, 154(f)–155(f), 156
    in midtarsal joint motion, 19
    in subtalar joint motion, 11, 12(f)

Ortalani's sign, in hip dislocation, in children, 234(f), 235
Orthotics, 307–326
    ankle-foot, 391–403. *See also* Ankle-foot orthoses (AFOs)
    anterior irritation from, correction of, 344–345, 346(f)
    for avascular necrosis, 67
    for calcaneal spur, 68
    for capsulitis, 68
    casting for, 297–298, 298(f)
    for children, 439t, 439–449, 440(f)–448(f)
        Blake inverted, 446, 446(f)
        gait plates, 447(f)–448(f), 447–449
        heel stabilizing, 442–443, 443(f)
        history of, 439
        prefabricated, 441(f)–442(f), 441–442
        Root functional foot, 443–445, 444(f)–445(f)
        triplane wedge, 440–441, 441(f)
        UCBL, 445(f), 445–446
    for clawtoe deformity, 69
    dorsal metatarsophalangeal joint pain from, correction of,
        345–346, 347(f)
    extrinsic corrections to, 302, 304(f)–305(f), 304–306
    fabrication process for, 298–302, 299(f)–303(f)
        errors in, 331(f), 331–332
    for first metatarsal-first cuneiform exostosis, 69
    first metatarsal head pain from, correction of, 346–348, 347(f)
    fitting, closed kinetic chain and, 336(f)
    functional, 106–107
    functional foot, diagnosing problems with, 327–348
    and ground reaction force, 347(f)
    for hallux extensus, 69
    for hallux limitus, 70
    for hallux valgus, 73
    for hammer toe deformity, 74
    heel cup irritation from, correction of, 341–342, 342(f)–344(f)
    heel slippage in, correction of, 338(f)–340(f), 338–339
    for interdigital neuroma, 75
    inverted technique in, 463–495. *See also* Inverted orthotic
        technique
    for lateral ankle instability, 75
    lateral edge irritation from, correction of, 342–344, 344(f)
    lower extremity, range of motion study for, 296–297
    materials for, 307–326, 311(t), 313(f)–314(f), 315(t), 316(f),
        317(t)
        classification systems, 311(t)
        closed cell expanded rubber as, 317
        comparison of, 315(t), 317(t), 318–323, 319(t)–322(t)
        cork products as, 317
        creep and, 313, 314(f)
        efficacy of, 308–311
        extrinsic posts in, 318
        force and, 312
        glass transition temperature and, 314, 315(t)
        hardness of, 315
        history of, 308
        Poisson's ratio and, 314–315
        polyethylene as, 314(f), 315(t), 316(f), 316–317, 317(t),
            321(t)–322(t)
        polypropylene as, 314(f), 315(t), 315–317, 316(f), 317(t),
            319(t)–322(t)
        processing of, 318
        resilience of, 322(t), 322–323
        response to dynamic load in, 321(t), 321–322
        selection of, errors in, 331(f), 331–332
        stiffness of, 315, 315(t)
        strain and, 312, 313(f)
        stress and, 312, 313(f)–314(f)
        stress-strain curve in, 313(f)
        tensile strength of, 314(f)
        thickness of, 315(t), 317(t), 318–319
        TL-2100 as, 315(t), 316–317, 317(t), 319(t)–322(t)
        viscoelastic polymers as, 317
        weight of, 319(t)–320(t), 319–321
    negative casting for, errors in, 325(f), 328–329
    for patellofemoral dysfunction, 76

plantar fascial irritation from, correction of, 339–341, 341(f)
    for plantar fasciitis, 76
    for plantarflexed first ray deformity, 77
    plantar foot-ground angle and, 337(f), 337–338
    for plantar tylomas, 83
    positive cast correction technique for, 300, 300(f)
    positive casting for, errors in, 329(f)–331(f), 329–331
    prescription form for, 298(f)
    rearfoot posts for, errors in, 332(f), 332–333
    for retrocalcaneal exostosis, 77
    semiweightbearing casting technique for, 305–306
    serial, 494, 494(t)
    for sesamoiditis, 77–78
    in shoes, problems with fit of, 333(f)–337(f), 333–338
    for sinus tarsi syndrome, 78
    for stress fractures, 79
    for tailor's bunion, 80
    for tendinitis, 82
    topcover for, 476(f), 484(f)
    varus wedge on, 473(f)
Osseus locking mechanisms, in midtarsal joint, 17–19,
    18(f)–20(f)
Osteomyelitis, and gait abnormalities, in children, 240
Outflare last shoe, for children, 437–438
Overcorrection modifications, in inverted orthotic technique,
    486–491, 487(f)–490(f), 488(t)

P

Pads, 367–389
    bunion, 383–385, 384(f)
    buttress, 282–283
    callus, 385(f), 385–386
    crescent, 383–386, 384(f). *See also* Crescent pads, palliative
    digital, 380–388. *See also* Digital pads
    hallux pinch callus, 385, 385(f)
    palliative
        adhesive tape as, 368–369
        butterfly sling as, 387–388, 388(f)
        cork as, 374
        digital pads as, 380–388
        Elastoplast as, 379–380, 380(f)
        felt as, 374
        foam rubber as, 374
        for heels, 378(f)–379(f), 378–379. *See also* Heel pads
        interdigital, 386(f)–386–387
        materials for, 374–375
        plantar, 375–379
        plastazote as, 374
        PPT as, 374
        purpose of, 368
        skiving accessories for, 373(f), 373–374
        Spenco as, 374–375
        sponge rubber as, 374
    for shoes, 356–359, 357(f)–358(f), 375, 375(f)
Paralysis
    of gluteus medius, in children, 228–229, 229(f)
    of quadriceps, in children, 229, 229(f)
Paralytic gait, in children, 228–230, 229(f)–231(f)
Parkinsonism, gait in, 176(f)
Patella
    position of, in biomechanical examination of children,
        247–248, 248(f)
    running injuries of, 122–123, 124(f)–126(f)
Patellofemoral dysfunction, 75–76
Pavlik harness, for hip dislocation in children, 236, 236(f)
Pedorthist, role of, 366
Pelvic crossed syndrome, 110
Pelvic level, in biomechanical examination of children, 247
Pelvic tilt syndrome, 101–105, 105(f)–107(f)
Pelvis, distortion, 106(f)
Perinatal history, in biomechanical examination of
    children, 244

Peroneal tendinitis, 81
Peroneus longus tendon, in gait, 26, 26(f)
Pes cavus, 61–62, 106
Pes planovalgus, 105–106
Pes planus, 60–61
Pes valgus, convex, congenital, in biomechanical examination
    of children, 267–268, 268(f)
Phasic gait
    double float, 161(f)
    double stance, 161(f)
Piriformis muscle, anatomy, 99, 101(f)
Planal dominance
    in midtarsal joint, 16(f), 16–17
    in subtalar joint, 9–11, 11(f)
Plantar aponeurosis, physiology, 23(f)
Plantar fascial accommodation, for orthotics, 340–341, 341(f)
Plantar fascial irritation, from orthotics, correction of, 339–341,
    341(f)
Plantar fasciitis, 76
Plantarflexion, 3(f), 3–4, 6(f)–7(f)
Plantar foot-ground angle, for orthotics, 337(f), 337–338
Plantar lesions, and gait evaluation, 156, 157(f)–158(f)
Plantar pads, 375–379
    accommodative, 376
    medial or long arch, 376, 376(f)
    metatarsal, 375(f), 375–376
    modified, 376(f)–378(f), 376–378
Plantar tylomas, 82–83
Plastazote, as palliative padding, 374
Plaster splints, for children, 434, 435(f)–436(f)
Poisson's ratio, and orthotic materials, 314–315
Polyethylene, for orthotics, 314(f), 315(t), 316(f), 316–317, 317(t),
    321(t)–322(t)
Polymers, viscoelastic, for orthotics, 317
Polypropylene, for orthotics, 314(f), 315(t), 315–317, 316(f),
    317(t), 319(t)–322(t)
Positive casting, 293(f), 294
    correction technique, 300, 300(f)
    in inverted orthotic technique, 478(f)–481(f), 478–481
    for orthotics
        errors in, 329(f)–331(f), 329–331
        preparation of, 329(f)–331(f), 329–331
Posture, and biomechanical examination, 144(f), 145
PPT, as palliative padding, 374
Pressure, measurement of, by computerized gait evaluation, 193
Pretibial muscles
    in active propulsion phase of gait cycle, 48
    in contact phase of gait cycle, 40(t), 40–41
    in midstance phase of gait cycle, 43
    in passive lift-off phase of gait cycle, 51(t), 52
    in swing phase of gait cycle, 55, 55(t)
Projection angles, in computerized gait evaluation, 196, 197
Pronated casting technique, for impressions, 292, 293(f)
Pronation, 105–106
    overcorrection, 472(f)
    subtalar joint, 11–12, 12(f)–13(f), 25(f)
        and chondromalacia patellae, 466(f)
Prone casting, for impressions, 290, 290(f)
Propulsion, first metatarsophalangeal joint and, 29–30, 30(f)
Pubis, biomechanics, 109

Q

Q angle
    in gait evaluation, 163, 165, 167(f)
    measurement, 124(f)
Quadratus lumborum, anatomy, 99, 100(f)

R

Radiography
    in hip dislocation, in children, 235(f), 235–236
    in juvenile hallux valgus, 275, 275(f)
    in metatarsus adductus, 272, 273(f)
Range of motion
    of ankle, in biomechanical examination of children, 260–264,
        261(f)
    in fifth ray, 32
    instruments for, in pediatric hip evaluation, 252(f), 252–254
    in metatarsophalangeal joints, 30–31, 32
    in midtarsal joint, 22
    study of, in lower extremities, for orthotics, 296–297
    in subtalar joint, 13
    of subtalar joint, in biomechanical examination of children,
        264–265, 265(f)–266(f)
Rays
    fifth, 31–32, 32(f)
    first, 23–27, 24(f)–26(f)
        anatomy, 24
        axis, 24, 24(f)
        biomechanical examination of, 137–138, 138(f)
        exostosis, 69
        and gait, 25–26, 26(f)
        hallux valgus in, 24–25, 25(f)
        hypermobile, 69
        kinetic chains in, 24–25, 25(f)
        and metatarsus primus adductus, 25
        physiology, 24(f)–26(f), 24–26
        plantarflexed deformity, 76–77
    fourth, 31
    running injuries of, 130
    second, 31
    stress fractures, 78
    third, 31
Rearfoot
    anatomy, 129(f)
    everted
        with everted forefoot, pathologic changes with, 91
        with inverted forefoot, pathologic changes with, 92
        with perpendicular forefoot, pathologic changes with,
            91–92
    perpendicular
        with everted forefoot, pathologic changes with, 90
        with inverted forefoot, pathologic changes with, 91
        with perpendicular forefoot, pathologic changes with, 90–91
    perpendicular to forefoot, with inverted calcaneus, patho-
        logic changes with, 89
    position, in gait evaluation, 165–168, 169(f)–170(f)
    running injuries of, 125–128, 129(f)
    valgus, 170(f)
    valgus in frontal plane, 62(f), 65
    varus, 170(f)
    varus in frontal plane, 62–63
Reciprocal innervation, Sherrington's law, 111
Reflexes
    muscle stretch, in neuromuscular examination, 214, 217–218,
        220(t)
    myotatic. See also Reflexes, muscle stretch, in neuromuscular
        examination
    superficial, in neuromuscular examination, 218–219, 220(t)
Resilience, of orthotics, comparison of materials in, 322(t),
    322–323
Resting calcaneal stance position, 143(f), 145
Retrocalcaneal exostosis, 77
Rhythmic phase, of walking, 33
Roberts brace, 442
Rocker soles, for shoes, 363–365, 364(f)
Romberg test, in neuromuscuoar examination, 220
Root functional foot orthosis, 443–445, 444(f)–445(f)
Rubber
    closed cell expanded, for orthotics, 317
    as palliative padding, 374
Running
    gait cycle of, evaluation of heel during, 120(f)
    shoes for, 452–453
        antipronation, 466(f)

Running injuries, 113–130
    clinic assessment, 114
    evaluation of shoes in, 118, 120(f)
    of foot, 125–130, 129(f)
    functional symmetry assessment in, 116–118,
        120(f)
    of hips, 116t, 118–122, 121(f)–122(f)
    history questionnaire for, 115(f)
    hospital assessment, 114
    iliotibial tract irritation from, 122
    of knee, 122–124, 124(f)–127(f)
    of leg, 124–125, 128(f)
    limb measurement in, 118, 121(f)
    low back, 114, 116(t), 116–118, 117(f)–119(f)
    motion analysis in, 116–118, 120(f)
    neurologic examination in, 116(t)
    office assessment, 114, 115(f)

S

SACH heels, for shoes, 365(f), 365–366
Sacroiliac joint, anatomy, 96–97, 97(f)–98(f)
Sacrum
    anatomy, 96–97, 97(f)–98(f)
    biomechanics, 109
Sagittal plane, functional disorders in, 65
Sagittal plane balance, and support moment, in com-
        puterized gait evaluation, 199–200
Scissors gait, 176(f)
Scoliosis, 166(f)
    in children
        Cobb's angle in, 239(f)
        and gait abnormalities, 239(f)–240(f), 239–240
Screening tests, spinal, 100–101, 102(f)–103(f)
Screw displacement axes, in computerized gait eval-
        uation, 196–197
Second ray. See Rays, second
Semiweightbearing casting technique
    for impression casting, 291–292, 292(f), 305–306
    for orthotics, 305–306
Sensors, for computerized gait evaluation, 153(f)
    calibration of, 185–186
Sensory evaluation, in neuromuscular examination,
        219–220, 220(f)
Serial orthotics, 494, 494(t)
Serial plaster immobilization
    for clubfoot, 417–419, 420(f)–422(f)
    for congenital foot deformities, 405–422
    for metatarsus adductus, 406(f)–414(f), 406–413, 409–413,
        411(f)–414(f)
        radiography in, 407(f)–408(f), 407–408
        technique, 409–413, 411(f)–414(f)
    for talipes calcaneovalgus, 416–417, 417(f)–419(f)
    for talipes equinoadductovarus, 417–419, 418–419,
        420(f)–422(f), 421(f)–422(f)
    for talipes equinus, 419–422
    for tibial position, 413–416, 415(f)–417(f)
Sesamoid, stress fractures of, 78–79
Sesamoiditis, 77–78
Sever's disease. See Calcaneus, apophysitis of
Shaffer plate, 442
Sherrington's law of reciprocal innervation, 111
Shoe inserts. See Orthotics
Shoes, 349–366
    for ankle-foot orthoses, 399–400
    athletic, 451–461. See also Athletic shoes
    for children, 434–439, 437(f), 437(t)
    closure systems for, 351
    construction of, 352–353, 353(f)–354(f)
    counter pad for, 357(f), 358
    crest pad for, 357(f), 358
    cuboid pad in, 358–359
    dancer's pad for, 357, 357(f)

    designs and styles of, 351–352
    evaluation, in running injuries, 118, 120(f)
    external modifications for, 359–366, 363(f)–365(f)
    fit of, 351(f), 351–352, 353(f)
    heel grip for, 357, 358(f)
    heel height differential of, and fit of orthotics, 334(f)–335(f),
        334–336
    heel spur pads for, 358, 359(f)
    history of, 350–351
    lifts for, 104–105
        for leg length discrepancy, 360–363, 363(f)
    longitudinal arch pads for, 357, 358(f)
    Morton's extension for, 358, 359(f)
    orthotics in, problems with fit of, 333(f)–337(f), 333–338
    padding for, 356–359, 357(f)–358(f), 375, 375(f)
    reverse Morton's extension for, 358, 359(f)
    rocker soles for, 363–365, 364(f)
    SACH heels for, 365(f), 365–366
    with splints, in children, 428
    stretching of, 355–356, 356(f)
    therapeutic uses of, 353–366, 354(f)–360(f), 363(f)–365(f)
    Thomas heel for, 365(f), 366
    tongue pads for, 357, 357(f)
    upper modificatoins of, 355–359
    wear of, in biomechanical examination of children, 246,
        247(f)
    wedge design of, 354(f), 354–355
Shortened extremities, in children, 230–232
Shoulder level, in biomechanical examination of
        children, 247
Shoulders, in gait evaluation, 162–163, 165(f)–166(f)
Sinus tarsi syndrome, 78
Sitting position, in biomechanical examination of children,
        245, 246(f)
Skiing, downhill, shoes for, 454–455, 455(f)
Skinfolds, in congenital hip dislocation, 233(f), 234
Skin rolling test, 100, 103(f)
Skiving, accessories for, 373(f), 373–374
Sleeping position, in biomechanical examination of children,
        245, 245(f)–246(f)
Sling, butterfly, as palliative padding, 387–388, 388(f)
Slit catheter, for compartmental pressure analysis,
        124–125, 128(f)
Soccer, shoes for, 455–456, 456(f)
Soleus, congenital equinus of, 260
Spastic gait, in children, 230, 231(f)
Spenco, as palliative padding, 374
Spica strap, for hallux fracture or sprain, 373
Spine, 95–112
    anatomy, 96(f)–101(f), 96–100
    biomechanics, 107–109, 108(f)
    curves, 96, 96(f)
    facet joints, 96, 97(f)
    functional pathology, 110–112
    lifting and, 101, 104(f)
    muscle imbalance in, 101
    musculoskeletal connections, 98–100, 99(f)–101(f)
    screening tests for, 100–101, 102(f)–103(f)
Splints
    buddy, for fracture or sprain, 372(f), 372–373
    for children, 428(t), 428–434, 429(f)–434(f)
        Brachman skate, 431, 432(f)
        Denis Browne, 428, 429(f)
        extent of correction in, 427
        factors affecting, 425–428
        fiberglass, 434, 435(f)–436(f)
        Filauer, 428, 429(f)
        Flexosplint, 431
        Friedman counter, 431
        Ganley, 430, 430(f)–431(f)
        Ilfeld, 236, 237(f)
        for impedance of subluxatory changes, 427–428
        Langer Counter Rotation, 431–432, 432(f)–433(f)
        plaster, 434, 435(f)–436(f)

shoes for, 428
  Uni-bar, 428, 430, 430(f)
Sports
  participation in, and biomechanical examination of
    children, 247
  shoes for, 451–461. *See also* Athletic shoes
Sprains, strapping and padding for. *See* Pads; *Strapping*
Spurs, calcaneal, 67–68
Squat test, 100, 102(f)
Stance measurements, in biomechanical examination,
    144–145
Stance phase. *See* Gait cycle, stance phase of
Step
  definition, 157
  in gait cycle, 35, 35(f)
Steppage gait, 174(f)
Stereometer, for measurement of motion, in computerized
    gait evaluation, 197–198
Straight leg raise test, 100, 102(f)
Strain, and orthotic materials, 312, 313(f)
Strapping
  palliative
    adhesive tape for, 368–369
    basket weave strap for, 371, 372(f)
    buddy splint for, 372(f), 372–373
    digital strap for, 372
    Gibney strap for, 371, 372(f)
    for hallux fracture or sprain, 373
    J strap for, 371–372
    Low Dye strap for, 369–371, 370(f), 372(f)
    materials for, 368–369
    skiving accessories for, 373(f), 373–374
  techniques for, 367–389
Stress, and orthotic materials, 312, 313(f)–314(f)
Stress fractures, 78–79
  of fibula, 79
  of fourth and fifth metatarsals, 78
  navicular, 78, 128
  of sesamoids, 78–79
  tibial, 79
Stress-strain curve, for plastic orthotic materials, 313(f)
Stride, definition, 157
Stride length, 35, 35(f)
Subtalar joint
  in active propulsion phase of gait cycle, 47, 47(t)
  anatomy, 8–9, 9(f)–10(f)
  axis of, 9, 10(f)
  biomechanical examination of, 139(f)–142(f), 141–143
  in contact phase of gait cycle, 39–41, 40(t)–41(t)
  interdependence with midtarsal joint, 16(f), 17
  ligaments, 10(f)
  loading response, 14(f)
  in midstance phase of gait cycle, 43, 43(t)
  motion of, kinetic chains in, 11–12, 12(f)–14(f)
  neutral position, 12–13
    in impression casting, 281(f)–283(f), 281–282
  palpation, 281(f)
  in passive lift-off phase of gait cycle, 51, 51(t)
  physiology, 9–13, 10(f)–14(f), 15
  planal dominance in, 9–11, 11(f)
  position, in gait evaluation, 165–168, 169(f)–170(f)
  pronation, 11–12, 12(f)–13(f), 25(f)
    and chondromalacia patellae, 466(f)
  range of motion, 13
    in biomechanical examination of children, 264–265,
      265(f)–266(f)
    in gait evaluation, 154, 155(f), 156, 157(f)
  supination, 11–12, 12(f)–13(f)
  in swing phase of gait cycle, 54, 55(t)
Supination
  of midtarsal joint, 14(f), 15
  of subtalar joint, 11–12, 12(f)–13(f)
Supinatus, of forefoot, 64–65
Supinatus foot impression casting technique, 292–293, 293(f)

Supporting structures, loss of, in childhood gait abnormal-
    ities, 232
Support moment, and sagittal plane balance, in computerized
    gait evaluation, 199–200

T

Tailor's bunion, 79–80
  palliative pads for, 385, 385(f)
Talipes calcaneovalgus
  in children, 265–267, 266(f)–267(f)
  serial plaster immobilization of, 416–417, 417(f)–419(f)
Talipes equinoadductovarus, serial plaster immobilization
    for, 417–419, 420(f)–422(f)
Talipes equinus, serial plaster immobilization for, 419–422
Talocalcaneal ligament, interosseous, anatomy, 8–9
Talus, dorsal view, 2(f)
Tarsal coalitions, in biomechanical examination of children,
    268–269
TBFR sequence, for gait evaluation, 161–163, 163(f)–171(f),
    165–169, 171
"Temporary Kirby," 490, 490(f)
Tendinitis, 80–82
  Achilles, gait and, 464(f)
Tendons, flexibility, measurement, goniometry for, 465(f)
Tennis, shoes for, 457–458, 458(f)
Thighs, biomechanics of, 123(f)
Third ray. *See* Rays, third
Thomas heel, for shoes, 365(f), 366
Tibia
  biomechanical examination of, 143(f), 144
    in children, 255–260, 256(f)–257(f)
  position
    in gait evaluation, 165, 168(f)
    serial plaster immobilization for, 413–416, 415(f)–417(f)
    vs. tibial torsion, 413–416, 415(f)–417(f)
  stress fractures of, 79
Tibial tendons, tendinitis, 81
Tibial torsion
  in biomechanical examination of children, 255–256,
    256(f)
  and malleolar position, 135(f)–136(f), 136–137
  vs. tibial position, 413–416, 415(f)–417(f)
Tibial torsion transformer, 434
Tibial valgum, in children, 260
Tibial varum, in children, 260
Tibiotalar joint. *See* Ankle
TL-2100, for orthotics, 315(t), 316–317, 317(t), 319(t)–322(t)
Tongue pads, for shoes, 357, 357(f)
Torqheel, circular, for children, 434
Torsion, femoral, 249
Torso-medius shoe, for children, 436–437, 438(f)
Tractograph
  in pediatric ankle measurements, 265(f)
  in pediatric hip measurements, 252, 252(f)
Transverse plane
  functional disorders in, 66
  in hip rotation, in biomechanical examination of children,
    249–251, 251(f)
Tremor, intention, exam for, 211
Trendelenburg gait, 176(f)
  in children, 225, 225(f)
Triplane wedge orthotics, for children, 440–441, 441(f)
Truss phenomenon, 22
Tuning fork test, in running injuries of leg, 125
Twister cables, for children, 432–433
Tylomas, plantar, 82–83

U

UCBL orthotics, 445(f), 445–446
Ultrasonography, in hip dislocation, in children, 236

Undercorrection modifications, in inverted orthotic technique, 490(t), 491–492, 492(f)
Uni-bar splint, 428, 430, 430(f)
Upper motor neuron, dysfunction, and gait abnormalities, 176(f), 176–177

V

Vacuum impression casting, 290–291, 291(f), 306
Valgus
    with everted rearfoot, pathologic changes with, 91
    forefoot, 170(f)–171(f)
        positive casting in, 479(f)
    in frontal plane, 62(f)–63(f), 65
    with inverted calcaneus, pathologic changes with, 89
    with perpendicular rearfoot, pathologic changes with, 90
    rearfoot, 170(f)
Valgus midsole wedge, 476(f), 488(f)
Varus
    with everted rearfoot, pathologic changes with, 92
    forefoot, 170(f)–171(f)
        negative casting in, 478(f)
    in frontal plane, 62(f)–63(f), 62–64
    with inverted calcaneus, pathologic changes with, 90
    with perpendicular rearfoot, pathologic changes with, 91
    rearfoot, 170(f)
        negative casting in, 478(f)

Varus wedges, 465(f), 473(f)
Version, femoral, 249
Vertical calcaneous, 62(f)
Vertical load
    in active propulsion phase of gait cycle, 46, 46(f)
    in contact phase of gait cycle, 37, 39(f)
    in midstance phase of gait cycle, 42, 42(f)
    in passive lift-off phase of gait cycle, 50, 50(f)

W

Walking, phases of, 33, 160(f)
Waveforms, comparisons of, in computerized gait evaluation, 192
Wedges
    common degrees of correction for, 493(t)
    midsole, valgus, 476(f), 488(f)
    varus, on orthotics, 465(f), 473(f)
Wheaton brace, 433(f)–434(f), 433–434
Whitman plate, 441–442, 442(f)
Whitman-Roberts plate, 442
Wick catheter, for compartmental pressure analysis, 124–125, 128(f)
Windlass effect, in midtarsal joint motion, 21–22, 23(f)
Wire-spring brace, for ankle-foot orthoses, 395, 395(f)